OXFORD MEDICAL PUBLICATION

Oxford Desk Reference
Toxicology

Oxford Desk Reference
Toxicology

Edited by

Professor D Nicholas Bateman

Formerly Professor of Clinical Toxicology and Consultant Physician
Royal Infirmary of Edinburgh and Formerly Director
National Poisons Information Service (Edinburgh Unit)
Edinburgh, UK

Dr Robert D Jefferson

Consultant Occupational Physician
Health Management Ltd., UK

Professor Simon HL Thomas

Consultant Physician and Professor of Clinical Pharmacology and Therapeutics
Newcastle Hospitals NHS Foundation Trust and Newcastle University
Medical Toxicology Centre and Director
National Poisons Information Service (Newcastle Unit)
Newcastle upon Tyne, UK

Dr John P Thompson

Senior Lecturer in Clinical Pharmacology
Institute of Molecular and Experimental Medicine, Cardiff University
and Director National Poisons Information Service
(Cardiff Unit), Cardiff, UK

Professor J Allister Vale

Director
National Poisons Information Service (Birmingham Unit) and
West Midlands Poisons Unit
City Hospital, Birmingham and School of Biosciences
University of Birmingham, Birmingham, UK

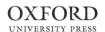
OXFORD
UNIVERSITY PRESS

OXFORD
UNIVERSITY PRESS

Great Clarendon Street, Oxford, OX2 6DP,
United Kingdom

Oxford University Press is a department of the University of Oxford.
It furthers the University's objective of excellence in research, scholarship,
and education by publishing worldwide. Oxford is a registered trade mark of
Oxford University Press in the UK and in certain other countries

© Oxford University Press 2014

The moral rights of the authors have been asserted

First Edition published in 2014

Impression: 1

Published in the United States of America by Oxford University Press
198 Madison Avenue, New York, NY 10016, United States of America

British Library Cataloguing in Publication Data
Data available

Library of Congress Control Number: 2014930243

ISBN 978–0–19–959474–0

Printed and bound by
CPI Group (UK) Ltd, Croydon, CR0 4YY

Oxford University Press makes no representation, express or implied, that the
drug dosages in this book are correct. Readers must therefore always check
the product information and clinical procedures with the most up-to-date
published product information and data sheets provided by the manufacturers
and the most recent codes of conduct and safety regulations. The authors and
the publishers do not accept responsibility or legal liability for any errors in the
text or for the misuse or misapplication of material in this work. Except where
otherwise stated, drug dosages and recommendations are for the non-pregnant
adult who is not breast-feeding

Links to third party websites are provided by Oxford in good faith and
for information only. Oxford disclaims any responsibility for the materials
contained in any third party website referenced in this work.

Dedication

To our teachers and patients.

Preface

Most physicians will see patients with poisoning. Their management is a common clinical problem, and appropriate assessment of potential severity, likely clinical features, and available treatments are key to optimal clinical care.

This book provides a source document for the theoretical and practical aspects of clinical toxicology and covers acute presentations to hospital following accidental or deliberate overdose; accidental exposure to natural toxins; effects of drugs of abuse; exposure to chemicals and radioactive substances particularly following workplace exposure or environmental release, including that by terrorists; and interpretation of the public health implications of poisoning, both incident management and epidemiology.

The book is designed to support the learning needs of doctors in training and will also provide an evidenced-based reference for those managing patients in clinical settings both in the UK and internationally. The authors have been chosen because of their expertise in the areas being addressed, which will ensure that the book is a valuable resource for all health professionals working with poisoned patients.

D Nicholas Bateman
Robert D Jefferson
Simon HL Thomas
John P Thompson
J Allister Vale
Spring 2014

Contents

Detailed Contents

List of Contributors

Professor D Nicholas Bateman
Formerly Royal Infirmary of Edinburgh
and National Poisons Information Service
 (Edinburgh Unit)
Edinburgh, UK

Dr Sally M Bradberry
National Poisons Information Service (Birmingham Unit)
 and West Midlands Poisons Unit
City Hospital
Birmingham, UK

Professor Nick Buckley
Medical Professorial Unit
Prince of Wales Hospital Clinical School
University of New South Wales
Randwick, Australia

Dr James M Coulson
Senior Lecturer in Clinical Pharmacology
Institute of Molecular and Experimental Medicine
Cardiff University
and Honorary Consultant
National Poisons Information Service (Cardiff Unit)
Cardiff, UK

Dr Paul Dargan
Toxicology Office
Guy's Hospital
London, UK

Professor Michael Eddleston
National Poisons Information Service (Edinburgh Unit)
Royal Infirmary of Edinburgh
and University of Edinburgh
Edinburgh, UK

Dr Ronald Goans
MJW Corporation
Clinton, TN, USA

Dr Jane Goddard
Department of Renal Medicine
Royal Infirmary of Edinburgh
Edinburgh, UK

Alison M Good
Formerly National Poisons Information Service
 (Edinburgh Unit)
Royal Infirmary of Edinburgh
Edinburgh, UK

Professor Alasdair Gray
Emergency Department
Royal Infirmary of Edinburgh
Edinburgh, UK

Dr Simon Hill
Newcastle Hospitals NHS Foundation Trust
Newcastle University Medical Toxicology Centre
and National Poisons Information Service
 (Newcastle Unit)
Newcastle upon Tyne, UK

Dr Geoffrey K Isbister
University of Newcastle School of Medicine and
 Public Health
Newcastle, Australia

Dr Robert D Jefferson
Occupational Health Department
Health Management Ltd, UK

Dr Liam Kevern
North Devon District Hospital,
Barnstaple, UK

Dr Ian J Lawson
Rolls-Royce plc
Derby

Dr Philip Masson
Department of Renal Medicine
Royal Infirmary of Edinburgh
Edinburgh, UK

Dr Robert L Maynard
Birmingham University
Birmingham, UK

Professor Bruno Mégarbane
Department of Medical and Toxicological Critical Care
Lariboisière Hospital
Paris, France

Dr Stephen G Potts
Department of Psychological Medicine
Royal Infirmary of Edinburgh
Edinburgh, UK

Dr Paul Rice
Biomedical Sciences Department
Dstl Porton Down
Salisbury, UK

Professor Philip A Routledge
Institute of Molecular and Experimental Medicine
Cardiff University
Cardiff, UK

Dr Tracy Ryan
Department of Psychological Medicine
Royal Infirmary of Edinburgh
Edinburgh, UK

Dr Kenneth J Simpson
Scottish Liver Transplantation Unit
Royal Infirmary of Edinburgh
Edinburgh, UK

Dr Roger Smyth
Department of Psychological Medicine
Royal Infirmary of Edinburgh
Edinburgh, UK

Dr Robby Steel
Department of Psychological Medicine
Royal Infirmary of Edinburgh
Edinburgh, UK

Dr HK Ruben Thanacoody
Newcastle Hospitals NHS Foundation Trust and
    Newcastle University Medical Toxicology Centre
and National Poisons Information Service
    (Newcastle Unit)
Newcastle upon Tyne, UK

Dr Alison Thomas
Institute of Molecular and Experimental Medicine
Cardiff University
and Honorary Consultant
National Poisons Information Service (Cardiff Unit)
Cardiff, UK

Professor Simon HL Thomas
Newcastle Hospitals NHS Foundation Trust and
    Newcastle University Medical Toxicology Centre
and National Poisons Information Service
    (Newcastle Unit)
Newcastle upon Tyne, UK

Dr John P Thompson
Institute of Molecular and Experimental Medicine
Cardiff University
and National Poisons Information Service (Cardiff Unit)
Cardiff, UK

Professor J Allister Vale
National Poisons Information Service (Birmingham Unit)
    and West Midlands Poisons Unit
City Hospital, Birmingham
and School of Biosciences
University of Birmingham
Birmingham, UK

Professor Heather Wallace
Department of Medicine & Therapeutics & Biomedical
    Sciences University of Aberdeen
Aberdeen, UK

Dr W Stephen Waring
Acute Medical Unit
York Hospital
York, UK

Professor David A Warrell
University of Oxford
Nuffield Department of Clinical Medicine
John Radcliffe Hospital
Oxford, UK

Professor Julian White
University of Adelaide
and Toxinology Department
Women's and Children's Hospital
Adelaide, Australia

Dr David Wood
Toxicology Office
Guy's Hospital
London, UK

Dr Laura Yates
UK Teratology Information Service
Newcastle Hospitals NHS Foundation Trust
Newcastle, UK

Symbols and Abbreviations

>	greater than
<	less than
~	approximate
α	alpha
β	beta
γ	gamma
ν	neutrino
2DPMP	desoxypirpradrol
5-HT	5-hydroxytryptamine (serotonin)
AACT	American Academy of Clinical Toxicology
AAPCC	American Association of Poisons Control Centers
ACE	angiotensin-converting enzyme
ACGIH	American Conference of Governmental Industrial Hygienists
Ach	acetylcholine
AChE	acetylcholinesterase
ACP	Advisory Committee on Pesticides
ACS	acute coronary syndrome
ADHD	attention deficit hyperactivity disorder
ADR	adverse drug reaction
AE	adverse event
AIN	acute interstitial nephritis
AIOH	Australian Institute of Occupational Hygienists Inc.
AKI	acute kidney injury
ALF	acute liver failure
ALS	Advanced Life Support
ALT	alanine aminotransferase
AMT	alpha-methyltryptamine
ANCA	antineutrophil cytoplasmic antibody
APAMT	Asia Pacific Association of Medical Toxicology
APD	action potential duration
API	active pharmaceutical ingredient
APTT	activated partial thromboplastin time
ARB	angiotensin-II receptor blocker
ARDS	acute respiratory distress syndrome
ARS	acute radiation syndrome
AST	aspartate aminotransferase
ATN	acute tubular necrosis
ATP	adenosine triphosphate
AUC	area under the curve
AV	atrioventricular
BEM	biological effect monitoring
BfR	Bundesinstitut fur Risikobewertung
BLL	blood lead level
BM	blood glucose monitoring
BOHS	British Occupational Hygiene Society
BSA	body surface area
BZ	3-quinuclidinyl benzilate
CAS	Chemical Abstracts Service
CAVHDF	continuous arterio-venous haemodiafiltration
CBRN	chemical, biological, radiation, or nuclear
CDC	Centers for Disease Control and Prevention
CHM	Commission on Human Medicines
CI	confidence interval
CIWA-Ar	Clinical Institute Withdrawal Assessment for Alcohol scale, revised
CK	creatine kinase
CKD	chronic kidney disease
CNS	central nervous system
CO	carbon monoxide
CO_2	carbon dioxide
COHb	carboxyhaemoglobin
COPD	chronic obstructive pulmonary disease
CPAP	continuous positive airway pressure
CPN	community psychiatric nurse
CPR	cardiopulmonary resuscitation
CRP	C-reactive protein
CSF	cerebral spinal fluid
CSF	chlorobenzylidenemalononitrile
CT	computed tomography
CTG	cardiotocography
CVVHDF	continuous veno-venous haemodiafiltration
CVVHF	continuous veno-venous haemofiltration
CYP	cytochrome P450
DFO	desferrioxamine
DIC	disseminated intravascular coagulation
DMA	dimethylarsinic acid
DMAP	4-dimethylaminophenol
DMHP	dimethylheptylpyran
DMPS	dimercaptopropane sulphonate
DMSA	dimercaptosuccinic acid
DMT	dimethyltryptamine
DNA	deoxyribonucleic acid
DOB	dimethoxybromoamfetamine
DOC	4-chloroamfetamine
D2PM	diphenylprolinol
DTPA	diethylenetriamine penta-acetate
DTs	delirium tremens

EAPCCT	European Association of Poisons Centres and Clinical Toxicologists	INR	international normalized ratio
		IPCS	International Programme on Chemical Safety
EASHW	European Agency for Safety and Health at Work	IPPV	intermittent positive pressure ventilation
		ISA	intrinsic sympathomimetic activity
EC	European Commission	IV	intravenous
EC_{50}	median effective concentration	LD_{50}	median lethal dose
ED_{50}	median effective dose	LDt_{50}	median lethal concentration and time
EEG	electroencephalogram	LET	linear energy transfer
EMA	European Medicines Agency		
EMA	electromagnetic	LEV	local exhaust ventilation
EPO	erythropoietin	LFT	liver function test
EPR	electron paramagnetic resonance	LH	luteinizing hormone
ERP	effective refractory period	LOAEL	lowest observed adverse effect level
ESR	electron spin resonance	LSD	lysergic acid diethylamide
EU	European Union	MAH	microangiopathic haemolysis
FBC	full blood count	MAOI	monoamine oxidase inhibitor
FDA	Food and Drug Administration	MBDB	N-methyl-1-(3,4-methylenedioxyphenyl-2-aminobutane
FEV_1	forced expiratory volume in 1 second		
FHF	fulminant hepatic failure	MDAC	multiple-dose activated charcoal
G6PD	glucose-6-phosphate dehydrogenase	MDEA	3,4-methylenedioxy-N-ethylamfetamine
GABA	gamma-aminobutyric acid	MDMA	3,4-methylenedioxymethamfetamine
GBL	gamma-butyrolactone	MHRA	Medicines and Healthcare products Regulatory Agency
G-CSF	granulocyte colony stimulating factor		
GFR	glomerular filtration rate	MMA	monomethylarsonic acid
GGT	gamma-glutamyl transferase	MSA	membrane stabilizing activity
GHB	gamma-hydroxybutyrate	MSDS	Material Safety Data Sheet
GI	gastrointestinal	N/L	neutrophil/lymphocyte
GN	glomerulonephritis	NAC	acetylcysteine
GP	general practitioner	NADH	nicotinamide adenine dinucleotide
GTN	glyceryl trinitrate	NADPH	nicotinamide adenine dinucleotide phosphate
HBO	hyperbaric oxygen	NAPQI	N-acetyl-para-benzo-quinone imine
HCG	human chorionic gonadotropin	NG	nasogastric
HD	haemodialysis	NHANES	National Health and Nutrition Examination Survey
HEAA	hydroxyethoxyacetate		
HEPA	high-efficiency particulate absorption	NHS	National Health Service
HF	haemofiltration	NICE	National Institute for Health and Care Excellence
HIET	hyper-insulinaemia euglycaemia therapy		
HIV	human immunodeficiency virus	NIOSH	National Institute for Occupational Safety and Health
HPF	haemoperfusion		
HPLC	high performance liquid chromatography	NMDA	N-methyl-D-aspartate
HSE	Health and Safety Executive	NMJ	neuromuscular junction
IARC	International Association for Research on Cancer	NMR	nuclear magnetic resonance
		NNH	number needed to harm
IC_{50}	median incapacitating dose	NNT	number needed to treat
ICD	International Classification of Diseases	NO	nitric oxide
ICRP	International Council on Radiological Protection	NOAEL	no observed adverse effect level
		NPDS	National Poisons Data System
		NPIS	National Poisons Information Service
IFN	interferon	NSAID	non-steroidal anti-inflammatory drug
IL	interleukin	O_2	oxygen
IM	intramuscular	OC	oleoresin capsicum (pepper spray)

ONS	Office of National Statistics		SD	standard deviation
OP	occupational physician		SIADH	syndrome of inappropriate antidiuretic hormone secretion
OP	organophosphorus			
PCB	polychlorinated biphenyl		SNRI	serotonin and norepinephrine reuptake inhibitor
PCC	premature chromosomal condensation			
PD	peritoneal dialysis		SPECT	single-photon emission computed tomography
PEEP	positive end-expiratory pressure ventilation			
			SSRI	selective serotonin re-uptake inhibitor
PHE	Public Health England		SUSAR	suspected unexpected serious adverse reaction
PMA	paramethoxyamfetamine			
PMMA	2,5-dimethoxy-4-chloroamfetamine		$t\frac{1}{2}$	half-life
PO	per os (orally)		T3	tri-iodothyronine
POEA	polyethoxylated amine		T4	thyroxine
PPE	personal protective equipment		TCA	tricyclic antidepressant
ppm	parts per million		THC	tetrahydrocannabinol
PSUR	periodic safety update report		THOR	The Health and Occupation Reporting network
PT	prothrombin time			
QA	quality assurance		TTX	tetrodotoxin
QC	quality control		U&Es	urea and electrolytes
RADS	reactive airway dysfunction syndrome		UKTIS	UK Teratology Information Service
RBC	red blood cell		WADA	World Anti-Doping Agency
RNA	ribonucleic acid		WBI	whole-bowel irrigation
SAE	serious adverse event		WHO	World Health Organization
SCBA	self-contained breathing apparatus		WRIH	work-related ill health

Scientific principles in clinical toxicology

Epidemiology of poisoning

Background

For an understanding of the epidemiology of poisoning it is necessary to understand the terminology used to describe events that may cause toxicity to a patient. Five centuries ago Paracelsus said that all things were potentially toxic, and that the key factor was the dose. This principle applies today.

Definitions

- Suicide: an intentional act resulting in death.
- Accidental poisoning: exposure to a poison resulting in symptoms arising from accidental action; common in young children, may occur in adults at home, workplace, or as a result of fire or transport accident.
- Deliberate poisoning: this forms part of the spectrum of self-harm (formerly termed parasuicide).
- Occupational poisoning: occurs in the context of employment.
- Environmental poisoning: refers to exposure resulting from presence of a chemical either in the air, food, or water.

Poisoning may be acute, that is following a single ingestion, or more chronic, following repeated exposure, such as may occur in an industrial setting. Similarly the effects of a poisoning may be acute, resulting in rapid onset of symptoms with rapid resolution, subacute in onset and offset, or chronic with persistent, and in some cases permanent, injury.

There are many thousands of events every day which could theoretically result in poisoning, these are accidental and rarely result in severe injury. The most common relate to medication errors and exposures resulting from exploratory behaviour by young children who place potentially toxic materials into their mouths.

In contrast, serious cases of poisoning resulting in hospital admission are less frequent but nevertheless an important part of healthcare. In the UK, most acute medical services will admit between 5 and 10% of their overall patients as a result of poisoning. The vast majority of these cases in adults result from deliberate self-harm. This problem of behaviourally induced self-harm also includes physical damage (e.g. cutting). For the physician and intensivist, however, the majority of cases in developed countries are due to drugs. These may be either prescription medicines, which are most common, or drugs of abuse—intentional, recreational, toxic drug combination, or contaminated product.

Poisoning exposure may also occur in the workplace in industrial accidents, or as a result of a 'chemical incident' in which more than one or two people are affected following exposure to a chemical. Most often this is due to an accidental event, for example, release of a chemical from an industrial site in a fire, a road traffic or rail accident involving industrial tankers, or very rarely deliberate release of a chemical secondary to terrorist activity. Homicidal poisoning is extremely rare.

Precise definitions of poisoning therefore become difficult. In general, medication errors are ignored, but statistical data often includes very low-level excess exposure to other materials that occurs accidentally. These are often products found in the home. Of course many mild events are never formally recorded by health service personnel or collected in national statistics. Indeed in the United Kingdom the majority of patients with suspected poisoning are seen and assessed in emergency departments or primary care and never admitted to a health facility. It is only data from actual hospital admissions that are collected for use in estimating hospital activity in relation to poisoning. Finally, mortality statistics are also collected and may be used in combination with other data sources in fuller analyses.

Poisons information services (see Poisons information services, pp. 12–13) collect information on the enquiries they receive. This will depend on the way in which the information is delivered (telephone or Internet), and what the enquirer can provide in respect to the potential toxin and the patient. Details of the circumstances (accidental or deliberate) and place the event occurred may also be acquired. It will thus be clear that the data collected by poisons information services and those from hospital activity statistics will be very different, since many enquiries do not result in hospital referral.

Data sources

Information on the causes of death relating to poisoning and self-harm is collected centrally in the United Kingdom for England and Wales and separately for Scotland. These data include the place of death and the agent(s) deemed responsible by the Coroner in England and Wales and the Procurator Fiscal in Scotland. Pathologists, who may not always have specialist toxicological training, advise them, and there are no uniform definitions to assist in determining precise causation. This can potentially result in death being attributed to the wrong agent, particularly in mixed ingestions. Care is therefore required in interpreting UK mortality data. Similar caveats also apply internationally.

UK health departments also collect information on hospital activity analysis which is coded and includes data on poisoning. The International Classification of Diseases (ICD) diagnostic codes used in these data extractions are quite wide and normally do not allow precise detail to be obtained on the actual agent used. For detailed information about, for example, the precise types of antidepressant taken in overdose, poisons information service data provides a more detailed breakdown, though it is not specifically linked to the case outcome data reflected in Health Department statistics. Other countries also collect data in various ways. Those without national health systems, such as the USA, tend to have less complete or readily accessible hospital data to link to specific population groups for detailed study.

Other sources of data are of course those derived from individual hospital units, or groups of hospitals working together. An excellent example of the latter is the collaboration around the Hunter Valley in Australia that comes from a defined population. This is also the strength of data from cities with only one emergency facility, such as Edinburgh in Scotland.

In some European countries it is possible to anonymize and 'data-link' individual patient data. In this way individual patient histories may be tracked anonymously from hospital admission data. This has been used, for example, to study psychological diagnosis, agents ingested, and long-term outcomes in patient cohorts. Such studies require careful ethical consideration but are probably the most powerful for examining longer-term effects of poisoning and the interaction of self-harm on further health.

Psychosocially the data linkage system described also allows estimates of the influence of deprivation on poisoning and self-harm. These are derived from the postcode address of the anonymized patient and statistically linked. This approach has, for example, been used to show that rates of paracetamol self-harm tend to be higher in lower social groups, and, more worryingly, that the mortality outcome is worse. Similar studies have been done elsewhere in the world and show similar trends.

Effects of age and gender

Thirty years ago self-harm was regarded by many as a disorder of young females. In the 21st century, females still exceed males in some age groups, particularly late teens and 20s, but poisoning increasingly affects men and women to the same extent. This disorder is unusual in medical practice in being most frequent in younger adults, with the highest incidence in individuals between the ages of 15 and 35 years. A worrying trend is the recognition of self-harm as a problem in older children, and it would appear the age affected has fallen over the past 20 years such that children as young as 10 years now present with self-harm.

Understanding the trends in this population is clearly important, and epidemiological data offers the best tool to track changes with time. These age groups are economically active and socially valuable, particularly in countries with rural economies, as they are often the main real or potential earners in families.

Agents taken by patients in different age groups also vary, and that is probably most related to materials readily available. Thus in the United Kingdom self-harm from poisoning in young adults is less often with prescription medication than in older patients, and often involves over-the-counter analgesics. This accounts for the limitation on prescription pack-size introduced by the UK government in an attempt to limit the severity of self-harm in this group.

Influence of local factors

Where good quality data is available the rates of self-harm in different populations across the world appear surprisingly similar. For example, the rates of self-harm in the two very different environments of the United Kingdom and Sri Lanka are very similar. The mortality rate is, however, far higher in Sri Lanka. The reasons for this are not the quality of medical care but the agents used in poisoning. In the UK the most common agent is paracetamol with a mortality rate estimated at around 0.5–1% overall. In Sri Lanka the commonest agents are pesticides, which have individual mortality rates as high as 60%. In the UK intensive care beds are rarely taken up by cases of poisoning, but in Sri Lanka poisoning with organophosphate pesticides is the commonest reason for intensive care occupancy.

Use of epidemiological data for public health gain

In the United Kingdom epidemiological data has been used to show the major change in agents ingested in self-harm in the 1980s when paracetamol became a dominant agent accounting for approximately 40% of admissions from poisoning in Scottish hospitals.

Poisons centre data may be particularly useful to study trends in use of drugs of abuse and in identifying new agents which present with unusual symptom patterns. It may also assist in identifying adverse effects from new formulations of commercial products, or adulteration of drugs of abuse by toxic agents such as quinine and levamisole. Using these data both to advise the public and physicians is important in improving public health.

Unusual patterns of symptoms thought due to poisoning may be an indication of adulteration of food supply. A recent example in Europe has been the substitution of different types of pine nut for the edible version, resulting in persistent taste disturbance. Similarly in North America an outbreak of food poisoning due to bacterial contamination of vegetables was detected by studying day-to-day variation in poison centre calls.

Understanding case fatality rates for different types of product in the same group, either pharmaceutical or pesticide, has resulted in legislation in many countries. Thus in Europe, showing that patients who ingested co-proxamol died prior to hospital presentation was key to its withdrawal from the market. This could only be shown by amalgamating data from three sources—national mortality statistics, hospital activity, and information from poison services on the rates of enquiry for different combination analgesics. In Sri Lanka, studying mortality rates for different pesticides identified more toxic insecticide products. Since these offered no agricultural advantage, removal from the marketplace was possible and self-harm death rates fell significantly.

Use of statistical data on poisoning is therefore important to improving public health, although politically this may sometimes be difficult to promote as some individuals still feel that patients should be held fully responsible for their actions in the circumstance of self-harm. In reality the data show that self-harm is a disorder affecting predominantly young adults who are economically and socially valuable. High mortality among these individuals, particularly in developing countries, presents a major and continuing public health problem for which epidemiological data are required.

Further reading

Bronstein A, Spyker D, Cantilena JR, et al. (2011). 2010 Annual report of the American association of Poisons Control Centers' National Poisons Data System (NPDS): 28th Annual Report. Clin Tox, 49:910–41.

Camidge DR, Wood RJ, Bateman DN (2003). The epidemiology of self-poisoning in the UK. Br J Clin Pharmacol, 56:613–19.

Dawson AH, Eddleston M, Senarathna L, et al. (2010). Acute human lethal toxicity of agricultural pesticides: a prospective cohort study. PLoS Med, 7:e1000357.

Hawton K, Bergen H, Simkin S, et al. (2009). Effect of withdrawal of co-proxamol on prescribing and deaths from drug poisoning in England and Wales: time series analysis. BMJ, 338:b2270.

Office for National Statistics (2012). Deaths Related to Drug Poisoning in England and Wales 2012. <http://www.ons.gov.uk/ons/rel/subnational-health3/deaths-related-to-drug-poisoning/2012/stb---deaths-related-to-drug-poisoning-2012.html>.

Basic mechanisms of poisoning

Background

The man often regarded as the father of modern toxicology, Paracelsus, made a statement that can be summarized as: 'all things are poisonous, but what makes a poison is the dose'.

As toxicology became more developed as a scientific discipline, toxicologists first became interested in the dose of a compound that killed. This led to the method of assessing toxicity of drugs and chemicals by the use of the LD_{50}. This is the dose resulting in death of 50% of the animals in a sample. This test is now outmoded on both humane and scientific grounds. The principle however is of interest in that it is based on a classical pharmacological dose–response relationship which often applies to other aspects of the way in which toxins exert their effects.

The LD_{50} plot consists of a log dose–probit mortality line. This has a parallel to the drug dose–response curve (see Figure 1.1) where the concept of 50% effective dose (ED_{50}) is replaced by the LD_{50}.

One fundamental problem with all animal testing is to be sure that the metabolic and physiological responses in the species examined resemble those of humans. The fact that there are differences in species, for example, the hamster is exquisitely sensitive to paracetamol, has led some animal rights campaigners to suggest that all animal experiments are therefore valueless. This claim cannot be allowed to pass unchallenged as it misrepresents the importance of knowing the basic mechanisms in any drug or chemical effect, which must be understood clearly in order to develop appropriate therapy. Such therapies may also of course be for animals as well as for humans.

A more appropriate measure for use in human toxicity assessment is the ED_{50}, which is the lowest dose producing a specific effect in 50% of those exposed. As a response in different people varies significantly, sometimes depending on drug metabolism or receptor sensitivity, it may be more useful clinically to consider the lowest possible toxic dose. In practice it is often only established following experience in clinical use. If it is clear that the basic physiology and mechanisms of toxicity are similar in animals it may be possible to extrapolate from animal data to humans.

Timeframes of poisoning

When faced with a patient who is potentially poisoned, the clinician needs to appreciate the importance of systemic dose as this is likely to affect the clinical pattern seen in the patient.

Most physicians will see patients poisoned acutely; however, clinical effects and toxicity may result from repeated doses of quantities that themselves are below a toxic threshold, with accumulation resulting in toxicity. Clinical features may also be acute, passing over a few hours; subacute, persisting for some days or possibly weeks; and chronic, in some cases being irreversible. The effects of the toxin may result in cellular changes that produce more chronic effects, or produce effects delayed beyond the initial onset of poisoning. One of the best recognized syndromes in the latter category is that of delayed polyneuropathy following significant organophosphate pesticide poisoning.

Clinical features in chronic poisoning will depend on the toxin and the organ involved.

Classification of poisons

There are many different ways in which to categorize poisons—this may be based on their origins, their chemical structure, or their modes of action and target organs. Poisons information services often categorize poisons based on their source, for example:

- pharmaceutical
- household product
- pesticide
- chemical
- cosmetic
- snake or other bite
- plant.

It may also be useful to understand the site of the poisoning, for example:

- home
- garden
- workplace
- school
- hospital or medical facility
- outdoors.

This approach may be useful when considering likely dose, or designing and planning preventative measures.

Mechanisms of toxic effect

The most useful clinical classification, presented here, relates to the mode of action of the toxin. Poisons produce their effects by a variety of mechanisms; these include:

- acting as caustic material (acids or alkalis) and generating non-specific tissue damage
- damaging lipid membranes (organic solvents)
- classical pharmacological processes interacting with specific receptors or ion channels
- acting as direct metabolic poisons on cell enzyme systems
- following biotransformation into toxic metabolites
- acting as mutagens or carcinogens altering cell nuclear mechanisms and resulting in malignancy
- acting as cytotoxics, primarily damaging rapidly dividing cells in the gut or bone marrow
- acting on cell organelles to cause damage, e.g. mitochondrial toxins
- triggering secondary biological processes (e.g. snake venoms)
- acting as teratogens causing damage to the developing embryo
- emitting radiation (radioisotopes) causing cell damage or cell death.

Many natural poisons have facilitated discoveries in medicine and pharmacology, since they have identified potential therapeutic targets for development as sites of action for commercial pharmaceutical agents. Biological organisms synthesize some of the most toxic agents known to man.

Time course of toxicity

Most drugs are designed to work shortly after administration. Caustic chemicals will also produce symptoms relatively quickly, secondary to non-specific tissue damage. Metabolic poisons will take longer to act, depending on the site at which they are targeted. Most hepatic toxins take at least 12–24 hours before features develop. Evidence of renal toxicity may take several days. Drugs which are mutagens or carcinogens will take far longer. To be subject to a teratogen the fetus requires to be exposed in the 1st trimester of pregnancy. Fetotoxic agents affect the developing baby later in pregnancy, for example, by interfering with placental function or the production of amniotic fluid. Long latency toxicity may also occur, the most dramatic being vaginal tumours in the daughters of mothers given oestrogen during pregnancy as a prophylactic against miscarriage.

Classification of toxic actions

When patients with an overdose are first seen it is useful to bear in mind the various mechanisms of toxicity that may be present, particularly in a mixed exposure. These will vary depending on the physicochemical properties, the biochemical properties, and the pharmacological properties of the poison.

Physicochemical properties

Caustic materials
Typically strong acids or alkalis that cause direct tissue injury from a local chemical reaction. Secondary effects may then occur due to the extent of the injury, physiological responses to it, and secondary metabolic disturbances that may follow from the chemical nature of the caustic material. An example would be ingestion of strong alkali causing initial tissue damage to the lining of the gut, with possible perforation and mediastinitis or peritonitis, in the case of recovery followed by local stricture formation and upper gastrointestinal (GI) obstruction.

Irritants
Patients often complain of symptoms from exposure to compounds causing irritation without overt tissue damage. Irritant effects are common as a cause of lachrymation, change in taste, and upper respiratory tract irritation, with cough and wheeze in susceptible subjects.

Pharmacological actions

Primary and secondary pharmacology
Pharmaceuticals are developed with the intention of achieving a specific therapeutic action and for most modern pharmaceutical products this is achieved by targeting a single receptor type. The dose used to achieve a clinical effect is determined by the interaction with this primary receptor. Many chemical compounds used as drugs lose this specificity for a single receptor as their dose increases. This is described in individual chapters in this book. Other older drugs have actions on several receptors. As an example, tricyclic antidepressants have a primary pharmacological action of altering uptake of monoamines into the presynaptic neuron, but secondary properties of these molecules include antimuscarinic receptor (anticholinergic) properties, sodium channel blockade ('membrane stabilizing') properties, histamine H_1 receptor antagonism, and alpha adrenoceptor antagonism. In overdose it is the combination of these different molecular properties that contributes to the clinical syndrome.

Understanding the difference between the therapeutic and toxic dose led to the concept of a 'therapeutic ratio' which gives a measure of the difference between the dose causing toxic effects and those causing therapeutic effects. For drugs like warfarin or insulin this number is low and underlies their potential toxicity in overdose.

Agonists, antagonists, and partial agonists

Pure agonists
These drugs stimulate a receptor. Examples would include epinephrine or norepinephrine. Such compounds can be inhibited by antagonists in a dose-dependent manner.

Antagonists
Drugs that act on a receptor block the effect of an agonist, but on their own have no intrinsic activity at the receptor site and are called pure antagonists. Beta blockers such as metoprolol or bisoprolol are examples. In overdose this type of drug will produce excess features to those seen from their therapeutic action at beta receptors. Thus bradycardia, hypotension, and negative inotropic effects on the myocardium are to be expected. In addition it can be normally assumed that if an agonist for that same receptor site is given in sufficient quantity, reversal of the effect of an overdose will occur. In practice it is often difficult to overcome the effect of a very large excess dose of an antagonist therapeutically, usually due to the quantity needed and the effects of that agent at other 'off-target' sites. Further cardiovascular support is therefore generally required in patients severely poisoned with beta blockers. Some beta blockers also possess secondary pharmacological properties which may complicate clinical management, for example, propranolol is a sodium channel blocker.

Partial agonists
Drugs that act on a receptor and block the effects of a full agonist, which if present without that agonist cause stimulation of the same receptor site, are termed partial agonists.

Most theories of drug action suggest that the rate of interaction between receptor and an agent acting on it determines the amount of response induced. Partial agonists therefore can be considered to be drugs that bind to receptor sites but interact slowly. Their molecular structure causes some stimulation of the receptor, and hence clinical response. This is in contrast to a pure antagonist. From a therapeutic perspective partial agonist drugs seem less attractive, but nevertheless some are used quite widely, for example, dihydrocodeine. When taken in overdose such compounds do not produce such a full pharmacological effect as a pure agonist. Thus the effects of dihydrocodeine are less severe than those of morphine. Partial agonist drugs are, however, more difficult to displace with an antagonist once they are bound to a receptor, and therefore the effect of the opioid antagonist naloxone on a molar basis is less for dihydrocodeine than morphine.

Dose–response
The differences between agonists, antagonists, and partial agonists may be described graphically. The normal relationship between a drug and receptor means that as the dose of the drug increases, the natural maximal response is achieved, such that a higher dose of agonist will not increase the effects seen. Plotted on semi-logarithmic graph paper, with the dosage in logarithms, a sigmoid curve is produced (Figure 1.1). Antagonists move the curve to the right, such that a higher dose of agonist is needed for the same agonist effect, but do not change the maximum response

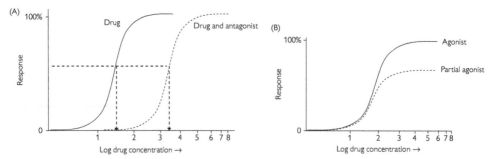

Fig 1.1 (A) Log dose–response curve showing the effects of a pure agonist and of an agonist–pure antagonist combination with shift of the dose–response curve to the right. The horizontal dotted line is the ED_{50}. Vertical arrows illustrate the effect of a pure antagonist on dose–response of an agonist. The parallel movement of the dose–response depends on dose of agonist and antagonist, and can be overcome by increased agonist dose. (B) The dose–response curves for a pure agonist and a partial agonist showing the difference in dose–response, and reduced maximum effect of a partial agonist. Note initial dose–response relationship is not parallel to the pure agonist.

possible (Figure 1.1A). Partial agonists produce a diminished response such that the sigmoid curve does not reach the same height, and the slope of the curve may also be less (Figure 1.1B).

In the presence of an agonist a partial agonist will tend to reduce the maximum response, moving the curve to the right and also often reducing its slope.

In poisoned patients such clear differentials in biological response are rarely seen, principally because most drugs in overdose tend to cause complex pathophysiological changes as well as often acting on more than one receptor site. Nevertheless these concepts assist an understanding of dosing and the therapeutic approach in the poisoned patient. In the presence of an antagonist larger doses of agonist will be required than normal. Similarly in the presence of an agonist larger doses of antagonist will be required. In the case of pure antagonists, increasing doses are unlikely to cause biological effects and dose limitation is determined merely by availability or lack of clinical response, which may indicate an incorrect first diagnosis, or multiple drug ingestion.

For drugs with several actions (i.e. complex primary and secondary pharmacological actions in overdose) a combination of treatments will be required to manage all aspects of the poisoning. This is why in overdose patients several different therapeutic actions may be required within a short space of time. For example, in antidepressant poisoning the central nervous system (CNS) actions may cause convulsions. Metabolic acidosis follows and will aggravate sodium channel blockade and cause cardiac arrhythmias. Therapy is therefore required to be targeted both against convulsions (benzodiazepines) and the myocardial membrane (administration of sodium bicarbonate). Understanding that the cardiac arrhythmias are due to sodium channel blockade is important, since standard antiarrhythmic therapy, such as lidocaine, will aggravate the clinical problem as lidocaine acts by sodium channel blockade.

Agonists or antagonists act at specific receptor sites but the extent of the clinical problem that results from this interaction will depend upon the precise nature of the receptor, and the organ in which it is sited. Thus beta-receptor antagonists and calcium channel antagonists affect the heart rate and force of myocardial contraction. This causes a decrease in cardiac output resulting in hypotension, a drop in organ perfusion, and secondary effects resulting from that, including acute renal injury, lack of CNS perfusion, and eventually death.

In overdose the importance of 'secondary' pharmacology becomes very relevant. The dose chosen for a therapeutic use is often designed to deliver a drug to a target receptor organ at a particular range of concentration. The effect of an overdose will be to change the concentration effect profile of the compound and introduce concentrations far in excess of those normally seen in therapeutic use. The molecular structure of most drugs mean that as concentrations change, the receptor interaction profile is altered to produce a clinical picture that results from the combined effects of all the receptors on which the drug is now acting.

Acting as direct metabolic poisons on cell enzyme systems

Cell metabolism is fundamental to energy production, synthetic processes, and is a potential target for toxins. Most compounds that work in this way cause injury to key organs such as the liver and kidney, as the cellular processes being altered are generic.

Examples of general metabolic poisons include carbon monoxide, cyanide, and iron.

Carbon monoxide competes with oxygen and effectively asphyxiates cells. Cyanide also interferes with mitochondrial cytochrome oxidase, and iron seems to work as a non-specific metabolic poison once taken up into cells, particularly liver, kidney, and brain.

Paraquat is actively taken up into cells and results in free oxygen radical generation. This causes a secondary fibrotic reaction in the lung to the damage being caused by paraquat, and this fibrosis is a common cause of death from hypoxia.

Biotransformation into toxic metabolites

In the case of some chemicals, conversion to a toxic metabolite is necessary to cause cell damage, and only when that is formed in excess does injury occur. Understanding the metabolic pathways of a poison is thus most useful where conversion to a toxic metabolite is a prerequisite for toxicity. Examples where such metabolic conversion to toxic metabolites occurs include paracetamol, methanol, and ethylene glycol.

New metabomic and genomic techniques are beginning to offer better insights. Research on this aspect of poisoning is an expanding area. Production of toxic by-products may cause immunological responses in susceptible patients, and these are related to genetic differences. For example, rare severe immunological toxicity to carbamazepine is believed to be due to this mechanism, and genomic studies are encouraging as a way forward in understanding basic mechanisms behind flucloxacillin-induced liver injury, and the differences in response to warfarin.

Biological toxins
These include toxins of both bacterial, animal, and plant sources. They have a variety of actions, depending on their source. Some are extremely specific in the receptor site they attack, for example, botulinum toxin (from botulism). Some act on cellular mechanisms to cause cell death, for example, ricin (from the castor oil plant) or amatoxin (*Amanita* species). Snake venoms act on several targets, often including a local inflammatory response and systemic features. In paralytic shellfish poisoning, the toxins in dinoflagellates in algal blooms are concentrated up the food chain and cause neurotoxicity in animals or humans eating shellfish in which they are concentrated. In scombroid poisoning, scombrotoxin is made by bacteria on fish after capture, and contains high levels of histidine which causes histamine effects after ingestion.

Mutagens and carcinogens
Mutagens are compounds which act on the DNA, affecting replication and transcription in a cell nucleus to cause damage and mutations. Since mutations are a basic mechanism underlying the onset of cancer, the effect is to increase cancer risk. A commonly used test for mutagenic potential is the Ames test, in which *Salmonella typhimurium* bacteria are exposed to a chemical and the occurrence of mutations evaluated. Many anticancer agents are mutagens, but their benefit in therapy outweighs the mutagenic risk. Carcinogens cause cancer, a common biological example is the fungus toxin aflatoxin B1 produced by *Aspergillus* growing on mouldy food crops. The compound benzo[*a*]pyrene, found in tobacco smoke is converted to a reactive metabolite, benzo[*a*] pyren-7,8-dihydrodiol-9,10-epoxide which underlies its carcinogenic potential. It also acts as an enzyme inducer, and may therefore affect the metabolism of other potential toxins (see Basic mechanisms of mutagenicity and carcinogenicity, pp. 8–9).

Cytotoxics
These primarily damage rapidly dividing cells in the gut or bone marrow. The mechanisms that follow include rapid necrosis or a slower programmed cell death (apoptosis). Cell death may also follow an immune response involving lymphocyte subgroups such as cytotoxic T cells.

Teratogens and fetotoxic agents
Teratogens cause damage to the developing embryo in the early weeks of gestation, and result in malformations. Fetotoxic agents affect the developing fetus, for example, affecting liquor production (see Management of the pregnant woman who is poisoned, pp. 48–51).

Radiation (radioisotopes)
Ionizing radiation causes cell damage and cell death, usually via damage to DNA. Mechanisms involve both cytotoxicity and, if not fatal, increased mutagenicity and carcinogenesis (see Chapter 15, pp. 357–379).

Other causes of 'toxic response'
A certain proportion of patients have symptoms that are not easy to explain using conventional toxicological assessments. Such patients develop symptoms which appear to occur at concentrations of chemicals that would not be expected to cause conventional toxic effects. Symptoms may, for example, be triggered by odour, particularly of chemical materials or perfumes. In rural environments odours emanating from sprayed crops or present in spray-drift may trigger symptoms. Such symptoms can cause acute anxiety and stress in patients who believe they have been poisoned. A full explanation and reassurance is essential in gaining trust and reducing consequent morbidity. It is important, however, to ensure that symptoms caused by low-dose exposure to chemicals are not due to specific immunological responses, as found, for example, in occupational asthma, or due to biological material present in the atmosphere, for example, toxins from mouldy hay.

Conclusion
Understanding the mechanisms by which a toxin acts is a key part to understanding its likely effects, time course, and potential therapies. Toxic agents may act in more than one way—ethylene glycol causes intoxication, but kills by conversion to toxic metabolites—and appreciating such complexities is crucial to the optimum care of patients.

Further reading
Hayes AW (2007). *Principles and Methods of Toxicology*, 5th edition. New York: Informa Healthcare.

Klassen CD (2008). *Casarett & Doull's Toxicology: The Basic Science of Poisons*, 7th edition. New York: McGraw Hill.

Timbrell JH (2008). *Principles of Biochemical Toxicology*, 4th edition. New York: Informa Healthcare.

Basic mechanisms of mutagenicity and carcinogenicity

Definitions

A mutagen is an agent that can alter the structure of the genetic material (DNA or RNA).

A carcinogen is an agent that will induce neoplastic transformation of cells either directly or indirectly.

There are many agents that cause cancer including chemicals, radiation, viruses (e.g. human papillomavirus and cervical cancer), and some anticancer drugs themselves such as etoposide and tamoxifen. While mutagens can also be carcinogens not all mutagens induce carcinogenesis and vice versa.

Mutagenicity

The classic test for mutagenicity is the Ames test, devised by Bruce Ames in the 1970s. This test uses a mutated strain of *Salmonella typhimurium*, which requires histidine for growth, and will not grow in its absence. When this strain is exposed to a mutagen the bacterium reverts to wild type and can grow on medium lacking histidine. Putative mutagens can therefore be easily detected by this simple test.

It is important to note that cells contain mechanisms that repair damaged DNA. If such systems are absent (genetically) or altered by drugs (e.g. antiviral agents) then cancers may be more likely.

Carcinogens are classified by their mode of action: genotoxic or non-genotoxic

Genotoxic carcinogens produce tumours by damaging DNA directly. This may be by forming an adduct with DNA as in the case of doxorubicin (Adriamycin®) or by causing DNA strand breaks which prevents normal DNA replication. Some carcinogens require activation before they become effective, e.g. polyaromatic hydrocarbons. Activation of these pro-carcinogens usually involves cytochrome P450 mixed function oxidases.

Non-genotoxic carcinogens do not affect DNA directly. There are several ways in which non-genotoxic carcinogens can work, for example, by increasing cell proliferation and thereby increasing the probability of mutation within the cell. Often these agents enhance the effects of genotoxic carcinogens. In this case, however, an initiated cell (see 'Initiation' subsection) is required.

Carcinogenesis

Carcinogenesis rarely occurs as the result of a single event, and is often a multi-step process (Figure 1.2). It requires multiple alterations to DNA, which accumulate with time, explaining why most of the solid tumour changes are associated with increased age of detection. The common changes that occur are amplification, mutation or deletion, or any combination thereof of a range of growth-related genes. The process involves three distinct and separate stages: initiation, promotion, and progression.

Initiation

Requires exposure in some way to a carcinogen. This will produce a change within the genetic material of the cell; these will often be simple mutations. This initiation event will most likely have no obvious effects, and an initiated cell can remain dormant for months, years, or even decades. Initiation is an additive and irreversible process.

Promotion

A second 'event' leads to increased proliferation of the initiated cell. This process is reversible and a

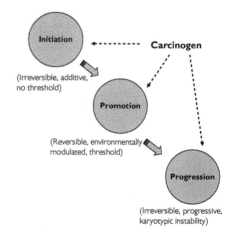

Fig 1.2 Multi-step carcinogenesis.

dose–response relationship exists. In other words, there is a threshold effect. It can be environmentally modulated by factors such as smoking and diet.

Progression

Results in complete neoplastic transformation, an irreversible process associated with complex changes to DNA and karyotypic instability. Often the changes at this stage result in the production of unusual proteins, for example, ectopic production of fetal proteins in adults. For example, α-fetoprotein is produced by some lung cancers and carcinoembryonic antigen is produced in colorectal cancer.

Carcinogenesis is therefore a progressive process requiring multiple 'errors' before a normal cell is converted into a cancer cell (Figure 1.3). This progression has been particularly well documented for colorectal carcinoma where the adenoma–carcinoma sequence was first outlined. As the normal cell moves through the sequence from adenoma I to II to III and to carcinoma, mutations accumulate in both tumour suppressor genes such as *APC*,

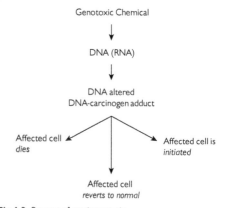

Fig 1.3 Process of carcinogenesis.

p53, and *DCC* and proto-oncogenes such as *K-ras*. In the main, proto-oncogenes are converted to oncogenes which usually means a loss of regulation of the 'normal' gene and continued, or over-expression, of the growth-promoting gene. Tumour suppressor genes are usually mutated such that they no longer produce the appropriate protein, or are deleted entirely. The net result of these changes is uncontrolled cell growth or neoplasia.

Characteristics of cancers

Cancer cells are essentially normal cells that have acquired certain altered characteristics that enable them to become malignant. It is the very fact that cancer cells are mutated forms of our own cells that makes cancers difficult to treat effectively. Chemotherapy normally exploits biochemical differences between the pathogen and the host to kill or remove the invader. In a patient with cancer there are a few biochemical differences in cancer cells, compared to normal cells, that can be exploited for therapeutic purposes. This results in many 'off target' or side effects that are common and well known in cancer treatments.

There are five key characteristics that differentiate cancer cells from normal cells:

1 Loss of growth controls—the ability to grow continuously and evade signals from growth suppressors.
2 Evade apoptosis and thus resist cell death.
3 Induce angiogenesis—providing the growing tumour with its own blood supply.
4 Invasion and loss of spatial relationships to other cells.
5 The ability to metastasize.

Loss of growth control

Normal cells respond to and release a range of growth factors which are used by neighbouring cells to continue cell proliferation. This is known as paracrine signalling, meaning between different cells. Normal cells continue to do this until a counter signal indicates cessation of growth. Cancer cells also have this paracrine signalling, but in addition cancer cells can release and respond to their own growth factors, known as autocrine signalling. This provides the cancer cell with a continuous supply of growth-promoting signals. This is often linked to the loss of anti-proliferative signals from tumour suppressors such as p53 and Rb.

Apoptosis is an altruistic form of cell death that allows a single cell to die in a controlled manner. Cell grow requires the cell to undergo an ongoing process of replication of DNA and synthesis of key regulatory proteins, a process known as the cell cycle. There are four phases in this cycle and between each boundary there are check points where cells can undergo a type of surveillance to ascertain any damage that may prevent normal cell cycling and division. In normality, a damaged cell can be programmed to undergo apoptosis and therefore be eliminated. In cancer, the cells have lost these critical gatekeeper functions and so can continue to grow harbouring mutations. Understanding the process of apoptosis and its regulation are key goals for oncology as this may provide novel targets for controlling cell death (and cell growth) which will have implications for treatment of patients not just with cancers but with other diseases where inappropriate cell death occurs, e.g. Alzheimer's disease.

Biomarkers

A biomarker is defined as a biochemical feature or facet that can be used to inform the clinician about the prognosis for the patient. In cancer, biomarkers can be used to detect exposure to a carcinogen, diagnose early disease,

and perhaps inform on mode of action of the carcinogen. A biomarker may also be an objective measure of the disease and its response to therapy. There are many types of biomarker: predictive, prognostic, mechanistic, safety, and surrogate. Safety biomarkers are commonly used as an indicator of toxicity, and are used in the drug development process. Biomarkers of response to therapy are particularly important in oncology where drugs with low therapeutic index are used routinely and non-responding individuals are relatively common.

Carcinogens

The complete list of carcinogens is beyond the scope of this section but the interested reader is referred to the International Association for Research in Cancer (IARC) who produce both categories and lists of known and suspected carcinogens:

- Class 1: definite (e.g. azathioprine, etoposide, diethylstilbestrol, vinyl chloride).
- Class 2A: probable (e.g. doxorubicin, cisplatin, dibenzo[*a,l*]pyrene, nitrogen mustard).
- Class 2B: possible (e.g. benz[*a*]anthracene, carbon tetrachloride, mitomycin C).
- Class 3: not classifiable (e.g. zidovudine, aciclovir, anthracene, cimetidine).

(Reproduced from International Agency for Research on Cancer, *World cancer report 2008*, IARC, Lyon, France, Copyright © 2008, with permission.)

Interestingly, a number of anticancer drugs fall into class 1 or 2A. This may prove problematic, for example, in adults treated with drugs such as etoposide in childhood.

Anticancer drugs

Most of the anticancer agents are cell poisons and as such affect any cell type, thus the major toxicity is in normal cells. The action of these drugs is mainly anti-proliferative and so they will affect any growing cell but especially rapidly growing cells, such as bone marrow and gastrointestinal cells. The majority of the standard anticancer drugs affect either DNA synthesis or function or the building blocks required for DNA replication. The next-generation agents are biologics and as such tend to be more selective albeit in a smaller and highly selected population of patients.

The standard anticancer drugs are most effective against cancers where the majority of the cells are in the cell cycle, e.g. leukaemias where 80% of cells are dividing compared to solid tumours where ~20% of the cells are dividing at any one time. Drugs fall into two broad categories: the cell cycle specific drugs, which only affect cells at a specific stage in the cell cycle (vincristine affects M phase), and the cell cycle non-specific agents such as the alkylating agents, which affect cells at any stage of growth.

Although there are a number of drugs that will prevent cell growth as yet there are few, if any, that specifically influence cancer metastases.

Further reading

Ames BN (1979). Identifying environmental chemicals causing mutation and cancer. *Science*, 204:587–93.

Elmore S (2007). Apoptosis: a review of programmed cell death. *Toxicol Pathol*, 35:495–516.

Hanahan D, Weinberg RA. (2000) The hallmarks of cancer. *Cell*, 100:57–70.

Hanahan D, Weinberg RA (2011). The hallmarks of cancer: the next generation. *Cell*, 144:646–74.

Vogelstein B, Fearon ER, Hamilton SR, *et al.* (1988). Genetic alterations during colorectal-tumor development. *N Engl J Med*, 319:525–32.

Drug handling in the poisoned patient—toxicokinetics

Background

The study of drug handling in patients during normal dosing is called pharmacokinetics. The term toxicokinetics has been derived to describe the handling of drugs and other toxins in overdose and poisoning. The word 'xenobiotic' is used to describe all foreign chemicals the body encounters, and through evolution organisms have developed techniques to change and remove such compounds. These processes are normally designed to make lipid-soluble compounds, which are usually more biologically active, more water-soluble, and thus suitable for excretion, normally in the urine, but also in bile. In the case of some xenobiotics and their metabolites, excretion may be by exhalation of breakdown gases (e.g. CO_2) in breath. The liver is the major organ involved in metabolizing xenobiotics, but drug metabolism may occur in many body systems, as drug metabolizing enzymes and drug transporter systems occur widely. Local toxicity may follow such reactions if they produce toxic metabolites.

Under normal circumstances the enzyme systems in man that are responsible for metabolism are present in excess amounts in proportion to the xenobiotic. This allows the same proportion of material to be metabolized per unit time no matter what the original quantity. This type of process is called 'first-order' metabolism and explains why in general the use of drugs therapeutically is relatively simple. Doubling the concentration of the drug will not affect the proportion removed over a fixed period and thus the concept most physicians find easiest, that of the plasma half-life, will be unaffected. If the enzyme system is saturated, a maximum amount (rather than proportion) is excreted and overall elimination will slow. This is termed 'zero-order' metabolism.

Useful definitions

Kinetics

- Half-life: the time for a plasma concentration to reduced by 50% (this assumes first-order kinetics). Units: time, e.g. 4 hours.
- Clearance: is a measure of the amount of plasma from which the quantity of drug removed in a fixed time period would be present. Units: volume/time, e.g. mL/minute (analogous to creatinine clearance).
- Apparent volume of distribution: uses the plasma concentration of a drug and its known dose to estimate the total volume into which that drug is apparently dissolved. For very water-soluble compounds this volume is low, approximating extracellular water (a few litres), whereas for lipid-soluble compounds this may be many times the actual volume of the patient, as drugs are sequestered into fat. Units: L or L/kg body weight.
- Bioavailability: the proportion of the dose reaching the systemic circulation. For intravenous administration this is 100%. For oral administration this may vary from virtually zero to 100% for different compounds, and is affected by solubility, uptake pumps in the gut wall, and first-pass metabolism. Units: percent.
- First-pass metabolism: the proportion of a drug metabolized while it is being transported via the portal circulation into the systemic circulation for the first time (the first pass). Usually much higher for lipid-soluble

drugs. May also be important when active metabolites are formed.
- Peak concentration: the maximum concentration achieved in plasma or blood, usually this is measured following oral dosing as with intravenous dosing peak is immediately after the injection. Units: concentration/volume, e.g. 10 mg/mL.
- Time to peak concentration: the time taken to reach the peak concentration. This is a useful measure following oral dosing as it may indicate when maximum effects of the drug are to be expected. Units: time.
- Modified (slow-release): for drugs with very short half-lives pharmaceutical companies may market preparations that slow the absorption, and hence prolong the effective action of a drug. Typical examples are morphine and other short-acting opioids, theophylline, and some calcium channel antagonists.

Drug metabolism

- First-order metabolism: metabolism in which a fixed proportion of drug is metabolized within unit time.
- Zero-order (saturation) metabolism: metabolism in which a fixed amount of drug is metabolized in unit time. In this situation it is not possible to calculate a drug's half-life since a different proportion of amount of drug in the body is eliminated as the total quantity reduces.
- Saturation kinetics: the pattern of drug metabolism that results from zero-order kinetics. Small increases in dose result in larger than expected increases in plasma concentration.
- Phase 1 metabolism: usually largely by hepatic enzymes (e.g. cytochrome p450, classified as CYP...) in which the structure of the drug is altered, normally by the addition of chemical groups which make it more water-soluble, or able to be conjugated. These metabolites are usually inactive, but may be more active (e.g. codeine to morphine by CYP2D6, see later in this list). Some metabolites may be very toxic, termed reactive metabolites (e.g. for paracetamol).
- Phase 2 metabolism (conjugation reactions): in which parent drug or phase 1 metabolite has groups such as sulfate or glucuronide attached, resulting in increased water solubility.
- Pharmaco- and toxico-genetics: the study of genetic influence on drug handling in dose and overdose.
- Polymorphic metabolism: metabolism by an enzymic pathway under genetic control in which discrete populations differentially express the gene. Consequently metabolism by that route is at different rates in different patients. In some cases this may result in an almost total lack of therapeutic effect in those lacking enzymes responsible for converting relatively inactive drug to more active drug (e.g. codeine to morphine by CYP2D6) or resulting in excess action of the drug because metabolism does not occur (e.g. inactivation of metoprolol by CYP2D6). If extra copies are present the opposite effect is seen (e.g. excess morphine from codeine). Expression of polymorphisms often varies in different racial groups.
- Drug transporters: specific molecular mechanisms by which drugs are pumped in and out of cells. These

transport processes are differentially expressed in different cell lines, and, for example, one reason why some malignancies are relatively resistant to anti-cancer drugs.

Since the half-life is constant in first-order systems, it would be the same after 1 or 10 g. Thus it is possible to calculate fairly easily that changing a dose from 1 to 10 g, while leaving the dosing interval unchanged, will produce a tenfold increase in average plasma concentration. For most overdose situations, therefore, the implications of these basic principles are that the concentration in the body will be proportionally higher, and the rate of decline in plasma concentration will often be similar to that of normal therapeutic doses. It may therefore be possible to estimate how long it may take for a particular drug to be eliminated.

The handling of drugs and toxins following overdose normally obeys the same principles as apply following normal dosing. However, as the dose of ingested material increases it becomes more likely that individual enzymes become saturated, or absorption delayed or perturbed.

Two classical examples of enzyme saturation at 'therapeutic' doses are for ethanol and phenytoin. For ethanol the dose range for enzyme saturation varies between approximately 5 and 15 g/hour in different individuals, with most being around 10 g/hour. Phenytoin metabolism also saturates within the therapeutic dosing range. Plotting plasma concentration against time on semi-log-linear graph paper will show a convex curve in drugs that have this type of metabolism. It is, however, important to be aware that a similar pattern may be caused by very slow absorption, and here it is the process of absorption that controls the plasma concentration, rather than the processes of elimination. This is often seen in overdose when large quantities are retained in the stomach.

Significance of toxicokinetics for techniques to alter drug elimination

The processes involved in drug handling are simply: absorption, distribution, metabolism, and elimination. It is theoretically possible to affect all these four processes, but it is important to understand the implications for overall toxicity.

Absorption may be reduced by binding material within the gut, with charcoal, or by increasing toxin removal from the gut using whole-bowel irrigation (WBI). Evidence of the clinical benefits of these techniques is limited, the first being very time-dependent, and the second really only potentially applicable for poisons that are absorbed slowly, classically modified-release formulations.

Distribution is generally a passive process but there is some active uptake of material into cells, although it is rare for an antidote to be targeted at cell transport processes. Binding of material within plasma by using chelation is one technique that is used to alter distribution of agents such as metals or digoxin.

It is possible to affect drug metabolism in two ways, induction or inhibition. Induction requires synthesis of new enzyme and takes several days. It is therefore not used therapeutically, but may be seen in individual patients who ingest drugs that increase their own metabolism ('auto-induction') such as carbamazepine. Inhibition of drug metabolism is used therapeutically in poisoning, for example, in the management of toxic alcohol ingestion to prevent formation of toxic metabolites.

Increasing the elimination of water-soluble drugs may be achieved by haemodialysis or haemoperfusion. In these systems drugs are extracted from blood passed over membranes or columns. The amount of drug removed is proportional to the flow rate on the system and its ability to cross the membrane. In haemodialysis the dialysate is water-based and it is only the most water-soluble compounds for which this technique is appropriate. Key to understanding the role of haemodialysis is the proportion of total drug clearance for which the kidney is responsible and which can be modified by artificial means. If the kidney only excretes 10% of total clearance it is clear that even doubling this will have little effect on the overall quantities of drug remaining in the body and exerting a toxic effect. Hepatic metabolism forms the principal route of drug elimination for most drugs and haemodialysis therefore has a limited role.

Unfortunately there are many claims in the literature of the benefits of these techniques, which do not bear close scrutiny. Toxic alcohols, salicylates, lithium, and valproate are examples where benefit can be shown.

Effects of poisoning on kinetics

One of the main problems facing the clinician managing a patient with poisoning is in understanding the effects that poisoning has on normal physiology, that will in turn change drug handling. Some simple examples include:

- delayed gut motility resulting in slow, or delayed absorption (virtually no absorption occurs from the stomach)
- impaired cardiovascular function affecting drug distribution and liver blood flow
- impaired hepatic function due to a hepatic toxin impairing drug metabolism (e.g. in paracetamol poisoning)
- renal failure (hypotensive or toxic) resulting in impaired renal excretion of parent drug, and/or accumulation of active metabolites and renal acidosis.

Studying kinetics

Relating blood concentrations of poisons to their effects is key in understanding how best to approach therapy, particularly that aimed at changing toxin elimination and handling. While complex statistical techniques using population kinetics have thrown new light on this aspect, important data can often be gleaned by careful analysis of results in individual patients. This means both studying blood and urine concentrations of parent drug, and also ideally metabolites, together with amounts from any elimination techniques applied. This should allow calculation of the impact (i.e. overall contribution) of a particular therapy. Determining whether saturation of metabolism or changes in metabolic pathways in overdose occurs can most effectively be done in individual patient studies.

Further reading

European Medicines Agency (1995). *ICH Topic S 3 A: A Guidance for Assessing Systemic Exposure in Toxicology Studies*. <http://www.ema.europa.eu/docs/en_GB/document_library/Scientific_guideline/2009/09/WC500002770.pdf>.

Rowland M, Tozer TN (2011). *Clinical Pharmacokinetics and Pharmacodynamics Concepts and Applications*. Philadelphia, PA: Wolters Kluwer.

Winter ME (2010). *Basic Clinical Pharmacokinetics*. Philadelphia, PA: Wolters Kluwer.

Poisons information services

Background

After 1945 there was a rapid expansion in the production of pharmaceuticals, industrial and household chemicals, pesticides, and other products resulting in an increase in the number of people exposed to such chemicals. A subsequent increase in accidental poisonings in children resulted and a rise in the number of suicides and, as then termed, parasuicides. Poisoning treatment centres for such patients were set up in various countries and poisons information centres began to appear. The first information centre was probably that in Chicago in 1953 and the first in Europe in the Netherlands in 1959.

UK services

In the UK in the 1960s there was considerable concern about poisoning resulting in the Atkins Report (1962) and the Hill Report (1968) which recommended setting up regional poisoning treatment centres. Poisons information centres and treatment centres were subsequently established. The poisoning treatment centre in Edinburgh, for example, provided medical and psychiatric treatment and was the home for an information centre. Poisons information centres in Belfast, Birmingham, Edinburgh, Leeds, London, and Newcastle provided information, mainly to medical professionals, about human and (from Leeds and London) animal poisonings. These centres grew and changed over the years and the National Poisons Information Service (NPIS) resulted. In 2003 this service was commissioned by the UK Health Protection Agency, now part of Public Health England (PHE) with units in Birmingham, Cardiff, Edinburgh, and Newcastle.

The information services initially gave advice by telephone to medical professionals. From 1983 the Edinburgh centre provided information via computer using Viewdata technology, initially to Scotland, but later expanding to serve registered users throughout the UK and also poisons centres in other countries. Registered users are generally emergency departments, other hospital departments, general practices, pharmacists, public health physicians, and other medical professionals. In 1999 the database TOXBASE® transferred to the Internet (<http://www.toxbase.org>) and is available as an app since 2012. Since 2000, telephone enquiries in the UK have fallen from more than 240,000 to just over 53,000 in 20012/13, while TOXBASE® sessions (logons) rose from over 100,000 to over 608,000 (Figure 1.4).

Most countries in the world now have one or more poisons information services and in all but two (UK and Netherlands) enquiries are answered from both medical professionals and members of the public, whereas in the UK and the Netherlands telephone enquiries are answered from health professionals only. In the UK information for the public is provided by NHS 111 or NHS Direct (England and Wales) and NHS 24 (Scotland), who use NPIS services, including TOXBASE®, to provide poisons information.

Poisons information internationally is usually available 24/7 by telephone, but several other countries have followed the UK and now provide information to health professionals via the Internet, including Australia and New Zealand, Sweden, and the Netherlands. In the UK information is provided:

- by access to the Internet poisons information databases TOXBASE® (registered users only)
- by telephone enquiry to the NPIS national service.

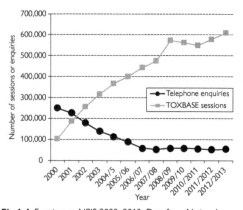

Fig 1.4 Enquires to NPIS 2000–2013. Data from National Poisons Information Service.

In the UK and the USA initial telephone information is provided by information staff (scientists, SPIs), pharmacists, and nurses. In some countries such services are always provided by qualified physicians, though this is much more expensive. The availability of consultant clinical support from poisons services varies in different countries depending on the model. Thus, in the UK further information in complicated and serious cases is available by telephone referral for discussion with an NPIS consultant clinical toxicologist (24-hour service).

Services provided by poisons services vary but in the UK include:

- information on ingredients, toxicity, features, and management for poisoning with thousands of agents:
  - chemicals which could be potentially be involved in terrorism
  - herbal products
  - household products
  - industrial chemicals
  - pesticides and other agrochemicals
  - pharmaceuticals
  - plants and fungi
  - snakes and venomous animals
  - substances of abuse
  - toiletries and cosmetics.
- advice in cases of poisoning, from specialists in poisons information
- advice on exposure to agents during pregnancy—UK Teratology Information Service (UKTIS)
- advice to government departments on poisoning issues
- chemical incident advice
- deliberate release advice
- e-learning for toxicology
- location of antidotes
- referral for discussion with a clinical toxicologist in serious cases
- tablet identification.

Internet poisons information

As the costs of providing 24-hour telephone information services increase, providers have sought other cost-effective alternatives. The largest is currently the UK service TOXBASE®.

TOXBASE® provides information on more than 14,000 agents, together with additional information on antidotes, nursing guides, and teratology information, and has more than 1.3 million hits per year. Alert boxes for triage are available for public access services, primary care, and ambulance services. Nursing guides are provided for use by emergency department nurses.

Information structure and content range from other international providers of on-line services varies.

Telephone services

Numbers of calls vary depending on the service provided. Thus the NPIS receives in excess of 50,000 telephone enquiries per annum, but over 600,000 Internet enquiries. The telephone call load is a low number compared to services taking public calls, but the overall enquiry rate per head of population is similar or exceeds that in other developed countries when measured per head of population.

Calls are normally recorded for clinical governance purposes. Specialists in poisons information who handle the poisons enquiries need to collect all relevant clinical information about the patient and the incident to ensure that the caller receives the best advice. Details of the calls are entered into case record databases for audit purposes and to improve further the management of poisoning.

The following details will generally be requested by any international poison service:

- The caller's full contact details including telephone number
- Patient details (age, gender, identifier, relevant medical history)
- Details of the case (agent, co-ingestants, route(s) of exposure, times of exposure, acute, chronic or staggered overdose)
- Patient's clinical condition, investigations carried out with results (including units)
- Management to date, including any antidotes used.

The NPIS conducts surveillance activities on behalf of the PHE, Medicines and Healthcare products Regulatory Agency (MHRA), and other government agencies on the toxic effects of agents and products in the United Kingdom, and additional information may be requested of enquirers about an agent or product of interest, or further follow-up carried out to check the outcome of the incident. Similar functions are conducted internationally.

At times of national emergency, or during heavy workload periods, some poisons centres have constructed automatic telephone systems to deal with the common enquiries. These use voice recognition software but have not been widely tested internationally.

Poisons centres

Poisons centres work collaboratively internationally, through academic groupings such as the European Association of Poisons Centres and Clinical Toxicologists (EAPCCT; <http://www.eapcct.org>) and the American Association of Poisons Control Centres (AAPCC). A worldwide listing is available (<http://www.who.int/gho/phe/chemical_safety/poisons_centres/en/>).

Most countries provide similar services and often take the majority of their enquiries from members of the public. Some, for example in France, are funded to provide pharmacovigilance, others provide combined services with medicines information. Annual reports are prepared, either individually or for cooperating centres.

Poisons information staff are involved in teaching and research. Staff attend and contribute to international congresses and are involved closely in the work of the World Health Organization (WHO), the International Programme on Chemical Safety (IPCS), and local state or national activity, e.g. in European Union (EU) member states and the European Commission (EC).

Poisons centre staff can provide experts in cases of unusual outbreaks as they have connections with centres in other countries via organizations such as EAPCCT, AAPCC, the Asia Pacific Association of Medical Toxicology (APAMT), and the American Academy of Clinical Toxicology (AACT). These hold annual meetings and promote research in clinical toxicology. International groups often cooperate in projects to produce consensus reports such as the position statements on gut decontamination, e.g. single-dose activated charcoal. Poisons centres also collaborate with the WHO International Programme on Chemical Safety (IPCS) INTOX project which provides help, particularly to poisons centres in the developing world.

Further reading

Chyka PA, Seger D, Krenzelok EP, et al. (2005). American Academy of Clinical Toxicology; European Association of Poisons Centres and Clinical Toxicologists. Position paper: single-dose activated charcoal. *Clin Toxicol*, 43:61–87.

Federal Institute for Risk Assessment (BfR) Annual reports. <http://www.bfr.bund.de/en/publication/annual_reports-62595.html>.

IPCS INTOX Programme: <http://www.who.int/ipcs/poisons/intox/en/index.html>.

James D, Adams RD, Spears R, et al. (2010). Clinical characteristics of mephedrone toxicity reported to the UK National Poisons Information Service. *Emerg Med J*, 28:686–9.

Mowry JB, Spyker DA, Cantilena LR et al (2013). 2012 Annual Report of the American Association of Poison Control Centers' National Poison Data System (NPDS): 30th Annual Report. *Clin Toxicol*, 51:949–1229.

National Poisons Information Service (2013). *National Poisons Information Service* – Annual Report 2012–13 <http://www.hpa.org.uk/Publications/ChemicalsPoisons/NationalPoisonsInformationServiceAnnualReports/>.

Pharmacovigilance

Background

Pharmacovigilance is the process by which:

1 use of medicinal products is monitored to identify previously unrecognized adverse effects or changes in the patterns of adverse effects both during clinical trials and during routine clinical use post-marketing
2 risks and benefits associated with the use of medicinal products is assessed to determine if regulatory action is required
3 information is provided to healthcare professionals and patients to optimize safe and effective use of medicines
4 impact of regulatory action is monitored.

Regulatory agencies

Within the European Union (EU), the regulatory agencies involved in pharmacovigilance consist of the European Commission (EC) as the competent authority and responsibility for medicinal products authorized centrally in the EU being devolved to the European Medicines Agency (EMA) and the competent authorities for regulation of medicines in the member states. The EMA supports the competent authorities in member states and provides a coordination role.

In the UK, the competent authority agency is the Medicines and Healthcare Regulatory Agency (MHRA) which coordinates pharmacovigilance via its advisory committee, the Commission on Human Medicines (CHM) and other expert advisory groups.

Adverse drug reactions and adverse events

- An adverse drug reaction (ADR) is an unwanted or harmful reaction experienced following the administration of a drug or combination of drugs under normal conditions of use, which is suspected to be related to the drug. This may be a known side effect of the drug or it may be new and previously unrecognized. The reaction may be dose-related and predictable from the known pharmacological actions of the drug or may be idiosyncratic.
- An adverse event (AE) is any undesirable event experienced by a patient whilst taking a medicine, regardless of whether or not the medicine is suspected to be related to the event.

The key word in both these definitions is 'suspected' and there is no requirement for proof of association when making reports.

ADRs are common and cause significant morbidity. It is estimated that in the UK, ADRs cause 6.5% of hospital admissions, of which 2% were fatal reactions. The overall annual cost of ADRs to the National Health Service (NHS) has been estimated to be £466 million.

Adverse drug reaction reporting

In clinical trials

Clinical trials involving medicinal products are subject to the safety reporting provisions of The Medicines for Human Use (Clinical Trials) Regulations 2004.

All serious adverse events (SAEs) and suspected unexpected serious adverse reactions (SUSARs) should be reported by the investigator to the trial sponsor who should then report to the MHRA. Any fatal or life-threatening reaction should be reported within 7 days of being informed and all others within 15 days.

Post-licensing

Following drug licensing, the marketing authorization holder for the drug is responsible for providing periodic safety update reports (PSURs), which summarize the worldwide safety experience with that medicinal product at specified time points after licensing. In addition for new drugs there is a requirement for marketing authorization holders (licensing holders) to produce risk management plans.

Although this is not a statutory obligation, healthcare professionals and patients can also voluntarily report adverse reactions using spontaneous adverse drug reaction reporting schemes such as the Yellow Card Scheme in the UK.

Yellow Card Scheme

The Yellow Card Scheme was introduced in the 1960s in response to the thalidomide disaster and was the first of its kind in the world. It has evolved from originally being just for physicians to a scheme that now takes reports from all healthcare professionals and patients. Yellow Cards can be completed in paper or electronic form to report any suspected adverse reaction, regardless of causality.

Reactions to licensed and unlicensed medicine, over-the-counter drugs, complementary and herbal medicines, radiographic contrast media, and blood products can be reported using the Yellow Cards.

It is particularly important to report the following:

- ALL reactions to new drugs and vaccines (marked with an inverted black triangle (▼) in the *British National Formulary* (BNF).
- SERIOUS reactions to established drugs and vaccines (including over-the-counter and herbal medicines), even if this is a well-recognized reaction.

  These include reactions which are fatal, life-threatening, disabling, incapacitating, resulted in or prolonged hospitalization, medically significant, and congenital abnormalities.
- ALL adverse reactions in children.
- ALL suspected delayed drug effects.

Data from the Yellow Card Scheme is entered into a database in MHRA using MeDRA (Medical Dictionary for Regulatory Activities)—an internationally accepted terminology for adverse event reporting.

Risk assessment

The Yellow Card database of suspected ADRs is used to generate signals for previously unidentified hazards or side effects which can then be evaluated with additional sources of evidence. These include:

- worldwide regulatory authorities, e.g. other adverse reaction databases such as Eudravigilance database maintained by the EMA which contain adverse reaction reports to medicines licensed across the EU and the WHO's international database maintained by the Uppsala Monitoring Centre.
- pharmaceutical companies
- morbidity and mortality databases
- worldwide published medical literature including case reports, clinical, and epidemiological studies.
- pharmaco-epidemiological studies.

Pharmaco-epidemiological studies

Pharmaco-epidemiological studies can be of a variety of types. Typically two designs are adopted; case–control studies or cohort studies.

Case–control studies—large prescription-based databases such as the Clinical Practice Research Datalink (CPRD) formerly known as General Practice Research Database (GPRD) can be used to compare adverse event rates in patients exposed to a drug (cases) compared to matched patients not exposed (controls). This is a more robust design than that of cohort studies, but is generally much more expensive.

Cohort studies follow groups of patients receiving a drug and attempt to evaluate toxicity. There is no formal control group. One example is the prescription-event monitoring or 'Green Form' scheme conducted by the Drug Safety Research Unit in Southampton. General practitioners are asked to complete a questionnaire (Green Form) to record all events in patients prescribed a particular drug over a specified time period.

In addition careful consideration of information from all sources may lead to identification of unexpected adverse reactions or increased frequency of adverse reactions in susceptible groups or in specific situations, e.g. in overdose. This type of approach is sometimes termed toxi-covigilance to differentiate it from pharmacovigilance.

Regulatory actions

Regulatory agencies will then consider what actions need to be taken to minimize risk and communicate this to healthcare professionals and the public.

The MHRA works closely with other regulatory authorities in the EU on these issues. The EMA has a Pharmacovigilance Working Party which advises the Committee for Medicinal Products for Human Use (CHMP) and the competent authorities in member states. An EU Rapid Alert and Incident Management System also exist to provide timely responses to new safety data. The European agencies also collaborate with other agencies across the world, including the Food and Drug Administration (FDA) in the USA.

Regulatory action may include:

- changes to warnings in the product information, i.e. Summaries of Product Characteristics (SPCs) or on the package label, i.e. patient information leaflets (PILs)
- restricting the indications for use
- changes in the specified dose
- changing the legal status, e.g. from over-the-counter to prescription only
- removal of the medicine from the market, if the risks outweigh the benefits.

These regulatory actions are communicated to healthcare professionals by:

1 posted letters (popularly known as Dear Dr letters) to all doctors and pharmacists
2 electronic cascade highlighting urgent warnings
3 publication in the monthly bulletin 'Drug Safety Update'
4 publication on the agency (MHRA or EMA) website.

Further reading

Aronson JK, Ferner RE (2005). Clarification of terminology in drug safety. *Drug Saf*, 28:851–70.

Clinical Practice Research Datalink: <http://www.cprd.com>.

Drug Safety Research Unit website: <http://www.dsru.org/pem>.

Drug Safety Update website: <http://www.mhra.gov.uk/Safetyinformation/DrugSafetyUpdate/index.htm>.

European Medicines Agency website: <http://www.ema.europa.eu>.

Eudravigilance website: <http://eudravigilance.ema.europa.eu/human>.

Hauben M, Aronson JK (2007). Gold standards in pharmacovigilance: the use of definitive anecdotal reports of adverse drug reactions as pure gold and high-grade ore. *Drug Saf*, 30:645–55.

Medicines and Healthcare Regulatory Agency Pharmacovigilance Learning module: <http://www.mhra.gov.uk/ConferencesLearningCentre/LearningCentre/pharmacovigilancelearningmodule>.

Pirmohamed M, James S, Meakin S, et al. (2004). Adverse drug reactions as cause of admission to hospital: prospective analysis of 18820 patients. *BMJ*, 329:15–19.

Uppsala Monitoring Centre website: <http://www.who-umc.org/>.

Wu TY, Jen MH, Bottle A, et al. (2010). Ten-year trends in hospital admissions for adverse drug reactions in England 1999–2009. *J R Soc Med*, 103:239–50.

Principles of surveillance of non-pharmaceutical poisoning (toxicovigilance)

Background

Health surveillance can be defined as an ongoing activity to detect changes in trends or distribution of a disease with the aim of preventing or controlling it. The majority of effort in surveillance of the toxic effects of chemicals has focused on pharmaceuticals. It is, however, obvious that the human population is exposed to many other potential toxins. Such exposures may be the result of specific events, for example: the use of pesticides in agriculture or in the home; exposures in the workplace to chemicals used in industry; or accidental exposures following chemical incidents. Toxic materials may also be present in the environment, or in water supplies.

While many manufacturers of commercial products will collect data on reports they receive of toxicity from the use of their products it is only in relatively rare cases that such material is systematically analysed over a range of products within the same category made by different manufacturers. Thus in the case of pesticides, for example, there are European directives requiring governments to undertake surveillance of the health effects of pesticides in their population. For most other commercial products this does not apply in the UK though individual European member states do have other arrangements, the best example being in Germany, where all chemical exposure health effects are required by law to be reported to a central government agency. This section will deal with the various techniques that can be applied to study the effects of non-pharmaceuticals on population or individual health.

Definitions

A short discussion on the epidemiology of poisoning and on pharmacovigilance is presented elsewhere in this chapter (see The epidemiology of poisoning, pp. 2–3 and Pharmacovigilance, pp. 14–15). It is important to differentiate surveillance from formal epidemiological academic studies. Table 1.1 offers a tabular explanation of the main differences.

Table 1.1 Comparison between surveillance and epidemiological research

Variable	Surveillance	Epidemiological studies
Data collection timescale	Ongoing	Limited
Method of data collection	Part of routine; wide population coverage	Special procedure; focused on smaller populations
Amount of data per case	Often limited	Generally detailed
Dissemination of information	Regular; supporting fast actions	Sporadic, infrequent reports or academic publications
Uses of data	Hypothesis generating; identifying a problem; monitoring trends	Hypothesis testing; characterizing a problem

Simple surveillance is a continuous process, and ideally should use routine data collection systems. Epidemiological studies are more focused to specific populations and time periods. They are often retrospective and further hypotheses on exposure effect may then be generated from associations discovered using statistical modelling. In contrast, surveillance systems require no a priori hypothesis and are designed to signal generate in much the same way used for pharmacovigilance systems such as the Yellow Card Scheme.

By their nature most health surveillance systems relating to poisoning tend to deal with acute exposures. Examining the chronic effects of acute exposures, or the effects of lower-dose chronic exposure, requires more subtle population measures that can be derived from population statistics. Thus to study occupational exposure to chemicals and cancer risk, for example, it is necessary to have information on occupation, duration of occupation, and ideally level of exposure (i.e. job type) that links to a health registry covering many years. This type of approach works more readily for increased incidence of rarer diseases. Thus scrotal cancer in chimney cleaners and bladder cancer in aniline dye workers are examples of diseases where surveillance systems could detect a disorder. Establishing the effects of coal mining on different lung disease than silicosis is a much more challenging problem due to the co-morbid effect of smoking, which is common in this population.

Types of surveillance systems

There are a number of sources of surveillance data within most countries. Examples within the United Kingdom would include:

- hospital activity analysis from the Office of National Statistics (ONS) in England and Wales, and from the Information and Statistics Division, part of NHS National Services Scotland
- poisons information services (NPIS in the UK) from their enquiry data
- manufacturers, who receive reports from members of the public and health professionals about their products
- occupational health schemes
- for pesticides, monitoring systems run by the UK Health and Safety Executive
- the Veterinary Product Committee 'blue card' scheme for human effects from use of veterinary medicines.

Worldwide a number of other systems operate and some of these will also be briefly mentioned in this section.

In order to appreciate and understand the roles of these various systems it is necessary to be aware of their limitations and the methodologies employed. It is useful to consider what the optimal surveillance system would actually look like and what data it would attempt to collect and collate (Table 1.2).

In practice no surveillance system operating is completely comprehensive, but some may be used together to gain a greater understanding. Thus it is relatively common to examine both poisons information material and

Table 1.2 Example of information required for surveillance systems

Category	Details
Agent(s)	Product name; active ingredients and co-formulants of toxicological significance; additional information, e.g. concentrate or dilute, spray or solid
Exposure details	Location; circumstance (e.g. deliberate, occupational, or accidental); amount: duration of exposure and time since ceased; biomarkers as appropriate
Patient details	Gender; age; weight; clinical features; severity score; medical history; occupation; geographic location; health record identifier
Investigation and treatment	Results of investigations and treatments given (e.g. decontamination, antidote use)
Outcomes: acute and/or chronic	Levels of medical intervention; results of investigations; health outcomes; organ damage; long-term sequelae

hospital activity analysis, although the best examples where this has been successful tend to be in the area of pharmacovigilance.

Each type of surveillance will now be described briefly together with their strengths and weaknesses.

NHS systems

Data are recorded for each episode of hospital care provided by the NHS. Each episode will have one or more codes applied that reflect a diagnostic category or procedural activity, and codes are linked to the ICD system. Data linkage has been available for episodes in Scotland for many years, and is being developed in England and Wales.

Codes are normally assigned by administrative staff, and are based on scrutiny of the clinical records after the hospital episode. Therefore, the quality of the coding process is influenced by the accuracy and ability of the administrative staff to interpret the clinical documentation in reaching the most appropriate codes to reflect that hospital episode. UK Hospital Episode Statistics (HES) does not currently collect information on the employment of patients. Collection and analysis of information on employment classification and health outcomes in this surveillance scheme would provide valuable data at little cost.

The strengths of this scheme are:
- Hospital data afford a very large number of reports of episodes of ill health of all types and from whatever cause (~13 million hospital admissions and 15 million hospital episodes annually are included).
- Detailed recording of the duration of hospital stay.
- There is a standardized format for coding. This makes it possible to compare regional data.
- Demographic data captured includes age, gender, and the patient's home postcode.

The weaknesses of the scheme are:
- The ICD coding structures used tend to deal with classes of compound in a diagnostic category rather than specific ingredients, making the study of many specific agents difficult.

- Quality of case definition cannot be confirmed (studies have indicated that coding may be inaccurate for a number of specific clinical diagnoses).
- The occupation of patients, which would provide valuable information on work-related exposures, is not recorded.
- Changes in coding processes or systems can make it difficult to understand data trends (ICD coding changes with updates).
- An admission might involve several hospital episodes owing to transfer of care between consultants; therefore, data will vary between hospitals where different practices exist for handover between consultants.
- There is no confirmation of the extent of any exposure.
- Symptoms that might be attributable to possible exposure are not captured in a systematic way.
- There has been no linkage between multiple hospital episodes for an individual patient.
- The outcomes of exposure cannot be attributed; e.g. toxin exposure, pneumonia, and death might all be coded for a single episode but this does not indicate a causal relationship.
- Symptoms attributable to chronic exposure are less likely to be recorded.
- Unlikely to cover long-term health effects unless used in epidemiological studies.
- The data are not collected in real time but normally assimilated days, weeks, or months later.
- Emergency department attendances that do not result in admission have not previously been recorded. However, some data may be available in the future from the experimental HES ED database.

Information is also collected on deaths, in England and Wales by the ONS, and in Scotland by the General Register Office (GRO). These datasets are derived from death certificates provided by medical practitioners, or in poisoning after inquests by coroners in England and Wales, and procurators fiscal in Scotland. These data may not be entirely reliable as a definitive cause of death in toxicological cases since the determination may be by jury under the instruction of non-medically trained coroner, or following advice from a pathologist without specific expertise in toxicology.

Public Health England (previously known as the Health Protection Agency) and Health Protection Scotland keep records of public health incidents involving chemicals for surveillance purposes, and carry out investigations as well as advising on public health approaches to management. These data are provided to local public health bodies and government. They are reliant on information reaching their networks and are closely linked to poisons information services in the UK.

Poisons information services

In the UK there is no routine system for monitoring exposures of biochemical effects of household products, chemicals, or pesticides, unless the patients are significantly symptomatic. The UK NPIS systems collect data that can be used to assist surveillance.

The strengths of this scheme are:
- Data are collected in real time with involvement of a clinician and therefore are of high clinical quality.
- Data are collected at a time very adjacent to exposure, and graded for severity. Treatment details are included,

and routine laboratory test results are collected as available.

- For telephone enquiries a WHO poisons severity score (PSS) is applied.
- Data are immediately available for analysis by NPIS.
- Appropriate ethical and anonymization procedures potentially allow data to be used for long-term research studies.
- The system acquires data concerning circumstances of exposure, site of use, and geographical location.
- Data may include specific information about both actives and formulations.
- Links to the UK Teratology Information Service give specific consideration to the few reported incidents involving pregnant women.
- Samples for specific analysis can be suggested near the time of exposure.

The weaknesses of this scheme are:

- There is relatively low collection of chronic (repeated or long term) data.
- Mild incidents where a patient may not access medical advice will not be recorded.
- Reporting via third parties (healthcare staff) may lead to more selective reporting.

This can be compared to data obtained by the US National Poisons Data System (NPDS), which is published in a more comprehensive format, and where all data is collected from phone calls to poisons centres. In contrast to the UK these units take calls from members of the public, which represents their main source of enquiries.

The strengths of this scheme are:

- Data collection is in real time from enquirers by telephone (US poison centres do not use online enquiry systems).
- The caller often receives active follow-up near to the time of exposure.
- Treatment details and laboratory data are available if medical staff make the enquiry.
- Data are available for real-time analysis (NPDS uses custom-built software to do this for incident alerting with Bayesian algorithms).
- Data on circumstances of exposure and product used are acquired.
- Data may include specifics of batch and formulation.
- Sample collection may be possible for medical enquiries.
- Data collection over more than 10 years allows time trend analysis.

The weaknesses of this scheme are:

- Majority of enquiries are from members of the general public causing potential for 'noise' in the data through duplicate reporting or inaccuracies.
- Use of the system by health professionals is variable across USA.
- There is no link to public health data sets.
- The system has very limited capability for detecting chronic effects.
- It is costly to operate.

Other UK surveillance systems

Other UK surveillance systems run by government sponsored agencies cover veterinary products and pesticides.

A recent EU directive has stressed the need for pesticide surveillance systems in all members of the EU.

UK pesticide systems

A number of approaches are used in detecting adverse health effects from pesticides. The longest established is the Pesticide Incident Appraisal Panel which is sponsored by the Health and Safety Executive (HSE). This examines case reports received by the HSE and investigated by their field inspectorate. The visits from these inspectors are often some days after actual exposure and information is therefore derived from the patient and their health professional if they have consulted one. The information is collated and assessed by the panel which produces annual reports based on its assessment of causality. These reports are also seen by the Advisory Committee on Pesticides (ACP) and used to inform licensing decisions the pesticide use. This system collects information on about 100 cases a year. Manufacturers are legally required to report any adverse effect reports to the ACP.

Professionals who use pesticides, for example, in agriculture and forestry, now have to undergo a certification programme, and a national register of certificate holders has been established, from which information on health effects can potentially be obtained going forward over time. This has not been tested yet but offers an opportunity for future use. The cohort will include several thousand individuals.

The NPIS has been conducting surveillance on pesticide-related ill-health following acute exposures reported by health professionals, using a structured questionnaire in order to obtain information on a larger cohort of patients. This project has been funded as a research tool, but in future may be incorporated into a national system to meet the requirements of the EU directive on pesticides. It has so far collected information over 10 years and a number of research publications have been produced in addition to regular reports to the HSE, the funding agency, which are also shared with the ACP. This system currently collects information on about 2000 exposures per annum. Since this information is close to the time of exposure, acute symptoms assessed, and biological samples obtained, the system provides information on pesticides of a similar type produced by the NPDS system described earlier.

UK veterinary product systems

Humans may become exposed to veterinary products during their use or afterwards, e.g. for products applied topically, such as flea sprays for domestic pets. In order to appropriately license such products for use by both professionals and members of the public the Veterinary Medicines Directorate (VMD) and the VPC have set up a system akin to the Yellow Card Scheme used for pharmacovigilance. In this case the cards are coloured blue and the system termed the 'blue card' system. Reports may be completed and returned to the VMD who analyse and present the data to the VPC. The system collects less than 100 cases per annum.

Industrial occupational health schemes

While individual companies often employ their own medical advisers, most are not large enough to undertake routine health surveillance in the workplace, pp. 388–389). (see also Medical surveillance

The Health and Occupation Reporting network (THOR) collects data on work-related ill health (WRIH)

in the UK and is run by the Centre for Occupational and Environmental Health at the University of Manchester. THOR is composed of a number of sister schemes that allow clinical specialists, occupational physicians (OPs), and general practitioners (GPs: THOR-GP) to report cases of WRIH. In all schemes, physicians are asked to (voluntarily) report new cases of disease seen in the previous month which in their opinion are work related.

For each reported case, the physician is asked to provide details on diagnosis, age, gender, geographical region, occupation, industry, and the associated causal agent. An estimate of the incidence of occupational disease or disorders in the UK based on medical specialist diagnoses can then be derived. The scheme has identified specific risks and tracked trends in occupational disease, relating them to interventions.

This scheme collects significant numbers of cases; more than 8000 cases related to skin disorders were reported to the scheme between 2002 and 2009. Between 2005 and 2009 almost 5500 cases were reported to THOR-GP.

International schemes of surveillance

Most countries have health surveillance schemes in place, although many apply to infectious disease rather than poisoning. In this section some specific examples illustrating the difference approaches to, and benefits of, surveillance will be highlighted briefly.

There are networks across the EU collaborating on surveillance, and these tend to concentrate on individual outbreaks of health problems, for example, related to imported products which contain potentially toxic material, or potential terrorist incidents.

In Sri Lanka pesticide poisoning has been a major problem for many years. By examining the numbers of deaths caused by individual pesticides in different groups, and particularly within the overall category of insecticides, determining which appear more toxic to humans, public health officials have been able to markedly reduce deaths by removing more toxic insecticides from the marketplace.

In Germany a system is in place through the Bundesinstitut fur Risikobewertung (BfR) Poison and Product Documentation Centre for reporting poisoning incidents associated with a wide range of chemicals. The list of notifiable substances is: biocides, pesticides, cosmetics, wood preservatives, any professionally used chemical, harmful chemical substances from the environment, and toxic plants and animals. The system is regulated under German law, and physicians are obliged to notify the BfR of any actual or suspected cases of poisoning. The approval holders or manufacturers are also required to provide information regarding formulations of products to support investigations.

BfR provides details of poisoning incidents to manufacturers and distributors to alert them to any issues related to their products. In the case of severe health problems the incident is notified immediately, in less severe health issues the notification comes in the form of an annual report. The reports are also available publicly.

There are a number of ways that incidents can be reported to BfR, including by using the official form for notifications of poisonings, physicians' letters or test results, telephone notifications, or written notifications submitted by post, fax, or email. All those submitting information including physicians are anonymous. Interestingly although the scheme is legally binding, the numbers of cases reported are significantly lower than the anticipated exposures in a population the size of Germany.

In the USA a number of agencies may be involved, both at national (federal) and state level. The main agency is the Centers for Disease Control and Prevention (CDC) which has its own systems, but also collects information from NPDS run by the US poisons information centres. CDC also runs a National Health and Nutrition Examination Survey (NHANES) which uses interviews, clinical examination, and samples of blood and urine for laboratory testing for 1 in 50,000 of a randomly selected group of US citizens. Information is collected, for example, on 219 environmental chemicals, including pesticides herbicides, and fungicides. These results do not appear to be clearly linked in the CDC analysis to health outcomes but provide more strategic information on the exposures of the population to individual compounds within the survey. Individual US states, for example, California for pesticides in fruit growing, have developed intensive surveillance systems for populations deemed at risk, including both workers and their families. These report to state legislatures.

Conclusion

A wide range of surveillance systems are in place nationally and internationally; however, none is comprehensive. It is important to understand the benefits of surveillance and also the potential witnesses of each system in order to better understand how to apply surveillance within populations. Readers are encouraged to study surveillance approaches to the areas in which they have interest.

Further reading

Barr DB, Wong L-Y, Bravo R, et al. (2011). Urinary concentrations of dialkylphosphate metabolites of organophosphorus pesticides: National Health and Nutrition Examination Survey 1999–2004. Int J Environ Res Public Health, 8:3063–98.

BfR. Notification of poisoning incidents. <http://www.bfr.bund.de/en/notification_of_poisoning_incidents-10143.html>.

Bronstein AC, Spyker DA, Cantilena LR, et al. (2012). 2011 Annual Report of the American Association of Poison Control Centers' National Poison Data System (NPDS): 28th Annual Report. Clin Toxicol, 50:911–1154.

Dawson AH, Eddleston M, Senarathna L (2010). Acute human lethal toxicity of agricultural pesticides: a prospective cohort study. PLoS Med, 7:e1000357.

NPIS Annual Reports: <http://www.hpa.org.uk/Publications/ChemicalsPoisons/NationalPoisonsInformationServiceAnnualReports/>.

Office for National Statistics (2012). Deaths Related to Drug Poisoning in England and Wales 2012. <http://www.ons.gov.uk/ons/rel/subnational-health3/deaths-related-to-drug-poisoning/2012/index.html>.

Persson HE, Sjoberg GK, Haines JA, et al. (1998). Poisoning severity score. Grading of acute poisoning. J Toxicol Clin Toxicol, 36:205–13.

PIAP reports: <http://www.hse.gov.uk/agriculture/resources/pesticides.htm>.

The Health and Occupation Reporting network (THOR) website: <http://www.medicine.manchester.ac.uk/oeh/research/thor>.

Clinical trial design

Clinical trials

Conventional studies of novel pharmaceuticals are performed in a sequential manner, but this is often unfeasible in clinical toxicology research. Therefore, the general approach to clinical trial design in toxicology involves an approach that is adapted from conventional drug safety studies. There are a number of unique methodological limitations.

Phase I studies

These typically involve a single ascending-dose design, including 'entry into human' studies. Minimal effective concentrations in animals or *in vitro* models are used to estimate the likely human dose by allometric scaling; the initial dose selected for entry to human studies is typically 100–1000-fold lower than the intended therapeutic dose. In each dose tier, eight to ten participants receive only a single administration; one or two are randomly allocated to placebo. Clinical, electrocardiographic (ECG), and laboratory safety data are reviewed before proceeding to the next dose tier in different participants. Basic pharmacokinetic data may be obtained, for example, concerning food interactions, but the main purpose is to assess tolerability and safety.

Phase II studies

Based on phase I data, a smaller number of doses are selected for phase II studies. These may involve multiple ascending-dose study design, where each participant receives multiple administrations of a particular dose. Phase II also includes 'proof of concept' studies, for example, demonstration that a novel antihypertensive might lower blood pressure. Phase II studies may involve both healthy subjects and patients. Dose-ranging studies establish the minimal effective dose, and maximal response is defined by no greater response despite a two- to threefold increase in dose.

Phase III studies

These extend beyond 'proof of concept' and evaluate the novel drug with reference to an established comparator in an appropriate patient group. This may involve, for example, examining the effects of a novel antidepressant in comparison to an existing treatment in patients with depression. Phase III also includes pertinent interaction studies and long-term outcome measures of safety and efficacy.

Phase IV research

Whereas phase I to III studies allow collection of sufficient data to support application for a Marketing Authorization, these data are limited to safety, tolerability, and efficacy in only several thousand people. Phase IV studies examine therapeutic usefulness and broader safety issues after marketing authorization. These involve drug exposure in large patient numbers, including long-term prospective clinical trials, and may reveal unexpected adverse effects or drug interactions. Post-marketing surveillance is undertaken by pharmaceutical companies concerning their own products, pharmacovigilance programmes (see Pharmacovigilance, pp. 14–16).

Unique considerations in clinical toxicology study design

Sources of data: case reports

Individual case reports may provide an important source of clinical outcomes after toxic exposure, particularly where patients have been exposed to an unusually high dose, or a novel agent with limited clinical data concerning toxicity. Patients that present after drug overdose do so in an uncontrolled manner and the opportunity to ascertain baseline function is lacking, in contrast to regulatory clinical trial design. It is impossible to have certainty regarding the time and quantity of drug(s) ingested, or prior use of other medications. These factors limit the interpretation of naturalistic case reports. Nonetheless, case reports may indicate toxic effects that were unexpected from effects of therapeutic doses, and indicate mechanisms of action not previously considered.

Sources of data: case series

Whilst individual case reports require very cautious interpretation, larger case series may be somewhat more informative. For example, across large patient series there is reasonable correspondence between patient reporting and qualitative and quantitative analytical measures of drug exposure. Evaluation of clinical outcomes across large groups of patients can help discern dose–toxicity relationships for particular agents, and allow comparison between the toxicity profiles associated with different agents. For example, excess cardiovascular mortality with dextropropoxyphene overdose compared to other opioid analgesics.

Assessment of toxicological effects

A fundamental challenge in clinical toxicology research is the lack of baseline clinical, ECG, and laboratory values. These may be estimated from data in the recovery phase if there has been a sufficiently long washout period, so that this might allow the magnitude of toxic responses to be determined. The primary manifestation of toxicity will depend on the particular agent, its mechanisms of action, and its known or anticipated toxic effects based on the basic pharmacological profile. For example, close electrographic monitoring would be appropriate for agents known to exert cardiotoxic effects. Likewise, the optimal duration of clinical observation is likely to be informed by the toxicokinetic properties of the particular agent, and the anticipated onset and duration of clinical effects. For example, hypotension is likely to occur within 2–4 hours of angiotensin-converting enzyme (ACE) inhibitor ingestion, whereas after thyroxine ingestion agitation and other effects might not occur until 12–36 hours later. In many cases, there is disparity between the duration of effect of therapeutic versus toxic drug quantities; for example, therapeutic dosages of short-acting insulin might be expected to last for several hours, whereas hypoglycaemia may persist for several days after massive overdose.

Comparison between groups

Greatest statistical efficiency is normally achieved using a cross-over clinical trial design, which is subject to less inter- and intra-subject variability and minimizes the participant numbers needed to attain statistical power. Patients would normally be allocated to treatment A followed by B after a suitable washout period, or B followed by A. However, the cross-over trial design is rarely feasible in clinical toxicology research, and parallel group design may be more appropriate. This involves random allocation to receive a particular treatment, and can be used to study an active treatment versus placebo, or compare different treatments. Inter- and intra-individual variation mean that very large participant numbers are needed to reach statistically significant conclusions. For example, 4629 patients were needed to achieve reasonable power in a study of single-dose or multiple-dose oral activated charcoal.

Dose versus toxicity

Toxic effects may be predictable from a known pharmacological mechanism of action, for example, hypotension due to calcium channel blockade. Conventional dose-titration studies involve sequential administration of higher and higher doses until a therapeutic response is achieved or adverse events occur, and this allows definition of the dose–response relationship. For certain drugs, increases beyond the therapeutic dose range produce little additional response, a so-called flattening of the dose–response relationship. However, other agents ingested in supra-therapeutic quantities may evoke a more profound response. Large patient series may define a clinically meaningful range of doses associated with moderate or severe toxicity. In some cases, this is a predictable extrapolation from therapeutic doses, for example, profound bradycardia and cardiac impairment after beta-blocker ingestion. In other cases, a toxic range may be defined for effects not normally encountered after therapeutic doses; for example, a higher rate of occurrence of seizures is observed after acute ingestion of more than 300 mg citalopram.

Toxicokinetic versus toxicodynamic data

A relationship is often sought between drug concentrations and pharmacological response, forming the basis of so-called pharmacokinetic-pharmacodynamic (PK-PD) modelling. There are many examples of where PK-PD correlation is poor, for example, antidepressants, analgesics, antiplatelet drugs, chemotherapy, and hormone therapies. Clinical responses persist beyond the period of drug exposure, and may be due to time taken to trigger an intracellular response or up-regulate receptor expression, development of tolerance, and inter-individual differences in drug response. Similarly, discrepancies exist between toxicokinetic data and toxicodynamic effects: laboratory confirmation of high drug levels may support the diagnosis but does not necessarily inform the likelihood of toxicity or outcome. Laboratory determination of drug concentrations are normally relied upon only if these correlate with poisoning severity and inform prognosis or need for antidote therapy, for example, carbamazepine, lithium, paracetamol, and salicylate concentrations.

Confounding factors

Naturalistic data in clinical toxicology are confounded by inaccurate dose reporting, co-ingestion of ethanol, and the coexistence of psychiatric or medical co-morbidities. In clinical practice, identification of the agent and dose is normally reliant upon patient self-reporting, although in clinical studies it may be desirable to measure drug concentrations. The effect of confounding by co-ingested drugs or ethanol may be minimized by selection of an appropriate control group with similar patterns of co-ingestion. Multivariate analyses attempt to address the effects of confounding factors, such as co-ingested agents, but these introduce a further source of error due to inappropriate weight applied to certain factors.

Regression to the mean is an important source of error if participants are selected on the basis of extreme physiological variables. For example, patients selected on the basis of abnormally low blood pressure are likely to show a time-dependent increase in blood pressure due to natural variation, rather than any specific intervention.

Ethical considerations

The ethical principles that underpin good clinical practice in the conduct of clinical trials are embodied in regulatory documents such as the European Clinical Trials Directive. There is a strong emphasis on protecting individual research participants, and patients that present to hospital after deliberate self-harm are a particularly vulnerable group. Patients are often unable to offer informed consent to study participation, due to intoxication, coma, distress, or psychiatric illness. The perception that informed consent is essential to clinical research has significantly hampered study in this patient group, and there has been slow progress towards developing new interventions and technologies. In some cases, it may be appropriate to seek the consent of a person close to the patient, where the decision is likely to reflect the patient's wishes. Alternatively, a legal representative may be able to provide informed consent on the patient's behalf.

Statistical considerations

The number of study participants should be based on a priori power calculations to allow statistically meaningful conclusions to be reached. Study design should take account of potential sources of bias where possible, for example, by using random treatment allocation rather than open label to minimize selection bias. Biological responses in a clinical toxicology context are not expected to be uniformly distributed, and should be assumed not to observe a normal distribution. Therefore, presentation of data should involve appropriate summary statistics, such as median and interquartile range or 95% confidence intervals, with comparison between groups using appropriate non-parametric tests. The rather ubiquitous Student's t-test should be reserved for comparison of data that observes a normal distribution!

Further reading

Afshari R, Maxwell SR, Webb DJ, et al. (2009). Morphine is an arteriolar vasodilator in man. Br J Clin Pharmacol, 67:386–93.

Eddleston M, Juszczak E, Buckley NA, et al. (2008). Multiple-dose activated charcoal in acute self-poisoning: a randomised controlled trial. Lancet, 371:579–87.

Gibbons RD, Amatya AK, Brown CH, et al. (2010). Post-approval drug safety surveillance. Annu Rev Public Health, 31:419–37.

Lee C, Lee LH, Wu CL, et al. (2006). Clinical Trials of Drugs and Biopharmaceuticals. Boca Raton, FL: CRC Press.

Muller PY, Milton M, Lloyd P, et al. (2009). The minimum anticipated biological effect level (MABEL) for selection of first human dose in clinical trials with monoclonal antibodies. Curr Opin Biotechnol, 20:722–9.

Waring WS, McGettigan P (2010). Clinical toxicology and drug regulation: a United Kingdom perspective. Clin Toxicol, 49:452–6.

Waring WS, Rhee JY, Bateman DN, et al. (2008). Impaired heart rate variability and altered cardiac sympathovagal balance after antidepressant overdose. Eur J Clin Pharmacol, 64:1037–41.

Study assessment and interpretation

Background

As a physician managing a poisoned patient it is important to be able to interpret and understand published work that may affect clinical decisions. Unlike most fields of medicine much of the practice of the management of poisoned patients is based on case reports or small studies in patients, rather than large clinical trials. These are often supported by data derived from work in animals. On some occasions it is necessary to use basic principles to decide treatment, even though there is no case material upon which to form a clear literature-based opinion. Thus a degree of pragmatism may be necessary, but where data is available it is important to be able to interpret it correctly.

One particular difficulty is that patients with poisoning rarely present soon after the poisoning episode, when it might be possible to obtain a clear series of blood tests or physiological observations that would assist in determining time-course and mechanistic relationships easily. Measurement of plasma concentrations for most toxins is impossible in an acute setting, and requires a formal research plan. Thus understanding the significance of any intervention in patient outcome becomes more challenging, since a clear risk assessment may not be readily applicable.

The literature base in clinical toxicology is usually formed from a series of different sorts of material; these will be briefly outlined, and some of the problems which apply to each will be discussed. It is useful to consider strength of evidence (Table 1.3).

Preclinical studies—normal volunteer studies

These studies are usually performed to establish 'proof of principle' and intended to study specific actions of a toxin (at low dose) or antidote. An example is the use of volunteer studies to examine efficacy of activated charcoal in reducing the bioavailability of a compound. Such studies show *potential* efficacy, but obviously the true dose of toxin cannot be administered to volunteers, and extrapolation from such studies may be unreliable if the toxin has pharmacological effects on the gut, which would be present at a higher dose than that used in an experimental situation. Thus this type of study is best used for hypothesis generation or to investigate specific physiological actions of an antidote or potential toxin.

Table 1.3 Example of levels of evidence

Evidence level	Category of evidence
A	Randomized controlled clinical trial, or meta-analysis
B	Non-randomized controlled trial or extrapolation from level A
C	Case-series study or extrapolations from level B studies
D	Expert opinion, ideally based on physiology, bench research, or first principles

Reproduced with permission from 'Acute Pain Management: Operative or Medical Procedures and Trauma'. AHCPR Clinical Practice Guidelines, No. 1. Acute Pain Management Guideline Panel. Rockville (MD): Agency for Health Care Policy and Research (AHCPR); 1992 Feb, Available from http://www.ncbi.nlm.nih.gov/books/NBK52152.

Clinical studies

Case reports

These may be the only data available for rare toxins and provide insights into toxic effects, and potentially beneficial treatments. The best types of report include information on toxin plasma concentrations over time, clinical features, and carefully documented effects of any treatment provided. Unfortunately many authors over-interpret data. A common example is in claiming benefits from extracorporeal removal of toxins. In this situation it is key to understand the proportional effect of dialysis or haemofiltration over and above the endogenous clearance of the toxin. Such calculations are rarely provided. For this reason merely showing that extraction of material is efficient across a dialysing membrane does not necessarily translate into a large difference in clinical benefit. In reality, recovery may be occurring at the normal rate.

Case series

These are an extension of case reports, and may provide more information on dose response across a population. Where treatment is given it may provide insights into benefits which should properly be then applied to a more formal clinical trial. It will be obvious that for rare poisons such studies are a major challenge. Very careful interpretation of claims in case series is therefore necessary. Application of population kinetic analysis methods to this type of scarce data usually produces a more informative result. If different therapies are applied to patients within the cohort it may be possible to show effects. Ideally pharmacological data should be linked to specific physiological variables, and cardiovascular or neurological effects are most easy to study in this way.

Comparative case series often compare historical control groups, but ideally should be collected concurrently. The key problem here is the change in other aspects of medical care that may affect outcome. In some clinical situations the benefits of treatment are thought so obvious that proper clinical trials are discouraged. This was the case when acetylcysteine was first introduced as a treatment for paracetamol poisoning. This effectively prevented dose ranging studies with the antidote to establish the optimum dose. Lack of such dose ranging studies in patients is common to many antidotes, and current recommendations are thus often empiric. For pharmacological antidotes the benefits may be rapid and easy to show, but for chelating agents or antibodies the outcome is delayed, and too often the surrogate marker of increased excretion or decrease in blood concentration is interpreted as an optimum response.

Controlled clinical trials

These are the best method of assessing clinical benefit, but the key problem in toxicology is acquiring adequate numbers of patients into such trials. Ethics committees are sometimes sensitive about the patient group, which is perceived to be vulnerable. The key feature for the clinician is, however, the appropriate endpoint. This may be difficult to establish, particularly for toxins that act on a number of sites. Use of surrogate endpoints is therefore relatively common and location may be misleading if not relevant to the mechanisms of actions causing death or major dysfunction.

Perhaps the most important message to give is that a statistically significant result may not indicate a clinically useful result. Similarly if very small numbers of patients have been studied a non-significant result may falsely suggest that treatment is ineffective. Ideally clinical trials are carried out using predefined patient groups, with estimated power calculations conducted based on the relevant clinical outcome. Data from previous studies or case series, indicating likely magnitude of clinical effects, aid this calculation. Over the past decade very large studies have been conducted in Sri Lanka which illustrate what can be done using this approach.

Key considerations are therefore:

- Use of an appropriate comparator group: retrospective control groups are less desirable but may be useful for very dramatically effective therapy, as was the case 40 years ago with acetylcysteine in paracetamol poisoning.
- Blinding and randomization: unfortunately many investigators forget the importance of this. Bias is a major problem in trials that are not blinded. Blinding may be to treatment, and/or outcome assessment. The crucial aspect is that the assessments are applied in a way which is not influenced by knowledge of the treatment being given. Changes in practice other than the treatment of being investigated, or changes in the epidemiology of the poisoning, may need to be considered when doing a clinical trial that may last several years. Sadly in toxicology very many studies cannot be evaluated as they are merely case series without adequate controls.
- Study power: adequate calculation of sample size in advance of the experiment is key to determining whether statistical errors may be present in the assessment. Two major errors apply: type A error, in which a false positive result is identified, and is usually caused by too small a sample size and random error; type B error in which a study is thought to be negative, when a larger experimental sample size is required, i.e. the study is 'underpowered'.
- Using the appropriate statistical test: simple data may be parametric or non-parametric in type, and observations may be done on several occasions. Applying the correct analysis is critical. The inexperienced researcher often picks on one paired grouping of data, and applies the wrong statistical analysis. Regrettably despite peer reviewing many studies still suffer from this problem.
- Using the correct endpoint: the most uncontentious endpoint in a clinical study is death. In practice most studies use 'surrogate' endpoints, measures that are intended to demonstrate biological change and assumed to equate to a long-term good or bad outcome. Mere evidence of reduction in concentration of the toxin in blood does not necessarily equate to improved survival.
- Analysis by number needed to treat (NNT) and number needed to harm (NNH) are useful in considering the clinical (as opposed to statistical) benefits of therapy.

Animal studies

Animal studies have traditionally been performed as baseline toxicity assessments to support the marketing of commercial products. The main reason for the studies is to ensure that the compounds are safe in use. Where hazards do exist, for example, in the case of pesticides, appropriate engineering processes or formulation change may be developed to reduce risk. Studies performed to support licensing often include material that is of interest to the clinician, but is usually not readily available,

particularly in Europe where issues of commercial confidentiality often prevent these data being seen. Studies to support a licence include short- and long-term toxicity, mutagenicity, carcinogenicity, and teratogenicity. There is data on the dose likely to cause harm in an animal, usually small rodents such as mice or rats.

The relative toxicity of the compound in animals may give some idea of possible toxicity in man. The clinician's main interest is in the likely *clinical* consequences, which is rarely fully reflected in the basic scientific data in animal studies. Information on the mode of death may, however, help; e.g. convulsions suggest CNS or cardiovascular toxicity. Short- and long-term toxicity studies in animals provide information on specific organ toxicity, usually obtained by examining blood test results, or histology. Animal data should include information on metabolism in animals, although not equivalent to man, it indicates main pathways of metabolism. This is particularly relevant to pharmaceuticals where drugs with similar structure tend to be handled alike. Effects often follow this pattern, thus ACE inhibitors cause hypotension and beta-blockers bradycardia. Animal data may also give an indication as to whether the onset or duration of these effects is similar to that of other drugs in the class and therefore whether delayed toxicity may occur.

Specific animal studies may be used to investigate more closely the mechanisms of action of the toxin or an antidote to support the use of an antidote for a particular poison. Unfortunately many studies are conducted by pre-treatment with an antidote prior to giving a toxin. This is different to the actual clinical situation and it is very difficult to know how to translate such studies to man. A much more realistic scenario is to give a toxin and subsequently treat with an antidote. This approach has been used in animal models to show intravenous lipid emulsion will reverse the effects of local anaesthetic agents on the cardiovascular system. This design of experiment is far more reliable than antidote pre-treatment.

It is also important to study the effect of the dose of toxin in such experiments. If a very high supra-lethal dose of poison is given followed by an antidote it will be difficult to show a benefit of therapy. Most antidotes work best within a range of effect where the poison is being given in a relatively small supra-toxic dose.

Understanding how the antidote is meant to work in clinical practice should help determine whether or not the animal data being presented is relevant to the human situation. Finally, the species being studied is important. Thus different rodent species differ very greatly in their susceptibility to paracetamol, with hamsters being exquisitely sensitive. It is therefore important to ensure the correct species has been used when interpreting data.

Further reading

Centre for Evidence Based Medicine (2009). *Levels of Evidence*. <http://www.cebm.net/index.aspx?o=1025>.

Cochrane database website: <http://www.cochrane.org/>.

GRADE Working Group (2004). Grading quality of evidence and strength of recommendations *BMJ*, 328:1490.

National Institute for Health and Clinical Excellence (2004). *Self-harm*. CG16. <http://www.nice.org.uk/CG016NICE guideline>.

Smyth RMD, Kirkham JJ, Jacoby A, et al. (2010). Frequency and reasons for outcome reporting bias in clinical trials: interviews with trialists. *BMJ*, 341:c7153.

Classification of psychiatric disorders and principles of treatment relevant to poisoning

Background

In the United Kingdom, as in other Western countries, the most common form of self-harm which presents to hospitals is self-poisoning. Since many, if not the majority, of those who self-harm meet criteria for one or more mental disorders, toxicologists, more so than other physicians, will encounter patients with mental health problems in their routine clinical practice.

For these clinicians a working knowledge of psychiatric diagnosis and treatment is useful in making preliminary diagnoses, guiding initial medical management, and communicating with psychiatric colleagues. Also, since many patients with a pre-existing psychiatric condition receive psychotropic medications which are often used in a self-poisoning episode, the rationale for psychotropic prescription in individual psychiatric conditions should be understood.

Classification and diagnosis in psychiatry

Diagnosis in psychiatry

In most branches of medicine, disease classification is by aetiology, or, where this is unknown, by pathology. While diagnoses are most often made clinically, they can subsequently be confirmed or refuted by objective tests—e.g. radiology, blood testing, biopsy, etc. Unfortunately, in psychiatry the aetiology and the pathological mechanisms of disease causation are often unknown or only partially understood and objective diagnostic methods are unavailable. For this reason, diagnosis in psychiatry is made via operational diagnostic criteria—where diagnoses are made according to explicitly stated, pre-agreed sets of symptoms with precise descriptions of the type, number, and duration of symptoms required for any particular diagnosis.

Operational classification

Two operational diagnostic classification systems for mental disorder are in common use worldwide: chapter V of the *International Classification of Diseases*, tenth revision (ICD-10), produced by the WHO, and the *Diagnostic and Statistical Manual*, fifth revision (DSM-5), produced by the American Psychiatric Association. The DSM-5 is an exclusively psychiatric classification system, while chapter V of ICD-10 is one chapter in a general medical classification covering all disease types. In this context *mental disorder* refers to mental illness, mental handicap, personality disorders, and substance use disorders.

Both these diagnostic schedules contain clearly defined clinical descriptions of mental disorders, together with explicit inclusion and exclusion criteria, and details of the type, number, and duration of symptoms required for diagnosis. The two classification systems are broadly similar without being completely compatible. Both continue to evolve: the DSM has recently been updated and the eleventh version of the ICD is currently under development. For non-psychiatrists, ICD-10 will be more familiar and will be the system used in this section and textbook.

Psychiatric diagnoses in ICD-10

ICD-10 divides psychiatric disorders into ten categories (see Table 1.4) within which are the individual disorders. Each disorder may be further defined by subtype, severity, or clinical course. There is no explicit 'hierarchy' of diagnosis but in clinical use there is an implicit hierarchy

Table 1.4 ICD-10 Classification of Mental and Behavioural Disorders

Category	Individual diagnoses
Organic disorders	Alzheimer's dementia, vascular dementia, other dementias, acute confusional state (delirium), mental disorders due to identifiable brain disease
Substance use disorders	Acute intoxication, harmful use of drugs or alcohol, drug or alcohol dependency, withdrawal states, drug- or alcohol-induced psychosis, drug- or alcohol-induced amnesic syndromes (e.g. Wernicke–Korsakoff syndrome), residual disorders (e.g. LSD flashbacks, alcohol-related dementia)
Psychotic disorders	Schizophrenia, schizotypal disorder, delusional disorder, acute psychosis, schizoaffective disorder
Affective (mood) disorders	Single-episode mania or depression, bipolar and unipolar depressive illness, cyclothymia, and dysthymia
Neurotic (anxiety-related) disorders	Phobic disorders (e.g. agoraphobia, social phobia), panic disorder, generalized anxiety disorder, obsessive–compulsive disorder, post-traumatic stress disorder, somatization disorder
Behavioural syndromes	Eating disorders (e.g. anorexia nervosa, bulimia nervosa), sleep disorders, sexual disorders
Disorders of personality and behaviour	Specific personality disorders (e.g. emotionally unstable (borderline) personality, dissocial personality, dependent personality), habit and impulse disorders, gender identity disorders, paraphilias
Mental retardation	Categorized as mild, moderate, severe, or profound depending on IQ and functional level
Disorders of psychological development	Specific developmental disorders of speech and language, specific developmental disorders of scholastic skills, pervasive developmental disorders (e.g. autism, Rett's syndrome)
Behavioural and emotional disorders of childhood	Attention deficit hyperactivity disorder (ADHD), conduct disorder, childhood anxiety disorders, tic disorders, enuresis/encopresis

Data from ICD-10 Classification of Mental and Behavioural Disorders <http://www.who.int/classifications/icd/en/bluebook.pdf>.

where a more serious diagnosis 'trumps' a lesser one—for example, a patient with active schizophrenia may well have prominent anxiety symptoms related to the presence of persecutory delusions, but would not be viewed as having an additional diagnosis of generalized anxiety disorder, even if the anxiety symptoms would, in isolation, have merited such a diagnosis.

Organic disorders

The organic disorders are those where the psychiatric symptoms can be directly related to gross structural brain abnormalities—in contrast to the (presumed) minor structural, or functional (i.e. neurochemical) abnormalities that lie behind other mental disorders. These disorders have the greatest overlap with neurological disorders, indeed many are also categorized *as* neurological disorders, with neurologists tending to deal with the motor and sensory aspects of the condition and psychiatrists with the cognitive, emotional, psychological, and behavioral aspects. The organic disorders include Alzheimer's dementia, vascular dementia, dementias related to other causes, acute confusional states, and psychiatric syndromes where there is a clear structural basis, e.g. hallucinations occurring after the development of a brain lesion such as a tumour—organic hallucinosis.

Substance use disorders

The substance use disorders are a range of characteristic psychiatric syndromes which directly relate to the ingestion of psychoactive substances. While the majority of these substances are illegal drugs, the greatest clinical importance by far in terms of numbers of patients affected and healthcare burden, are those disorders related to alcohol use. People take alcohol and illicit drugs for their brain effects, with the aim of producing a desirable alteration in mental state such as reduction of anxiety, euphoria, increased alertness, etc. They may, however, have undesirable effects, both acutely and when taken for a prolonged period. These are in addition to the physical health consequences of drug ingestion, overdose, or habitual use. The exact effects on mental state are drug specific; nonetheless a number of characteristic clinical syndromes are recognized.

Acute intoxication is a combination of physical and mental health features characteristic to the drug ingested and dependent on the dose taken, the degree of habituation, and the route of ingestion. In harmful use (also known as abuse), use of the substance persists despite negative consequences and attempts to stop. More severe than harmful use is dependency, where there is a development of psychological and/or physical dependency, increased tolerance to the drug's effects, physical withdrawals, and reinstatement of drug use after abstinence. In patients with established drug dependency, attempted abstinence can be followed by withdrawals that may be complicated by the development of delirium or seizures. Finally a number of drugs are associated with psychotic disorders and residual disorders, where psychiatric symptoms persist beyond the period of use of or withdrawal from the drug. This group includes alcoholic hallucinosis, Korsakoff's psychosis, and the 'flashbacks' occasionally seen in previous users of LSD.

Psychotic disorders

The psychotic disorders are characterized by the presence of psychotic symptoms as their core feature. These symptoms are qualitatively abnormal, rather than the quantitative abnormalities seen in the mood and anxiety disorders. The major psychotic illness (and in many ways the exemplar) is schizophrenia; other psychotic illnesses include delusional disorders, schizoaffective disorder, and acute psychotic episodes.

The main psychotic symptoms are delusions, hallucinations, and thought disorder. Delusions are abnormal beliefs, held with absolute subjective certainty, which are not amenable to reason or contradiction by argument. While they are often bizarre and absolutely improbable this is not always the case. Hallucinations are abnormal perceptions where there is an internal perception without an external object in the 'real' world. They can occur in any modality of perception, but in schizophrenia auditory hallucinations are the most common and are a diagnostic feature. Thought disorder is a breakdown in the normal connections between the flow of ideas in conscious thought and is often reflected in jumbled or incoherent speech.

Mood disorders

Mood disorders are those disorders where the central clinical feature is pathological disturbance of mood—either lowering of mood (depression), or elevation of mood (hypomania and mania). Depressive and manic illnesses are clinical syndromes where the core mood features are joined in depression by anhedonia (loss of the ability to experience pleasure), anergia, and deterioration in sleep, appetite, concentration, and libido; and in mania by over-activity, increased subjective speed of thought, increased rate of speech, and grandiose ideas, which may amount to delusions. Illness severity varies from mild (symptoms but without functional impairment), to moderate (functional impairment), and severe (functional loss). Severe depression and severe mania can be complicated by psychotic features (e.g. delusions and hallucinations) which are usually mood-congruent (e.g. delusions of poverty or terminal illness in depression; delusions of special powers or wealth in mania). Recurrent episodes are referred to as *unipolar disorder* (depressive episodes only) or *bipolar disorder* (aka manic depression) where there are both manic and depressive episodes.

Anxiety disorders

The anxiety (or neurotic) disorders have as a common feature the experience of the psychological and physiological effects of excess anxiety. Anxiety is of course a normal and adaptive response but in the anxiety disorders it occurs with pathological frequency, with insufficient stimulus, or in association with other features of mental disorder. The anxiety disorders include panic disorder, generalized anxiety disorder, the phobias (specific, social, and agoraphobia), obsessive–compulsive disorder, post-traumatic stress disorder, and the dissociative and somatization disorders.

Behavioural syndromes

The behavioural syndromes are a more diverse group of disorders where the characteristic abnormality is disordered behaviour, but where there are also mental state abnormalities and disturbed patterns of thinking. It includes anorexia nervosa, bulimia nervosa, other eating disorders, non-organic sleep disorders, and non-organic sexual dysfunction.

Personality disorders

The personality disorders are an occasionally contentious category of disorders where the abnormalities of mental state do not occur as discrete episodes, but are present in continuous form from adolescence onwards. Common to all personality disorders are that the abnormalities are seen in multiple areas of psychological functioning and behaviour, are present from late adolescence and persist through adult life, and cause distress to the individual and impair personal and social function and inter-personal relationships. The individual personality disorders include paranoid personality, schizoid personality, dissocial personality, and emotionally unstable (borderline) personality. The last of these will be familiar to toxicologists because of its strong association with repeat self-poisoning (the tendency to self-harm being one of its defining characteristics).

Mental retardation

The formal title of this group of disorders remains 'mental retardation' in ICD-10 but is now universally referred to as 'learning disability'. This group of disorders includes a very wide range of underlying illnesses including chromosomal abnormalities, pre- or intrapartum brain injury, and storage diseases. Their point in common is reduction in IQ below two standard deviations (SDs) from the human mean, i.e. below 70. Mental handicap is further subdivided into mild (50–69), moderate (35–49), severe (20–34), and profound (below 20). Progressively lower IQ is associated with progressive impairment in overall function and eventually the ability to self-care and develop language skills. Patients with mental handicap have increased risk of other mental disorders, which may be difficult to diagnose due to communication difficulties and differences in clinical presentation.

Developmental and childhood behavioural disorders

Deliberate (rather than accidental) self-harm is rare in children and so those psychiatric disorders only seen in childhood will be more rarely seen by toxicologists. They include autism and Asperger's disorder, ADHD, conduct disorder, and specific developmental and behavioural disorders.

The association of psychiatric diagnoses with self-harm

The majority of individual mental disorders are associated with an increased risk of both self-harm and suicide, with recurrent mood disorders and schizophrenia having particularly high rates of completed suicide. In any cohort of patients seen after self-poisoning, patients with mental disorders will be significantly over-represented. This coexistence of self-harm and mental disorder can arise by a number of mechanisms:

- Self-harm or attempted suicide as a result of abnormal mental state—e.g. a patient with severe depression taking an excess of antidepressants in an attempt to die or a patient with acute psychosis taking an overdose in response to hallucinations urging them to do so.
- Self-harm as a habitual behaviour used by patients with chronic disorders as a means of symptom control—particularly in patients with personality disorders.
- Self-poisoning with recreational drugs—patients with drug problems may self-poison due to inadvertent overdose or misidentification of the substance taken.
- Accidental with associated mental disorder—patients with learning disability or with dementing illnesses may be at increased risk of accidental overdose of medications.

An individual episode of self-poisoning may be a marker of as-yet-undiagnosed mental disorder, or, in patients with pre-existing mental disorder, it may be a marker of a relapse or worsening of the disorder. Patients with an episode of self-poisoning have a subsequently raised risk of further self-harm and of future death by completed suicide, with diagnosis and appropriate treatment of underlying mental disorder being a major potentially modifiable risk. Because of this a full psychosocial assessment of the patient following self-harm is mandatory. Toxicologists should liaise closely with psychiatric colleagues regarding the psychiatric assessment and treatment of these patients once the acute poisoning has been appropriately managed. Local arrangements will usually exist allowing shared working, collaboration, and smooth transfer of care to appropriate services.

Psychiatric drug treatments

Background

Drug treatments are used in mental disorders to control acute symptoms, as prophylaxis in conditions prone to recurrences, and for detoxification/maintenance in substance misuse conditions. The currently available drug treatments for mental disorders are often ineffective or only partially effective. Even when effective symptomatically, drug treatments are rarely curative and may not be disease modifying. Despite these caveats, psychotropic drug treatment is undoubtedly effective in treating the symptoms of many types of mental disorder and preventing recurrent episodes in vulnerable patients. Additionally, rates of completed suicide are found to be lower in effectively treated patients and conversely completed suicide is associated with inadequacy of drug treatment. In the management of mental health conditions, drug treatment should always be one part of a comprehensive treatment plan, involving psychological and social and rehabilitative and supportive elements.

Antidepressants

Antidepressant drugs are indicated for the treatment of major depressive episodes and as prophylaxis against depressive relapse. They may also be useful in the treatment of neurotic disorders, eating disorders, and in managing chronic pain. They should not be first-line drugs in the treatment of mild depression. They are clearly effective although compliance is often poor. Their mode of therapeutic action remains uncertain but all have the effect of increasing neurotransmitter availability in the postsynaptic cleft by either reuptake inhibition or breakdown inhibition. Only oral preparations are used clinically and may take 3–4 weeks to achieve therapeutic action when effective. In choosing an individual drug the factors considered are previous effectiveness in an individual, tolerability, risk in overdose, and side effect profile.

Antipsychotics

Antipsychotics are used in the treatment of acute psychoses (including schizophrenia) and maintenance of remission in patients with psychotic illnesses. They are also used in the treatment of manic illnesses, of psychotic features in severe depression, and are used in lower doses as anxiolytics, and for symptom control in delirium and in dementia. They have specific antipsychotic effects as well as undoubtedly beneficial anxiolytic and anti-arousal actions. All clinically effective antipsychotics are dopamine antagonists with D2 receptor specificity, with the exception of clozapine—a fact which may help to explain its unique clinical effectiveness in otherwise treatment-resistant patients.

Drug choice is again based on consideration of previous effectiveness, tolerability, and side effect profile. If a drug is successful in treating an episode of acute psychosis it is continued at that dose as a prophylaxis for at least 6–12 months, with lifelong treatment advised in some patients. Antipsychotic drugs are associated with a range of undesirable effects, including extra-pyramidal side effects, akathisia, acute dystonias, excess sedation, and weight gain which may limit ongoing compliance, particularly if patients are otherwise well. In some patients with poor compliance, or disorganization, antipsychotics may be given by depot preparation. Although not therapeutic drugs in mental health, patients with psychosis will often be prescribed anticholinergics—e.g. procyclidine, orphenadrine, to counteract extra-pyramidal side effects.

Mood stabilizers/antimanic agents
The carbonate or citrate salts of lithium are used in the treatment of acute manic episodes and in the maintenance of normal mood following remission. They also have a role in prophylaxis in unipolar depression and as an adjunct to antidepressant treatment. Lithium salts have a narrow therapeutic window necessitating blood level monitoring. Anticonvulsants (primarily carbamazepine and valproate) also have mood stabilizing and antimanic actions and are used for these purposes where lithium is not well tolerated or ineffective. There is a clear risk of 'rebound' mania following discontinuation of mood stabilizers, particularly if this is rapid, so these drugs should not be rapidly discontinued without advice and arrangements for close psychiatric follow-up.

Anxiolytics/hypnotics
Benzodiazepines replaced barbiturates in clinical practice following their introduction in the 1960s due to the latter's narrow therapeutic safety window. The benzodiazepines are clinically effective drugs which should be used with caution because of the risk of the development of tolerance, dose escalation, and iatrogenic dependency. They remain effective and useful drugs when appropriately prescribed and are useful for short-term management of severe anxiety, as short-term hypnotics, as sedative agents in severe behavioural disturbance, as an adjunctive treatment in depressive illness, and in management of withdrawal states, particularly from alcohol.

Cognitive enhancers
Acetylcholinesterase inhibitors are occasionally used as cognitive enhancers in dementia. These drugs are not curative or disease modifying. They are used in mild to moderate Alzheimer's disease and can be at least partially successful in stabilizing or even partially reversing cognitive and functional decline. Disease progression is unaffected and they are discontinued when ineffective or when the dementia has progressed so far that minimal improvement is functionally meaningless.

Substitute prescribing
Opiates, benzodiazepines, and occasionally amfetamines are prescribed to individuals dependent on these substances to facilitate medically supervised detoxification or, more commonly, as a substitute for illicit consumption as a 'harm-reduction' measure. The patient's account of the prescribed dose should always be checked with the prescriber and/or dispenser before being prescribed in hospital. The out-of-hospital prescription should be cancelled while the hospital is providing the prescription.

Prescribing after an episode of self-harm
Following an episode of self-harm one concern is often how to reduce the risk of further, perhaps more serious, self-harm, arising from the patient's possession of potentially toxic psychotropics. In some cases the self-harm episode will prompt a change in treatment itself. In other cases steps can be taken to reduce the risk—e.g. by dispensing smaller amounts of medication more frequently, or moving to medication supervision. In general the previous psychotropics should be restarted, at the previous dose, once the treatment of the poisoning episode allows. There should be no changes to the patient's psychotropic prescription without discussion with the psychiatrist managing the case.

Further reading
American Psychiatric Association (2013). *Diagnostic and Statistical Manual of Mental Disorders*, 5th edition. Arlington, VA: American Psychiatric Publishing.

Hawton K, Van Heeringen K (2009). Suicide. *Lancet*, 373:1372–81.

National Institute for Health and Clinical Excellence (2004). *Self-harm: The Short-term Physical and Psychological Management and Secondary Prevention of Self-harm in Primary and Secondary Care*. CG16. London: NICE.

National Institute for Health and Clinical Excellence (2011). *Self-harm: Longer-term Management*. CG133. London: NICE.

Skegg K (2005). Self-harm. *Lancet*, 366:1471–83.

Tournier M, Molimard M, Cougnard A, et al. (2005). Psychiatric disorders and their comorbidity in subjects with parasuicide by intentional drug overdose: prevalence and gender differences. *Psychiatry Res*, 136:93–100.

World Health Organization (1992). *International Statistical Classification of Diseases and Related Health Problems*, 10th revision. Geneva: World Health Organization.

Risk assessment and principles of occupational exposure assessment

Background

Risk assessment is something we do each time we cross the street, drive a vehicle, participate in sport, or purchase new equipment for the home. For each event we have assessed the associated risks and deemed them acceptable. The process is no different in the workplace except that the health and safety of populations of workers, and the corporate well-being of the employing business, is dependant on the actions taken. The following gives a brief overview of the principles involved and the reader is guided to other sources of information for a more detailed discussion of this topic. For additional information see Principles of industrial hygiene and toxic hazards in the workplace pp. 382–387.

The purpose of risk assessment

Risk assessment is the structured and systematic procedure that is dependent on the correct identification of hazards and an appropriate estimation of the risks arising from them, with a view to making risk comparisons for purposes of their control or avoidance (see <http://www.hse.gov.uk/risk/>). It also provides the link between the scientific knowledge of the risks and the risk reduction measures that can be taken, which can be both qualitative and quantitative. If performed well the process will reduce the uncertainty in a process but will never make it disappear. There is no such thing as a risk-free environment in the workplace (or anywhere else).

In occupational settings the purpose is to enable a valid decision to be made about any measures that are deemed necessary to control exposure to substances and events hazardous to health arising in the workplace.

These broadly fall into the following categories:

- *chemical*, e.g. cyanide, hydrofluoric acid, asbestos
- *biological*, e.g. HIV, hepatitis B
- *psychological*, e.g. stress
- *physical*, e.g. noise, vibration, radiation.

However, this section will concentrate on chemical hazard assessment in the UK, but the principles are the same for all hazards and translate to other countries.

Definitions

Hazard

A source or situation with a potential for harm in terms of human injury or ill health, damage to property, damage to the environment, or a combination of these.

Simple examples include: chemicals, electricity, working with ladders, etc.

Risk

Is the combination of the likelihood and consequence of a specified hazardous event occurring together with an indication of how serious the harm could be.

The process of risk assessment

This should be kept as simple as possible so that non-specialists are able to perform risk assessments in the workplace. A successful tool used in the UK is the five-step model outlined here as an exemplar. Other counties have their own systems, requirements and frameworks, e.g.

NIOSH (National Institute for Occupational Safety and Health; USA), DOSH (Department of Occupational Safety and Health; Malaysia), EASHW (European Agency for Safety and Health at Work; EU):

1 Identify the hazards.
2 Decide who might be harmed and how.
3 Evaluate the risks and decide on precautions.
4 Record your findings and implement them.
5 Review your assessment and update if necessary.

(Reproduced from the 'Five steps to risk assessment', Health and Safety Executive <http://www.hse.gov.uk/pubns/indg163.pdf>, licensed under the Open Government Licence v2.0, <http://www.nationalarchives.gov.uk/doc/open-government-licence/version/2/>.)

In many organizations, the risks are well known and the necessary control measures are easy to apply. In others it will be more complicated.

The first stage is to identify the hazard. This may result from an inspection of the process in question, or may be suggested by the signs and symptoms of disease in exposed people. As regards chemicals in the workplace and their assessment, knowledge of the toxicological properties of the chemical in question is clearly important. It must be noted that of the 6,000,000+ chemicals in use worldwide less than 5% have good toxicological data available and a small proportion of that data relates to the human experience. A useful starting place is to have access to the Material Safety Data Sheet (MSDS), which should be available with any chemical used in the workplace. MSDS information may include instructions for the safe use and potential hazards associated with a particular material or product. There is also a duty to properly label substances on the basis of physicochemical, health, and/or environmental risk. Labels can include hazard symbols such as the EU standard black diagonal cross on an orange background, used to denote a harmful substance. This labelling system, in the EU, is under change and review due to the phased implementation of the REACH regulations. In the UK, the Chemicals (Hazard Information and Packaging for Supply) Regulations 2009—known as CHIP 4 Regulations—impose duties upon suppliers, and importers into the EU, of hazardous materials, however these are to be replaced in the near future by the Classification, Labelling and Packaging (CLP) regulations. Full copies of these regulations are available on UK government websites. The Control of Substances Hazardous to Health 2002 (COSHH) Regulations govern the use of hazardous substances in the workplace in the UK and specifically require an assessment of the use of a substance. Regulation 12 requires that an employer provides employees with information, instruction, and training for people exposed to hazardous substances. This duty would be very nearly impossible without the MSDS as a starting point.

Chemical exposures can lead to a variety of toxic effects including:

- duration of exposure (acute or chronic)
- site of tissue damage (local or systemic)
- effect in relation to time (immediate or delayed)
- reversibility of effect or not

Table 1.5 Principal workplace controls that reduce worker hazard, ordered in accordance with a general hierarchy (abbreviations are explained in the text)

Control measure	Explanation
Elimination	Complete removal of the hazard so no risk arises
Specification	Work process redesigned so hazards are 'designed out' or fully considered as regards prevention
Substitution	One type of hazard is substituted for another, e.g. man-made mineral fibres replaces asbestos. Note that the change may lead to new hazards
Segregation	Is it possible to segregate in space (e.g. isolated area in the workplace) or time (e.g. at night when fewer people are exposed)?
Engineering control measures	**LEV**—control at the source by extracting contaminated air close to its emission source and removing it from the workplace, e.g. HCN gas in a fume hood.
	Dilution ventilation—this can be used with low toxicity contaminant, which is diluted by the normal workplace air, e.g. vapors from organic liquids or use of high-efficiency particulate absorption (HEPA) filters
	Noise control—reducing the noise produced by either maintaining of the equipment, sourcing low noise alternatives, or using acoustic booths or screen to isolate the noise
Personal hygiene	This is having adequate welfare facilities and arrangements for eating/drinking/washing on site or off site depending on the hazards
Information, instruction, and training	It is vital that both workers and managers have adequate information on hazards and risks and methods of control
Good housekeeping	Keep the workplace clear, clean, and tidy to prevent workplace contamination
PPE	This is asking workers to wear special clothing and protective devices during the time they are exposed to the hazard. This is only done after due consideration to all the other control measures and **is not** a first-line control measure
Reduced time exposure	Control the exposure by removing them from the hazard, e.g. working with radiation sources

- target organ, e.g. hepatotoxicity with carbon tetrachloride
- nature of toxic effect (functional, biochemical, or morphological)
- specific effect, e.g. carcinogenesis, mutagenesis

The second stage is to analyse the risk, i.e. quantify exposure to the hazard and compare with a tolerability standard, e.g. occupational exposure limit (OEL) HSE (UK) or recommended exposure level (REL) NIOSH (USA).

Having assessed the risk the next stage is to decide on the best strategy for prevention or control. It is also import to record any decisions made (steps 3 and 4). A wide range of options will hopefully be available to achieve adequate control depending on the case. These range from a complete redesign of a process to eliminate the hazard, to the installation of local exhaust ventilation (LEV) system and a worker having to wear personal protective equipment (PPE). These are outlined in Table 1.5.

The list of controls in Table 1.5 is often called the 'general hierarchy of control' and is listed in order of desirability, i.e. the control measures outlined at the top of the table take precedence to the ones lower down the table. However, in a specific risk situation, it is advisable to consider all options but not necessarily to weight each similarly.

Regulatory provisions, in different countries, may preferentially require control at source or by engineering controls, where this is thought to be reasonably practicable, before other methods are considered i.e. in the UK this would be the COSHH and the Control of Noise at Work Regulations 2005.

The final stage is to review an assessment and update if necessary. This is part of an audit cycle and continual improvement and is considered as part of a dynamic risk assessment and leads to adequate risk management as outlined in Table 1.5. As things change and new information becomes available such as the toxicological profile of a new chemical, or new information on an old one, then the risk assessment process will start again.

Further reading

Baxter PJ, Aw T-C, Cockcroft A, et al. (eds) (2010). *Hunter's Diseases of Occupations*, 10th edition. London: Hodder.

BSI. (2008). *Guide to Achieving Effective Occupational Health and Safety Performance. BS 18004:2008*. London: BSI.

Gardner K, Harrington JM (2005). *Occupational Hygiene*, 3rd edition. Oxford: Blackwell.

Sadhra SS, Rampal KG (eds) (1999). *Occupational Health Risk Assessment and Management*. Oxford: Blackwell Science Ltd.

General management of the poisoned patient

Assessment and general management

Background

The assessment and general management of an acutely poisoned patient in a healthcare facility involves the following four steps:

- Immediate assessment of ventilation and circulation, and their correction if abnormal.
- History taking.
- Physical examination.
- Arranging appropriate toxicological and non-toxicological investigations.

Ventilatory impairment

Assessment

Pulse oximetry can be used to measure oxygen saturation. The displayed reading may be inaccurate when the saturation is below 70%, when peripheral perfusion is poor, and in the presence of carboxyhaemoglobin or methaemoglobin. Even when ventilation is satisfactory on presentation, it must be reassessed periodically because deterioration is well recognized (e.g. after ingestion of a sedative drug). If the patient has an arterial oxygen saturation of less than 95% (by pulse oximetry), is comatose (Glasgow Coma Scale score <8), and/or the laryngeal (gag) reflex is absent, arterial blood gases should be measured. Only measurement of arterial blood gases indicates the presence of both hypercapnia and hypoxia. Ventilatory insufficiency is present if arterial partial pressure of oxygen ≤9 kPa on air and/or arterial partial pressure of carbon dioxide ≥6 kPa.

Management

Food, vomit, secretions, and dentures should be removed from the patient's mouth and pharynx, and the tongue prevented from falling back. The patient should be nursed with their head down in the left lateral position to minimize the risk of aspiration of the gastric contents into the lungs. If these measures do not lead to an improvement in ventilation, consideration should be given to intubation and assisted ventilation if the central respiratory depression cannot be reversed by administration of a specific antidote, such as naloxone.

Circulatory impairment

Assessment

Pulse, blood pressure, and temperature (core and peripheral) should be measured to assess cardiovascular function. An ECG should be undertaken in moderately or severely poisoned patients, particularly when a drug with a cardiotoxic action (e.g. a tricyclic antidepressant that produces QRS prolongation) has been ingested.

Although hypotension (systolic blood pressure <80 mmHg) is a recognized feature of acute poisoning, the classical features of shock (tachycardia and pale, cold skin) are seen rarely because only a minority of patients are severely poisoned.

Hypotension and shock may be caused by the following:

- A direct cardiodepressant action of the poison (e.g. β-blockers, calcium channel blockers, tricyclic antidepressants).
- Vasodilation and venous pooling in the lower limbs (e.g. ACE inhibitors, calcium channel blockers, phenothiazines).
- A decrease in circulating blood volume because of gastrointestinal losses (e.g. profuse vomiting in theophylline poisoning), increased insensible losses (e.g. salicylate poisoning), increased renal losses (e.g. poisoning due to diuretics), and increased capillary permeability.

Hypotension may be exacerbated by coexisting hypoxia, acidosis, and dysrhythmias.

Management

Young patients are generally not at risk of cerebral or renal damage unless their systolic blood pressure falls below 80 mmHg. In people over 40 years old, it is preferable to maintain systolic blood pressure above 90 mmHg. As a first step, the patient should be placed in a head-down position (the foot of the bed should be elevated by 15 cm). If this simple measure fails to produce improvement, plasma volume should be expanded by infusion of a crystalloid solution.

In more severe cases, consider echocardiography to assess myocardial function, and/or invasive haemodynamic monitoring to confirm that adequate volume replacement has been administered. These patients should be managed in a high dependency area. The use of inotropic or vasopressor (vasoconstrictor) sympathomimetics may be indicated if hypotension is resistant to volume repletion.

The choice of drug depends on the cause of hypotension. If due to cardiac depression, an inotropic sympathomimetic should be given, such as dobutamine 2.5–10 micrograms/kg/minute (paediatric dose 2–20 micrograms/kg/minute) or dopamine 2–5 micrograms/kg/minute (paediatric dose 3–20 micrograms/kg/minute).

If hypotension is due to vasodilation, a vasopressor should be used such as norepinephrine 40 micrograms (base)/mL at 0.16–0.33 mL/minute according to response via a central venous line (paediatric dose 20–100 nanograms (base)/kg/minute). Norepinephrine may raise blood pressure at the expense of perfusion of vital organs, particularly the kidneys.

A few drugs when taken in overdose, e.g. cocaine and amfetamines, may produce systemic hypertension. If this is mild and associated with agitation, a benzodiazepine may suffice. In more severe cases, there may be a risk of arterial rupture, particularly intracranially. To prevent this, intravenous isosorbide dinitrate 2–10 mg/hour up to 20 mg/hour if necessary (not recommended in children), or glyceryl trinitrate 10–200 micrograms/minute by intravenous infusion (paediatric dose 0.2–0.5 micrograms/kg/minute) should be administered until blood pressure is controlled. Alternatives include an α-adrenergic blocking agent such as phentolamine 2–5 mg intravenously repeated as necessary (not recommended in children), or sodium nitroprusside 0.5–1.5 micrograms/kg/minute by intravenous infusion (increased in steps of 500 nanograms/kg/minute every 5 minutes until there is a satisfactory response; maximum dose 8 micrograms/kg/minute); this is not recommended in children.

History taking

Adults

About 80% of adults who have ingested an overdose are conscious on arrival at hospital and the diagnosis of self-poisoning can usually be made from the history. In unconscious patients, a history from friends or relatives is helpful, and the diagnosis can often be inferred from tablet bottles or a 'suicide note' brought by the paramedics, or made by exclusion of other causes. Self-poisoning must always be considered in the differential diagnosis in any patient with an altered consciousness level.

Acutely poisoned patients may be emotionally and psychiatrically distressed, and require competent, sympathetic assessment if essential information is not to be missed. It is pertinent to try to establish the nature of the substance taken, the amount involved, the route, and time of exposure, so that the clinical course can be anticipated and the risk assessed.

Statements about the nature and amount of what has been taken should be regarded with clinical suspicion, however, because these are often inconsistent with laboratory analysis of blood or urine. Patients may not use generic drug names, and it is important to clarify the specific preparation involved because the composition of formulations with similar names can differ.

Furthermore, self-poisoning is often an impulsive act involving swallowing the contents of the first bottle or blister pack that comes to hand; sometimes, the drugs used may have been prescribed for another individual. Few patients count the number of tablets taken; the amount is often estimated in unquantifiable terms such as 'handfuls' or 'mouthfuls', though the patient may be able to recall the number of strips or packets. When the time of exposure is important (e.g. paracetamol poisoning), the accuracy can be improved by relating events to activities of daily life (e.g. the time of a television programme).

Children

Very young children may be found eating potential poisons, or with tablets or other materials around their mouth or on their clothing. Most such exposures occur in the home either because medicines have not been stored in a safe place or have been taken out of their original container. Such episodes may occur particularly when parents are inattentive or neglectful as at times of family crises.

In those under 5 years of age the exposures are clinically serious in less than 1%, probably because younger children typically ingest small amounts of a toxic substance as they are being inquisitive and not trying to induce self-harm. However, the ingestion of some drugs including antipsychotics, antimalarials, anti-arrhythmics, calcium channel blockers, essential oils, iron, methyl salicylate, opiates/opioids, tricyclic antidepressants, and theophylline can cause severe poisoning after very small exposures.

A clear history is unlikely to be obtained from the child or older witnesses. Statements about amounts taken are usually unreliable because the quantities present in containers before such incidents are often unknown.

Psychological history and assessment are also of great importance and dealt with in other sections in this chapter.

Physical examination

Physical signs are particularly important when trying to elucidate the cause of unexplained coma. A diagnosis of acute poisoning can never be made on the basis of a single physical sign, but there are typical clusters of signs that make a diagnosis of poisoning with specific drugs very likely (Table 2.1). Head injury should be excluded as a contributing or causative factor in comatose patients.

General observations may reveal useful information. For example, solvents or alcohol may be smelt on the breath, track marks may reveal undisclosed illicit substance abuse, atypical bruising may warn of domestic or other violence, and the stigmata of alcoholic liver disease may be revealed.

Skin blisters

Skin blisters may be found in poisoned patients who are, or have been, unconscious. Such lesions are not diagnostic of specific poisons, but are sufficiently common in poisoned patients (and sufficiently uncommon in patients unconscious from other causes) to be of diagnostic value. Bullous lesions should be left intact until they burst, to reduce the risk of infection. De-roofing should be performed when the blister bursts; a non-adhesive dressing is then applied.

Neurological signs

The Glasgow Coma Scale (GCS) is the most commonly used method to assess the degree of impairment of consciousness. A GCS of ≤8 (not obeying commands, not speaking, not eye opening) should prompt careful respiratory assessment, particularly if the laryngeal (gag) reflex is lost. In poisoned patients, an initial GCS ≤8 has been claimed to be both a good and a poor predictor of the need for intubation. The AVPU (alert, responsive to verbal stimulation, responsive to painful stimulation, and unresponsive) responsiveness has also been employed and corresponds well to GCS when assessing level of consciousness in the poisoned patient.

With the exception of transient inequality of pupil size, lateralizing neurological signs effectively exclude a diagnosis of acute poisoning unless they can be explained by a pre-existing illness. The usual features of pyramidal tract involvement (hypertonia, hyper-reflexia and

Table 2.1 Common clusters of features that may be diagnostic

Feature cluster	Likely poisons
Coma, hypertonia, hyper-reflexia, extensor plantar responses, myoclonus, strabismus, mydriasis, sinus tachycardia	Tricyclic antidepressants, antihistamines less commonly, thioridazine, orphenadrine
Coma, hypotonia, hyporeflexia, plantar responses flexor or non-elicitable, hypotension	Barbiturates, benzodiazepines, and alcohol combinations. Severe tricyclic antidepressant poisoning
Coma, miosis, reduced respiratory rate	Opioid analgesics
Nausea, vomiting, tinnitus, deafness, sweating, hyperventilation, vasodilatation, metabolic acidosis	Salicylates
Restlessness, agitation, mydriasis, anxiety, tremor, tachycardia, convulsions, arrhythmias	Sympathomimetics
Hyperthermia, tachycardia, delirium, agitation, mydriasis	Ecstasy (methylenedioxymethamphetamine – MDMA), amfetamines, cocaine
Blindness (usually with other features)	Quinine, methanol
Miosis and hypersalivation	Organophosphorus and carbamate insecticides, nerve agents

extensor plantar responses) are commonly found in tricyclic antidepressant poisoning, and with other drugs with marked anticholinergic actions (e.g. the older antihistamines). However, all of these signs may be abolished in deep coma.

Decerebrate and decorticate movements of the limbs often occur in unconscious poisoned patients, but in most cases there is no irreversible brain damage and the patient recovers fully. Acute dystonic movements (including acute torticollis, orolingual dyskinesias and oculogyric crises) are also produced; these are usually caused by metoclopramide, or less commonly by haloperidol, droperidol, prochlorperazine, or trifluoperazine. Choreoathetosis has been reported as a rare presenting feature of poisoning with organophosphorus insecticides.

Inequality of the pupils is not uncommon in poisoned patients. Widely dilated pupils that react poorly to light may be caused by poisons with anticholinergic actions (e.g. tricyclic antidepressants), sympathomimetic effects (e.g. amfetamines), or which cause blindness (e.g. quinine, methanol). Miosis is usually caused by opioid analgesics or poisons with cholinergic or anticholinesterase actions (e.g. organophosphorus insecticides, nerve agents). The degree and speed of reaction of the pupils to light is of no clinical value.

Ocular movements

Strabismus, internuclear ophthalmoplegia, and total external ophthalmoplegia have been described in acute poisoning, with impairment of consciousness caused by various drugs that act on the brain. Transient and variable strabismus (usually with the optic axes divergent in the horizontal plane) have been attributed to phenytoin, carbamazepine, and tricyclic antidepressants. Dysconjugate, roving eye movements may also be seen if both eyes are observed for a period of time, and occasionally there may be total external ophthalmoplegia, even in patients in whom consciousness is no more than minimally impaired.

Dysconjugate eye movements may become apparent only when the oculovestibular reflexes are examined using caloric stimuli, and have been reported in poisoning with tricyclic antidepressants, phenothiazines, benzodiazepines, barbiturates, and ethanol. Instillation of ice-cold water into an ear should make both eyes turn to the irrigated side; failure of one eye to deviate suggests internuclear ophthalmoplegia and disturbed function of the medial longitudinal fasciculus.

Oculocephalic and oculovestibular reflexes

Loss of these reflexes is usually regarded as evidence of severe brainstem damage and brain death. In acute poisoning, however, such a conclusion is not justified. Overdose with carbamazepine, phenytoin, and tricyclic antidepressants can be associated with loss of these reflexes, but patients recover completely.

Visual impairment

Visual impairment is associated most commonly with quinine and methanol poisoning.

Convulsions

Convulsions caused by, for example, tricyclic antidepressant drugs can usually be controlled with intravenous diazepam 10 mg (child 100–300 micrograms/kg) or lorazepam 4 mg (child 100 micrograms/kg), once hypoxaemia and acidosis have also been corrected. Additional anticonvulsant therapy, muscle relaxation, and mechanical ventilation may be required if this is unsuccessful (see also sections in Chapter 3, pp. 63–94).

Hypothermia

A core temperature below 35°C, measured in the rectum or ear, may be recorded in deeply unconscious patients who have been exposed, particularly in cold weather, for several hours. Placing the patient in a room with moistened air at a temperature of 27–29°C and covering him or her with a foil space blanket to minimize heat loss is the best way to treat hypothermia. Local radiant heat should not be used.

Fluid, acid–base and electrolyte balance

Patients who are vomiting should be given fluids intravenously to replace gastrointestinal losses (see also Acid–base and electrolyte imbalance in the poisoned patient, pp. 75–76 for more discussion on electrolyte disturbance). Severe and clinically significant hypokalaemia (e.g. that caused by β2-agonist poisoning) should be corrected by infusing potassium to prevent arrhythmias.

Metabolic acidosis is a common complication of severe poisoning and is a characteristic feature of severe poisoning due to ethylene and diethylene glycols, methanol, and salicylates. After correction of hypoxia and hypotension, infusion of sodium bicarbonate may be necessary.

Hypoglycaemia may follow an overdose of insulin, sulphonylureas, or ethanol, and may occur in liver failure due to paracetamol. It is initially corrected by infusing 10% dextrose (see also Antidiabetic drugs, pp. 152–153 for management of antidiabetic agents).

Toxicological investigations

Measurement of the concentration of a specific poison in the blood, or toxicological screening of blood or urine, can be used to establish a diagnosis of poisoning. It is neither possible nor necessary to measure the concentration of every agent in biological fluids. Emergency measurement of the blood concentration of the poisons shown in Box 2.1 is useful in ensuring appropriate clinical management.

The plasma paracetamol concentration should be measured in all unconscious poisoned patients—multiple drug overdoses are common and paracetamol is one of the drugs most often involved, particularly in Europe. It is important to diagnose an overdose of paracetamol at a stage when administration of antidotes might prevent liver damage and death. In contrast, routine requests for salicylate concentrations cannot be justified. Salicylate poisoning seldom causes coma and it is unlikely that clinically significant concentrations will be present in patients without the typical signs of salicylism (see Salicylates, pp. 124–127).

Box 2.1 Poisons for which emergency measurement is essential

- Carboxyhaemoglobin
- Ethanol (when monitoring treatment in ethylene glycol and methanol poisoning)
- Ethylene glycol
- Iron
- Lithium
- Methanol
- Paracetamol
- Salicylate
- Theophylline.

Box 2.2 Non-toxicological investigations

- Serum sodium (e.g. hyponatraemia in ecstasy poisoning)
- Serum potassium (e.g. hypokalaemia in theophyl-line poisoning; hyperkalaemia in digoxin poisoning, rhabdomyolysis, haemolysis)
- Plasma creatinine (e.g. renal failure in diethylene and ethylene glycol poisoning)
- Blood sugar (e.g. hypoglycaemia in insulin and severe untreated paracetamol poisoning, hypogly-caemia and hyperglycaemia in salicylate poisoning)
- Serum calcium (e.g. hypocalcaemia in ethylene gly-col poisoning)
- Serum alanine aminotransferase (ALT)/aspartate aminotransferase (AST) activities (e.g. increased in paracetamol poisoning)
- Serum phosphate (e.g. hypophosphataemia in paracetamol-induced renal tubular damage)
- Acid–base disturbances, including metabolic acidosis
- Red blood cell (RBC) cholinesterase activity (e.g. organophosphorus insecticide and nerve-agent poisoning)
- Whole-blood methaemoglobin concentration (e.g. in nitrite poisoning)

Non-toxicological investigations

Blood and urine

Information about the nature of poisons ingested can occasionally be obtained from standard haematological and biochemical investigations, and from arterial blood gas analysis (Box 2.2). Brown discoloration of the urine may be caused by the presence of haemoglobin (if there is intravascular haemolysis), myoglobin secondary to rhabdomyolysis, or metabolites of paracetamol. Crystals may be prominent after an overdose with primidone or ingestion of ethylene glycol.

Radiology

Routine radiology is of little diagnostic value. It can be used to confirm ingestion of metallic objects (e.g. coins, button batteries) or injection of globules of metallic mercury. Rarely, hydrocarbon solvents (e.g. carbon tetrachlo-ride) may be seen as a slightly opaque layer floating on the top of the gastric contents with the patient upright, or outlining the small bowel. Some enteric-coated or sustained-release drug formulations may be seen on plain abdominal radiographs, but, with the exception of iron salts, ordinary formulations are seldom seen.

Radiography may have a limited role in confirming iron overdose in children, but more widespread use in acute poisoning is restricted by the fact that most adult patients are women of child-bearing age. Ingested packets of illicit substances may be discernible on a plain radiograph, but CT or MRI is more reliably able to detect such objects.

Radiology may be particularly helpful in confirm-ing some of the complications of poisoning, for exam-ple, aspiration pneumonia, non-cardiogenic pulmonary oedema (salicylates), bronchiolitis obliterans (nitrogen oxides), acute respiratory distress syndrome (ARDS), pulmonary fibrosis (paraquat).

ECG

Routine ECG is of limited diagnostic value, though it should be undertaken in those ingesting potentially cardiotoxic drugs; continuous ECG monitoring may be appropriate in such patients. Sinus tachycardia with pro-longation of the PR and QRS intervals in an unconscious patient should prompt consideration of tricyclic antide-pressant overdose. With increasing cardiotoxicity, it may be impossible to detect P waves, and the pattern then resembles ventricular tachycardia. Overdose with cardiac glycosides or potassium salts also induces characteristic ECG changes. Q–T interval prolongation is a recognized adverse effect of several drugs in overdose (e.g. quetia-pine, terfenadine and quinine) and predisposes to ven-tricular arrhythmias, notably torsades des pointes.

Further reading

Bradberry SM, Vale JA (1995). Disturbances of potassium home-ostasis in poisoning. *J Toxicol Clin Toxicol*, 33:295–310.

Chan BS, Ali DR (2006). Glasgow coma scale and its relationship to intubation in patients with poisoning. *Clin Toxicol*, 44:763.

Chan B, Gaudry P, Grattan-Smith TM, et al. (1993). The use of Glasgow Coma Scale in poisoning. *J Emerg Med*, 11:579–82.

Delk C, Holstege CP, Brady WJ. Electrocardiographic abnormali-ties associated with poisoning. *Am J Emerg Med* 2007; 25:672–8.

Jones A (2012). Metabolic effects of poisoning. *Medicine*, 40:55–8.

Kelly CA, Upex A, Bateman DN (2004). Comparison of con-sciousness level assessment in the poisoned patient using the alert/verbal/painful/unresponsive scale and the Glasgow coma scale. *Ann Emerg Med*, 44:108–13.

Olson KR, Pentel PR, Kelley MT (1987). Physical assessment and differential diagnosis of the poisoned patient. *Med Toxicol*, 2:52–81.

Pohjola-Sintonen S, Kivistö KT, Vuori E, et al. (2000). Identification of drugs ingested in acute poisoning: correlation of patient his-tory with drug analyses. *Ther Drug Monit*, 22:749–52.

Tenenbein M (2009). Do you really need that emergency drug screen? *Clin Toxicol*, 47:286–91.

Thomas SHL, Watson ID (2002). Laboratory analyses for poi-soned patients. *Ann Clin Biochem*, 39:327.

Decontamination

Background

Decontamination involves the removal of drug or other chemical from a patient before it is absorbed. External decontamination refers to the removal of chemical from the patient's skin, hair, eyes, and any wounds. Gastrointestinal (GI) decontamination involves the use of emesis, gastric lavage, or the administration of activated charcoal and/or a cathartic. Occasionally, whole-bowel irrigation (WBI) has been employed, particularly if the poison involved (e.g. iron) is not adsorbed by activated charcoal, or is in a modified (slow-release) formulation, for which delayed absorption may be theoretically reduced by expulsion from the gut.

The aims of decontamination are:

• to prevent on-going exposure to the patient, thereby reducing the absorbed dose
• to reduce the risk of secondary contamination of healthcare facilities and staff (particularly for more hazardous chemicals).

Skin decontamination

Skin decontamination methods include:

• removing the chemical by washing the skin with soap and water or by using adsorbents such as Fuller's earth
• inactivating the chemical, e.g. using hypochlorite solution to inactivate organophosphorus compounds.

The evidence base for these methods is limited. Furthermore, as skin decontamination does not reduce the damage that is caused by chemicals that have already been absorbed, it is important that skin decontamination is undertaken as soon as possible after exposure has occurred.

Full skin decontamination traditionally has involved the 'rinse–wipe–rinse' method:

• Rinse 1. The patient is drenched under the shower. This removes particulate matter and water-soluble substances.
• Wipe. Detergent solution (10mL in a bucket of water) is applied with a soft brush/sponge. This removes organic chemicals.
• Rinse 2. The patient is drenched again under the shower. This removes the detergent and chemicals.

Particular attention should be paid to the patient's face and the process should be repeated if there is any visible, residual contamination. Wounds should be irrigated thoroughly.

Water should be lukewarm; there is a risk of inducing hypothermia if it is too cold. Water that is too warm may promote transcutaneous absorption of chemical.

Eye decontamination

Irrespective of the chemical involved, it is imperative that immediate irrigation of the whole eye is undertaken with water. A suspended litre bag of intravenous sodium chloride solution with an infusion line works well for irrigation. During transportation of the casualty, irrigation should be continued and on reaching hospital a topical anaesthetic should be applied to enable the patient to open the eye lids; use of a lid speculum may be necessary.

Removal of particulate matter with fine forceps or a moistened cotton wool-tipped application (bud) should be undertaken; the upper eye lid should be everted to ensure particles under the lid are removed. The use of special buffered solutions offers no advantage over water and is likely to delay irrigation. Attempts at neutralization are inappropriate as ocular damage is likely to be increased.

Except in minor cases, irrigation with water should continue for at least 15 minutes and for longer in severe cases. The pH of the conjunctival sac/eye surface can be tested with a pH paper and after alkali exposure the pH should be maintained at 7 for several hours by continuous irrigation with water or the use of an irrigating contact lens. Systemic analgesics may be required, particularly if irrigation is prolonged.

Normal assessment of visual acuity, epithelial damage (slit lamp examination with fluorescein staining) and intraocular pressure should be undertaken. In all severe cases an ophthalmologist must assess the magnitude of the damage and the requirement for further treatment.

Gastrointestinal decontamination

GI decontamination has been an historical cornerstone in the management of poisoned patients to prevent the absorption of ingested poisons. However, GI decontamination is no longer employed routinely since the publication of Position Statements by the American Academy of Clinical Toxicology and the European Association of Poisons Centres and Clinical Toxicologists (see 'Further reading').

The commonest method used to reduce GI absorption is single-dose activated charcoal. However, the largest clinical trial of no decontamination versus single-dose activated charcoal failed to show clinical benefit, though most ingestions in this study performed in Sri Lanka were not pharmaceuticals (see 'Single-dose activated charcoal' subsection).

Single-dose activated charcoal

Rationale

Single-dose activated charcoal therapy involves the oral administration or instillation by nasogastric tube of an aqueous preparation of activated charcoal after the ingestion of a poison. Activated charcoal adsorbs a wide variety of poisons in the GI tract, thereby decreasing absorption and reducing or preventing systemic toxicity.

Volunteer studies

The results of 122 comparisons with 46 drugs indicate considerable variation in the absolute amount of charcoal used (0.5–100 g) and the time of administration. When activated charcoal was administered 30 minutes after drug administration, there was a mean reduction of absorption of 51.7% (n = 7), and at 60 minutes after drug administration, the mean reduction was 38.4% (n = 16).

In 48 studies involving 26 drugs, using at least 50 g of activated charcoal, the mean reduction in absorption was 47.3% (n = 3) when charcoal was administered 30 minutes after dosing; the mean reduction at 60 minutes was 40.0% (n = 12). These volunteer studies demonstrated that the reduction of drug absorption decreases to values of questionable clinical importance when charcoal is administered at times greater than 1 hour after the ingestion of a poison. However, these values do not take account of the influence of food in the stomach and the presence of a poison that may delay gastric emptying.

Clinical studies

In the largest study reported of 4632 patients, 50.5% had ingested pesticides whilst 35.6% had ingested yellow oleander seeds. Patients were randomized to receive no charcoal (1554), a single dose of charcoal (1545), or six doses of charcoal (1533). Outcomes were available for 4629, and mortality did not differ significantly between the groups. No significant differences were noted for patients who took particular poisons, were more severely ill on admission, or who presented early.

One study of symptomatic patients who received activated charcoal and some form of gastric evacuation (gastric lavage, syrup of ipecacuanha, gastric aspiration) showed that patients receiving gastric aspiration and activated charcoal were less likely to be admitted to an intensive care unit than patients who received activated charcoal and either lavage or syrup of ipecacuanha.

Complications
Considering the widespread use of single-dose activated charcoal, there are relatively few reports of activated charcoal-related adverse effects in the literature. The majority of adverse events are not related to the appropriate use of activated charcoal, but are a complication of aspiration or the direct administration of charcoal into the lung. Aspiration of charcoal containing povidone has led occasionally to major respiratory problems.

There are no reports of GI obstruction, constipation, or haemorrhagic rectal ulceration associated with single-dose activated charcoal therapy.

Conclusion
There are no satisfactorily designed clinical studies assessing benefit from single-dose activated charcoal to guide the use of this therapy in drug ingestion. Single-dose activated charcoal should not be administered routinely in the management of poisoned patients. Based on volunteer studies, the administration of activated charcoal may be considered if a patient has ingested a potentially toxic amount of a poison (which is known to be adsorbed to charcoal) up to 1 hour previously. Although volunteer studies demonstrate that the reduction of drug absorption decreases to values of questionable clinical importance when charcoal is administered at times greater than 1 hour, the potential for benefit after 1 hour cannot be excluded. There is no evidence that the administration of activated charcoal improves clinical outcome. Unless a patient has an intact or protected airway, the administration of charcoal is contraindicated.

Gastric lavage

Rationale
Gastric lavage involves the passage of an orogastric tube and the sequential administration and aspiration of small volumes of liquid with the intent of removing toxic substances present in the stomach.

Volunteer studies
Five volunteer studies provide insufficient support for the clinical use of gastric lavage: Three were performed less than 20 minutes after dosing; two were undertaken at 60 minutes. The recovery of marker was highly variable when lavage was undertaken less than 20 minutes after dosing. When gastric lavage was performed at 5 minutes, the mean recovery of a thiamine marker was 90%; when it was performed at 10 minutes, the mean recovery of a cyanocobalamin marker was 45%; and when it was undertaken at a mean time of 19 minutes, the mean recovery of a 99mTc-labeled marker was 30.3%. In the studies performed at 60 minutes after dosing, the mean reduction in the area under the curve (AUC) was 32% in one study, and in the second study, the mean reduction in

salicylate excretion was 8%. Other studies suggested that tablet debris may be found in the stomach after lavage and that lavage may propel material into the small intestine, increasing the possibility of enhanced drug absorption.

Clinical studies
Clinical studies have not confirmed the benefit of gastric lavage alone even when it was performed less than 60 minutes after poison ingestion, and there is the possibility that drug absorption may be enhanced by its use. In one study, benefit from lavage was shown in a small subset (n = 16) of obtunded patients in whom lavage was undertaken and activated charcoal administered less than 60 minutes after ingestion; there were only three patients in the comparison group who received charcoal alone. Small group sizes and selection bias limit the conclusions that can be drawn from this study.

In a similar although larger study, benefit from gastric lavage was not confirmed regardless of the time post ingestion. Although anecdotal reports indicate that occasionally impressive returns are achieved, there is no strong clinical evidence to support the view that, overall, gastric lavage benefits the poisoned patient.

Complications
The potential complications of gastric lavage are well documented, although serious sequelae are uncommon. Aspiration pneumonia is particularly likely to ensue if petroleum distillates have been ingested or lavage is carried out in a patient with depressed airway protective reflexes without an endotracheal tube *in situ*. In one study in 257 patients with self-poisoning the odds ratio for the development of aspiration pneumonitis when gastric lavage was performed in unconscious non-intubated patients was 2.7 (95% confidence interval (CI) 0.8–9.3). However, aspiration has been reported in alert patients even when hydrocarbons were not involved. Aspiration pneumonia has also been reported in patients who have been intubated prior to gastric lavage.

Laryngospasm has been observed particularly when a semiconscious patient has resisted the procedure, either intentionally or as a consequence of the agent ingested. In a group of 42 patients the mean (±SD) PaO_2 fell significantly (p < 0.001) from 95 ± 13 to 80 ± 19 mm Hg during lavage. This fall was significantly greater in conscious than unconscious patients, in smokers than in non-smokers, and was most marked in male smokers aged 45 years or older. In one study of 42 patients, the mean (±SD) pulse rate rose significantly (p < 0.001) from 92 ± 19 to 121 ± 23 bpm. There was a greater rise in the pulse rate in conscious than unconscious patients. Atrial and ventricular ectopic beats were also observed and transient ST elevation developed during lavage in two patients, one of whom had a history of previous myocardial infarction.

Perforation of the oesophagus and gut has been reported rarely.

Small conjunctival haemorrhages are observed commonly and are particularly likely to occur in those who are not fully cooperative with the procedure.

Conclusion
Gastric lavage should not be employed routinely in the management of poisoned patients. Based on experimental and clinical studies, it is unlikely that gastric lavage would be of value longer than 1 hour post-ingestion. Unless a patient is intubated, gastric lavage is contraindicated if airway protective reflexes are lost. It also is contraindicated if a hydrocarbon with high aspiration potential or corrosive substance has been ingested.

Syrup of ipecacuanha

Rationale

Syrup of ipecacuanha contains two alkaloids, emetine (methylcephaeline) and cephaeline, which induce vomiting theoretically removing ingested poisons from the stomach. These alkaloids stimulate gastric mucosal sensory receptors which activate the vomiting centre in the brain. They also directly stimulate the chemoreceptor trigger zone in the area postrema in the brain. Emesis is non-invasive, uses a physiological mechanism, and consumes little staff time.

Volunteer studies

Eleven volunteer studies have investigated the value of syrup of ipecacuanha in preventing the absorption of marker substances. In these studies, the recovery of material was highly variable, although generally the amount of ingested material removed by syrup of ipecacuanha-induced emesis depended on the elapsed time between dosing and the onset of emesis. If syrup of ipecacuanha was administered 5 minutes after dosing, the mean recoveries in two studies using a ^{99m}Tc marker were 54.1% and 83%. In two other studies, the mean plasma concentrations for various drugs were reduced to 21–48% of control. A study using paracetamol as a marker showed a 67% reduction in bioavailability if syrup of ipecacuanha was administered within 5 minutes. When syrup of ipecacuanha was administered at 10 minutes after dosing, the mean recoveries in two studies were 28.4% (cyanocobalamin marker) and either 46.9% or 47.2% (cobalt marker).

Syrup of ipecacuanha administered at 30 minutes after dosing resulted in a mean recovery of 59% of the ^{99m}Tc-labelled human albuminsucralfate marker. In another study, in which ipecac was given at 30 minutes, the mean plasma concentrations of three drugs (paracetamol, tetracycline, aminophylline) were 70–107% of control. When syrup of ipecacuanha was administered at 60 minutes, the mean AUCs were 79% and 62%. When mean total urine salicylate excretion was measured over 48 hours in volunteers administered syrup of ipecacuanha 60 minutes after aspirin dosing, 70.3% (control 96.3%) and 55.6% (control 60.3%) of the administered aspirin dose were recovered. In another study, the mean recovery of marker at 60 minutes was 44%.

Other studies suggested that tablet debris may be found in the stomach after administration of syrup of ipecacuanha and that it may propel material into the small intestine, increasing the probability of enhanced drug absorption.

Clinical studies

In a study in children with non-toxic paracetamol concentrations, the mean plasma paracetamol concentrations decreased from 33.1 mg/L (2.40 mmol/L) to 15.7 mg/L (1.14 mmol/L), a 52.6% reduction, when emesis was induced 59 minutes after ingestion. Two clinical studies showed no benefit on patient outcome from the administration of syrup of ipecacuanha before activated charcoal compared with activated charcoal alone, regardless of the time of syrup of ipecacuanha administration. Most studies excluded the use of syrup of ipecacuanha in life-threatening intoxications, so it is difficult to determine the benefit of syrup of ipecacuanha in more severely poisoned patients.

Adverse effects

The most common adverse effects of using syrup of ipecacuanha are diarrhoea, lethargy and drowsiness, and prolonged (>1 hour) vomiting. The last-mentioned effect renders the patient at risk for aspiration and, in small children, volume and electrolyte imbalance.

Conclusion

Syrup of ipecacuanha should not be administered routinely in the management of poisoned patients. There is no evidence from clinical studies that syrup of ipecacuanha improves the outcome of poisoned patients, and its routine administration in the emergency departments should be abandoned. In addition, syrup of ipecacuanha may delay the administration or reduce the effectiveness of activated charcoal, oral antidotes, or WBI. Syrup of ipecacuanha administration may increase the risk of complications in a patient who has a decreased level of consciousness, has an impending loss of consciousness, has ingested a corrosive substance or hydrocarbon with high aspiration potential, is elderly or debilitated, or has a medical condition that may be compromised further by the induction of emesis.

Cathartics

Cathartics are the least validated of the GI decontamination techniques. The two general types of osmotic cathartics used in poisoned patients are saccharide (sorbitol) and 'saline' (magnesium citrate, magnesium sulfate, sodium sulfate) agents. Cathartics alone have been administered with the intent of decreasing the absorption of substances by accelerating their expulsion from the GI tract. Sorbitol improves the palatability of activated charcoal by imparting a sweet taste and by masking the grittiness of the charcoal.

Volunteer studies

Magnesium sulfate did not alter significantly (p >0.10) the serum concentrations of lithium and salicylate when administered 30 minutes after dosing. Sodium sulfate did not significantly change the recovery of urine paracetamol and its metabolites (87% ± 8.3% (mean ± SD)) compared with control (89.6% ± 10.7%). After the administration of sorbitol, urine salicylate recovery (95.9% ± 14.4%) was not significantly reduced compared with control (100%). The mean peak plasma theophylline concentration (7.8 mg/L (42.9 micromol/L)) was significantly (p < 0.001) greater in volunteers given sorbitol than in the control group (5.5 mg/L (30.5 micromol/L)). The mean time to peak concentration was significantly (p < 0.01) shorter (11.38 hours) in the sorbitol group than in the control group (16 hours). There was no difference in the mean AUC_{0-24} hours between the sorbitol (116.6 mg/L/hour (647.1 micromol/L/hour)) and control (97.6 mg/L/hour (541.7 micromol/L/hour)) groups. In another study, sorbitol did not alter significantly the AUC of theophylline whether administered at 1 hour (142.2 mg/L/hour (789.2 micromol/L/hour)) or at 6 hours (124 mg/L/hourr (688.2 micromol/L/hour)) after dosing compared with control (152.8 mg/L/hour (848 micromol/L/hour)).

Clinical studies

No clinical studies have been published to investigate the ability of cathartics to reduce the bioavailability of drugs or to improve the outcome of poisoned patients.

Complications

Potential complications of administering cathartics include nausea, abdominal cramps, vomiting, transient hypotension, dehydration, hypernatremia in patients receiving a sodium-containing cathartic, and hypermagnesaemia in patients receiving a magnesium-containing cathartic.

Conclusion

The administration of a cathartic alone has no role in the GI decontamination of a poisoned patient.

Whole-bowel irrigation

Rationale

WBI involves the use of large volumes of polyethylene glycol isosmotic solution, administered with the theoretical intention of flushing the bowel, enhancing elimination of poison from the gut. WBI is accomplished through the enteral administration of large amounts (infants and children 9 months–6 years old, 500 mL/hour; children 6–12 years old, 1000 mL/hour; children >12 years old and adults, 1500 to 2000 mL/hour) of an osmotically balanced polyethylene glycol electrolyte solution, which induces a liquid stool. WBI has the theoretical potential to reduce drug absorption by decontaminating the entire GI tract by physically expelling intraluminal contents. The concentration of polyethylene glycol and electrolytes in polyethylene glycol electrolyte solution causes no net absorption or secretion of ions, so no significant changes in water or electrolyte balance occur.

Volunteer studies

Ten volunteer studies investigated the value of WBI in reducing the absorption of ingested drugs. Three studies involving dosing with ampicillin, delayed-release aspirin, and sustained-release lithium showed significant reductions in bioavailability of 67%, 73%, and 67% (all $p < 0.05$). In a study designed to evaluate whether WBI enhanced the excretion of drugs during the post-absorptive phase, WBI did not reduce the bioavailability of aspirin. Two studies involving aspirin are difficult to interpret because one lacked a control (no treatment) arm and because both the duration and the total volume of WBI were less than in other studies. A study of WBI using coffee beans as a marker failed to show enhanced expulsion from the GI tract. A study using delayed-release paracetamol preparation along with a capsule containing radiopaque markers failed to demonstrate a significant reduction of paracetamol absorption, although simultaneously ingested radiopaque markers progressed further through the gut during whole bowel irrigation.

Clinical studies

No controlled clinical studies have been performed. Twenty-one anecdotal reports of the use of WBI in 29 patients have been published. Nine patients ingested iron, and 19 ingested other agents (e.g. sustained-release verapamil, delayed-release fenfluramine, latex packets of cocaine, zinc sulfate, lead oxide, and arsenic). No conclusions regarding the efficacy of WBI can be gleaned from these observations.

Complications

Nausea, vomiting, abdominal cramps, and bloating have been described when WBI is used.

Conclusion

WBI should not be used routinely in the management of poisoned patients. No controlled clinical trials have been performed, and there is no conclusive evidence that WBI improves the outcome of poisoned patients. There are insufficient data to support or exclude the use of WBI for potentially toxic ingestions of iron, lead, zinc, or packets of illicit drugs; WBI remains a theoretical option for these ingestions. WBI is contraindicated in patients with bowel obstruction, perforation, and ileus and in patients with haemodynamic instability or compromised unprotected airways. WBI should be used cautiously in debilitated patients or in patients with medical conditions that may be compromised further by its use.

Further reading

Barceloux D, McGuigan M, Hartigan-Go K, et al. (2004). American Academy of Clinical Toxicology and European Association of Poisons Centers and Clinical Toxicologist position paper: cathartics. *J Toxicol Clin Toxicol*, 42:243–53.

Chyka PA, Seger D, Krenzelok EP, et al. Position paper: single-dose activated charcoal. *Clin Toxicol*, 43:61–87.

Clarke SFJ (2010). Medical management of chemical incidents. In: Baker D, Fielder R, Karalliedde L, et al. (eds), *Essentials of Toxicology for Health Protection: A Handbook for Field Professionals*, pp. 71–86. Didcot: Health Protection Agency.

Eddleston M Juszczak E Buckley NA, et al. (2008). A randomised controlled trial of multiple dose activated charcoal in acute self-poisoning. *Lancet*, 371: 579–87.

Krenzelok EP, McGuigan M, Lheureux P, et al. (2004). American Academy of Clinical Toxicology and European Association of Poisons Centers and Clinical Toxicologist position paper: ipecac syrup. *J Toxicol Clin Toxicol*, 42:133–43.

Kulig K, Vale JA (2004). American Academy of Clinical Toxicology and European Association of Poisons Centers and Clinical Toxicologist position paper: gastric lavage. *J Toxicol Clin Toxicol*, 42:933–43.

Tenenbein M, Lheureux P (2004). American Academy of Clinical Toxicology and European Association of Poisons Centers and Clinical Toxicologist position paper: whole bowel irrigation. *J Toxicol Clin Toxicol*, 42:843–54.

Vale JA (1994). Chemical incidents: diagnosis and treatment of eye, skin and respiratory injuries. In: *Health Aspects of Chemical Incidents: Proceedings of a Symposium*, 14 and 15 April 1993. Utrecht: AZU.

Principles of enhanced elimination in the poisoned patient

Background

Procedures to increase the elimination of drugs and/or chemicals are used in only a minority of patients with features of severe poisoning. They are used for a small number of specific drugs/chemicals, as an adjunct in individuals with clinical or biochemical features of severe poisoning in whom appropriate gut decontamination, antidotes, and other supportive care techniques have been used. There are four different broad categories of techniques that may be used to enhance the elimination of toxins in the poisoned patient, these are:

- multiple-dose activated charcoal (MDAC)
- manipulation of urinary pH: urinary alkalinization
- extracorporeal techniques such as peritoneal dialysis, haemodialysis, continuous haemofiltration/haemodiafiltration, and haemoperfusion
- chelation to increase excretion of heavy metals.

Chelation is dealt with in detail in Chapter 10 (pp. 265–287) on metal toxicity. Essentially chelators increase urinary clearance of metals.

Note: urinary acidification is no longer recommended in the management of the poisoned patient.

Kinetic factors

Pharmacokinetic and toxicokinetic principles are important in determining whether an enhanced elimination technique is likely to have a significant impact on overall removal of a toxin from the body. These are:

- volume of distribution
- protein binding
- intrinsic clearance.

If a drug has a large volume of distribution (e.g. >1–2 L/kg) an enhanced elimination technique will have no significant impact on the total body burden of the substance because the technique only clears drug that is present in the blood compartment. For the same reasons, substances with high protein binding have a low concentration of free drug/chemical present, which limits the amount available for removal. It is important to note that protein binding of drugs can become saturated in overdose and therefore protein binding of drugs at therapeutic doses cannot be used to predict protein binding in overdose. Finally, these techniques are only likely to have a significant impact on increasing elimination of drugs that have low endogenous clearance rates (<4 mL/min/kg) and long half-lives.

There are other kinetic principles that are important in determining the whether a drug is suitable for increased elimination by multiple-dose activated charcoal or urinary manipulation and these are considered in the following subsections.

Multiple-dose activated charcoal

MDAC involves the repeated administration (more than two doses) of activated charcoal. MDAC may be given for two reasons: (1) to decrease absorption of toxins that are slowly absorbed from the GI tract (see Decontamination, pp. 36–39) or (2) to increase the elimination of toxins that have already been absorbed. In the latter case, MDAC increases elimination of drugs by interrupting the enteroenteric (and/or enterohepatic) recirculation of toxins that have already been absorbed. These are eliminated through the biliary tract into the duodenum, and are then partly reabsorbed in the terminal ileum. MDAC prevents this recirculation by adsorbing toxin as it passes through the small intestine, thereby preventing reabsorption in the terminal ileum.

Evidence for the use of MDAC

Animal and human volunteer studies have shown that MDAC increases the elimination of a number of drugs. The only data in poisoned patients comes from uncontrolled case reports and case series. Data from these studies suggests that MDAC should be considered in the management of significant ingestions of carbamazepine, dapsone, phenobarbital, quinine, and theophylline. However, in the absence of controlled trials it is not possible to determine whether MDAC has a significant impact on morbidity or mortality in these poisonings. It seems to have no effect in oleander or pesticide poisoning.

Contraindications

- If the patient's airway is not intact or protected.
- Intestinal obstruction or ileus.

MDAC regimen

Charcoal should be given at a dose of 50 g in adults and 1 g/kg in children every 4 hours. The duration will depend on the indication and this is discussed in the individual subsection covering each of the drugs for which MDAC is used. If vomiting is a problem, anti-emetics should be used. Charcoal given at a dose of 12.5 g hourly in adults (0.25 g/kg in children) or 25 g 2-hourly (0.5 g/kg in children) may be better tolerated. It is important that bowel sounds are elicited before each dose of charcoal; patients with ileus should not receive further doses of charcoal.

Adverse effects

MDAC is generally well tolerated. Charcoal is unpalatable and vomiting can occur. Charcoal can cause constipation and this may be more likely in patients who are drowsy and bed bound; however, routine use of laxatives is not currently recommended.

Urinary alkalinization

Urinary alkalinization involves the administration of sodium bicarbonate to increase urine pH to 7.5–8.5. This can be used to increase the renal elimination of drugs that are weak acids and for which renal elimination is the major contributor to total body clearance of the drug. Urinary alkalinization involves manipulation of urine pH, *not* diuresis; forced alkaline diuresis is no longer recommended as it can cause significant fluid and electrolyte imbalance.

Urinary alkalinization works by increasing the proportion of drugs that are weak acids (drugs with a low pKa) that are in the ionized form in the renal tubular lumen. This decreases reabsorption of the drug from the renal tubule back into the blood, thereby 'trapping' the drug in the tubule and increasing renal elimination.

Evidence for the use of urinary alkalinization

Urinary alkalinization increases the elimination of a number of drugs and chemicals including chlorpropamide, diflunisal, fluoride, mecoprop, methotrexate, phenobarbital, and salicylates. However, there is limited evidence for its use in the management of poisoning with most of these and it is generally only considered in the management of moderate–severe salicylate poisoning (see Salicylates, pp. 124–127 for discussion). This is based on studies in volunteers and one clinical study in salicylate poisoned patients which demonstrated an increase in salicylate clearance with urinary alkalinization. There have been no controlled studies which have investigated whether urinary alkalinization has an impact on outcome in salicylate poisoning.

Urinary alkalinization regimen
Plasma creatinine and electrolytes, arterial blood gas, and urinary pH should be checked before starting urinary alkalinization. It is important to correct hypokalaemia since urinary alkalinization will worsen hypokalaemia and it can be difficult to achieve adequate urinary alkalinization in patients who are hypokalaemic. Sodium bicarbonate administration should ideally be through a central line, but can be given peripherally if required. The dose of sodium bicarbonate should be 225 mmol ((225 mL of 8.4%) over 60 minutes or 1.5 L of 1.26% over 2 hours)) in adults, 1 mL/kg 8.4% bicarbonate diluted in 0.5 L 5% dextrose or normal saline given at 2–3 mL/kg/hour in children. Further bolus doses or an infusion of sodium bicarbonate may be required to maintain the urinary pH at 7.5–8.5. The urinary pH should be checked every 30–60 minutes and arterial blood gases and serum potassium concentration checked every 1–2 hours. Plasma salicylate concentration should be repeated 1–2-hourly to ensure that treatment has been effective.

Adverse effects
The main risks of urinary alkalization are fluid and electrolyte imbalance. Alkalaemia can occur; arterial pH should be kept below 7.50 (ideally 7.45). Hypokalaemia is also common and patients are likely to require supplemental potassium, and guided by regular monitoring of serum potassium concentrations. Hypocalcaemia occurs rarely.

Extracorporeal techniques
The extracorporeal techniques that may be used in the management of the poisoned patient include peritoneal dialysis, haemodialysis, continuous veno-venous haemofiltration/haemodiafiltration (continuous veno-venous haemofiltration (CVVHF), continuous veno-venous haemodiafiltration (CVVHDF)) and haemoperfusion. Peritoneal dialysis is no longer recommended as it is too slow to significantly impact on toxin clearance in a clinically meaningful time-frame.

Haemodialysis, CVVHF/CVVHDF, and haemoperfusion, involve inserting a double-lumen catheter into a large vein (femoral or internal jugular/subclavian) and pumping blood through an extracorporeal circuit. The device within the extracorporeal circuit varies with technique. In haemodialysis toxins are removed by diffusion across a dialysis membrane into the dialysate which runs countercurrent to the blood circuit; in haemofiltration the toxin is removed by convection, with substances smaller than the pore size of the filter membrane being removed with plasma water; CVVHDF involves a combination of drug removal by filtration (convection) and dialysis (diffusion). In haemoperfusion an adsorbent such as charcoal is used to remove the toxin. Haemoperfusion is rarely performed now as the cartridges required are not widely available and modern dialysis techniques are able to clear drugs for which haemoperfusion was previously used.

Evidence for the use of haemodialysis and CVVHF/CVVHDF
There have been no controlled studies investigating the role of these techniques in the management of the

poisoned patient. Recommendations are therefore based on the kinetics of the drugs/chemicals involved and case reports/case series. Some of these reports have provided data on clearance of the toxins involved, and also the impact of the extracorporeal technique on total body elimination which is vital in understanding the potential efficacy of the techniques. Normally CVVHDF, but particularly CVVHF, are less efficient than haemodialysis.

In view of the limited evidence for the use of these techniques, it is recommended that clinicians discuss cases with a poisons centre/clinical toxicologist before considering use of an extracorporeal technique in the management of a poisoned patient. Currently, haemodialysis should be considered in cases of severe poisoning related to lithium, salicylates, and toxic alcohols (methanol, ethylene glycol, diethylene glycol, and isopropanol). It may also play a role in certain circumstances in the management of other poisonings including bromide, carbamazepine sodium valproate, and phenobarbital. Haemodialysis is generally preferred to CVVHF/CVVHDF but if haemodialysis is not available, or the patient is too unstable to transfer to a specialist centre for haemodialysis preferably CVVHDF can be considered in severe poisoning with the earlier mentioned agents. CVVHF is least effective, and ideally not used.

Extracorporeal techniques may also be needed for the management of other complications of poisoning including acute kidney injury, severe metabolic acidosis, or severe electrolyte disturbances.

Adverse effects
The adverse effects of haemodialysis and CVVHF/CVVHDF in the poisoned patient are the same as those that can occur when these techniques are used for renal replacement therapy in acute kidney injury and end-stage renal disease. These include line-related complications (e.g. sepsis, bleeding, thrombosis), bleeding related to the anticoagulation required, increased elimination of drugs used therapeutically (e.g. fomepizole or ethanol being used in methanol/ethylene glycol poisoning), and hypotension related to the pressure required to drive the extracorporeal circuit and/or excessive fluid removal. It can be difficult to establish haemodialysis in severely poisoned patients and CVVHDF (or CVVHF) may be better tolerated in these patients.

Further reading
American Academy of Clinical Toxicology; European Association of Poisons Centres and Clinical Toxicologists (1999). Position statement and practice guidelines on the use of multi-dose activated charcoal in the treatment of acute poisoning. *J Toxicol Clin Toxicol*, 37:731–51.

Eddleston M, Juszczak E, Buckley NA, et al. (2008). A randomised controlled trial of multiple dose activated charcoal in acute self-poisoning. *Lancet*, 371:579–87.

Garlich FM, Goldfarb DS (2011). Have advances in extracorporeal removal techniques changed the indications for their use in poisonings? *Adv Chronic Kidney Dis*, 18:172–9.

Ghannoum M, Nolin TD, Lavergne V, et al. (2011). Blood purification in toxicology: nephrology's ugly duckling. *Adv Chronic Kidney Dis*, 18:160–6.

Holubeck WJ, Hoffman RS, Goldfarb DS, et al. (2008). Use of haemodialysis and haemoperfusion in poisoned patients. *Kidney Int*, 74:1327–34.

Proudfoot AT, Krenzelok EP, Vale JA (2004). Position paper on urine alkalinization. *J Toxicol Clin Toxicol*, 42:1–26.

Antidotes

An antidote is a remedy to counteract the effects of a poison. Antidotes are usually considered to be specific molecules, but usually the definition is broadened to include complex mixtures, such as snake antivenins, non-specific therapies used in the management of poisoning, or non-specific therapeutic agents such as activated charcoal.

In order to treat poisoned patients properly it is important to understand the role and mechanism of action of antidotal therapies (Table 2.3). It is often assumed by the inexperienced that there is an antidote to every poison. This is of course far from the case, and the major improvements in the management of poisoning over the past 60 years have resulted as much in understanding when not to intervene, particularly with non-specific treatments such as stimulants, as when to treat.

Antidotes may be:

- targeted exactly at one toxic mechanism, removing the active poison from its site of action, usually by bringing about chemical detoxification of the poison
- antidotes that act specifically at pharmacological receptors, on enzymes or bind specifically to other macromolecules
- antidotes that act by specific binding, chelation, or non-specific binding
- antidotes that act on other receptors than targeted by the poison but act to improve outcome. They may be designed to specifically alter the effect of a toxin by acting on a distant site, or serve to improve the general physiological status of the patient without specifically addressing the mechanism of action by which these changes are caused.

Table 2.3 Antidote actions with examples and targets

Action	Example antidote	Target
Chelating agents	Desferrioxamine	Iron
	Dicobalt edetate	Cyanide
Antibodies	Anti-digoxin FAB	Digoxin
Methaemoglobin formation (secondary detoxification)	Sodium nitrate	Cyanide
Enzymic co-substrate	Sodium thiosulfate (rhodanase)	Cyanide
Inhibition of formation of toxic product	Ethanol Fomepizole	Methanol Ethyleneglycol
Enzyme-toxin complex	Oxime	Organophosphate pesticides
Reaction with toxic metabolite	Acetylcysteine	Paracetamol
Pharmacological receptor antagonist	Naloxone Flumazenil	Opioids Benzodiazepines
Pharmacological receptor agonist	Salbutamol Norepinephrine	β-blocker α-blocker
Symptomatic (functional) action	Diazepam Dobutamine	Anticonvulsant inotrope

Chelating agents and immunological products

The most simple and most easily understood mode of antidotal action is direct chemical or physicochemical reaction between an antidote and a poison to form a product that is less toxic. By mouth this could in theory prevent absorption, or if given parenterally promote more rapid excretion.

Activated charcoal is the most commonly used agent to prevent absorption, but there must be direct physical contact with a compound that can be bound by it to be effective (Decontamination, pp. 36–39). It is very non-specific in its binding characteristics. Most patients unfortunately present too late for this to make a major difference as absorption has already occurred (see Decontamination pp. 36–39).

Other agents are less effective orally as the binding may dissociate (e.g. desferrioxamine), or the antidote itself is a target for enzyme attack in the gut (antibodies).

In contrast to activated charcoal, parenteral chelating agents are generally more specific in their mode of binding:

- Antibodies may be directed against a specific molecule (e.g. Fab antibodies for digoxin) while having less efficacy against similar molecules, other cardenolides in the case of digoxin antibody (Digoxin, pp. 142–145).
- Chemical chelating agents bind metal ions, rarely just a single metal, and other toxic groups—e.g. Cyanide (see Cyanide, pp. 229–231).
- Antibodies may be derived against venoms or toxins derived from animals or plants in a more complex mixture (anti-toxins and anti-venins). Such products are derived by immunizing animals with low doses of toxin to produce high-titre antisera (Chapter 12, Poisoning due to fungi, plants and animals, pp. 297–314).

Even for chelating agents the mode of action resulting in the therapeutic benefit may be complex. Thus while the antidote–toxin complex may be less toxic than the free metal, changes in distribution may cause mobilization of the toxin from critical sites of action may occur before increased elimination. Often these processes occur at once.

Metal chelating agents are rarely specific to a particular metal and they often result in excretion of other metals which may have important roles as enzyme cofactors. Indiscriminate use of chelating agents for small increases in heavy metal concentration is therefore not only unwarranted but potentially hazardous. It is also most important to understand the effects of individual chelating agents and their targets. Redistribution of toxin to more sensitive tissues, such as brain, may occur as a compound is taken from a site where it has been distributed, bound and is less toxic, into blood from where it may subsequently differentially partition. This is a potential hazard when treating mercury poisoning. It is therefore very important to use the appropriate antidote based on kinetic or efficacy data, rather than in vitro binding.

Toxicity of many metals results from reaction with sulfhydryl groups, and the active binding sites of some chelating agents therefore contain sulfhydryl groups. Penicillamine, a monothiol used to bind copper is an example. This also will chelate a variety of other metals, including lead.

Other chelating agents have other types of active site. Calcium ethylenediaminetetraacetate (Calcium edetate) chelates lead and zinc and can be also used in acute cadmium poisoning. Desferrioxamine is a compound of natural origin that binds iron and aluminium.

The net affinity (conditional stability) constants of metal complexes can be misleading as indices of efficacy. The beneficial action of chelating agents is often the result of a combination of effects, including detoxification by complexation, mobilization, and elimination.

In order to detoxify effectively, chelating agents must gain access to the tissue were the metal is exerting its action. In the case of mobilization, the process must occur in a toxicologically desirable direction; that is, away from the critical site of toxic action of the metal. Unfortunately, net affinity constants cannot predict the extent to which chelation occurs *in vivo*, or whether mobilization of the metal occurs in a beneficial direction. Thus penicillamine is a more effective mobilizing agent in mercury poison than diethylenetriaminepentaacetate (DTPA) whereas the corresponding affinity constants would suggest the opposite. It is likely that water solubility of the chelated complex is important in successful chelation therapy. The ideal chelator should have sufficient affinity for the agent of interest, ideally be sufficiently water-soluble to take by mouth, and, be sufficiently lipid-soluble to distribute to sites of accumulation of the metal.

Some chelating agents themselves contain potentially toxic compounds that are neutralized in complex with the toxin. Examples include the cobalt-containing cyanide antidote dicobalt edetate, and the iron chelator desferrioxamine. Both cause hypotension if given in excess in the absence of toxin. This demonstrates the importance of using chelating agents for appropriate clinical indications, and shows why there is still research into safer antidotes; for example, hydroxocobalamin in cyanide toxicity. For hydroxocobalamin a balance is struck between safety in use, dosing volume, time and ease of administration, and speed of expected efficacy.

Immunological antidotes such as antisera have long been used to treat poisoning with toxins of biological origin, such as botulinum toxin and toxins in snake venom. This appears an attractive option for poisons where no antidotes of sufficient efficacy and safety are available. Thus, monoclonal antibodies have reportedly been successful in experimental poisoning by the organophosphorus nerve agent soman.

In the best-known example of immunotherapy for poisoning with a drug, poisoning with digoxin, whole antibodies are not used, instead poisoning with this cardiac glycoside is treated with Fab antibody fragments. Fab fragments have the advantage that they can be eliminated by glomerular filtration through the kidney, and are less immunogenic than whole antibodies (see Digoxin, pp. 142–145). Although immunotherapy can in theory be used to treat any poisoning where detoxicating antibodies can be made against a toxin, in practice the size of the dose of poison makes the approach of limited practical value for most clinical poisonings as huge amounts of antibody would be required to treat most pharmaceuticals. This approach is only practical for potent toxins.

Toxin redistribution
The redistribution of a toxin with the bloodstream will reduce its concentration at the site where it exerts its clinical effect. This is an extension of the concept of chelation. Chelating agents facilitate excretion as well as redistribution. The agents considered under this category

merely change distribution. An example is the use of agents that cause methaemoglobinaemia to increase the concentrations of that molecule in blood in order to bind the toxin cyanide.

This group of compounds are in themselves inactive but result in formation of a compound that is an antidote. The best examples are the methaemoglobin-forming antidotes, used in cyanide poisoning. Methaemoglobin is a form of haemoglobin in which the iron has been oxidized from Fe^{++} to Fe^{+++}. Methaemoglobin is unable to carry oxygen reversibly in the way that haemoglobin does but it has a high affinity for cyanide and sulphide. The most widely available methaemoglobin producer is sodium nitrite. The more recently introduced 4-dimethylaminophenol (DMAP) is used in Germany. Sodium nitrite and DMAP produce methaemoglobin, but in different ways, the former somewhat more slowly. It is important that these antidotes are not used in excess since this will reduce the oxygen-carrying capacity of blood and cause tissue hypoxia.

Methaemoglobin caused by agents such as local anaesthetics can be converted back to haemoglobin by methylthioninium chloride (methylene blue).

Use of intravenous lipid emulsion as an antidote was initially based on evidence in local anaesthetic overdose where it appeared to change the intravascular distribution of the toxin and reduce its concentration at the receptor site on the myocardium (the sodium channel). This concept of redistribution of drug by differential solubility in fat is in effect a type of chelation, although binding is less tight, and ultimately drug will be re-released. The concept is based on the very high lipid solubility of many drugs, and a temporary reduction in free active compound in plasma while distribution to fat-containing peripheral tissues occurs. This is possibly not the only action of lipid, which has effects on cellular energy production and the mitochondria, but lipid solubility of drugs, as measured by water-octanol coefficients, may be an indicator of potential efficacy. Further research is needed to establish the exact role of this therapy.

Antidotes that act on the poison via enzyme catalysed reactions
The existence of enzymatic pathways can be theoretically be exploited in several ways by:
- increasing detoxification—by co-substrates, provision of enzyme or enzyme induction
- inhibiting formation of toxic metabolites—enzyme inhibitors
- exogenous supply of an alternative substrate
- acting on a toxic metabolite to neutralize it
- acting to change binding of an enzyme–toxin complex, enabling re-activation of the enzyme.

To increase detoxification co-substrates can be used, but will usually only be effective if the rate of reaction of that particular metabolic pathway is co-substrate-limited. Alternatively the amount of enzyme present can be increased. Increasing the amount of endogenous enzyme requires new protein synthesis and is normally too slow for use in therapy. Some drugs induce their own metabolism (auto-induction), and elimination becomes more rapid over a few days. This is seen with carbamazepine and barbiturates.

Where poisoning results from metabolism of an indirectly acting poison to a toxic metabolite it may be possible to reduce conversion by either use of a competitive substrate or direct enzyme inhibitor.

Co-substrates

The rhodanese reaction accelerates the rate of cyanide transulphuration to thiocyanate, which is considerably less toxic than cyanide. Rhodanese is a mitochondrial enzyme, while sodium thiosulfate administered intravenously remains largely extracellular. Because of the slow nature of the fall in cyanide blood levels that are observed after the use of sodium thiosulfate, the main use of this cyanide antidote has been as a second-line antidote to one of the methaemoglobin formers (see later in section and Cyanide, pp. 229–231) such as sodium nitrate or DMAP.

Exogenous enzymes

Exogenous enzymes suffer from the disadvantage of being potentially foreign proteins, but have nevertheless been used experimentally as antidotes. Thus, in an attempt to place rhodanese in the extra-cellular space, the use of intravenous bovine heart rhodanese accompanied by sulphur-containing cyanide antidotes has been studied in animals.

Another antidote studied has been cholinesterase in the treatment of anticholinesterase poisoning. As yet efficacy data only exists in animal models.

Inhibition of toxic metabolite formation

An enzymatic method of detoxification, only applicable to indirectly-acting poisons, is the inhibition of the formation of a toxic metabolite. Clinically this approach is adopted to target the active site of the enzyme alcohol dehydrogenase and thus to inhibit the formation of toxic metabolites in methanol poisoning and ethylene glycol poisoning. Two agents are in use, ethanol (a preferential substrate) and fomepizole (4-methylpyrazole), which competitively inhibits alcohol dehydrogenase (see Ethanol and methanol pp. 236–238 and Ethylene and diethylene glycols pp. 240–241).

Antidotes that act on a toxic metabolite of the poison

Compounds may require metabolism before they become toxic. In theory any therapy that affects this metabolism could reduce toxicity, but direct neutralization of the toxic metabolite is often a more logical approach, and this is used in the management of paracetamol (acetaminophen) poisoning. Paracetamol is converted into a toxic intermediate N-acetyl-p-benzoquinone imine (NAPQI). This is normally bound by glutathione, an essential amino acid which is rapidly exhausted in paracetamol poisoning. When the glutathione is exhausted the NAPQI binds to other sulphydryl groups causing cell damage and death. A number of antidotes were trialled in the 1970s, but the most effective and least toxic was acetylcysteine (see Paracetamol, pp. 116–121). This compound is now widely used for acute liver injury of various aetiologies, but efficacy data is less strong for this use.

Antidotes that react with an enzyme–poison complex

The interaction between anticholinesterase pesticides and nerve agents on the active site of acetyl-cholinesterase results, over time, in structural change in the enzyme molecule known as ageing (see Organophosphorus insecticides, pp. 298–300). A number of oxime compounds have been developed which prevent this process. Their efficacy varies depending on the toxin to which the patient has been exposed, and the compounds may be given both as treatment following exposure and in prophylaxis prior to exposure to protect the active enzyme from damage.

Antidotes that act pharmacologically

This group of antidotes effectively works by binding to receptors, classically as agonists or antagonists, competing with or displacing a toxin at a specific receptor site. Such receptor interactions may occur at classical pharmacological receptors, or to binding sites on macromolecules which are less well characterized. This rather artificial distinction may be clinically useful.

Antidotes that act at pharmacological receptors—agonists and antagonists

Classical antagonist antidotes include naloxone (for opioids) and flumazenil (benzodiazepines). These agents bind to the receptor, but do not stimulate it. Agonists act on receptors to stimulate an action, and include adrenergic compounds such as epinephrine and norepinephrine in the management of beta-blocker poisoning. These are discussed in more detail in Basic mechanisms of poisoning, pp. 4–7. Many receptor systems are linked to second messenger chemicals in the cell that act as multiplier systems to amplify the signal caused by the drug–receptor interaction. One of the best recognized is cyclic AMP, the second messenger at beta-adrenergic receptors. Cyclic AMP is targeted by glucagon in the management cardiac effects of beta-blockers.

Antidotes that act to change binding to receptor sites

The best example of this concept is oxygen use to manage carbon monoxide poisoning. Carbon monoxide is toxic by virtue of its tight binding to haemoglobin and other cellular components. Carbon monoxide is displaced competitively by oxygen, reducing its toxicity and increasing its elimination. Increasing the partial pressure of oxygen (hyperbaric therapy) increases the carbon monoxide elimination further, but the clinical benefits remain uncertain (Carbon monoxide, pp. 219–220).

The use of sodium bicarbonate to increase the pH of blood in tricyclic antidepressant poisoning is an example of the binding affinity of a toxin for a receptor being changed. The binding of tricyclics to the sodium channel is pH dependent across physiological pH, being less in a more alkaline environment. Hence the target of a pH of 7.5 in patients with severe tricyclic antidepressant overdose and cardiotoxicity (see Antidepressants, pp. 100–103).

Antidotes working on secondary toxin effects

In clinical management of poisoning, antidotes do not necessarily work at the same receptor as that at which the toxin acts. Atropine is an anticholinergic drug acting on muscarinic cholinergic receptors. However, this drug is used as an antidote for organophosphate and carbamate anticholinesterase poisoning, substances whose major action is not directly on the cholinergic receptor. The anticholinesterases bind to the enzyme acetylcholinesterase, and poisoning is a consequence of accumulation of acetylcholine, the normal substrate for the enzyme. It is this effect which is antagonized by atropine (see Organophosphorus insecticides, pp. 298–300).

Symptomatic (functional) antidotes

There are a number of antidotes that are used symptomatically in poisoning and are difficult to classify. In some cases, further research may show these to have actions that belong to one of the earlier mentioned groups. An example is the use of diazepam to treat convulsions in a wide range of poisoning; and in the case of organophosphate poisoning an additional benefit is reduction in muscle fasciculations. Diazepam acts allosterically on the gamma-aminobutyric acid A ($GABA_A$) receptor. The GABA system is an inhibitory neurotransmission system and the agonist effect of diazepam is to treat or prevent convulsions that may occur in organophosphate poisoning.

The wide range of inotropic and vasopressor drugs used in poisoning that impairs cardiac function or cardiac output is a further example of this approach.

Principles of use of antidotes

When using any antidote it is important to understand the principles underlying use of this type of therapy.

- Firstly it is important to appreciate the mechanism of action and time of response. Thus pharmacological antagonists can be monitored and their response is normally rapid. Indeed it is essential that when the toxin is uncertain, close monitoring of the effects of the antidote is conducted. Failure to respond to an adequate dose of antidote is often an indication to look for an alternative diagnosis than that initially considered.
- Secondly it is important to understand what component of response to monitor. This may be a physiological variable, an absolute concentration of parent or metabolite, or a biochemical marker of the secondary organ toxicity. For antidotes that act on metabolic pathways dosing will often be dependent on the dose of the toxin. There is often the need for repeat toxin measurement in such cases. Sometimes the actual site of interaction is impossible to measure directly, as in the case of acetylcysteine in paracetamol poisoning. Here excess antidote is administered with monitoring being based on hepatic function as a measure of efficacy after a number of hours of therapy.
- Thirdly it is important to understand how much antidote to administer under specific clinical situations. Use of excess antidote, or inappropriate use of antidote may be potentially hazardous. Metal chelating antidotes also remove essential metals. Adverse anaphylactoid reactions to acetylcysteine are more likely in those with lower plasma concentrations of paracetamol. In determining the use of an antidote it is therefore necessary to ensure that the risk–benefit balance is favourable.
- Fourthly it is important to understand the appropriate duration of therapy, and the times at which therapy should be monitored. This means an understanding of the mode and duration of the effect of the toxin and the antidote are required. Depending on the method of administration of the poison the antidote may be given after the peak plasma concentration has been achieved, or before it. In the case of metabolic

poisons the antidote may prevent the formation of toxic metabolites, and thus knowing how long the parent toxin stays in the body, and at what concentrations it becomes non-toxic, will determine length of treatment. Pharmacological antidotes such as naloxone and flumazenil have far shorter half-lives than the drugs that are used to antagonize. Close monitoring of response and repeated dosing is therefore necessary.

- Fifthly it is important that an appropriate target for treatment is chosen. In the case of opioid addicts it is not necessary, or appropriate, to fully reverse the effect of the opioid. All that is required is for the patient to be safe, breathing adequately, with an adequate airway, with an adequate pulse and blood pressure. In the case of digoxin poisoning it is unnecessary to completely neutralize the digoxin, but merely sufficient to prevent features of toxicity. In the case of snakebite it is important to understand the particular features of an envenomation that will respond to the antidote being given. Thus repeated dose of antidote will have no benefit on the outcome of coagulopathy secondary to consumption of clotting factors induced by snake venom. In patients suffering heavy metal poisoning the key component is removal from exposure. Chelation therapy should not be used as a treatment to enable workers in unsatisfactory environments to remain at work and avoid health and safety measures.
- Sixthly it is important to be certain that the indication for treatment is appropriate. This may seem self-evident, but there is sometimes a feeling that something must be done because a result is 'abnormal' rather than a careful balance of risk versus benefit. In recent years a number of 'health scares' have, for example, developed around low-level mercury exposure associated with mercury amalgams. Although there is no evidence of health damage from this exposure, clinicians managing poisoning will meet patients who have been persuaded, often by uninformed practitioners, that antidote treatment is required. It is importance that such patients are treated respectfully and sensitively but given the correct advice.

Further reading
Bateman DN, Marrs TC. Antidotal studies. In: Ballantyne B, Marrs TC, Syversen T (eds), *General and Applied Toxicology*, 3rd edition, pp. 809–22. Chichester: John Wiley & Sons Ltd.

Eddleston M, Juszczak E, Buckley NA (2008). Multiple-dose activated charcoal in acute self-poisoning: a randomised controlled trial. *Lancet*, 371:579–87.

Good AM, Kelly CA, Bateman DN (2007). Differences in treatment advice for common poisons by poisons centres – an international comparison. *Clinical Toxicol*, 45:234–9.

Isbister GK, Kumar VV (2011). Indications for single-dose activated charcoal administration in acute overdose. *Curr Opin Crit Care*, 17:351–7.

Drug and alcohol withdrawal

Background
Regular use of drugs which act on receptors in the central nervous system may lead to adaptive changes resulting in the development of a withdrawal syndrome when the drug is discontinued.

This is seen with a number of drugs including ethanol, nicotine, caffeine, opioids, benzodiazepines, barbiturates, gamma-hydroxybutyrate (GHB), and selective serotonin re-uptake inhibitors (SSRIs).

Mechanisms
Mechanisms of neuroadaptation to chronic exposure to ethanol and benzodiazepines include:
- altered gene expression of the GABA$_A$ receptor
- post-translational modification via receptor subunit phosphorylation
- receptor endocytosis
- modification of receptor subtypes.

For example, in a naïve person, consumption of ethanol causes intoxication by acting as a GABA$_A$ receptor agonist and antagonist at the N-methyl-D-aspartate (NMDA) subtype of the glutamate receptor. With continuous ethanol use, there is a change in the GABA$_A$ subunit type causing reduced sensitivity to sedating effects of ethanol and up-regulation of NMDA subtypes causing increased wakefulness. The loss of the tonic effects of ethanol on these receptors leads to symptoms of withdrawal.

Acute alcohol withdrawal
It is estimated that 24% of adults in the UK drink excessively and alcohol-related problems are a major cause of morbidity and mortality.

An abrupt reduction in alcohol intake in a person with alcohol dependence may lead to the development of an acute alcohol withdrawal syndrome.

Clinical features
Uncomplicated alcohol withdrawal
Early symptoms are manifestations of autonomic hyperactivity and can arise as early as 6 hours after cessation of alcohol intake. These symptoms generally peak between 12 and 30 hours and subside by 48 hours.

They include: anxiety, tremor, sweating, tachycardia, hypertension, and psychomotor agitation.

Assessment of symptoms of acute alcohol withdrawal may be done using a validated scoring system such as the revised Clinical Institute Withdrawal Assessment for Alcohol scale (CIWA-Ar).

Complicated alcohol withdrawal
Alcohol withdrawal seizures or 'rum fits' occur in about 10% of patients, usually within 12–48 hours. These are most commonly generalized isolated tonic–clonic seizures with a short post-ictal period and may be the presenting feature of acute withdrawal. Status epilepticus occurs rarely.

Auditory hallucinations develop in about 25% of patients with acute alcohol withdrawal.

Alcoholic hallucinosis characterized by persistent hallucinations which are classically visual or tactile (e.g. sensation of ants crawling on the skin) may develop in a small proportion.

Delirium tremens (DTs) occur in <5% of patients with alcohol withdrawal. Symptoms start 2–5 days after cessation of drinking and may last for up to 2 weeks. Untreated, it is associated with a mortality rate of 10–15%. The manifestations are much more severe: tremor, sweating, tachycardia, hypertension, agitation, confusion, hallucinations, hyperpyrexia, ketoacidosis, and may lead to cardiovascular collapse.

Risk factors for development of DTs include:
- history of alcohol withdrawal seizures
- history of DTs
- clinical features of alcohol withdrawal with blood ethanol concentration >1000 mg/L.

Wernicke–Korsakoff syndrome
Wernicke's encephalopathy results from degenerative changes in the mammillary bodies from thiamine deficiency. It may develop acutely or evolve over a period of days.

It comprises a triad of:
- ophthalmoplegia (nystagmus, VIth nerve palsy)
- cerebellar ataxia (affecting trunk and lower extremities mainly)
- confusion (apathy, disorientation, memory impairment).

Korsakoff's psychosis generally develops after an episode of Wernicke's encephalopathy and results from changes in the dorsomedial thalamus. It is characterized by profound retrograde and anterograde amnesia but with relatively preserved intellectual ability such that the patient often confabulates to mask their memory impairment.

Patients at risk of developing Wernicke–Korsakoff syndrome include:
- alcohol-related liver disease
- acute alcohol withdrawal
- malnourishment
- hospitalization for acute illness.

Management of alcohol withdrawal
1 Nurse in a well-lit and reassuring environment.
2 Give prophylactic thiamine to all patients (orally for low-risk and parenterally for high-risk groups). Continue parenteral thiamine for at least 5 days in patients with Wernicke's encephalopathy.
3 Check BMs to exclude hypoglycaemia. Note that administration of dextrose may precipitate Wernicke's encephalopathy in severely thiamine-deficient individuals. Administer thiamine as well as dextrose to correct hypoglycaemia.
4 Consider and exclude other organic causes for clinical features, e.g. infection, subdural haematoma, hepatic encephalopathy.

Seizures are often self-limiting. Recurrent seizures may be treated with long-acting benzodiazepines (e.g. diazepam). Phenytoin is less effective in preventing recurrence.

Sedation with long-acting benzodiazepines, e.g. diazepam or chlordiazepoxide, is used for features of autonomic hyperactivity. Diazepam is available parenterally; avoid mixing benzodiazepines and use a regimen with which you are familiar

Regimens for parenteral diazepam include:
- fixed dose reducing regimen, e.g. starting at 20 mg four times daily, reducing the frequency and dose over a number of days

- symptom-triggered regimen, e.g. 20 mg given up to hourly, based on symptoms
- front-loaded regimen, e.g. 50–100 mg every 2–4 hours until sedated then smaller doses every 4–6 hours as needed.

The symptom-triggered regimen is associated with reduced number of doses and reduced duration of treatment and is preferable if staff trained in assessment of acute alcohol withdrawal using a validated scale such as the CIWA-Ar are available.

Carbamazepine is as effective as benzodiazepines and is a suitable alternative.

Benzodiazepine withdrawal

The mechanisms and clinical features of benzodiazepine withdrawal are very similar to those of acute alcohol withdrawal. Evidence for management is poor. It is reasonable to treat with long-acting benzodiazepines acutely. Short-acting benzodiazepines tend to be associated with increased risk of habituation. In chronically habituated patients more complex drug rotating regimens may be used.

Gamma-hydroxybutyrate withdrawal

The clinical features are similar to the alcohol withdrawal syndrome but features are more prolonged and autonomic features less prominent.

Early (<24 hours): insomnia, tremor, confusion, nausea and vomiting.

Late (>24 hours): tachycardia, hypertension, agitation, seizures and/or myoclonic jerks and hallucinations (both auditory and visual).

Management

Benzodiazepines are the first-line treatment for managing acute GHB withdrawal. The same protocol as for acute withdrawal may be used initially but response should be monitored carefully. In severe cases, very high doses of benzodiazepines may be required (e.g. 10–20 mg at 2–4-hourly intervals). Baclofen is a specific GABA$_B$ receptor agonist and is anecdotally more effective in more severe cases.

Patients with extreme agitation who are not responding to high doses of benzodiazepines should be managed in a critical care setting. Barbiturates (e.g. sodium thiopental) or propofol have been used in such cases.

Opiate withdrawal

Chronic opioid use leads to:
- down-regulation of the mu-receptor subtype which is responsible for the physical symptoms of opioid withdrawal

- adaptive neuronal changes in the limbic system affecting the dopaminergic reward pathway which is responsible for the psychological dependence.

Clinical features

- Autonomic: sweating, yawning, sneezing, piloerection, rhinorrhoea, flushing, dilated pupils, tremor.
- GI: vomiting, diarrhoea, abdominal cramps.

The physical symptoms of opioid withdrawal can be assessed objectively using the Objective Opiate Withdrawal Scale. These are rarely serious although distressing to the patient ('going cold turkey').

A neonatal abstinence syndrome has also been described in neonates born to mothers addicted to opioids. Presenting symptoms usually occur within the first 48–72 hours after birth, but may present after 2–4 weeks in the case of methadone use. Symptoms may be assessed using the Finnegan Neonatal Abstinence Scoring System.

Management

- Reassurance that symptoms are not life-threatening.
- Give paracetamol or non-steroidal anti-inflammatory drugs (NSAIDs) for pain.
- Give loperamide for diarrhoea.
- Consider use of short acting z-drugs, e.g. zopiclone for insomnia.

Referral to a specialist drug addiction service is required for management of psychological dependence and opioid detoxification. Pharmacological treatments for chronic dependence include opioid substitutes such as methadone or buprenorphine, or an alpha-2-adrenergic agonist, e.g. lofexidine. These agents are often used to reduce craving and are less effective in achieving abstinence from opioid use. A partial agonist such as dihydrocodeine in doses of 60 mg may also be a useful interim measure.

Sublingual buprenorphine and clonidine have been used successfully in the management of neonatal abstinence syndrome.

Further reading

National Institute for Health and Clinical Excellence (2010). *Alcohol-Use Disorders: Physical Complications*. CG100. London: NICE.

National Institute for Health and Clinical Excellence (2007). *Drug Misuse: Opioid Detoxification*. CG52. London: NICE.

Sullivan JT, Sykora K, Schneiderman J, et al. (1989). Assessment of alcohol withdrawal: the revised Clinical Institute Withdrawal Assessment for Alcohol scale (CIWA-Ar). *Br J Addict*, 84:1353–7.

Tarabar AF, Nelson LS (2004). The gamma-hydroxybutyrate withdrawal syndrome. *Toxicol Rev*, 23:45–9.

Management of the pregnant woman who is poisoned

Background

Poisoning in pregnancy is uncommon, and evidence-based guidance regarding the management of the poisoned pregnant patient is therefore usually limited or unavailable. Furthermore, studies of fetal and maternal outcome following maternal poisoning are often highly confounded as a result of frequent co-ingestion of multiple substances, high rates of elective termination of pregnancy following self-poisoning, and the significant number of cases lost to follow-up. The information presented in this section is based on the published literature and data collected over the past 20 years by the UK National Poisons Information Service (NPIS) and UK Teratology Information Service (UKTIS).

Epidemiology of poisoning in pregnancy

Poisoning in pregnancy can be acute or chronic and may occur as a result of:
- deliberate self-harm (usually acute)
- accidental overdose (usually acute)
- illicit drug use (acute or chronic)
- therapeutic errors (usually acute)
- occupational exposure (usually chronic)
- environmental exposure (usually chronic).

Rates of deliberate self-harm and use of drugs or chemicals in attempted suicide have increased in recent years, with women aged 15–29 years commonly involved in episodes of self-poisoning. In the UK, poisons centres receive up to 300 enquiries per year regarding poisoning in pregnancy, including accidental or deliberate overdose and substance abuse. These account for about 5% of all poisoning enquiries, but represent only a very small percentage of maternities in the UK each year (>700,000). Although uncommon in pregnancy, suicide remains a leading cause of maternal death in the UK and elsewhere.

Risk factors

Risk factors for intentional self-poisoning in pregnancy include:
- younger maternal age
- unplanned pregnancy
- first pregnancy
- first or second trimester of pregnancy
- lower socioeconomic status
- incomplete high school education
- maternal mental illness
- concomitant substance abuse
- lack of social support
- domestic abuse or violence
- inappropriate withdrawal of regular psychiatric medication due to fears of fetal effects.

Substances involved

In the UK, the ten most common substance groups involved in poisoning reported to poisons centres between 2005 and 2010 were:
- pharmaceuticals (63%) especially paracetamol, antidepressants, ibuprofen, iron salts, codeine
- household products (12%), e.g. detergents, kettle descalers
- drugs of abuse (10%), e.g. cocaine, ecstasy
- industrial chemicals (4%)
- carbon monoxide (3%)
- agrochemicals (3%)
- heavy metals (2%)
- other gases (1%)
- smoke inhalation (1%)
- unknown substance (1%).

Pharmacology in pregnancy

Physiological changes associated with pregnancy affect the pharmacokinetic properties of drugs. Because of this, enhanced therapeutic drug monitoring may be indicated.

Absorption

This may be affected by the increase in gastric pH, while progesterone-related slower gastric emptying may delay peak drug concentrations after oral ingestion.

Distribution

Distribution is accelerated due to increased cardiac output. Total body water is increased by 20% and plasma volume by 50% by the third trimester, affecting distribution volumes and steady-state plasma concentrations of water-soluble drugs. Increases in body fat may also increase total distribution volume for lipid-soluble drugs. For drugs bound by plasma albumin, decreased plasma albumin concentration and binding affinity may result in higher free drug concentrations as a proportion of total drug concentration. Toxicity may therefore occur if doses are increased without taking this effect into account.

Metabolism

Metabolism may be unpredictable due to altered hepatic blood flow and variable effects of pregnancy on hepatic enzyme activity. Activities of the cytochrome p450 isoenzymes CYP1A2, CYP2C19 and of N-acetyltransferase 2 (NAT2) are reduced while CYP2A6, CYP2C9, CYP2D6, CYP3A4 and uridine diphospho-glucuronosyltransferases have increased activity, especially in later pregnancy. These changes may affect plasma drug concentrations in therapeutic doses. For example, lamotrigine concentrations fall during pregnancy, and this is associated with an increased risk of seizure.

Excretion

Pregnancy is associated with an increase in glomerular filtration amounting to 40–65% resulting in increased clearance of renally excreted drugs or metabolites, such as penicillins, atenolol, digoxin, metformin, lithium, and morphine glucuronides. Renal tubular secretion of drugs via P-glycoprotein (P-gp) is also increased in late pregnancy, contributing to increased clearance of drug substrates, for example, digoxin.

Placental transfer

Most therapeutic drugs are transferred via the placenta to the fetus, with transfer *increased* for dugs with the following characteristics:
- low molecular weight (e.g. <600D)
- high lipid solubility
- un-ionized drugs—weak bases are ionized in the relatively acidic fetal circulation and may become trapped
- low protein binding—maternal plasma albumin concentrations are higher than in the fetus and placental transfer of highly bound drugs will conversely be reduced
- active transport of drugs towards the fetus by placental membrane transporters, such as P-gp.

Principals of teratogenicity

A teratogen is any agent that results in structural or functional abnormality in the offspring following maternal exposure in pregnancy. Teratogenic effects of a compound may vary significantly between species and adverse developmental outcomes observed in animals can therefore not be assumed to be the same following human exposure, although for some teratogens, consistent cross-species effects have been observed.

The nature of a teratogenic effect depends primarily on the timing during gestation at which exposure occurs. Exposure to a teratogen at any stage of pregnancy may potentially result in pregnancy loss or fetal demise. The main structural modelling of most fetal organs (e.g. heart, lungs; limbs) occurs during weeks 2–8 after conception and a teratogenic exposure during this susceptible developmental period may therefore result in one or more major malformations of the organs undergoing development. For example, systemic exposure to isotretinoin between the 15th and 40th day after conception (week 4–8 of pregnancy) is associated with risk of central nervous system (microcephaly), ear (anotia, absent auditory canals), eye (microphthalmia), cardiac and limb defects. The first 2 weeks after conception, prior to implantation, have been referred to as the 'all or nothing' period, during which a teratogenic exposure is proposed to result either in miscarriage or to have no effect at all. Although epidemiological human data suggests that, for most agents, exposure during this period is not associated with an increased risk of malformation, caution needs to be applied as factors such as uncertainty regarding timing of conception (e.g. menstrual cycle irregularity, inaccurate maternal recall), long half-life of a drug (e.g. retinoic acid derivatives), and more recent research showing considerable inter-individual variability in growth and developmental stage of human embryos, may result in false reassurance being given.

Conversely, exposures after the first trimester confer a risk of functional abnormality and impairment of fetal growth, although development of the central nervous system continues well beyond the first trimester. Thus alcohol at any stage of pregnancy may be associated with neurodevelopmental and/or behavioural problems in the offspring.

Exposure in late pregnancy may be associated with specific fetal or neonatal effects that necessitate urgent delivery of the fetus or treatment of the neonate to counteract potentially fatal effects of the compound. The effect of a teratogen is usually dose dependent, but may be moderated by maternal and/or fetal genetic factors, inter-individual variation in drug metabolism, underlying maternal disease, and synergistic interactions with other maternal exposures (e.g. alcohol, therapeutic medications).

Features of maternal toxicity that may impact on fetal well-being

Maternal toxicity is likely to be a major determinant of adverse fetal effects following poisoning. Features of particular importance are listed here. Management should be directed at minimizing these effects as far as possible:

- cardiovascular: hypotension/hypertension, tachycardia/bradycardia, arrhythmia
- central nervous system: sedation/coma, convulsions
- respiratory: respiratory depression, hypoxia
- metabolic: alkalosis/acidosis
- GI: nausea, vomiting, diarrhoea, GI bleed, fluid and electrolyte imbalance.

Management of the pregnant woman who is poisoned

A potential pitfall in the management of the poisoned pregnant patient is failing to treat the mother adequately due to concerns about adverse effects of the treatment on the fetus. The unborn child is, however, susceptible not only to the action of the toxic compound(s) involved, but also the effects of impaired oxygen and nutrient transfer as a consequence of maternal toxicity. It is thus imperative that the maternal condition is optimized and that, where clinically indicated, antidotes and other interventions are not withheld on account of pregnancy. In most situations, the recommended immediate management of the pregnant patient is the same as for the poisoned non-pregnant patient.

Mother

Pregnancy should be excluded, where appropriate by pregnancy testing, in all women of childbearing potential presenting with suspected poisoning. Optimization of the maternal condition is an immediate priority, but consideration should be given to fetal well-being during any interventions and procedures.

- Assess maternal condition and stabilize—in later pregnancy resuscitate in left tilt using a wedge to avoid compression of the aorta and inferior vena cava by the gravid uterus.
- Where available, seek specific advice from a teratology or poisons specialist service. In the UK, UKTIS works in concert with the NPIS to provide around-the-clock case-specific advice (Table 2.4).
- In most cases it is recommended that the poisoned pregnant patient is treated as one would a non-pregnant patient.
- Where available, review by the perinatal psychiatry team should be considered if self-harm occurs in the context of any complex underlying psychiatric disorder.
- Document exposure and management in the maternity record as well as in hospital notes.

Fetus

Once the maternal condition has been stabilized, seek early obstetric/fetal medicine input as fetal monitoring (e.g. cardiotocography (CTG) in cardiotoxic drug poisoning), or a specific fetal intervention may be indicated. For example, expedited delivery by emergency caesarean section may be indicated when premature closure of the ductus arteriosus has occurred following NSAID overdose. Detrimental fetal effects of the maternal poisoning may require additional

Table 2.4 Teratology information service networks

Service	Contact details
UK Teratology Information Service (UKTIS)	<http://www.uktis.org www.toxbase.org> Tel.: 0844 892 0909
European Network of Teratology Information Services (ENTIS)	<http://www.entis-org.eu>
American Organization of Teratology Information Services (OTIS)	<http://www.otispregnancy.org>
Motherisk (Canadian Teratology Information Service)	<http://www.motherisk.org>

fetal or neonatal monitoring or treatment later on, even after the mother has made a full recovery.

Critical factors in assessing the risk of maternal poisoning to the fetus include stage of pregnancy (obtain accurate last menstrual period), half-life of the drug/chemical involved in the exposure, and the presence of maternal toxicity (effect on transfer of oxygen and nutrients to fetus).

Use of antidotes

Most antidotes and other medicines used in the treatment of poisoning cross the placenta and their safety in pregnancy is often poorly documented, especially for those used infrequently. Because fetal well-being is dependent on maternal health, however, it is likely that treatments that improve the outlook for the mother are also beneficial to the fetus.

Fetal outcome following poisoning in pregnancy

This depends on the poison ingested, the effects of maternal toxicity, the gestation at which exposure occurs, and the effects of factors such as maternal illness and co-ingestion of other substances. The risk that exposure will occur during a critical stage of pregnancy is increased for chronic poisoning, but doses are often higher in episodes of acute poisoning and the potential of exceeding a threshold above which adverse effects are observed is therefore more likely in the latter situation.

Data on fetal outcome following poisoning in pregnancy are severely limited by the small numbers of cases for individual substances, uncertainty regarding the degree of poisoning, and inter-study design, in addition to being heavily confounded as described previously. Some studies report an increased risk of miscarriage following overdose periconceptually or in early pregnancy, and of preterm birth, low birth weight, congenital malformation, or fetal death following poisoning in pregnancy. These findings are not consistently replicated, however, with no increase in adverse pregnancy outcome being demonstrated by others. Accurate documentation of exposure, management, and materno-fetal outcome, and reporting of such exposures to registries such as that held by the UKTIS is thus crucial for the development of evidence-based guidance on optimal management of poisoning in pregnancy and risks of adverse fetal outcomes.

Specific poisons

Some substances are of particular relevance to pregnancy, either because they are frequently encountered, have important maternal or fetal effects, or require the use of specific antidotes.

Paracetamol

Paracetamol overdose during pregnancy is associated with a risk of hepatotoxicity in the mother, as in the non-pregnant patient. It is not known if pregnancy is a risk factor for enhanced paracetamol hepatotoxicity in the mother; some clinicians use lower thresholds for treatment with antidotes during pregnancy although there is no specific guidance on this. There is also a risk of fetal hepatotoxicity due to metabolism of paracetamol by the immature fetal liver and fetal hepatotoxicity and intrauterine death have been recorded after maternal paracetamol poisoning.

Given soon after paracetamol overdose, acetylcysteine (NAC) is highly effective for preventing hepatotoxicity and there is no evidence that this is not also the case in pregnancy. NAC crosses the placenta, but the available limited evidence does not suggest an increase in fetal risk from the use of NAC. Indeed, delay in administration of NAC has been associated with an increased risk of fetotoxicity.

It is therefore recommended that NAC should be used in the treatment of paracetamol poisoning in pregnancy as in the non-pregnant patient. The pre-pregnancy weight should be used for calculating ingested paracetamol dose in mg/kg and standard paracetamol nomograms employed to determine the need for an antidote. The dose of NAC should be calculated using actual maternal weight at the time of poisoning, up to a ceiling of 110 kg, as in the non-pregnant patient.

NSAIDs

There is no conclusive evidence of adverse fetal effects following use of NSAIDs in usual therapeutic doses during early pregnancy. Reports of increased rates of fetal cardiac defects and spontaneous abortion have not been confirmed. Therapeutic use of NSAIDs in later pregnancy, however, may cause fetal renal impairment with associated oligohydramnios, premature closure of the ductus arteriosus, and possible increased risk of persistent pulmonary hypertension of the newborn (PPHN).

Following acute NSAID overdose, evidence of adverse fetal effects is scanty and conflicting. In one series of ibuprofen overdoses the rate of miscarriage was within the expected range, incidence of congenital malformations was higher than expected, and no cases of neonatal renal dysfunction were reported; however, the numbers of exposures at the critical times for these outcomes were low. No increase in abnormal outcomes was observed in another prospective study of ibuprofen overdose which included a cohort of pregnant women, although again numbers were small. A recent analysis of cases of ibuprofen overdose in the third trimester (n = 16) identified two cases of premature closure of the ductus arteriosus following a single exposure.

Management of NSAID overdose in pregnancy should be as in the non-pregnant patient, although enhanced fetal monitoring may be justified, especially following third trimester exposure, where early obstetric consultation is recommended in view of the risk of premature closure of the fetal ductus arteriosus

Iron

Iron is commonly available to women during pregnancy and as a result is not infrequently taken in overdose under these circumstances. Information on the effects of iron overdose during pregnancy is limited, especially following first trimester exposure, and the consequent risk of fetal malformation is unknown. Most available data relates to iron overdose in the second and third trimesters and does not suggest an increased risk of adverse fetal outcomes if the mother is treated as a non-pregnant patient.

There are several case reports describing the use of desferrioxamine in pregnancy for treatment of iron overdose and for haematological conditions such as thalassaemia, the latter involving chronic exposure throughout pregnancy. These limited available data do not suggest that desferrioxamine use is associated with an increased risk of congenital malformations or other adverse fetal effects, while untreated iron poisoning may have severe maternal and fetal consequences in the absence of appropriate antidotal treatment. Therefore, it is recommended that if desferrioxamine is indicated for the management of iron overdose, it should not be withheld on account of pregnancy.

Lead

Chronic lead poisoning may occur in pregnancy as a result of occupational or environmental exposure. Pica is more common in early pregnancy and this increases risk of raised blood lead levels (BLLs). Use of ethnic cosmetics or lead-glazed ceramics may also be responsible. Lead poisoning is more common with social deprivation, poor housing, urban environment, and in immigrant or ethnic populations.

Placental transfer of lead results in cumulative fetal uptake and increases with increased maternal plasma lead concentration. Mobilization of maternal lead stores from bone to blood during pregnancy contributes to fetal exposure.

Lead poisoning during pregnancy has several adverse effects on pregnancy outcome including higher risks of spontaneous abortion, maternal hypertension, impaired fetal growth, premature rupture of the membranes and premature delivery, and neurodevelopmental effects on the fetus. Congenital malformations have also been reported in some studies, but risks appear to be increased for some minor rather than for major malformations.

Neurodevelopmental effects are related to maternal BLL, but there is no safe threshold below which these do not occur. Intellectual impairment has been demonstrated in association with maternal BLLs <10 micrograms/dL.

Investigation and general management of lead poisoning during pregnancy is the same as in the non-pregnant patient. Prevention of further exposure and appropriate iron, folate, calcium, and zinc supplementation are important (see Lead pp. 276–277).

The indications for and safety of chelating agents for treating lead poisoning in pregnancy are uncertain. Sodium calcium edetate is likely to cross the placenta. Teratogenic effects have been reported in animal studies but these appear to be prevented by zinc supplementation. There are several case reports of successful use in pregnancy but evidence of efficacy in lowering fetal BLLs is limited. Dimercaptosuccinic acid (DMSA) is also likely to cross the placenta and teratogenic effects have been reported in some animal studies. Furthermore, lead concentrations in fetal liver and bone may increase following use as a result of redistribution. Other animal studies of lead poisoning, however, have suggested beneficial effects from DMSA including improved fetal growth. Evidence of use in human pregnancy is very limited.

Discussion with a specialist is strongly recommended for all pregnant women with possible lead poisoning. The current UK recommendation is that all adults with a BLL ≥50 micrograms/dL should be considered for chelation therapy, including women who are pregnant. Intravenous sodium calcium edetate is the preferred chelation agent in pregnancy. Where maternal chelation therapy has been used, neonatal BLLs should be measured as further chelation of the neonate may be required.

Toxic alcohols and glycols

Patients with severe poisoning following exposure to toxic alcohols or glycols such as ethylene glycol or methanol are at risk of life-threatening complications that may be prevented by appropriate therapy, including use of antidotes. There is very little information available on the adverse fetal effects of this type of poisoning, or on the safety of antidotes, but it is likely that the severity of maternal toxicity will be a major factor determining fetal outcome. It is therefore appropriate to use the same management for pregnant as for non-pregnant women (see Ethanol and methanol, pp. 236–238).

Fomepizole is the preferred antidote for use in pregnancy, particularly in the first trimester as the alternative antidote, ethanol, is a known teratogen associated with neurodevelopmental abnormalities following exposure at any stage of pregnancy. If fomepizole is unavailable or considered inappropriate, however, then ethanol should be used because any risk of adverse effects is likely to be far outweighed by the risks of untreated ethylene glycol poisoning.

Carbon monoxide

Carbon monoxide is a common cause of death from poisoning and pregnant women may be exposed accidentally or as a consequence of an act of self-harm.

Carbon monoxide is readily transferred to the fetus via the placenta, and carbon monoxide poisoning during pregnancy has been associated with intrauterine fetal death and neurological deficits in surviving infants. Severe fetal effects are usually associated with features of severe maternal toxicity. There is no persuasive evidence that subclinical carbon monoxide exposure in the mother is associated with adverse fetal outcomes.

Hyperbaric oxygen (HBO) therapy is advocated by some clinicians for the management of carbon monoxide poisoning, although use is controversial and this treatment is not recommended by poisons services in the UK (see Carbon monoxide, pp. 219–220). Concerns about the potential adverse fetal effects of carbon monoxide exposure have prompted some to use a lower threshold for recommending HBO in patients who are pregnant. There is no specific evidence to support or refute this approach. Clinical reports involving small patient numbers have not identified any specific maternal or fetal hazards from use of HBO therapy.

Further information

Teratology information services (TISs) are available in many countries and can provide information on the fetal effects of therapeutic, and in some cases toxic, exposure to drugs and chemicals in pregnancy. A few TIS work in collaboration with poisons centres and are also able to offer advice on the management of poisoning in pregnancy. Details of the key international teratology networks are shown in Table 2.4.

Further reading

Bailey B (2003). Are there teratogenic risks associated with antidotes used in the acute management of poisoned pregnant women? *Birth Defects Res*, 67:i.

Czeizel AE (2011). Attempted suicide and pregnancy. *J Inj Violence Res*, 3:45–54.

Flint C, Larsen H, Nielsen GL, et al. (2002). Pregnancy outcome after suicide attempt by drug use: a Danish population-based study. *Acta Obstet Gynecol Scand*, 81:516–22.

Gentile S (2010). Suicidal mothers. *J Inj Violence Res*, 3:90–7.

McClure CK, Katz KD, Patrick TE, et al. (2011). The epidemiology of acute poisonings in women of reproductive age and during pregnancy, California, 2000–2004. *Matern Child Health J*, 15:964–73.

McClure CK, Patrick TE, Katz KD, et al. (2011). Birth outcomes following self-inflicted poisoning during pregnancy, California, 2000 to 2004. *J Obstet Gynecol Neonatal Nurs*, 40:292–301.

Palladino CL, Singh V, Campbell J, et al. (2011). Homicide and suicide during the perinatal period: findings from the National Violent Death Reporting System. *Obstet Gynecol*, 118:1056–63.

Riggs BS, Bronstein AC, Kulig K, et al. (1989). Acute acetaminophen overdose during pregnancy. *Obstet Gynecol*, 74:247–53.

Psychiatric risk assessment and management of the patient with self-harm

Background

Self-harm is one of the most common reasons for presentation to hospital. Self-harming behaviours are not restricted to any particular gender, age group, or social background. Nor are they restricted to individuals with mental disorder. The motivation behind acts of self-harm varies from patient to patient and there can be an extensive array of ongoing risks (not just suicide). Such a breadth of presentations precludes a one-size-fits-all approach to assessment and management. Instead, patients who have self-harmed need to be approached without preconceptions, the clinical assessment needs to be wide-ranging, and the management plan needs to be tailored to the individual. This section offers a practical framework upon which bespoke assessments and management plans can be assembled.

Assessment of risk

Cohort studies show that 15–20% of patients presenting to hospital with self-harm return following another episode of self-harm within a year. Approximately 1% die through suicide within a year and 5–10% ultimately commit suicide. As a general rule, the more closely the patient resembles the typical profile of those who die by suicide, the greater the risk of completed suicide. Whilst this section deals primarily with risks of further acts of self-harm and of completed suicide, it is important to remain vigilant for other potential risks, for example, if the patient has children are the children at risk of neglect, emotional harm, or even death? The approach described here can be adapted to the assessment of other identified risks. The clinical assessment should cover four broad areas:

- *demographic* risk factors
- *diagnosis* (both psychiatric and 'physical');
- *actions* leading to the current presentation
- *indications of intent* elicited during the clinical interview.

Pertinent information from these four areas is then amalgamated into a formulation, which offers an explanation as to why this person self-harmed in this particular way at this particular time and acknowledges the immediate and long-term implications.

Demographic risk factors

As already mentioned, the more closely the patient resembles the typical profile of those who die by suicide, the greater the risk of completed suicide. In clinical practice this means generating an actuarial estimate of risk by collating demographic information about the patient and comparing it with known population risk factors (in the same way as an insurance company would use age, gender, occupation, etc. to determine a life insurance premium). Table 2.5 compares some recognized population risk factors for completed suicide with those for self-harm. The most important demographic risk factor is age. Elderly patients presenting with self-harm are at considerably higher risk of completed suicide than are younger patients. They are also more likely to be suffering from a mental disorder such as depression. It is therefore usually advisable to discuss older self-harm patients with colleagues in psychiatry.

Table 2.5 Demographic risk factors for suicide and self-harm

Death from suicide	Presentation with self-harm
Male > female	Female > male
Old > young	Young adult
Widowed, separated, single	Unmarried
Living alone/social isolation	Interpersonal crisis
Low income or unemployed + certain occupations (doctors, farmers, etc.)	Low income or unemployed
Family history of suicide	Recent self-harm by peer

Diagnosis

Many psychiatric and non-psychiatric conditions are known to be associated with an increased risk of suicide. Table 2.6 shows the relative risks associated with major psychiatric diagnoses and with a selection of non-psychiatric diagnoses.

Diagnosis is clearly a key component of risk assessment as well as a guide to clinical management, however, it is important to bear in mind that the majority of people

Table 2.6 Relative risk of suicide associated with various diagnoses: expressed as multiples of the population risk (~1 suicide per 100,000 patient years in the UK although it varies with gender, age, etc.)

Diagnosis	Relative risk of suicide
Previous suicide attempt	×40
Psychiatric diagnoses	
Anorexia nervosa	×25
Severe depression	×20
Bipolar affective disorder	×15
Recreational opiate use/dependence	×14
Anxiety disorders	×10
Schizophrenia	×8
Personality disorder	×7
Alcohol dependence/harmful use	×6
Learning disability	×0.9
Other selecteded diagnoses	
Haemodialysis	×14
Head & neck neoplasm	×11
HIV	×6.5
Epilepsy	×5
Systemic lupus erythematosus	×4.5
Renal transplantation	×4
Spinal cord injury	×4
Multiple sclerosis	×2.5

Data from Harris EC, Barraclough B. Suicide as an outcome for mental disorders. A meta-analysis. British Journal of Psychiatry. 1997;170:205–228.

presenting following self-harm do not meet the criteria for any diagnosis. The clinician may therefore have to resist the temptation to stretch the boundaries of the closest diagnostic category simply because it offers a least bad fit. This can be a particular challenge in services that require clinicians to record a code for every clinical contact. Helpfully, ICD-10 includes descriptive codes for 'Intentional self-harm' (X60–X84) and for 'Injury, poisoning and certain other consequences of external causes' (S00–T98).

Actions

Common sense tells us that someone who chooses a method of self-harm that they know is highly likely to prove fatal (such as jumping from a tall building) probably intends to die, whereas someone who chooses a method that they know is likely to prove harmless (such as swallowing five vitamin pills) probably does not. However, it is important to remember that most people have limited medical knowledge so there is often a marked discrepancy between perceived/intended risk and actual risk. This is particularly true for self-harm by medication overdose where most people have almost no awareness of whether the substance they are ingesting is innocuous or potentially lethal. The substances used in self-harm overdoses correlate more closely with availability and trends in prescribing than with suicidal intent. Hence the questions that are key to the assessment of *toxicological risk*—'What has been ingested, in what quantity, and when?' are of almost no value in assessing *suicide risk*.

In order to ascertain the psychological significance of an act of self-harm one has to understand the context. The simplest way to do this is to invite the patient to take you through an autobiographical timeline from at least 24 hours before the act, through the build-up to the act, the act itself, and the aftermath (including how they came to be in hospital). Of course, the patient may not be willing or able to provide a coherent account of what happened so a corroborative history often proves invaluable.

By following the patient's timeline it is usually possible to build up a picture of where their self-harming thoughts came from, of what caused them to act on these thoughts, of what they actually did, and of what they expected would be the outcome. This picture provides an insight into the patient's motivation at the time of the act, which is fundamental to the assessment of risk.

It is important to remember that suicidality is not an all-or-nothing phenomenon but is a spectrum ranging from a passive ambivalence about life: 'I wouldn't mind if I were killed by bolt of lightning tomorrow', to a settled determination to carry out a specific suicide plan: 'At the first opportunity I am going to drive to the Forth Road Bridge and throw myself off'. Self-harming thoughts often emerge from a sense of entrapment, that is, the patient feels caught in a situation that they can do nothing about, (such as an unhappy relationship, debt, or illness). The thoughts can often be understood as a hypothetical 'escape plan'—either escaping into the finality of death, or escaping from isolation by securing help through an act that communicates distress. When assessing a patient who has self-harmed, it is often possible to identify a specific triggering event that caused hypothetical thoughts to be translated into actions.

Table 2.7 illustrates how an examination of behaviour before, during, and after an act of self-harm can help to reveal the motives behind the act.

Table 2.7 An illustration of behaviours consistent with an intention to die and with an intention to communicate distress

Timeline	Actions indicating an intent to die	Actions indicating an intent to communicate distress
Before the act of self-harm	Final acts in anticipation of death, e.g. putting financial affairs in order, writing considered suicide notes, etc.	Impulsive response to an argument or short-term crisis
	Evidence of planning, e.g. researching methods of suicide, storing up tablets, etc.	Hastily produced, emotionally charged suicide note
		Absence of planning
The act of self-harm	High perceived lethality	Low perceived lethality
	Precautions against being found, e.g. remote location, usual contacts known to be away, etc.	Steps taken to ensure one is found and 'saved', e.g. tablets taken in front of someone, empty medication packets left in conspicuous place, phoning or texting a friend, etc.
	'Violent' method, e.g. firearm, jump from height, hanging, drowning	Opportunistic method, e.g. tablets that happened to be in the house
After the act of self-harm	Patient discovered by chance	Steps to secure medical assessment e.g. calling emergency services
	Steps taken to evade medical assessment or treatment	Overt displays of distress, particularly in front of friends and relatives
	Denial of the act or down-playing of its significance	

Interview

The often complex motives that give rise to acts of self-harm can intrude upon the clinical interview. For example, the patient whose determined suicide attempt has, in his eyes, been obstructed by well-meaning but misguided medical staff is likely to underplay or even deny his suicidality in the hope that he will be discharged home where he can make another (successful) attempt. Whereas the patient whose impulsive, non-suicidal overdose was provoked by a desire to end her husband's infidelity through demonstrating to him how unhappy it has made her is likely to overstate the seriousness of the act until she has secured a commitment from him to change his ways. Hence, direct questions such as 'Do you still want to die?' may invite misleading answers. A more subtle approach is required.

As already outlined, the simplest way to construct the clinical interview is to build it around an autobiographical timeline. This approach lends itself to exploration of the underlying stressors and triggering events as well as the motives behind the act: 'What did you think would happen when you took the tablets?' and of the patient's reflections at the time of the interview: 'Now that you are in hospital recovering, how do you feel about what happened?'. Furthermore, it is relatively easy to extend the timeline into the future thereby revealing the patient's immediate and longer-term plans: 'What are your plans when you leave hospital/for the next few days/for the longer term?'.

Sometimes there are inconsistencies or contradictions in the patient's account that make it difficult to determine the underlying motivation. Once again, the autobiographical timeline is a useful tool, highlighting apparent inconsistencies and providing an opportunity to explore these without resorting to overt confrontation. For example: 'Yesterday you made a determined attempt to end your life yet today you are telling me you are glad to be alive. What happened in between that caused you to change your mind?'. Sometimes such inconsistencies reflect a change in circumstances such that the patient no longer feels trapped: 'I thought I would lose my business but my partner has just shown me a letter from the bank pledging ongoing support'. Sometimes they reflect genuine ambivalence on the part of the patient: 'I didn't really care whether I lived or died'.

Sometimes, despite careful and skilled questioning, the interviewer is faced with a patient who refuses to answer or whose stated intentions appear to contradict the history. For example, the patient may have taken an impulsive overdose that they knew to be harmless before presenting themselves to the emergency department yet they are now saying that they firmly intend to commit suicide by throwing themselves in front of a train. Conversely, the patient may have been found by chance in the aftermath of a carefully planned, potentially fatal overdose yet is reporting bright mood and positive plans for the future. Faced with this dilemma most experienced clinicians would base their risk assessment primarily upon the patient's actions whilst at the same time trying to make sense of the patient's current stance (e.g. the patient may be attempting to secure or to avoid hospital admission). There is no foolproof technique for solving this problem. Experienced clinicians will often admit to relying upon clinical intuition or 'gut feeling'. Less experienced clinicians should seek senior review. Table 2.8 shows some of the topics that are covered during the clinical interview and how the patient's response informs the risk assessment.

Quantifying risk

A comprehensive clinical assessment covering the four broad areas described earlier (demographics, diagnosis, actions, and interview) should help to determine the nature of any ongoing risk—completed suicide, further non-fatal acts of self-harm, risks to others, etc. Whilst there are limits to how precisely one can predict such outcomes in individual cases, the information obtained during the assessment ought to allow some sort of risk estimation. Conventional psychiatric practice is to describe risk as 'high', 'moderate', or 'low' and to separate 'immediate' and 'long-term' risk.

It is helpful to contextualize any such estimates with a summary of the worrying and reassuring features in the presentation. Hence a risk assessment might conclude: 'This was an impulsive overdose precipitated by a marital row. Mrs Jones took the tablets in front of her husband and now regrets her actions and acknowledges that she did not intend to die. She has positive plans for the future. The risk of completed suicide is therefore low and her current presentation does not suggest a risk to others. However, whilst the immediate risk of further

Table 2.8 An illustration of how information elicited during the clinical interview can inform risk assessment

Topic	Responses indicating high suicide risk	Responses requiring further exploration	Responses indicating low suicide risk
Factors that lead to self-harm	Stressors remain and patient appears unable to engage in problem-solving (patient feels trapped or powerless)	Stressors remain and patient appears to be prematurely dismissing any proposed solutions	Stressor now resolved or patient is actively seeking solutions (patient feels empowered)
The act of self-harm	Unconvincing or muted statement of regret (particularly in the context of actions that indicated an intent to die—see Table 2.7)	Discrepancy between the act and the patient's statements about it (e.g. act of high perceived lethality yet patient minimizing its significance)	Sincere statement of regret (particularly in the context of an impulsive act)
The future	No plans for the future	Stated plans are unrealistic	Realistic and considered plans for the future
Suicide	Sincere statement of suicidal intent (or unconvincing denial)	Overt threats of suicide: 'If you send me home I'll do it again' (particularly in the context of actions that indicated an intent to communicate distress)	Sincere relief at being alive supported by compelling explanation (e.g. 'I couldn't put my children through that')

acts of self-harm is low, the fact that this is Mrs Jones' 5th such presentation in 4 years suggests that the long-term risk of further acts of self-harm is high'.

Management of risk

As mentioned in the background to this section, the sheer diversity of self-harm presentations precludes a one-size-fits-all approach to risk management. The management plan must be tailored to the individual patient, acknowledging his or her unique circumstances. This section is necessarily brief and is therefore limited to an outline of the principles of risk management followed by some practical advice for clinicians. For a more comprehensive review of this area the author would recommend NICE Clinical Guideline 16: 'The short-term physical and psychological management and secondary prevention of self-harm in primary and secondary care'.

Principles of risk management

1 Ensure the immediate *safety* of the patient, staff and others.

2 Conduct a clinical *assessment* (see earlier subsections 'Demographic risk factors', 'Diagnosis', 'Actions', and 'Interview').

3 Use the information gathered during the clinical assessment to *characterize* and *quantify* specific risks (e.g. risk of self-harm, self-neglect, suicide, homicide, risk to children, risk to spouse, etc.).

4 For each specific risk, identify *contributory factors* and ameliorate these.

5 For each specific risk, identify *protective factors* and maximize these.

Practical advice for clinicians

• The traditional clinical skills of diagnostics and therapeutics are often of limited use in the management of patients presenting following self-harm (remember, whilst diagnosis remains a key component of assessment, the majority of patients do not fit the criteria for any diagnosis). This can cause even experienced clinicians to feel under-skilled and powerless, sometimes resulting in unwarranted prescribing born of frustration and an urge to 'do something!' The solution is to adopt a pragmatic approach—*'What can I do that will help this person?'*.

• Information from relatives can form a valuable part of the assessment (e.g. by corroborating or refuting the patient's account of events leading to hospitalization). Ideally one should obtain the patient's consent before speaking with relatives but, strictly speaking, this is only necessary if the clinician is disclosing information that the patient has given in confidence—*you don't need the patient's permission to listen to what relatives have to say.*

• Suicidal thoughts often emerge from a sense of entrapment. For many patients drawing up a *problem list* (incorporating, e.g. relationship difficulties, job worries, debt, etc.) helps get into perspective problems that were previously seen as insurmountable and provides a starting point for *problem-solving.*

• Sometimes the problems are clinical (e.g. poorly controlled pain, depression, or other psychiatric disorder etc.) allowing the assessing clinician to make full use of his or her knowledge and training. However, often the problems lie beyond the clinician's expertise, in which case his or her input will be limited to guiding the patient towards appropriate services (e.g. relationship counselling, employment advisors, Citizens Advice Bureau, etc.). Most hospitals maintain a database of such services to allow clinicians to *provide patients with relevant contact details.* In many cases this includes providing contact details for emergency services such as the Samaritans.

• Whilst services such as those mentioned in this list may provide expert advice, most people get day-to-day support from friends and family rather than from professionals. It is important to clarify the patient's existing social supports. In the aftermath of self-harm, relationships may be strained. Patients may be reluctant to burden others with their problems or to admit what has happened. However, it usually makes sense to *encourage the patient to make full use of the support available from friends and family.*

• Ultimately, the only person who can ensure the patient's future safety is the patient. It is often useful to encourage self-reflection by asking, *'If you were ever to feel like that again what might you do differently?'*. This question can generate simple but effective actions such as entering the Samaritans' phone number as a mobile phone 'contact', ensuring there are no old tablets in the house etc.

• Although patient autonomy is paramount, most countries have legislation to ensure the welfare of patients who are unable to make decisions for themselves (see also legal aspects in UK Health law and competency and its application to the poisoned patient, pp. 59–62). Some of the most challenging self-harm cases are those where the patient's capacity to make decisions (and therefore the boundary of clinical responsibility) is unclear. In theory a clinician must always respect the autonomy of a patient with capacity, up to and including their right to make unwise decisions. However, when self-harm is involved the stakes can be frighteningly high. Faced with such a situation the only prudent option is to *seek senior advice.*

Further reading

Harris EC, Barraclough B (1997). Suicide as an outcome for mental disorders. A meta-analysis. *Br J Psychiatry*, 170:205–28.

Hawton K, Zahl D, Weatherall R (2003). Suicide following deliberate self-harm: long-term follow-up of patients who presented to a general hospital. *Br J Psychiatry*, 182:537–42.

National Institute for Health and Clinical Excellence (2011). *The Short-Term Physical and Psychological Management and Secondary Prevention of Self-Harm in Primary and Secondary Care.* CG16. London: NICE.

Owens D, Horrocks J, House A (2002). Fatal and non-fatal repetition of self-harm. Systematic review. *Br J Psychiatry*, 181:193–9.

Management of vulnerable, violent, and disturbed patients

Background
Emergency departments and acute medical admission wards often see toxicology patients whose behaviour is disturbed and risk-laden. Safe management requires careful attention to the manifestations and causes of the behavioural disturbance, and the risks arising. This can prove challenging: what follows is a framework intended to assist clinicians.

Manifestations
Clinicians deploy familiar sets of questions, often very quickly, in assessing acute medical presentations The same should apply to behavioural disturbance, which can take many forms, covering a wide range of severity, and so requires different approaches. The first set of questions should quickly narrow down the nature of the behavioural disturbance:

Speech and vocalizations
Is the patient:
- talking normally?
- shouting and swearing, understandably or incoherently?
- screaming, grunting?
- quiet and unforthcoming?
- mute?

Mobility
Is the patient:
- sitting/standing/lying still?
- pacing restlessly within their own bed area?
- intruding into other clinical areas?
- trying to leave; purposefully or otherwise?

Aggression
Is the patient:
- verbally aggressive (i.e. shouting at staff)?
- making verbal threats to staff or others (including himself)?
- physically aggressive incidentally when trying to leave?
- deliberately armed with a weapon, improvised objects to throw or strike with knife, gun, etc.?

Co-operation with investigation and treatment
Is the patient
- refusing observation, blood tests, X-rays?
- too agitated for investigations?
- spitting out or refusing to take medication?
- pulling out IV lines, urinary catheters, ECG leads, etc.?

A rapid assessment of the nature and level of behavioural disturbance via these questions will allow an initial risk assessment and suggest likely causes and management approaches, as well as guide the urgency of response.

Immediate risk management
If initial screening suggests imminent risk to life and limb of the patient or others the immediate priority switches to risk management, including calls to hospital security, the police, and additional clinical staff, to gain control of the situation while further assessment proceeds.

Clinicians are not obliged to run excessive risks in order to gain control: it may be right to stand aside and allow an aggressive man to leave if the risks of harm arising from restraining him are substantial and acute. The next step would be to inform the police: further medical management can be undertaken once control has been achieved and behaviour controlled.

Causes
Once the immediate risks are assessed and managed, attention should focus on the likely causes of the behavioural disturbance. These can be considered under the broad headings of medical, psychiatric, and criminal (though there will be overlap).

Medical
The abnormal mental state and disturbed behaviour may be:
- induced by the agent to which the patient has been exposed
- arise from other intoxicants the patient has taken, either recreationally or with the intent of self-harm
- manifestations of withdrawal from alcohol or other psychotropic agents.

Delirium (see Delirium (acute confusional state), pp. 89–90) is common in acute medical wards, and often presents as abnormal mental states and disturbed behaviour. There are many mechanisms by which a toxicological exposure could result in medical problems that in turn case delirium (aspiration pneumonia, seizures, hepatic encephalopathy, hypoxic or hypoglycaemic brain damage, etc.). Delirium is diagnosed more commonly than single underlying causes are identified: the absence of a clear cause does not obviate the diagnosis, which is made on clinical grounds.

It is also possible that the patient's baseline behaviour is chronically disturbed, but aggravated by the stress of hospitalization (as in some cases of dementia, learning disability, or chronic psychosis,)

Psychiatric
Some psychiatric disorders are strongly associated with self-harm, suicide, and death by misadventure. A smaller range of disorders is less strongly associated with risk to others. It is therefore important to assess behavioural disturbance in toxicology patients for evidence of an underlying primary psychiatric disorder—which is clearly likely when the toxicological exposure is self-inflicted.

People who have taken an overdose in an attempt to end their lives may regret survival, resist admission, refuse treatments, and seek to leave. There is usually little risk to others, though the risk to the patient is clearly direct, proximate, and severe.

Patients with psychotic illnesses such as schizophrenia may exhibit disturbed behaviour which is related to hallucinations or delusions, though these may also occur with intoxication, withdrawal, delirium, or dementia. The mood disturbance of a manic relapse of bipolar disorder may manifest as motor restlessness, agitation, irritability, and disruptive behaviour. When extreme, it too can present with hallucinations and delusions.

When the delusions are paranoid (with beliefs that hospital staff intend harm), patients may make risky escape attempts, prove fearful when approached by clinicians, and hit out in 'self-defence'.

Criminal

Where assessment makes it clear that the patient's disturbed behaviour does not arise from an underlying medical or psychiatric cause, it follows that he retains capacity for his decisions and responsibility for the consequences of his actions. Continued disturbed behaviour may therefore constitute one or more criminal offences (assault, threatening behaviour, criminal damage, breach of the peace, etc.). The criminal law applies just as much in hospital as the street, an airport, or any other public place.

Assigning causes

Information

The key to understanding the causes of behavioural disturbance is information from and information about the patient. When the patient is local and known to services, pursuing the latter is usually more rapidly productive than the former if the patient is uncooperative. Review of electronic and paper records, phone calls to relatives, GPs, out-of-hours GP services, local psychiatric services, social workers, and neighbouring hospitals can proceed in parallel with attempts to interview and examine the patient, and can prompt the patient to be more forthcoming.

Example: 'I understand you are in follow-up with Dr X in psychiatry. When are you next due to see her?'.

It is important to maximize the information available for the current episode. If a blood level or scan result is awaited, chase the lab or call radiology. For patients brought via police or ambulance to the emergency department, the initial incident reports from paramedics and police officers can be revealing.

Approach

Whatever the diagnosis, it will be necessary to approach a patient who may be frightened, angry, suicidal, aggressive, or desperate to leave: if only to try to explain, defuse the situation, and secure cooperation with a management plan.

This requires a careful of balancing of risk and benefit, and even when a security and police presence is at hand, should be as unthreatening as possible, in a bid to establish rapport. Simple empathic statements can be remarkably effective in de-escalating tense stand-offs and gaining cooperation.

Examples: 'I can see that you are scared, but we mean you no harm', 'You are obviously angry. If we can talk about that I may be able to help', 'I have asked the police to be nearby to keep us all safe'.

Remove potential ligatures (tie, ID lanyard, stethoscope) and weapons (pen, reflex hammer) from your clothing.

Interview

Any interview should be brief, aiming to assign a medical or psychiatric cause for the behaviour, or to exclude them and so assign a criminal cause.

Risks

The nature, severity, and acuity of the risks need to be clarified.

Risks may be direct:
• further self-harm
• suicide

• deliberate violence to others
• destruction of ward fabric (doors, windows, furniture, equipment)
• disruption of ward ambience.

Or indirect:
• via refusal of investigation and treatment
• via self neglect if allowed to leave
• provoking violence or exploitation by others (e.g. if verbally abusive or sexually disinhibited).

They may be immediate, short term, or remote. The harms to which the patients are exposed range from minor to moderate to life threatening.

Vulnerable patients

Vulnerability can be unobtrusive and be aggravated by the ward environment: quietly suicidal or cognitively impaired patients can slip out of a ward while attention is devoted to their noisier but lower-risk fellow patients.

Case mix

Risk minimization requires attention to the best allocation of patients within the ward, including the use of single rooms, and prioritization for moving patients elsewhere or discharging them home. For example, avoid placing in neighbouring beds frightened adolescent girls and noisy disruptive middle-aged men in severe alcohol withdrawal.

Interventions

Clearly understanding the nature of the risks and the causes of behavioural disturbance leads to confidence in choosing for the range of interventions, which include the following:

• Environmental measures: single room; reduced levels of stimulation; locked door (if using the Mental Health Act); additional nursing staff, e.g. 1:1 nursing, hospital security presence.
• Medication: antipsychotics (e.g. haloperidol) for psychotic symptoms and associated agitation in psychosis, delirium, drug intoxication, and as adjunct in severe alcohol withdrawal. (Note: anticholinergic agents or diazepam should be available in case an antipsychotic induces an acute dystonia in a drug-naïve patient.) Benzodiazepines (diazepam, midazolam, lorazepam) for alcohol withdrawal and non-specific sedation.

While there are protocols which guide drug treatments in this area, they are usually condition-specific and not universally adopted. For example, alcohol withdrawal can be managed under both fixed dosing or symptom-triggered schedules: each with its advantages and disadvantages (see Drug and alcohol withdrawal, pp. 46–47). There are also guidelines on emergency sedation in specifically psychiatric causes of disturbed behaviour. These were developed primarily for psychiatric settings but they may have application in an acute medical setting.

No protocol can cover all foreseeable clinical situations: the choice of drug, dose, and route of administration will be very different if the patient is a frail and medically unwell elderly lady with dementia, as compared to an athletically built young man now floridly psychotic due to cocaine misuse.

The following are suggested initial therapies. Agitated adults can be sedated with oral or IV diazepam (0.1–0.3 mg/kg body weight). If ineffective consider oral (5–10 mg) or parenteral (2–10 mg) haloperidol, 0.5–2 mg (oral or IV) initially in the elderly. Baclofen is being explored for its value in severe withdrawal from alcohol and GBL/GHB.

In children seek specialist paediatric advice. It is better to manage agitation without sedation and exclude other causes (e.g. hypoxia, infection, hypoglycaemia and raised intracranial pressure). Consider nursing in a dark and quiet environment with a close relative present; seek expert paediatric advice. If required, for children over 3 years buccal (3–5 years: 5 mg; 5–10 years: 7.5mg; 10–16 years: 10 mg) or IV midazolam (150–200 micrograms/kg body weight) is generally the most appropriate drug for managing agitation and requires specialist paediatric care.

Investigation and treatment of underlying cases of delirium is covered in Delirium (acute confusional state), pp. 89–90.

Legal aspects

These matters are dealt with in UK Health Law and Competency and its Application to the Poisoned Patient, pp. 59–62, but in brief a combination of common law, incapacity legislation, and mental health legislation may need to be used to justify keeping a disturbed patient in hospital and treating him against his will, for both his medical and psychiatric needs.

This most commonly arises in people requiring an acetylcysteine infusion for paracetamol poisoning. In the extreme, it may be necessary simultaneously to use: hospital security, police, handcuffs, and parenteral sedation under common law to gain control of acute severe behavioural disturbance; the relevant mental health act to authorize detention in hospital: and incapacity legislation to authorize continued infusion in a patient rendered incapable by sedation.

Discharge

Some disturbed behaviour is best dealt with by avoiding intervention via:

- agreed discharge
- allowing self-discharge as medically reasonable
- removing the patient (hospital security)
- having the police remove the patient.

It is important in these cases to ensure communication with the GP and other community agencies, and, where appropriate, the family. Where patients are removed to police custody it may be necessary to liaise with the forensic medical examiner or equivalent.

Matching intervention with need and risk

Clinical judgement is required to match the level of intervention with the level of need, and the range and severity of the risks associated with both intervening and deciding not to. The extreme measures referred to in the paracetamol case described earlier would only be justified if there was clear evidence of a level of poisoning likely to cause significant and potentially lethal liver damage.

In general, the more severe, direct, and proximate the risk, the greater the level of intervention which may be ethically justified and legally defensible. The corollary is that a decision not to intervene may itself be subject to subsequent legal challenge. A guiding principle for clinicians might be to ask by whom they would prefer to be

sued: a surviving patient angry at receiving an unwanted intervention, or a grieving family distressed that no intervention was undertaken. Following two simple precepts readily assuages any anxiety provoked by considering this dilemma:

1 Consult as widely as possible in the time available (family, nursing staff, psychiatry, peers, and seniors).
2 Document the decisions made and the reasons for making them.

It is easier to defend a well-documented decision taken carefully, after wide consultation, but with an adverse outcome, than it is a hasty, ill considered, and poorly recorded decision that leads to a near miss.

Clinical governance

Incidents of severe behavioural disturbance, especially if associated with adverse outcomes for the patient or others, or 'near misses,' should be subject to critical incident review or root cause analysis under the policies and procedures of the hospital. If staff or other patients have been injured or distressed, there may be a need for debriefing. Informal team meetings are best held within a day or so and should not be delayed for formal processes to work through.

If disturbed behaviour clearly arises from a criminal cause, there should be a low threshold for having the patient arrested and charged, and hospital management should be expected to support staff members in making statements and attending court.

Less serious incidents should be logged and reviewed in the prevailing clinical governance arrangements. Only by doing all of this can preventable causes of recurring behavioural disturbance be addressed and corrected. Hospital cultures such as 'it goes with the territory' need to be challenged.

Conclusion

The foregoing implies a sequential approach—in practice much of this work proceeds in parallel, via an approach adapted to the clinical realities of the behavioural disturbance, the setting, and the treatment need. Clinicians encountering these cases need to be able to think on their feet in the face of pressure, and work flexibly yet thoroughly to ensure safe effective care.

Further reading

Daeppen JB, Gache P, Landry U, et al. (2002). Symptom-triggered vs fixed-schedule doses of benzodiazepine for alcohol withdrawal: a randomized treatment trial. Arch Intern Med, 162:1117–21.

Hecksel KA, Bostwick JM, Jaeger TM, et al. (2008). Inappropriate use of symptom-triggered therapy for alcohol withdrawal in the general hospital. Mayo Clin Proceed, 83:274–9.

National Institute for Health and Clinical Excellence (2005). Violence: The Short-Term Management of Disturbed/Violent Behaviour in In-Patient Psychiatric Settings and Emergency Departments. CG25. London: NICE.

National Institute for Health and Clinical Excellence (2011). Alcohol Dependence and Harmful Alcohol Use. CG115. London: NICE.

Taylor, D, Paton C, Kapur S (2009). Acutely disturbed and violent behaviour. In: The Maudsley Prescribing Guidelines, 10th edition, pp. 417–24. London: Informa Heathcare.

UK health law and competency and its application to the poisoned patient

Background

Patients who take deliberate drug overdoses, or self-harm in other ways, may often refuse medical intervention. In liberal democracies such as the UK, the treating clinicians must consider whether a patient's refusal in these circumstances is a competent one, as if it is, they must respect it. If it is not, then they have a duty of care to act in that person's best interests. They will also need to arrange for an assessment of the intent behind the act of self-harm, so that risk can be evaluated, and to determine whether a mental disorder is present requiring treatment, and, if so, the mental disorder assessor will need to consider that individual's willingness or otherwise to accept such treatment, and whether this is a situation where compulsory detention for assessment and/or treatment for a mental disorder may be required.

The laws governing psychiatric care vary from country to country. This section describes the legal frameworks that guide such decisions for adults in England and Wales and in Scotland. It is based on information in the *Oxford Handbook of Psychiatry*, but for interested readers there are larger psychiatric texts and legal texts to which the reader is referred.

In the context of the management of poisoning, physicians need to be aware of four key aspects. These are:

- law relating to capacity and incapacity
- law relating to medical treatment decisions
- laws regulating the detention and treatment of patients with mental disorder
- laws and regulations regarding confidentiality.

(Reproduced from David Semple and Roger Smyth, *Oxford Handbook of Psychiatry*, 3rd edition, pp. 874–875, with permission from Oxford University Press.)

Psychiatrists also need to be aware of criminal law in relation to mentally disordered offenders, but this is not normally an issue for the management of acute poisoning in general hospitals.

Although separate legislation has been enacted affecting England and Wales, Scotland, and Northern Ireland over recent years the policies regarding healthcare of mental illness have been moving towards a common basis. The legal documentation supporting present approaches to management is complex, but a number of key principles affect the way in which patients should be managed, although these may not be specifically applicable when resolving clinical dilemmas. It is important to be aware of the difference between the legal aspects of detention of patients in hospital for clinical care and for their own safety, as opposed to the legal situation regarding the imposition of physical treatment. Detention under the mental health regulations does not necessarily itself permit physical treatment, more likely common law will allow, and medical ethics dictate, the physical treatment be imposed in the patient's best interest. The key test that applies in many instances is that of capacity.

What is capacity?

Capacity is a legal concept that concerns an individual's ability to understand what is being proposed and the consequences of refusing or accepting the advice given, the ability to weigh these in the balance to reach a decision, and to communicate that decision. This could include alternative forms of communication, such as sign language, blinking an eye, or squeezing a hand, when verbal communication is not possible.

It is important to note that no other person can consent on behalf of an incompetent adult, but the views of relatives are helpful in reflecting what the patient would have chosen if in a position to decide.

Legal framework

Common law

This is generally defined as the body of law arrived from previous decisions of the courts. This contrasts with statute law, law created by legislative bodies. Common law thus includes long-established custom and practice, clarification of the meaning and extent of statute law by courts, and finally statements of the law by judges' rulings on cases where there is no directly applicable existing law that fits precisely to the case. Common law is therefore dynamic, and changes as more cases come before the courts and judgments are made. Doctors should therefore try to keep up to date with current debate in decisions affecting their own speciality and their own geographical area. As common law is case based it will depend on the legal jurisdiction in which the patient is cared for. If in doubt clarification should be sought from senior colleagues, hospital legal advisers, or medical professional bodies, particularly in potentially contentious cases.

The principles of common law are not written in statute and so the physician needs to be aware of the general principles that apply (the following is derived from the *Oxford Handbook of Psychiatry*):

1 **To act in accordance with the patient's wishes**. This is a fundamental principle of the doctor–patient relationship, and in general patient's autonomy should be respected and only acted against in very limited circumstances.

2 **Presumed capacity**. Adults over the age of 18 years are presumed to have such capacity unless there is evidence to the contrary, as assessed on the balance of probabilities.

3 **The 'reasonableness' test**. This is a consideration often used in law to test what a hypothetical 'reasonable man' would do in the circumstances. As applied to medical decisions this refers to a 'reasonable doctor'.

4 **Act in the patient's best interests**. In emergency situations it is often impossible to obtain consent, for example, in unconscious patients, here it is accepted that the doctors overriding duty is to preserve life.

5 **The doctrine of necessity**. This provides a defence against potential criminal charge of assault by giving no-consensual treatment. Doctors may give emergency treatment to preserve life and prevent significant deterioration in health.

6 **Act in accordance with a recognized body of opinion**. The law accepts that medicine is not an exact science, and that in any situation several courses of action may be reasonable. However, there is an expectation that any treatment decision would be considered suitable by a body of professional opinion, in law this is known as the 'Bolam test'.

7 Act in a logical and sensible manner. This expands the Bolam test and adds the concept that medical decisions must be logically defensible themselves in the circumstances.

8 Consider use of applicable law. Doctors should consider whether the provisions of any existing law provides guidance and/or additional protection for the patient. Urgent treatment should not, however, be delayed under this circumstance.

9 Court intervention. In difficult circumstances following appropriate local senior medical and legal consultation it may be appropriate to apply to a court for specific ruling.

The three key judgments that affect medical decision making and treatment decisions are: the Gillick case, which refers to decisions by minors; the Bolitho case, which expanded on the 'Bolam test' and added the concept of negligence in regard to treatment that is deemed illogical by a judge even if it passes the 'Bolam test'; and finally the case of Ms B, which dealt with the decision of a patient with serious illness on artificial ventilation for that to be withdrawn, when her medical carer at the time did not feel able to comply with this decision.

Incapacity acts
Separate Incapacity Acts apply to England and Wales and Scotland. No such act exists in Northern Ireland. These Acts apply to individuals above the age of 18 years and are worded differently in the different countries. They are divided into four components:

- **The principle of capacity**; covering aspects such as autonomy, wishes, acting in the best interests of the patient, and restricting the freedom of the individual as little as possible.
- **Assessment** of incapacity in England and Wales or capacity in Scotland. These are perversely opposite sides of the same question. Namely does the patient understand what is being asked and why; do they understand this in terms of how the information is relevant to them; are they aware of the alternative choices available; do they understand the risks and benefits; and do they have sufficient memory to retain the relevant information; can they 'weigh in the balance' potentially life and death issues being discussed, and communicate that decision. In an emergency situation, where the patient may be in pain, extremely emotionally aroused, under stress, or intoxicated, the lack of ability to adequately carry out such judgements, as compared to when they are calm and sober, is an important assessment criterion.
- **Areas covered by the act**. These include powers of attorney, guardianship and court-appointed deputies, and advance directives. Most importantly for healthcare professionals both Acts provide protection from liability when providing routine medical care, and in Scotland a certificate of incapacity is signed to authorize these actions.
- **Bodies with powers under the Act.** In England and Wales this is the Court of protection and the Public Guardian. In Scotland the office of the Public Guardian, the mental welfare commission for Scotland, the sheriff's court, and local authorities are the relevant bodies.

Mental Health Acts
Different mental health acts apply in England and Wales, Scotland, and Northern Ireland. Although different in wording, framework of delivery, and to some extent local interpretation framework, the principles are similar.

The principles of the Mental Health Act in England and Wales are that:
- Decisions are taken with a view to minimizing the harm done by mental disorder, and maximizing the safety and health of patients and/or protecting the public from harm.
- Interventions without the patient's consent must be the least restrictive alternative available.
- Decision-makers must recognize and respect the different needs, values, and circumstances of each patient. Wherever practical will they should consider the patient's wishes and feelings and respect those.
- When planning and developing care, patients, their carers, and family members should be involved as far as practicable.
- Resources should be used in the most effective, efficient, and equitable way.

Definitions
Each individual Act defines mental disorder and readers are referred to the acts and standard psychiatry texts for more detailed discussion on these aspects.

Individuals named in the Acts
In addition other important definitions in the Acts refer to the following:
- Doctors who are approved to act as having special experience in the diagnosis and treatment of mental disorder (Approved Doctor in England and Wales, or Approved Medical Practitioner in Scotland).
- The responsible clinician; the consultant in charge of the patient's care.
- Approved mental health professionals (AMHP) in England and Wales, or mental health officers (MHO) in Scotland, who are often social workers or psychiatric nurses with special experience in care of individuals with mental disorder, and are specifically appointed under the Acts.
- A nearest relative or 'named person' (Scotland) to be consulted.

Various procedures of review and second opinions are in place, including the Mental Health Act Commission (MHAC), Mental Health Review Tribunal's (MHRT), and a second opinion appointed doctor (SOAD) in England and Wales. Similar supporting structures are in place in Scotland.

Compulsory measures
The mental health acts define three different types of detention. Most doctors who manage poisoning will only be involved in emergency detention, often used in accident and emergency departments or medical wards while further assessment is made, and treatment administered under common law. These detention orders ideally should involve an AMHP in England or MHO in Scotland, but under certain circumstances patients may be detained without these individuals being initially involved. In England and Wales, and also Scotland, there are facilities to detain patients under short-term detention for up to 28 days, intended for assessment the more complex disorders or admission for treatment where this is deemed necessary. The last two types of detention order require action from a psychiatrist with appropriate training under the Acts. Other aspects covered in the Acts include after-care

following detention and supervised community treatment. Detailed discussion of these is outside the scope of this textbook.

Consent to treatment

It has been a fundamental principle that patients should consent to medical treatment. Normally patients decide which treatments they undergo and which they refuse. If they are competent to make the decision this right is retained even when refusal of treatment could result in death or major adverse health impact. The key aspect of consent is capacity to make decisions, and secondly consent must be informed in the sense that the patient understands both the details and implications proposed treatment. Consent also implies that this is given freely and not under duress.

Capacity

Capacity is at present deemed to be a property of adults and present throughout the lifespan. It may be lost either temporarily or permanently. The law assumes capacity, but capacity may be lost in the context of poisoning, for example, due to the effects of drugs or other toxins, or be impaired because of the psychiatric condition or mental state contributing to an episode of self-harm. Assessment of capacity is essentially made on the balance of probabilities. In the clinical scenario it is important to understand this is not an 'all or nothing' ability and it may be possible to have capacity to make some decisions, but not others. Incapacity law currently generally divides this property into that regarding financial and that regarding welfare decisions. Capacity needs to be assessed in respect of each decision made and the patient's ability to assess and understand alternative courses of action and their merits and risks. It is also necessary to remember the decisions and to have sufficient ability to communicate them adequately.

Providing patients with sufficient information to facilitate consent and informed treatment is a further aspect of consent. This includes the provision of information on the likely risks and adverse effects of treatment and of withholding for avoiding treatment. Such questions must be answered honestly and relevant information should not be withheld unless disclosure is deemed to cause the patient serious harm.

Generally, consent is implied for many procedures, for example, venepuncture, in that the patient does not object to, and proceeds to cooperate with, the procedure undertaken. For more complex procedures, for example, surgery, formal consent is mandatory and needs to be recorded on a consent form.

Advance statements (advance directives)

These are normally statements prepared while patients have the capacity to make decisions which will then apply when such capacity has been lost. These are sometimes known colloquially as 'living wills', and generally indicate a patient's wishes in specific aspects of health management. These are formal legal documents, and, for example, a suicide note would not normally constitute an adequate advance statement that could give a legal indication of appropriate management. Key aspects of the decision in the advance statement is applicability to the circumstances the patients now find themselves in, and that there is no reason to believe the patient may subsequently change their mind. It is

possible to act against an advance statement, although where possible the patient's known wishes should be taken into account. It is also necessary to consider the common law principle of 'best interests'. This aspect is particularly challenging in the management of patients with overdose where risk to life is brief but may be clear, and where an antidote may easily prevent further harm when given in a relatively non-invasive manner. Many experienced physicians who deal with such patients use common law or a capacity act to support decisions made in the best interest of the patient at a time when their mental state is disturbed because of an acutely stressful event. Decisions on treatment in such cases need careful discussion with both physicians and psychiatrists involved.

Treatment without consent

Normally treatment can, and should, only proceed with a valid consent. There are four situations where treatment may continue without consent, each has appropriate legal safeguards:

- treatment undertaken under common law
- treatment under the provisions governing capacity acts
- treatment under the provisions of the mental health acts
- treatment authorized by a court.

Common law

The necessity to treat provides a doctor with a defence against assault when non-consensual treatment is given. An example is where therapy will include sedation in a patient with acute behavioural disorder. Here there is a danger of physical harm to the patient, or others, secondary to a psychiatric cause, and the doctor has to act against the patient's wishes in order to carry out their duty of care. Treatment is therefore under common law even though the patient may also fulfil criteria for emergency detention under mental health legislation.

Treatment under an incapacity act

These acts determine a legal framework to provide care for incapable adults. The acts define incapacity and establish both processes and safeguards that regulate the decision-making necessary on behalf of such incapable patients.

Treatment under a mental health act

This normally applies to patients with mental disorders that are clearly defined and diagnosed, for example, psychosis. It is important to note that the majority of patients with formal mental disorder receive treatment with their own consent. The mental health acts differ in each country but essentially allow for detention in hospital and the compulsory treatment of mental disorder. Very specific restrictions apply to the use of certain treatments, for example, prescription medication compulsorily beyond a certain period. They also include appeal processes and an oversight system reviewing treatment of detained patients. It is important to note that generally treatment of unrelated medical disorders cannot be authorized under a mental health act, and here the doctor treating the patient has to revert to treatment under common law or an incapacity act.

Authorization by a court

This is very unlikely in the context of the management of poisoning because of the timeframes involved in establishing a court order. Detailed discussion is outside the scope of this textbook.

Case examples

The following cases illustrate scenarios that may be useful when considering management of patients with poisoning.

Case 1

A 26-year-old man has been admitted to the emergency department from the city centre where he has been aggressive to passers-by and to police. When questioned he appears convinced that medical staff are secret police officers, and violently resists attempts to calm him by speaking to him in a quiet environment.

Comment

It is clear that this man is not acting normally and is a danger to himself and others. There is insufficient time to perform a formal psychiatric assessment and it is clear that he lacks capacity as he is disorientated and unable to comprehend his situation. He can be treated under common law with appropriate restraint and administration of medication sufficient to remove his aggression and sedate him. If this patient had suffered life-threatening injury requiring urgent surgery then that may also be legally applied under common law. It would not, however, be appropriate to undertake a non-urgent surgical procedure, for example, removal of an offensive tattoo.

Outcome

The patient was physically restrained, given intramuscular haloperidol and a benzodiazepine (lorazepam). Pulse was elevated at 140 bpm and he was pyrexial at 40° C. He was actively cooled and given further doses of benzodiazepine. The next morning his mental state was settled and 2 days later he was discharged from hospital well.

Case 2

A 19-year-old young woman has taken a large overdose of paracetamol washed down with alcohol following an argument with her boyfriend. She has written a suicide note following this event stating she wishes to die and to have no treatment, and then calls an ambulance. In hospital she refuses to have any treatment stating that her suicide note constitutes an advance directive.

Comment

An advance directive is a formal legal document that requires a witness confirming the patient is competent to make the decisions recorded at the time the directive is written. In this case acute mental distress in the context described would be sufficient cause for concern that such a situation did not exist, and to come to the conclusion that the suicide note was not immediately relevant to the care she should receive. In view of the relative urgency of the situation the patient's competence should be assessed bearing in mind the consumption of alcohol and the emotional disturbance precipitating the overdose.

It is often useful to involve other family members, or in this case even the boyfriend, in an attempt to engage the patient and gain consent. However, this patient can be treated under common law or a capacity act and most experienced clinical toxicologists are familiar with this scenario on a regular basis. Discussion of the risks, implications of treatment, and nature of the outcome from lack of treatment, particularly the delay to death, will often persuade the patient to change their minds. Most patients are unfamiliar with the duty of care that doctors have in a situation where lack of treatment it is likely to result in an extremely poor outcome. Here the balance is being threatened with legal action by the patient for potentially saving the life, or by other family members for failing to act in a patient who is acutely disturbed following an emotional event.

Outcome

This patient was unusual in refusing care despite the intervention of her boyfriend and her mother. Both were of the view that she should have antidote treatment, and a decision was therefore made to treat the patient under common law. Unusually she still resisted treatment despite the implications being explained. An intravenous dose of benzodiazepine was therefore administered to permit treatment. On discussion 24 hours later the patient thanked the medical staff for their attention and the fact that they had prevented her potential death.

Case 3

A 25-year-old woman presents with the third episode of self-harm in 5 days. On this occasion she has ingested a number of her mother's tablets, including some antibiotics, seven cetirizine and 30 × 75 mg aspirin. This followed an argument with her parents about her boyfriend. She has a community psychiatric nurse (CPN) whom she sees for 'bipolar disorder' but the patient is not on any regular medication. Her CPN is on holiday. She wishes to self-discharge but her parents are adamant she should be detained in hospital. Should she be held against her will?

Comment

The decision here is based on a simple assessment of her risk from the ingestion and mental state. The overdose is unlikely to be toxic. Detention in hospital is unwarranted if she is competent and has no underlying major psychiatric disease, and it is almost certain she will have had a psychiatric assessment in her recent presentations. Detention is unjustified and warnings about potential symptoms to trigger return are sufficient. The reasons for this decision will need to be discussed with her parents, and in due course her CPN.

Outcome

The patient returned home following explanation to her and her parents, and despite her parents' anxiety. A discussion was also held on the next available working day with her CPN, who described a manipulative personality who was dependant on the CPN for support. The CPN felt that failing to gain admission for this overdose could be a potentially useful message for the patient and aid behaviour modification. There were no adverse events and management of her psychiatric state continued in the community.

Further reading

Adults with Incapacity Act Scotland 2000. <http://www.legislation.gov.uk/asp/2000/4/contents>.

David AS, Hotopf M, Moran P, et al. (2010). Mentally disordered or lacking capacity? Lessons for managing serious deliberate self harm. *BMJ*, 341:c4489.

General Medical Council (2008). *Consent: Patients and Doctors Making Decisions Together*. London: GMC.

Kapur N, Clements C, Bateman N, et al (2010). Advance directives and suicidal behaviour *BMJ*, 341:c4557.

Mental Health Act 2007. <http://www.legislation.gov.uk/ukpga/2007/12/contents>.

Semple D, Smyth R (2009). *Oxford Handbook of Psychiatry*, 2nd edition. Oxford: Oxford University Press.

Common complications of poisoning

Cardiovascular toxicity

Background

Many poisons produce toxic effects on the cardiovascular system. The management of specific poisons is discussed elsewhere in this book, but it is helpful to have a general overview of the strategic approach to patients with features suggesting a toxin has caused adverse cardiovascular effects. Supportive care directed at the observed clinical features is particularly important since it may not be obvious either which poison is involved, or in the case of a mixed ingestion, which of the agents taken is responsible for the clinical features observed.

The cardiovascular system, for the purposes of this discussion, is considered to consist of the heart and the peripheral blood vessels. Failure of oxygenation may be a feature of pulmonary oedema or other causes of pulmonary impairment and in poisoning management is generally directed to the lungs by using appropriate ventilation techniques, while any cardiac defect is managed.

Cardiovascular assessment

Assessment of the cardiovascular system in people with suspected poisoning follows the same pattern as for any other condition. This will include measurement of pulse rate and rhythm, blood pressure and pulse pressure, and an assessment of peripheral perfusion. An important factor in poisoning is the rapid change in cardiovascular status that may occur as a toxin is absorbed and exerts its effects. It is therefore important to tailor the monitoring of patients, both in extent and frequency to the clinical status of the patient and/or the toxin ingested.

Some toxins produce electrophysiological abnormalities that may be reflected on the 12-lead ECG, such as heart block, PR, QRS, or QT interval prolongation (Figure 3.1). Most automated ECG machines use internal computer algorithms to provide estimates of these intervals, but since the morphology of an ECG may change

with poisoning these algorithms can sometimes provide misleading data.

Urgent echocardiographic assessment of cardiac function may be particularly useful in determining whether a patient is hypotensive because of a primary myocardial problem or toxin-associated vasodilation. Hypotension should be assessed in the context of the patient being treated and their expected normal physiological status. Blood pressure falls in most patients during sleep, and thus a systolic blood pressure of 90 mmHg in a patient who is otherwise clinically well with good peripheral perfusion has very different implications from the same blood pressure in a patient who is awake and has a tachycardia, is peripherally shut down, and/or has ECG abnormalities. Each patient therefore needs careful individual assessment when considering intervention.

Cardiac resuscitation

In contrast to almost all other causes of cardiac arrest, in poisoning, the patient is generally physiologically well prior to the event and does not have cardiorespiratory co-morbidity. Prolonged resuscitation can result in success and should therefore be the norm in this patient population. In the event of cardiac arrest in hospital, or witnessed out-of-hospital cardiac arrest with bystander CPR, resuscitation should be continued for at least 1 hour. Prolonged resuscitation for cardiac arrest is recommended as recovery with good neurological outcome may occur. Use of automated external cardiac massage, where this is available, can be useful.

Abnormalities of pulse rate

In poisoning, either bradycardia or tachycardia may be encountered. These should only be treated if the clinical condition of the patient indicates that physiological compromise is present or likely.

Bradycardia

Sinus bradycardia is a feature of poisoning with some agents. Most patients will tolerate heart rates as low as 45 beats/minute without compromise to cardiac output. For symptomatic bradycardia, e.g. associated with hypotension and poor cardiac output, give atropine intravenously (usual doses 0.4–1.2 mg for an adult or 0.02 mg/kg for a child). Repeat doses may be necessary, but for longer-acting agents this may cause atropine poisoning. Dobutamine or isoprenaline may be considered if bradycardia is associated with hypotension. In refractory cases, or in patients with heart block, temporary pacemaker insertion may be required; external pacing may be used as an alternative.

Tachycardia

Rapid heart rate in poisoning may be regular, sinus tachycardia, or due to an atrial or ventricular arrhythmia. In overdose, extreme sinus tachycardia is often associated with agitation following ingestion of sympathomimetic recreational drugs such as cocaine (see Cocaine, pp. 186–187). Management here is targeted at the increased arousal and heart rate will decline as this settles. Specific cardiovascular measures are therefore rarely required. In the context of extreme tachycardia due to excess direct sympathomimetic effects, consideration may be given to using a beta-blocker, or if due to an atrial arrhythmia, cardiac acting calcium

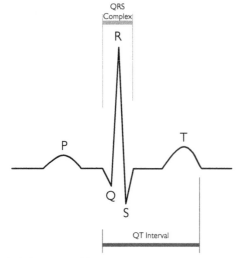

QRS
Complex

R

P

T

Q

S

QT Interval

Fig 3.1 A normal ECG trace illustrating the relevant intervals.

antagonist or even adenosine. It is important not to cause more physiological disturbance by giving excess intervention, and short-acting agents such as the beta antagonist esmolol may be used in order to avoid aggravating toxicity and assess response prior to using longer-acting agents. Use of beta-blockade for sympathomimetic cardiotoxicity remains controversial as it may result in increases in blood pressure as a result of unopposed alpha stimulation. Specialist advice should be sought.

Abnormalities of cardiac rhythm

Poisoning with cardiotoxic drugs can lead to rapid changes in heart rhythm. Therefore patients with suspected cardiovascular toxicity should have continuous cardiac monitoring. QRS and QT Intervals, measured on the 12-lead ECG (Figure 3.1), may indicate the risk of some tachyarrhythmias occurring and regular 12-lead ECGs should also be performed under these circumstances (initially 2–4-hourly, or as indicated by the clinical condition).

Check serum potassium, magnesium, and calcium concentrations in all patients who have ingested a potentially cardiotoxic dose of drug. Check venous or arterial gases and correct any hypoxia or acidosis. Replace electrolytes as necessary to keep within the high normal range.

QRS duration prolonged

The normal QRS duration is 40 to 120 msec. Most young adults will have a QRS duration of less than 100 msec. Prolongation of the QRS interval reflects reduced conduction velocity in the bundle of His and within the ventricular myocardium resulting from sodium channel blockade. Toxic doses of sodium channel blocking drugs, for example, class 1 antiarrhythmic drugs or tricyclic antidepressants (see Antidepressants, pp. 100–103 and Antidysrhythmic drugs, pp. 138–139) therefore increase the QRS duration and the extent of this is related to the risk of ventricular arrhythmia. A QRS duration of greater than 160 msec suggests severe cardiotoxicity with a very high risk of ventricular tachycardia; but arrhythmias may occur with lesser degrees of QRS prolongation. QRS prolongation and the arrhythmias that result are best treated by correction of hypoxia and acidosis. Consider immediate administration of 50 mmol sodium bicarbonate, with subsequent further doses titrated to achieve a pH of 7.5 (max 7.55). The volumes for different concentrations of sodium bicarbonate needed to achieve a dose of 50 mmol in adults depend on concentration, but ideally use 8.4% solution in a bolus. Caution is required if the solution is to be given by a peripheral venous line as it is irritant to veins and can cause pain or local necrosis in cases of extravasation; for rapid correction administer over 20 minutes, otherwise administer at a rate of 1 mmol/minute. Recheck acid–base status after administration of sodium bicarbonate. Monitor electrolytes since there is a risk of hypokalaemia and possibly hypernatraemia if substantial amounts of bicarbonate have been administered.

Drugs that exacerbate sodium channel blockade (class 1a—quinidine, disopyramide, procainamide, phenytoin and class 1c—flecainide, propafenone) should be avoided after poisoning with sodium channel blocking drugs and in the presence of increased QRS width, expect on specialist advice (Table 3.1).

QT interval prolongation

The QT interval is important because it reflects the duration of ventricular repolarization. QT interval

Table 3.1 Examples of drugs and other substances that may prolong QRS duration

Class	Examples
Anti-arrhythmic drugs:	
Class 1a	Quinidine
	Procainamide
	Disopyramide
Class 1c	Flecainide
	Propafenone
	Moricizine[a]
Class 3	Amiodarone
Class 2[b]	Propranolol
	Betaxolol
	Pindolol
	Acebutolol
Anticonvulsants	Carbamazepine
Antidepressants	Tricyclic antidepressants
	Maprotiline[a]
	Citalopram
	Venlafaxine
Drugs of misuse	Cocaine
Others	Aconite
	Amantadine
	Barbiturates
	Daunorubicin
	Diphenhydramine
	Propoxyphene

[a] Not licensed for use in the UK.
[b] Beta adrenoceptor antagonists which have membrane stabilizing (local anaesthetic) activity.

prolongation reflects blockade of potassium channels in the heart and, especially when extreme, is associated with the ventricular arrhythmia torsade de pointes. QT interval shortens as heart rate increases and formulae have been developed to provide QT intervals corrected for heart rate (QTc). An example is the Bazett formula ($QTc = QT/\sqrt{RR}$ interval). These formulae are inaccurate at extremes of heart rate and in particular may produce erroneously long QTc estimates in patients with tachycardia. It may be simpler and more reliable to plot the measured (uncorrected) QT interval against the heart rate using the nomogram in Figure 3.2.

Automatic ECG machines include algorithms for measuring QT interval which can be useful for detecting abnormalities, but are often unreliable in poisoning, particularly at the extremes of heart rate or in the presence of other ECG changes which may affect the accuracy of measurements. Machine readings should therefore be verified manually, especially when these suggest abnormality.

Torsade de pointes is generally associated with a corrected QTc interval of greater than 500 msec. If this is present, or the QT-heart rate nomogram indicates a risk of torsade de pointes, particularly in the presence of other risk factors such as frequent ectopics or underlying structural heart disease, consider administration of 8 mmol magnesium sulfate IV over 10–15 minutes. This may need repeating once, depending on response and

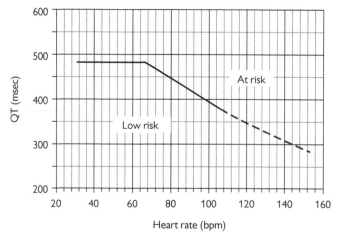

Fig 3.2 QT nomogram illustrating relationship between heart rate and uncorrected QT interval and likely risk of arrhythmia (torsade de pointes) (do not use the QTc interval calculated by some ECG machines). If above the nomogram then patient may be at risk. The dashed line reflects uncertainty of risk at higher heart rates. Reproduced from WikiTox Open Source Clinical Toxicology Curriculum, <http://curriculum.toxicology.wikispaces.net/Cardiotoxic+drugs>, with permission from Geoff Isbister.

magnesium concentration. Torsade de pointes and VT/VF preceded by prolonged QT should also be treated with magnesium. Torsade de pointes may also respond to increasing the underlying heart rate, through atrial or ventricular pacing or by isoprenaline (isoproterenol) infusion to achieve a heart rate of 90–110 beats/minute.

Drugs that prolong the QT interval (e.g. amiodarone, quinidine) are likely to worsen QT prolongation and may precipitate torsade de pointes. They should only be used on specialist advice (Table 3.2).

Abnormalities of blood pressure

Hypertension

In the context of poisoning, hypertension may be due to anxiety or agitation or reflect sympathetic stimulation with vasoconstriction, which may be accompanied by increased cardiac output. Many patients simply require reassurance and observation and pharmacological intervention is unnecessary. In agitated adults, hypertension may settle once a central sedative such as diazepam has been given. If hypertension persists and is severe, intravenous nitrates will lower blood pressure in a controlled fashion. Glyceryl trinitrate, starting at 1–2 mg/hour and gradually increased (maximum 12 mg/hour) until blood pressure is controlled. Calcium antagonists such as nifedipine, verapamil, or diltiazem are an alternative as second-line therapy.

Phentolamine, labetalol, or sodium nitroprusside are options for patients with hypertension without any evidence of cardiac ischaemia, but may cause a rapid fall in blood pressure.

Hypotension

This may be due to vasodilatation, pump failure, or a combination. Correct hypotension, initially by adequate fluid resuscitation with a crystalloid. Treat any brady- and tachyarrhythmias appropriately. Poisoned patients with fluid-resistant hypotension can deteriorate extremely

rapidly and should be referred as appropriate to the local critical care team.

In the context of poisoning, inappropriate vasodilatation is the most common cause of hypotension. This can usually be managed with intravenous fluids, but in extreme refractory cases, associated with poor organ perfusion and reduced urine output, vasopressor agents may be required. Options are norepinephrine, metaraminol, phenylephrine, and ephedrine

Reduced cardiac output is a common toxic effect of poisons with negative inotropic effects, such as calcium channel blockers or beta-blockers, and is associated with fluid-resistant hypotension. Inotropes such as dobutamine, epinephrine, glucagon, and dopamine may be required, as well as any other specific treatments directed at the poison involved.

Reduced cardiac output and vasodilation frequently coexist in severe or mixed poisoning, and both vasopressors and inotropes may be needed. Invasive vascular monitoring and echocardiography may help identify the specific mechanisms operating in a particular patient.

In severe cases of myocardial suppression, especially in the context of calcium channel blocker poisoning, high doses of insulin infused with dextrose can improve myocardial contractility, and improve systemic perfusion, hyper-insulinaemia euglycaemic therapy (HIET). It seems particularly useful in the presence of acidosis. Check plasma glucose and potassium before commencing insulin/dextrose therapy and if plasma glucose less than 10 mmol/L, give 50 mL of 50% dextrose. If serum potassium is less than 2.5 mmol/L correct before starting insulin/dextrose; give 20 mmol potassium IV over 30 minutes and recheck electrolytes. Once hypokalaemia is corrected give insulin 1 unit/kg as a bolus followed by an infusion of 0.5–2.0 unit/kg/hour titrated to clinical response. The rate may be increased by 2 unit/kg/hour every 10 minutes to a maximum of 10 unit/kg/hour if no increase in cardiac output or clinical improvement is

Table 3.2 Examples of drugs and other substances that may cause QT interval prolongation or torsade de pointes

Class	Examples
Anti-arrhythmic drugs:	
Class 1a	Quinidine
	Procainamide
	Disopyramide
Class 3	Amiodarone
	Sotalol
	Dofetilide[a]
Antipsychotic drugs	Pimozide
	Chlorpromazine
	Haloperidol
	Quetiapine
	Ziprasidone[a]
Antidepressants	Tricyclic antidepressants
	Lithium
	SSRI antidepressants
	Venlafaxine
Antimicrobials	Erythromycin
	Clarithromycin
	Azithromycin
	Moxifloxacin
	Itraconazole
	Ketoconazole
	Pentamidine
	Quinine
	Chloroquine
	Halofantrine[a]
	Amantadine
Anticancer chemotherapy	Arsenic trioxide
	Vandetanib[a]
Opioids	Methadone
	Propoxyphene
Others	Organophosphorus compounds
	Tacrolimus
	Fluoride
	Sevoflurane

[a] Not licensed for use in the UK

initially seen. Maintain 10% dextrose during insulin therapy and check capillary blood glucose every 20 minutes during dose changes, then hourly. When the insulin infusion rate is stable, check potassium hourly.

If cardiotoxicity is unresponsive to these treatments, consider the use of intravenous lipid emulsion. The role of lipid is not well defined, but appears effective in local anaesthetic poisoning, and for some other lipid-soluble drugs. A dose of 1.5 mL/kg of 20% Intralipid® is given as an intravenous bolus, followed by 0.25–0.5 mL/kg/min for 30–60 minutes to an initial maximum of 500 mL. The bolus can be repeated once or twice for persistent cardiovascular collapse or asystole. The infusion rate should be titrated against clinical response.

In specialist centres, mechanical cardiovascular support may be an option for patients with severe refractory poisoning. This may involve use of a balloon pump, left ventricular assist devices, and/or extracorporeal membrane oxygenation.

Further reading

Engebretsen KM, Kaczmarek KM, Morgan J, et al. (2011). High-dose insulin therapy in beta-blocker and calcium channel-blocker poisoning. Clin Toxicol, 49:277–83.

Jamaty C, Bailey B, Larocque E, et al. (2010). Lipid emulsions in the treatment of acute poisoning: a systemic review of human and animal studies. Clin Toxicol, 48:1–27.

Weinberg GL, VadeBoncouer T, Ramaraju GA, et al. (1998). Pretreatment or resuscitation with a lipid infusion shifts the dose-response to bupivacaine-induced asystole in rats. Anesthesiology, 88:1071–5.

Weinberg GL (2010). Treatment of local anesthetic systemic toxicity (LAST). Reg Anesth Pain Med, 35:188–93.

Respiratory tract management in poisoning

Background

Maintaining a patent and adequately protected airway and providing sufficient oxygenation and ventilation are essential for the management of any critically ill patient. Poisons can directly or indirectly damage the respiratory tract, which may result in inadequate oxygenation and ventilation leading to respiratory failure. Clinical management decisions should be directed both by the patients' immediate condition and their predicted course. Knowledge of the poisons involved assists such predictions.

Approach to the critically ill patient

A stepwise approach should be adopted which involves; preparation for the patient's arrival, ABCDE approach to identification and treatment of immediately life-threatening problems, dealing with less immediate issues, and transfer to a place of definitive care. Throughout the process continuous reassessment allows the detection of any deterioration.

Preparation and setting

Patients in whom airway obstruction or respiratory compromise are predicted should be treated by experienced practitioners in an area with advanced airway management and resuscitation facilities. The importance of calling early for appropriately experienced senior help cannot be overstated.

Airway

If a patient has normal speech then their airway is not immediately endangered. Additional sounds accompanying breathing may indicate partial airway obstruction.

- Stridor is caused by partial obstruction of the larynx, trachea, or main bronchi.
- Gurgling indicates the presence of excess fluid in the airway: vomit, blood, or secretions.
- Snoring noises result from partial obstruction of the airway by pharyngeal soft tissues.

The silent airway indicates either apnoea or if it is accompanied by paradoxical chest and abdominal wall movements complete airway obstruction.

In an unresponsive patient inspect the mouth and clear any secretions or other foreign matter with a Yankauer suction catheter. Well-fitting dentures should be left in place to preserve normal airway anatomy. The airway should be opened with either a head tilt, chin lift, or jaw thrust manoeuvre.

In patients who do not have an intact gag reflex an oropharyngeal airway may be used in order to maintain airway patency. A patient tolerating an oropharyngeal airway is likely to be not protecting their airway and should be considered for intubation unless the underlying cause is easily reversible, e.g. an opiate overdose. A nasopharyngeal airway is an alternative, particularly if it is not possible to open a patient's mouth. Nasopharyngeal airways may cause trauma to the nasal cavity resulting in bleeding and further airway compromise; they should be used with caution in patients taking anticoagulants.

Once a patient's airway has been opened they should be given supplemental oxygen via a facemask in order to achieve an SpO_2 of greater than 94%.

Breathing

The assessment of breathing commonly takes place intercurrently with that of the airway. Cyanosis is a late sign of hypoxia and therefore a patient may be significantly hypoxic in the absence of cyanosis.

Look for signs of respiration: fogging of the facemask indicates some respiratory effort, this may be inadequate. Observe chest wall movement, count respiratory rate with your palm resting on the patient's sternum. Auscultate the chest for breath sounds and any additional sounds.

Measure SpO_2 with a pulse oximeter. If there is diagnostic uncertainty, potential exposure to CO, or a methaemoglobin-generating agent perform blood gas analysis. The normal range of SpO_2 by pulse oximeter in healthy adults is 94–98%. Falsely high readings will be obtained where a patient has abnormal haemoglobin such as methaemoglobin or carboxyhaemoglobin. Falsely low readings may result from nail varnish, dark skin pigment, poor peripheral perfusion, and excessive movement. If spontaneous ventilation is inadequate or absent then a bag-mask technique should be used for assisted ventilation.

Circulation, disability, and environment

Decisions regarding airway and ventilatory management will be influenced by peripheral perfusion, pulse rate and rhythm, and blood pressure. In a profoundly shocked patient where the cause is not rapidly reversible early intubation and ventilation may be indicated.

The initial approach culminates with an assessment of conscious level, pupils, peripheral neurology, and temperature. This may give clues as to the cause of respiratory insufficiency. Pinpoint pupils may suggest opiate or gamma-butyrolactone toxicity.

Decision to intubate

Initial management of a critically ill patient's airway should be with basic techniques, as outlined earlier. Intubation should be considered only when an appropriately trained person is present. A patient should be intubated when the danger of them remaining unintubated exceeds the risks associated with intubation, for example:

- failure to ventilate with non-invasive techniques
- marked upper airway oedema, for example, due to anaphylaxis or burns
- unconsciousness with vomiting or a high risk of passive aspiration
- the requirement for prolonged respiratory support.

Treating reversible causes of airway obstruction or ventilatory failure may avoid intubation. Some reversible causes are:

- seizures
- opiate toxicity
- dysrhythmias
- bronchospasm
- anaphylaxis
- hypoglycaemia

Mechanisms of respiratory tract compromise

Poisons impair respiratory tract function through a combination of direct and indirect mechanisms.

Caustics and direct airway damage

Rapid airway assessment is a priority in patients who have ingested or inhaled caustic substances. Urgent intubation may be required with respiratory distress as this suggests impending obstruction. Endoscopy will evaluate airway damage and may facilitate intubation in patients with significant injuries or oedema.

Damage to the lower respiratory tract may occur from inhaling toxic gases. Industrial toxins (e.g. chlorine and hydrogen sulphide) cause bronchospasm, non-cardiogenic pulmonary oedema, and adult respiratory distress syndrome. The immediate management of these problems involves administering bronchodilators and ensuring adequate oxygenation. Use of positive airways pressure either non-invasively or via an endotracheal tube may be required in order to achieve this. Inspired gases should be humidified for patients suffering from irritative symptoms.

Inhalation of cadmium and other heavy metal fumes from industrial activity can result in a severe chemical pneumonitis. Over several days progressive hypoxia and failure of gas exchange can occur. The benefit of administering corticosteroids in this situation is uncertain. Despite mechanical ventilation patients may die due to respiratory failure.

Sedation and airway compromise

Central nervous system depressants (e.g. opiates, benzodiazepines, gamma-hydroxybutyrate) can cause deep sedation, particularly when they are taken in conjunction with alcohol. Patients may be unable to maintain the patency of their own airway and will lose protective airway reflexes. In patients who are lightly sedated laryngospasm is more of a risk.

Antidotes such as naloxone (opiates) or flumazenil (benzodiazepines) should be considered for patients who are suspected of having specific agent toxicity (see Benzodiazepines, pp. 108–109 and Opioid analgesics, pp. 128–129 for detailed advice); however establishing a clear airway should take precedence over their administration.

It is widely accepted that even in a situation where a patient has adequate respiratory function, unless the cause is rapidly reversible, a GCS of 8 or less mandates intubation for the purpose of airway protection. However it has been proposed that clinical assessment by experienced medical staff is a better determinant of the need for intubation, and that poisoned patients whose GCS is 8 or less may be safely managed in a well-monitored ward environment.

ß-blockers and bronchospasm

ß-blocking drugs inhibit cyclic adenosine monophosphate. Blockade of the β_2 receptor results in bronchospasm, resulting in wheeze, dyspnoea and hypoxia. Other effects of β_2-blockade are hypoglycaemia and smooth muscle constriction. As propranolol is non-cardioselective it is particularly likely to cause bronchospasm. In large doses cardioselective drugs such as atenolol are likely to also have significant β_2 activity.

Specific airway support in ß-blocker poisoning involves administration of supplemental oxygen and a nebulized agonist such as salbutamol. Severe bronchospasm may be treated with intravenous aminophylline. Advanced ventilatory strategies may be required if there is gas trapping in the lungs. Treatment of bradycardia and hypotension due to β_1-blockade is initially with glucagon, which promotes the production of myocardial cyclic adenosine monophosphate.

Poisons that cause hypoventilation

Hypoventilation occurs when respiratory rate and tidal volume are inadequate to maintain oxygenation and carbon dioxide removal from the blood. Toxicological causes of hypoventilation can be divided into:

- decreased central respiratory drive—commonly due to ethanol, opiates, benzodiazepines, and tricyclic antidepressants
- respiratory muscle weakness caused by neuromuscular blocking drugs, electrolyte abnormalities, organophosphates, and botulinum toxin
- bronchospasm due to ß-blockers, scombroid poisoning, irritant gas inhalation and anaphylactoid reactions
- chest wall rigidity, which may be caused by fentanyl toxicity or tetanus.

Clinical examination together with blood gas analysis should be used to assess ventilatory sufficiency and the need for respiratory support.

Poisons causing hyperventilation

This may be caused by either direct stimulation of respiration or in response to increased metabolic demand or metabolic acidosis.

Respiratory stimulants include cocaine, amphetamines, methylxanthines, and anticholinergics. Salicylates cause both direct respiratory stimulation and hyperventilation in response to metabolic acidosis.

Toxicological causes of metabolic acidosis include:

- lactic acidosis due to corrosive or cellular toxicity
- renal failure
- ingestion of excess acid or toxic alcohols
- rhabdomyolysis
- rapid infusion of large volumes of normal saline.

Metabolic acidosis is usually at least partially compensated for by hyperventilation. Inability to mount a hyperventilatory response to a metabolic acidosis can result in rapid decompensation with respiratory failure.

Prevention of nosocomial poisoning

Whilst managing a patient's airway the practitioner's face will be directly adjacent to the patient's. If a patient coughs or vomits, which is common in cases of poisoning, the practitioner will be contaminated. Off gassing in nerve agent poisoning may cause mild to moderate toxicity in emergency department staff (see Nerve agents, pp. 342–344). Similarly exposure to blood and secretions can result in the transmission of blood-borne viruses. In order to prevent secondary poisoning patients must be decontaminated and personal protective equipment should be used. A gas scavenging system should be used to collect harmful exhaled gases.

Further reading

Chan B, Gaudry P, Grattan-Smith TM, et al. (1993). The use of Glasgow Coma Scale in poisoning. J Emerg Med, 11:579–82.

Donald C, Duncan R, Thakore S (2009). Predictors of the need for rapid sequence intubation in the poisoned patient with reduced Glasgow coma score. Emerg Med J, 26:510–12.

Fernandez MA, Sanz P, Palomar M, et al. (1996). Fatal chemical pneumonitis due to cadmium fumes. Occup Med, 46:372–4.

Geller RJ, Singleton KL, Tarantino ML, et al. (2001). Nosocomial poisoning associated with emergency department treatment of organophosphate toxicity – Georgia, 2000. J Toxicol Clin Toxicol, 39:109–11.

Renal failure

Background

Nephrologists are involved in the care of poisoning and drug-related clinical presentations for three principal reasons:

1 Kidney injury due to drugs and other toxins is common. Kidney injury encompasses a wide range of renal disorders including tubular dysfunction, interstitial nephritis, glomerular disease, and urinary tract syndromes, and may be both acute and chronic.

2 Prompt, effective management of acute kidney injury (AKI) can minimize drug toxicity by facilitating drug elimination by the kidneys. Metabolic, electrolyte, and fluid-related side effects of drug or toxin toxicity may require active intervention and toxin elimination by means of extracorporeal treatments.

3 Extracorporeal techniques may remove toxins thus limiting potential toxic effects, including those on the kidney.

Drug-induced kidney injury

The kidneys are the principal route of excretion for many drugs. The high rate of drug delivery to the kidneys (which receive 20% of cardiac output) results in a high concentration of drugs within the tubular fluid and medullary interstitium. This makes the kidneys particularly prone to drug- and toxin-induced injury. Diagnosis rarely requires a kidney biopsy.

Acute tubular injury

Drugs and toxins may cause acute tubular necrosis (ATN) either secondary to the generalized effects of severe poisoning or as a result of direct nephrotoxicity.

Generalized effects

Systemic cardiovascular collapse can arise from overdose of most classes of drugs. The resultant reduction in effective circulating volume, hypotension, and secondary renal hypoperfusion causes ischaemic acute tubular injury. Certain drugs can inhibit normal compensatory changes in intraglomerular perfusion pressure in response to a reduction in renal blood flow by specifically inducing intra-renal vasomotor changes. For example, non-steroidal anti-inflammatory drugs (NSAIDs) inhibit prostaglandin-mediated afferent renal arteriolar dilatation, whilst angiotensin-converting enzyme (ACE) inhibitors and angiotensin-II receptor blockers (ARBs) prevent efferent arteriolar constriction. Both of these mechanisms cause relative renal hypo-perfusion and a reduction in glomerular filtration rate (GFR) often in the presence of a preserved systemic blood pressure.

Direct effects

Less frequently, tubular damage may result from a direct nephrotoxic effect of drugs or their metabolites (see Table 3.3). Additionally, many drugs may provoke haemolysis or rhabdomyolysis. The release of haemoglobin, methaemoglobin, or myoglobin into the peripheral circulation causes AKI as haemoglobin has a direct toxic effect on tubular cells and myoglobin release from striated muscle causes both intraluminal cast obstruction and tubular damage.

Some drugs result in kidney damage by forming crystalline deposits which causes interstitial inflammation, obstruction, and tubular injury. This particularly happens in states of volume depletion. For example, oxalate

Table 3.3 Mechanisms of drug-induced Acute Tubular Necrosis

Action	Causative toxin
General	
Systemic hypotension	Diuretics, antihypertensives, analgesics, sedatives, tricyclic antidepressants, anticonvulsants
Reduced intrarenal glomerular pressure	ACE inhibitors, ARBs, NSAIDs
Local	
Nephrotoxic ATN	Aminoglycosides, paracetamol, salicylate, heavy metals, phenoxyacetate herbicides, contrast media agents, NSAIDs, cisplatin, antiviral drugs; interferon alpha, foscarnet
Myoglobinuric ATN	Barbiturates, amfetamines, methadone, statins, cocaine, heroin, carbon monoxide, snake/arthropod/insect venoms
Haemaglobinuric ATN	Copper sulfate, sodium chlorate, lead poisoning, insect venoms
Crystalluric ATN	Ethylene glycol, thiazides, anti-retrovirals; tenofovir, indinavir, antivirals; aciclovir

ATN: acute tubular necrosis; ACE: angiotensin converting enzyme; ARB: angiotensin II receptor blocker; NSAID: non-steroidal anti-inflammatory drug.

crystals are commonly seen in cases of ethylene glycol poisoning, and uric acid crystals with ethanol, thiazide diuretics, and any chemotherapeutic agent triggering the tumour lysis syndrome.

Recognition and management

In-hospital AKI is attributable, at least in part, to drugs in up to 35% of cases, most frequently involving ACE inhibitors, antibiotics, NSAIDs, diuretics, and contrast media agents. Predisposing factors include advanced age, pre-existing chronic kidney disease (CKD), dehydration, and chronic liver disease. Management of AKI is generally symptomatic and supportive in nature whilst spontaneous excretion or metabolism of the drug occurs. This may involve correction of fluid, electrolyte, and acid–base derangements. In addition, general measures used to prevent the effects of a drug or toxin in overdose should be considered

Tubulopathies

Chronic drug ingestion is associated with a number of tubular syndromes. The Fanconi syndrome is associated with consumption of first-generation tetracyclines, 6-mercaptopurine, and herbal medicines. This is characterized by multiple tubular defects and is phenotypically variably expressed with hypophosphataemia, hypokalaemia, vitamin D deficiency, glycosuria, amino-aciduria, hypercalcaemia, and renal tubular acidosis. After removing the offending agent, treatment is by oral supplementation with potassium chloride salts, sodium bicarbonate for correction of acid–base status, and replacement of phosphate/vitamin D to prevent hyperparathyroidism. Nephrogenic diabetes insipidus can be caused by lithium, demeclocycline and antiretrovirals (cidofovir, foscarnet, didanosine).

Acute interstitial nephritis (AIN)

Any drug may provoke an immune-mediated reaction, independent of dose, producing AIN. Patients present

Table 3.4 Drugs associated with acute interstitial nephritis

PPIs	Omeprazole, pantoprazole
Antibiotics	Amoxicillin, ciprofloxacin, erythromycin, nitrofurantoin, rifampicin
NSAIDs	Aspirin, indometacin, naproxen, ibuprofen, phenazone[a]
Diuretics	Indapamide[a], furosemide, triamterene
Analgesics	Antipyrine[a], noramidopyrine[a], antrafenin[a]
Others	Allopurinol, captopril, phenobarbital, carbimazole

NSAID; non-steroidal anti-inflammatory drug.

[a] Not licensed for use in the UK

with renal impairment, (up to 40% are dialysis dependent), proteinuria (60%), haematuria (50%), eosinophilia (40%), and general symptoms of arthralgia, fever, and rash (40%). Definitive diagnosis requires renal biopsy. Treatment involves discontinuation of the likely offending agent, and consideration of a short course of oral steroids. Drugs commonly implicated in AIN are listed in Table 3.4.

Glomerulopathies

Glomerular diseases are classified by clinical presentation and characteristic histological features on renal biopsy (Table 3.5). Both the nephritic and nephrotic syndromes are associated with drugs and toxins. Treatment of glomerular syndromes depends on the underlying glomerular lesion. In addition to removal of the offending agent, general principles include strict blood pressure control, cholesterol-lowering therapy, and anti-proteinuric strategies with ACE inhibitors, ARBs, and calcium channel blockade. Immunosuppressive regimens are occasionally used in cases of immunologically mediated rapidly progressive glomerulonephritis.

Chronic kidney disease

Chronic interstitial nephritis with progressive loss of renal function can result from prolonged use of some drugs or the misuse of others. Analgesics, NSAIDs, herbal medicine, lithium, and calcineurin inhibitors are all associated with chronic renal scarring and CKD.

Table 3.5 Drugs associated with glomerular disease

Syndrome	Drug/toxin	Glomerular lesion
Nephrotic	Gold	Membranous glomerulonephritis (GN)
	Penicillamine	
	IV heroin	Focal segmental glomerulosclerosis
	Pamidronate	
	Interferon alpha	Minimal change
	NSAIDs	
	Poison ivy and oak	
Nephritic	Ciclosporin	Microangiopathy
	Oral contraceptive	
	Mitomycin C	
	Hydralazine	Lupus-like GN
	Procainamide	
	Infliximab	Crescentic GN
	Propylthiouracil	

Urinary tract syndromes

These range from atropine-induced urinary retention, to papillary necrosis (analgesics and NSAIDs) and renal calculi where certain drugs can precipitate to form stones. For example, acute nephrocalcinosis can result following the administration of oral phosphate-containing bowel purgatives due to the precipitation of calcium phosphate stones. Herbal medicines containing aristocholic acid are also linked with urinary tract carcinoma which may present with acute obstructive uropathy.

Supporting drug elimination in drug toxicity

Kidney injury reduces the clearance of drugs and toxins that would normally be excreted by the kidneys. Patients with renal dysfunction are therefore especially at risk of drug accumulation and toxic side effects, e.g. nephrotoxicity associated with high doses of penicillins and antiviral agents. When toxic levels occur, specific measures may be required to remove drugs, depending on the clinical severity of signs and symptoms, the drug ingested, plasma drug levels and baseline renal function measures used include:

- supporting recovery of native renal function to facilitate drug elimination
- diuresis at controlled urinary pH
- extracorporeal circuits: haemodialysis (HD), haemofiltration (HF), haemoperfusion (HPF)
- peritoneal dialysis (PD).

Some systems combine different modalities, such as haemodiafiltration.

Recovery of native renal function

The optimal way to remove a drug that is renally excreted is to maximize kidney function. Restoration of baseline renal function by appropriate fluid volume management and cessation of any drugs implicated in renal dysfunction is therefore paramount and aims to facilitate renal drug elimination and minimize the duration of symptomatic drug toxicity. Pre-emptive recognition of 'at-risk' patients allows appropriate drug dose adjustments, drug discontinuation, and optimal fluid management.

Diuresis at controlled urinary pH

Non-ionized drugs are lipid soluble and will diffuse through cell membranes relatively easily, thereby permitting passive tubular reabsorption of filtered drug by the kidney. Conversely, in the ionized state, drugs are poorly reabsorbed. For weak acids and alkalis, the ratio of ionized to non-ionized drug can therefore be significantly altered by manipulating the urinary pH. Alkaline urine enhances the urinary excretion of weak acids such as salicylate, phenobarbital, and phenoxyacetate herbicides. Whilst this can be achieved by administration of isotonic (1.26%) sodium bicarbonate, aiming for a urine pH of 7.5–8.5, forced alkaline diuresis is no longer advocated for salicylate poisoning due to issues with fluid overload. The only commonly occurring clinical scenario in which urinary alkalinization is used is in the treatment of rhabdomyolysis, as myoglobin is more soluble in alkaline urine. For weak alkalis such as amfetamine, acidification of urine with ammonium chloride can enhance excretion. Again, this approach is no longer used in clinical practice as amfetamines can cause rhabdomyolysis and an acidic urine will enhance myoglobin precipitation in the tubules.

Extracorporeal treatment of acute poisoning

Extracorporeal therapies (HD, HF, and HPF) to remove drugs and toxins are used in only 0.2% of all poisonings and, even in patients admitted to an intensive care unit with acute drug poisoning, only 1% require such treatments. The key issues in utility are the kinetic properties of the toxin and flow, and extraction rates on the relevant equipment (see Drug handling in the poisoned patient—toxicokinetics, pp. 10–11). While no absolute clinical contraindication to therapy exists, cardiovascular collapse may preclude its practical usage.

Indications include:

• ingestion of lethal dose for which supportive care is insufficient, i.e. clinical condition worsening despite maximal supportive care; hypoventilation, hypotension, hypothermia
• rate of extracorporeal clearance exceeds that of endogenous hepatic/renal clearance, e.g. impaired clearance of toxic compound due to coincidental liver/renal dysfunction (acute or chronic).

Haemodialysis

Drugs and toxins with a small volume of distribution, which are water-soluble and of low molecular weight are removed by HD by diffusion, e.g. lithium. HD is also indicated when AKI complicates poisoning, for correction of electrolyte imbalance (hyperkalaemia), severe metabolic acidosis, hyper- and hypothermia, and volume overload. It may also be combined with other strategies, e.g. in methanol overdose, where ethanol or fomepizole may be administered to competitively bind alcohol dehydrogenase thereby inhibiting formation of toxic methanol metabolites, HD then removes the unbound methanol. HD is generally reserved for cases which have not responded to conservative therapy where there is severe metabolic acidosis and plasma methanol levels greater than 500mg/L.

Haemofiltration

HF generates convective transport of solute through the dialysis membrane and allows flux of larger-molecular-weight molecules up to 40,000 Da. It is occasionally used in overdoses of valproate, vancomycin, hirudin, and metal-chelating complexes (e.g. desferrioxamine).

Haemoperfusion

In HPF, blood passes through an adsorbant cartridge in the extracorporeal circuit. Commonly used sorbents included activated charcoal, ion exchange resins, and non-ionic exchange macroporous resins. These are able to bind protein-bound and lipophilic drugs and toxins such as paraquat and amanita phalloides. The main complications include mild thrombocytopaenia, mild leucopenia, hypocalcaemia, hypoglycaemia, hypothermia, and

Table 3.6 Suggested drug threshold for considering extracorporeal removal

Haemodialysis		Haemoperfusion	
Drug	Threshold	Drug	Threshold
Lithium	>4 mmol/L	Phenobarbital	>150 mg/L
Ethanol	>5 g/L	Paraquat	Clinical
Methanol	>500 mg/L	Theophylline	>40 mg/L
Salicylate	>800 mg/L	Phenytoin	>30 mg/L

clotting of the cartridge. This approach is very rarely used today.

Continuous extracorporeal therapies

For drugs with a large volume of distribution, continuous dialysis prevents a rebound in the drug serum concentration following cessation of a standard intermittent HD treatment. Strategies to optimize removal of such drugs include slowing the pump speed or dialysate flow rate and performing an extended (8–10 hour) haemodialysis session, or carrying out two consecutive 4–6-hour intermittent treatments. Table 3.6 shows which form of extracorporeal therapy preferentially removes drugs in overdose, and the threshold plasma levels at which to consider such therapies.

Peritoneal dialysis

PD is only approximately 10% as effective as high-flux HD at drug/toxin removal and is therefore only used when vascular access is problematic or HD contraindicated, most commonly used in the paediatric population. It has little or no role in managing acute poisoning due to its slow and low rates of toxin removal.

Further reading

Barratt B, Harris K, Topham P (eds) (2009). Acute kidney injury (AKI). In: Barratt B, Harris K, Topham P (eds) *Oxford Desk Reference of Nephrology*, pp. 317–88. Oxford: Oxford University Press.

Barratt B, Harris K, Topham P (eds) (2009). Pharmacology and drug use in kidney disease. In: Barratt B, Harris K, Topham P (eds) *Oxford Desk Reference of Nephrology*, pp. 689–716. Oxford: Oxford University Press.

Bellomo R, Kellum JA, Ronco C. (2012). Acute kidney injury. *Lancet*, 380:756–66.

Davison AM, Cameron SJ, Grunfeld JP, et al. (eds) (2005). Acute renal failure. *Oxford Textbook of Clinical Nephrology*, 3rd edition, pp. 1435–1630. Oxford: Oxford University Press.

Parazella MA (2003). Drug-induced renal failure: update on new medications and unique mechanism of nephrotoxicity. *Am J Med Sci*, 325:349–62.

Mukherjee A (1974). Drug induced renal disease. *Int Urol Nephrol*, 6:225–31.

Hepatic failure

Background

The liver is the organ involved in metabolism of many ingested drugs and other substances. Hence, drug-induced liver injury is relatively common. A large variety of clinical and histological manifestations are reported ranging from the acute panacinar haemorrhagic necrosis induced by paracetamol overdose to chronic fibrosis and cirrhosis that may occur with long-term use of methotrexate. Given these protean manifestations of drug-induced hepatotoxicity, this section will focus on the most dramatic and rapidly fatal clinical picture which is acute (fulminant) liver failure. For descriptions of clinical presentation and management of other manifestations of drug-induced liver injury the reader is referred to other specialist text.

Acute (fulminant) liver failure

Definition

Acute (fulminant) liver failure (ALF) occurs following the sudden loss of hepatocellular function resulting in jaundice, coagulopathy, and encephalopathy. In the original definition, Trey and Davidson described ALF as 'a potentially reversible condition with an onset of hepatic encephalopathy within 8 weeks of the onset of first symptoms in the absence of pre-existing liver disease'. To avoid the subjective bias of 'symptoms', the original definition has been revised using jaundice as first symptom, and classify ALF as 'hyperacute', 'acute', and 'subacute' liver failure referring to a jaundice-to-encephalopathy time of 0–7, 8–28, and 29–84 days respectively.

Aetiology

The causes of ALF are dependent on geographical location, drug-induced ALF is more common in the developed world. The most common agent implicated in ALF is paracetamol. Overdoses of iron may also result in ALF. Many agents cause ALF (Box 3.1)

Clinical features

Obesity, hepatitis C (HCV) infection, and coexistent liver disease are risk factors for the development of ALF in those exposed to potentially hepatotoxic drugs. Chronic ethanol ingestion, fasting or starvation, unintentional ingestion, and delayed presentation are specific factors that increase risk of ALF following paracetamol ingestion.

Gastrointestinal

Initial clinical features are often non-specific. Nausea, vomiting, and right upper quadrant abdominal pains are frequently observed. Jaundice may be mild. The liver is usually impalpable. Ascites and portal hypertension may develop in subacute injury. Serum transaminases are elevated, very high concentrations being characteristic of paracetamol overdose. Variable elevation of bilirubin also occurs. Increases in serum alkaline phosphatase (ALP) and gamma-glutamyl transferase (GGT) are modest. Marked elevations of GGT compared with ALP can be indicative of enzyme induction as occurs with prolonged alcohol excess. Albumin concentrations fall as part of the negative acute phase response. Liver synthetic failure is manifest by increasing coagulopathy; the prothrombin time and factor V levels are particularly affected, and carry prognostic significance. Problematic bleeding is uncommon unless platelet count is also reduced. Hypoglycaemia is common in advanced cases. Reduced hepatic clearance contributes to lactic acidosis and hyperammonaemia.

Box 3.1 Causes of acute hepatic failure

- Drug overdose:
  - paracetamol
  - iron
- Idiosyncratic reaction to drugs:
  - antibiotics
  - anticonvulsants
  - NSAIDs
  - antidepressants
  - statins
  - halothane anaesthetics
  - illicit drugs
  - cocaine
  - ecstasy
- Fungi:
  - Amanita phalloides
  - Amanita virosa
  - Amanita verna
- Industrial chemicals:
  - carbon tetrachloride
  - 2-nitropropane
  - dimethylformamide
  - yellow phosphorus
- Herbal and traditional remedies:
  - germander
  - kava-kava

Cerebral

Hepatic encephalopathy defines the syndrome of ALF. The four-point scale used cannot be directly aligned to the Glasgow Coma Scale (GCS).

- Grade 1 encephalopathy: mild mental slowing, confusion and asterixis.
- Grade 2 encephalopathy: increasing confusion, drowsiness and occasionally aggressive agitation.
- Grade 3: coma but easily roused, no sensible conversation.
- Grade 4: unconscious and unrousable.

Data from Conn H, Lieberthal M. *The hepatic coma syndromes and lactulose*. Baltimore: Williams & Wilkins; 1979. p. 7.

Focal neurological deficit is unusual, but unilateral or bilateral extensor planter responses are common. Increasing hepatic encephalopathy is associated with increased risk of cerebral oedema. Cerebral oedema is a common cause of death in patients with ALF and grade 4 encephalopathy. Clinical features of raised intracranial pressure (hypertension, bradycardia, and pupillary abnormalities) are late manifestations. Intracranial pressure and cerebral perfusion pressure can be measured with extradural pressure monitors to allow early identification and intervention. Such monitoring may be complicated by intracranial haemorrhage; studies have not shown survival benefit.

Cardiovascular

Tachycardia, vasodilatation, and hypotension are common. Cardiac arrhythmias and subclinical myocardial injury may occur.

Respiratory

Hyperventilation is common, especially in patients with acidosis. Acute lung injury and ARDS can occur. Pneumonia is a common complication in ventilated patients.

Renal

Oliguria and anuria are common, especially following paracetamol overdose. Acute renal failure is common and also associated with worse outcome. Hypophosphataemia can occur.

Immune function

Features of a systemic inflammatory response are common, with pyrexia or hypothermia increased WBC. Immunoparesis increases risk of systemic bacterial and fungal infection.

Management

Indications for specialist referral

ALF is a complex rapidly progressive and potentially fatal condition. Early discussion and transfer to units able to provide emergency liver transplantation is to be encouraged. Transfer of patients with hepatic encephalopathy can be problematic and precipitate further clinical deterioration; experienced staff should accompany such patients. Indications for transfer to specialist units include:

- prothrombin time greater than the number of hours after the overdose
- prothrombin time greater than 50 seconds or INR greater than 5
- persistent acidosis
- hypoglycaemia
- renal failure
- hepatic encephalopathy.

Cause-specific intervention

N-acetylcysteine (NAC) is highly effective in preventing ALF following paracetamol overdose. There is some evidence that NAC is also effective in limiting complications in patients with established hepatotoxicity and ALF following paracetamol overdose. A recent US study also concluded that NAC improved non-transplant survival in patients with non-paracetamol ALF, but only when introduced early in the clinical course and with lower grades of hepatic encephalopathy.

Organ support

Patients developing ALF are best managed in a high dependency/intensive care setting, with close monitoring of organ functions. Fluid resuscitation is essential, although the optimum type of fluid and goals for therapy are not well defined. Norepinephrine is the vasopressor of choice. Terlipressin studies have produced variable results. Continuous haemofiltration methods are most commonly used to provide renal support. Mechanical ventilation may be instituted because for respiratory failure or hepatic encephalopathy. Conventional treatments for hepatic encephalopathy such as lactulose are ineffective in the setting of ALF. Recently the importance of ammonia in the cerebral complications of ALF has led to study of agents that reduce circulating ammonia. Cerebral oedema is treated with mannitol infusion. Limited controlled hyperventilation, moderate hypothermia, indometacin and thiopentone infusion can be utilized in resistant cases. Risk of systemic infection dictates the use of prophylactic antibiotics in many liver units. Glucose replacement, phosphate infusion, and hypertonic saline have all been used to treat the metabolic abnormalities observed in ALF.

Liver support devices and plasmapheresis

Artificial liver assist devices have received much attention in or charcoal to remove toxins. Bioartificial devices include porcine or human hepatocytes to add synthetic functions. Meta-analyses of these devices have shown no survival benefit in patients with ALF. Similar data are reported with plasmapheresis.

Liver transplantation

Emergency liver transplantation for ALF is widely accepted as a life-saving treatment in carefully selected individuals. Initial survival is generally poorer compared with transplantation for chronic liver disease, but 1-year survivals of between 65% and 80% are reported. Auxiliary liver transplantation (in which part of the native liver is left in situ and liver transplant performed, then removed after regeneration of the native liver) has not found widespread application. However, auxiliary transplantation may be more applicable in patients with paracetamol induced ALF, for in this condition complete regeneration of the liver is more likely to occur. Long-term outcomes are good, repeat overdoses of paracetamol are rarely reported.

Utilization of liver transplantation relies on accurate prognostication of the clinical course of ALF. In the United Kingdom this is determined using the 'King's College criteria'. These 'criteria' predict a risk of death greater than 90% and are as follows:

For paracetamol overdose

- Arterial pH less than 7.25 more than 24 hours after the overdose and after fluid resuscitation.
- Coexisting serum creatinine greater than 300 micromol/L, grade 3–4 hepatic encephalopathy, prothrombin time greater than 100 seconds (INR > 6.5). Or two of these three criteria with evidence of deterioration (e.g. increasing intracranial pressure or inotropic requirements) in the absence of clinical sepsis.
- Arterial lactate greater than 3.5 mmol/L on admission or arterial lactate greater than 3.0 mmol/L after adequate fluid resuscitation.

For other causes

- Any aetiology and degree of hepatic encephalopathy with PT greater than 100 seconds (INR > 6.5).
- Any three of the following five clinical features:
  - unfavourable aetiology (hepatitis A and B are favourable aetiologies, all others are defined as unfavourable)
  - age less than 10 or greater than 40 years
  - jaundice to encephalopathy interval greater than 7 days
  - prothrombin time greater than 50 seconds (INR > 3.5)
  - bilirubin greater than 300 micromol/L.

Other 'transplant criteria' are applied in other parts of the world. Non-paracetamol cause-specific indications for liver transplantation have been developed but the studies are often based on small numbers of cases.

Further reading

Bernal W, Auzinger G, Dhawan A, et al. (2010). Acute liver failure. Lancet, 376:190–201.

Ichai P, Samuel D (2008). Etiology and prognosis of fulminant hepatitis in adults. Liver Transplant, 14(Suppl 2):S67–79.

Polson J, Lee WM (2005). AASLD position paper: The management of acute liver failure. Hepatology, 41:1179–97.

Sass DA, Shakil AO (2005). Fulminant hepatic failure. Liver Transplant, 11:594–605.

Stravitz RT, Kramer AH, Davern T, et al. (2007). Intensive care of patients with acute liver failure: recommendations of the U.S. Acute Liver Failure Study Group. Crit Care Med, 35:2498–508.

Wendon J, Lee W (2008). Encephalopathy and cerebral edema in the setting of acute liver failure: pathogenesis and management. Neurocrit Care, 9:97–102.

Acid–base and electrolyte disturbances in the poisoned patient

Background

Acid–base and electrolyte disturbances are common in patients with severe poisoning. It is important that they are picked up and managed early as they can increase the risk of severe morbidity and mortality.

Acid–base disturbances

Metabolic acidosis

This is the most common acid–base disturbance seen in the poisoned patient. The arterial blood gas will show a pH less than 7.40, a low bicarbonate, and a significant base deficit (negative base excess); in addition, the pCO_2 may be low due to respiratory compensation (although this may not always be present, particularly if the patient has ingested a drug that causes central nervous system depression). The causes of a metabolic acidosis in the poisoned patient are:

- ingestion of drugs/substances that are acids, e.g. salicylates, hydrochloric acid
- substances that have acidic metabolites, e.g. ethylene glycol, methanol
- drugs that impair mitochondrial function, e.g. metformin, high-dose paracetamol, cyanide, sodium valproate; this results in a type A, or primary, lactic acidosis
- a type B, or secondary, lactic acidosis related to poor tissue oxygen delivery—this may be due to cardiorespiratory depression, impaired oxygen carrying capacity, or recurrent seizures
- substances that result in a keto-acidosis, e.g. ethanol, isoniazid
- impaired excretion of acids related to renal dysfunction either as a result of direct toxin-related renal failure or renal failure secondary to hypotension.

Anion and osmolal gaps

Measurement of the anion and osmolal gaps can be used to help determine the cause of a metabolic acidosis.

The normal anion gap ($[Na^+] - (HCO3^- + Cl^-)$) is 12 ± 4. Most toxicological causes of a metabolic acidosis are associated with a high anion gap. This occurs when the acid is paired with an unmeasured anion (e.g. lactate, glycolate, formate, salicylate, keto-acids). A normal anion gap metabolic acidosis occurs when there has been a gain of both H^+ and Cl^- ions, or a loss of HCO_3^- and retention of Cl^-. Toxicological causes of a normal anion gap acidosis include poisoning with acetazolamide, chloride containing acids (e.g. hydrochloric acid), colestyramine, magnesium chloride, ammonium chloride, toluene or topiramate, and renal tubular acidosis.

The osmolal gap is the difference between the laboratory-measured serum osmolality and the calculated osmolality. There are many difference formulae available for the calculated osmolality and there is little evidence to determine which of these is best. The formula most widely used is: $2 \times [Na^+] + [Urea] + [Glucose] + [Ethanol\ mg/dL\ /\ 3.7]$

A normal osmolar gap is often quoted as being less than 10 mOsm/L. However, a number of studies have shown normal/baseline osmolal gaps ranging from −15 to +20 mOsm/L and in some studies up to one-third of patients have a baseline osmolal gap greater than 10 mOsm/L.

Toxicological causes of a high osmolal gap include alcohols (toxic alcohols (methanol and ethylene glycol), ethanol, isopropanol, propylene glycol), mannitol, glycerol, acetone, and sorbitol. In addition, a high osmolal gap may be seen in a wide range of other condition including alcoholic/diabetic ketoacidosis, lactic acidosis, shock, and multi-organ failure. As a result of both this, and the reasons already outlined, it is important to interpret the osmolal gap with caution in the management of the poisoned patient with a metabolic acidosis.

Respiratory acidosis

This is also commonly seen in the poisoned patient. The arterial blood gas will show a pH of less than 7.40 and high pCO_2. A respiratory acidosis is caused by respiratory compromise which may be due to:

- central depression of respiratory drive—toxicological causes of this include poisoning with opioids, gamma-hydroxybutyrate, gamma-butyrolactone, ethanol, benzodiazepines, and other CNS depressants such as antipsychotics and tricyclic antidepressants
- peripheral impairment of respiratory function due to changes in respiratory muscle function—causes of this include organophosphates, strychnine, botulinum toxin, paralytic shellfish
- impaired gas exchange at an alveolar level within the lungs—causes of this include smoke inhalation, pulmonary oedema (cardiogenic or non-cardiogenic).

Metabolic alkalosis

Metabolic alkalosis secondary to poisoning is rare. The arterial blood gas will show a pH greater than 7.40, a high bicarbonate, and positive base excess. Metabolic alkalosis may be caused by urinary acid loss (e.g. diuretics, liquorice, magnesium deficiency), gastrointestinal acid loss (e.g. prolonged vomiting), alkali ingestion/administration (e.g. milk-alkali syndrome, excess use of antacids), renal bicarbonate retention (e.g. due to hypochloraemia, hypokalaemia).

Metabolic alkalosis results in decreased ionized calcium, which can result in weakness, tetany, or arrhythmias. Metabolic alkalosis also shifts the oxygen dissociation curve to the left, impairing tissue oxygenation; this is exacerbated by respiratory compensation for the metabolic alkalosis which results in hypoventilation.

Respiratory alkalosis

Respiratory alkalosis in the poisoned patient results from stimulation of the central respiratory centre and therefore an increase in the respiratory rate. The arterial blood gas will show a pH greater than 7.40 and a low pCO_2. The most common cause is salicylate (aspirin) poisoning, other causes include poisoning with caffeine/other methylxanthines and nicotine.

Electrolyte disturbances

The electrolytes most commonly affected in the poisoned patient are potassium and sodium. Changes in serum potassium concentrations can be particularly important because of the critical role that potassium plays in many cellular processes.

Disturbance of the serum concentration of other electrolytes is less common.

Hypokalaemia

Hypokalaemia is the most common electrolyte disturbance seen in the poisoned patient, most often due to gastrointestinal loss related to vomiting and/or diarrhoea. Other causes include renal potassium loss which can occur in: metabolic alkalosis; paracetamol poisoning; therapeutic and supratherapeutic use of loop and/or thiazide diuretics; increased sodium-potassium ATPase activity (e.g. due to beta-2 agonists such as salbutamol, theophylline, caffeine); competitive potassium channel blockade (e.g. poisoning with barium, quinine, chloroquine and hydroxychloroquine); and intracellular shift of potassium (e.g. insulin poisoning, sodium bicarbonate).

Mild hypokalaemia (serum potassium ~3.0mmol/L) can cause generalized weakness and malaise, lower serum potassium (<2.0mmol/L) is rare but can be associated with significant weakness that can proceed to areflexic paralysis. Cardiac manifestations of hypokalaemia are important in the poisoned patient, particularly with cardiotoxic or pro-arrhythmic drug poisoning. ECG changes such as non-specific ST-segment and T-wave changes and prominent U waves may be seen. Crucially hypokalaemia increases the risk of arrhythmias.

Management of hypokalaemia involves potassium supplementation—this may be given orally or intravenously depending on the degree of hypokalaemia and the clinical situation. In patients with significant hypokalaemia who have co-ingested a cardiotoxic, proarrhythmic drug intravenous potassium supplementation is generally required.

Hypokalaemia is a useful marker of severity in chloroquine poisoning, but over-aggressive reversal of hypokalaemia in chloroquine poisoning can be associated with adverse outcomes—this is discussed in more detail in Chloroquine, pp. 162–163.

Hyperkalaemia

Hyperkalaemia is less common than hypokalaemia in poisoning. It may occur as a secondary phenomenon due to AKI, rhabdomyolysis, or a severe metabolic acidosis. Primary hyperkalaemia related to inhibition of sodium-potassium ATPase activity can occur in poisoning with cardiac glycosides such as digoxin, digitoxin (not licensed for use in the UK), and yellow oleander (see Digoxin, pp. 142–145). Hyperkalaemia may occur with both therapeutic use and overdose with ACE inhibitors, ARBs, NSAIDs, spironolactone, amiloride, trimethoprim, and potassium salts. Hyperkalaemia can occur in fluoride poisoning due to activation of potassium channels.

Gastrointestinal symptoms (nausea, vomiting, ileus) can occur in potassium salt overdose, but these do not usually occur in hyperkalaemia from other causes (unless the drug/chemical causing hyperkalaemia also results in gastrointestinal symptoms, e.g. digoxin poisoning).

Hyperkalaemia can cause adverse cardiac effects; ECG abnormalities include peaked T waves, QRS prolongation, PR interval prolongation, and decreased P wave amplitude; in severe hyperkalaemia the ECG can resemble a sine wave pattern and there is an increased risk of ventricular tachyarrhythmias.

Management of hyperkalaemia depends on the cause and is summarized in more detail in the individual sections detailing with the drugs/chemicals that cause hyperkalaemia. However, as a general rule management involves administration of drugs that increase transit of potassium into the intracellular space (e.g. insulin-dextrose, sodium bicarbonate) and of calcium chloride (or gluconate) to decrease the risk of arrhythmias. Calcium should be used in cardioactive steroid toxicity after senior advice as there is a theoretical risk of arrythmia. If the hyperkalaemia is caused by total body accumulation of potassium (e.g. renal failure) gastrointestinal exchange resins such as calcium resonium may be used.

Hypernatraemia

Is relatively uncommon in poisoning coming in three types:

- hypovolaemic: as in severe hyperglycaemia, or extreme sweating
- euvolaemic: as with excess vasopressin
- hypervolaemic: inappropriate use of IV fluids or ingestion of hypertonic sodium salts or solutions.

Features are non-specific and include lethargy, weakness and irritability. Very high elevation of sodium causes fits and coma

Management is cautious replacement of fluid, usually using normal saline. Too rapid correction can cause cerebral oedema.

Hyponatraemia

Clinically significant hyponatraemia is relatively uncommon in the poisoned patient. The commonest cause is due to inappropriate ADH secretion preventing free water clearance. ADH is released by serotonin and drugs acting on this receptor are the commonest cause. Typically stimulants (MDMA) or antidepressants (see Amfetamines and related compounds, pp. 182–183). This is generally euvolaemic.

Large water intake with increased ADH release can rapidly drop serum sodium causing initially vague symptoms, reduced consciousness and seizures. Serum sodium must be corrected carefully as there is a risk of central pontine myelinolysis with over enthusiastic treatment.

Other causes are prolonged vomiting (hypovolaemic), cirrhosis or nephrotic syndrome (hypervolaemic). Hypertriglyceridaemia causes a laboratory analytical interference falsely suggesting hyponatraemia.

Hypocalcaemia

Hypocalcaemia can occur in ethylene glycol poisoning due to complexing of calcium with the oxalate metabolite of ethylene glycol (see Ethylene and diethylene glycols, pp. 240–241). Severe hypocalcaemia can also occur in hydrofluoric acid poisoning (both topical exposure and oral ingestion)—this can lead to complications such as tetany and arrhythmias. Management is by replacement with IV calcium salts (see Hydrofluoric acid, pp. 247–248). Hypocalcaemia may be a complication of the use of the chelation agent calcium sodium edetate. Calcium should be replaced judiciously intravenously.

Hypercalcaemia

This rarely occurs, but may, for example, be secondary to vitamin D intoxication. Other rare causes may include theophylline, lithium and thiazide overdose, excess vitamin A, and rhabdomyolysis from any cause. Management is by fluid replacement and stopping toxin ingestion.

Further reading

Bradberry S, Vale JA (1995). Disturbance of potassium homeostasis in poisoning. *J Toxicol Clin Toxicol* 33:295–310.

Judge BS (2006). Differentiating the causes of metabolic acidosis in the poisoned patient. *Clin Lab Med* 26:31–48.

Rhabdomyolysis and compartment syndrome

Muscle toxicity

Myopathy

Certain drugs and toxins are capable of provoking acute muscle injury. Although this is collectively considered to be drug-related myopathy, there is a spectrum of clinical manifestations. Minor toxicity may cause vague symptoms such as muscle ache and weakness that resolve after drug cessation. More severe injury may result in more severe weakness.

Myositis

This term is used to denote more significant myopathy and implies a degree of pain. There may be mild-to-moderate clinical symptoms, accompanied by tenderness of the affected muscle groups. Serum creatine kinase (CK) activity is usually elevated.

Rhabdomyolysis

In more severe toxicity, serum CK activity is substantially elevated. There is no universally accepted definition, and a variety of different cut-off values for CK have been proposed in different settings: more than 500 U/L, more than fivefold higher than the normal reference limit and more than tenfold higher than the normal reference limit. Rhabdomyolysis may also be distinguished from less severe muscle injury by the presence of metabolic disturbances secondary to myocyte disruption including myoglobinuria, hyperkalaemia, hypocalcaemia, metabolic acidosis, hyperuricaemia, and AKI.

Risk factors for acute muscle toxicity

Around 80% of myopathy may be attributable to drugs or toxins, and the most commonly implicated are opioids, benzodiazepines, selective serotonin reuptake inhibitors, and antipsychotics. Sedative agents including ethanol are capable of diminishing deep pressure reflexes, thereby rendering the patient more susceptible to pressure necrosis. Examination findings give clues to the diagnosis, for example, tenderness on palpation of affected skeletal muscles, neuropraxis, or evidence of pressure injury to the skin such as fluid-filled vesicles, so-called 'coma blisters'.

Patients who have been lying on top of a limb against a raised object, such as a paving edge, for a prolonged period are at particular risk of severe local damage. A high index of suspicion is needed in such cases.

Muscle injury in clinical toxicology

In poisoned patients muscle injury results from the following principal causes:

- Excess muscle activity to a point where muscle damage occurs. This is often exacerbated, or possibly caused, by hyperpyrexia resulting from the heat generated by muscle contraction.
- Pressure injury caused by prolonged immobility in an unconscious patient who has consumed a CNS depressant drug.
- Pressure injury following injection intramuscularly or in the vicinity of the muscle susceptible to compartment pressure resulting from secondary infection or a primary chemical response to an unphysiological solution (often acidic in the case of opioid users).

- A direct drug effect on the muscle cell membrane, particularly, for example, snake toxins or statins.
- A complication of severe electrolyte disturbance caused by the poisoning, severe hypokalaemia, and hypophosphataemia being potential examples.

Rhabdomyolysis may also be due to an indirect effect of drug ingestion due to acute dystonia or generalized seizures, or metabolic complications such as hypovolaemia or hypokalaemia. Rhabdomyolysis is also a feature of the serotonergic syndrome, a rare but recognized complication of drugs capable of enhancing serotonin pathways, particularly when multiple agents are co-ingested (see Serotonin syndrome, pp. 79–80). Other recognized causes of rhabdomyolysis include tetanus, mushroom poisoning, and direct injury from intramuscular drug injection. Snake bites may cause rhabdomyolysis due to local trauma and the effect of myotoxins present in certain venoms, such as that of the tiger snake of southern Australia.

Pathophysiology of rhabdomyolysis

Crush injury was first described in victims of World War II, and direct muscle trauma causes intracellular contents to readily enter the circulation, including myoglobin, urate, and phosphate, causing inflammation and renal ischaemia.

Certain drugs and toxins are associated with more subtle injury, for example, selective binding to skeletal muscle serotonin receptors increases myocyte membrane permeability without complete cellular disruption. This allows CK to diffuse from the myocyte into the circulation across a very high gradient, whereas other intracellular constituents might remain intact. Such a mechanism would help explain the poor correlation between serum CK activity and risk of AKI. Isoenzyme data suggest that injury is specific to skeletal muscle, rather than cardiac or smooth muscle types.

Muscle injury results in changes in serum calcium and phosphate. Depending on the severity of the muscle injury, and the primary cause, calcium and phosphate may rise or fall. Elevation in CK is the major indicator of muscle damage used clinically it is important to remember to our say this particular enzyme in anyone who is suspected to be or may potentially be at risk of muscle injury.

Other enzymes may rise in severe muscle injury, for example, transaminases, and may cause confusion diagnostically.

Rhabdomyolysis causes a typical urinary discolouration, with the urine turning a red brown colour. This will test positive on many dipsticks as blood. Rhabdomyolysis rarely causes significant renal injury on its own, in the absence of other precipitant factors such as hypotension when the CK level is less than 10,000 IU.

Treatment of rhabdomyolysis

The main approach is supportive care, including close monitoring of temperature, blood pressure, and urine output. Causative drugs should be stopped, for example, pre-existing statin or fibrate therapy. Electrolyte imbalance, such as hypokalaemia, should be corrected. Hypovolaemia should be corrected, because this may worsen acute tubular necrosis. Intravenous bicarbonate administration would for theoretical reasons protect against renal impairment by solubilizing urate and other intracellular constituents to avoid microcrystal formation within the renal tubules. However, insufficient clinical data exist to allow evaluation of the benefit or harm of this approach.

Renal replacement therapy should be considered in patients that develop AKI and oliguria, severe metabolic acidosis, or hyperkalaemia despite conservative treatment.

Compartment syndrome

Compartments are defined by connective tissues that do not permit stretch. A small degree of muscle swelling can cause a major rise in pressure. This arises most commonly from prolonged limb compression, but is a recognized complication of drug-related myopathy and intravenous drug injection.

Mechanisms

Raised pressure within the compartment is associated with diminished capillary blood flow and tissue ischaemia. Increased pressure causes impaired venous and lymphatic drainage of the injured area, thereby predisposing to further swelling and oedema and worsening ischaemia. As compartment syndrome develops, there is progressive ischemia of the muscles and nerves eventually causing necrosis and irreversible damage.

Management

Compartment syndrome requires a high degree of suspicion, and may normally be diagnosed on the basis of clinical examination findings. Urgent surgical review is needed. The diagnosis may be confirmed by direct measurement of intra-compartment pressure greater than 30 mmHg. Treatment requires emergency fasciotomy to relieve compartment pressure. Hyperbaric oxygen is an adjunctive therapy that improves wound healing and may lessen the need for repeated fasciotomy surgery. Conservative measures including limb elevation and NSAIDs are used to treat chronic compartment syndrome, but are ineffective for acute compartment syndromes.

Further reading

Collinge C, Kuper M (2010). Comparison of three methods for measuring intracompartmental pressure in injured limbs of trauma patients. *J Orthop Trauma*, 24:364–8.

McDonald S, Bearcroft P (2010). Compartment syndromes. *Semin Musculoskelet Radiol*, 14:236–44.

Possamai L, Waring WS (2007). Acute myopathy in a patient with oesophageal stricture. *Age Ageing*, 36:698–9.

Scop J, Little M, Jelinek GA et al (2009). Sixteen years of severe Tiger snake (Notechis) envenoming in Perth, Western Australia. *Anaesth Intensive Care*, 37:613–18.

Sanai T, Matsui R, Hirano T, et al. (2006). Successful treatment of six patients with neuroleptic malignant syndrome associated with myoglobulinemic acute renal failure. *Ren Fail*, 28:51–5.

Tóth AR, Varga T (2009). Myocardium and striated muscle damage caused by licit or illicit drugs. *Leg Med*, 11(Suppl 1):S484–7.

Waring WS, Sandilands EA (2007). Coma blisters. *Clin Toxicol*, 45:808–9.

Waring WS, Wrate J, Bateman DN (2006). Olanzapine overdose is associated with acute muscle toxicity. *Hum Exp Toxicol*, 25:735–40.

Wilhelm K, Curtis J, Birkett V, et al. (1994). The clinical significance of serial creatine phosphokinase estimations in acute ward admissions. *Aust N Z J Psychiatry*, 28:453–7.

Wilson AD, Howell C, Waring WS (2007). Venlafaxine ingestion is associated with rhabdomyolysis in adults: a case series. *J Toxicol Sci*, 32:97–101.

Serotonin syndrome

Background
The serotonin syndrome is a potentially fatal reaction resulting from drug interactions or intentional overdose involving drugs acting on central and peripheral serotonergic receptors. The syndrome results from excess intrasynaptic serotonin and encompasses a spectrum of clinical features ranging from minor symptoms to death.

Onset of symptoms occurs within minutes to hours after starting therapy with a second serotonergic drug, increasing the dosage of current serotonergic therapy, or following overdose, with up to 60% of patients presenting to hospital within 6 hours. An increasingly common scenario is the use of illicit 'designer drugs' acting on serotonin receptors (see Amfetamines and related compounds, pp. 182–183 and Psychedelic agents, pp. 192–193).

Clinical features
The serotonin syndrome classically as described in Sternbach's classification was originally described in psychiatric patients, who are receiving therapeutic doses a serotonergic agent. Three features are required, including physical and mental state changes. Subsequently Australian clinical toxicologists developed the Hunter score based on experience in acute poisoning and more useful clinically in this patient group (Table 3.7).

When examining patients these features may have different incidence. Thus examining the three main domains one finds:

- *Alteration of mental status:* around 40% of patients have evidence of altered mental status ranging from agitation, confusion, delirium, hallucinations to drowsiness and coma.
- *Neuromuscular hyperactivity:* around 50% of patients have evidence of neuromuscular hyperactivity including profound shivering, tremor, teeth grinding, myoclonus, ocular clonus, inducible or spontaneous clonus, and hyper-reflexia.
- *Autonomic instability:* around 40% of patients have evidence of autonomic instability including dilated pupils, diarrhoea, profuse sweating, flushing, tachycardia, hypertension, or hypotension.

In severe cases, hyperthermia, rhabdomyolysis, renal failure, and disseminated intravascular coagulopathy may develop.

Table 3.7 Diagnostic criteria of serotonin syndrome

Hunter serotonin toxicity criteria
In the presence of a serotonergic agent:
Any of:
a. Spontaneous clonus
b. Inducible or ocular clonus *and* agitation or diaphoresis
c. Tremor *and* hyper-reflexia
d. Hypertonia *and* hyperpyrexia (temperature exceeding 38° C) *and* ocular/inducible clonus

Reproduced from EJC Dunkley et al. (2003). The Hunter Serotonin Toxicity Criteria: simple and accurate diagnostic decision rules for serotonin toxicity, *QJM: An International Journal of Medicine*, 96(9):635–642, by permission of Oxford University Press.

Biochemical abnormalities associated with the serotonin syndrome include metabolic acidosis, elevated creatine kinase and transaminase activity, and renal impairment.

Diagnosis
There is no reliable test to make the diagnosis. It should be suspected in any patient taking serotonergic agents who display some of the clinical features, in particular if they have spontaneous clonus and hyper-reflexia.

Several diagnostic criteria have been developed to aid diagnosis and the most commonly used are Sternbach's criteria and the Hunter serotonin toxicity criteria (Table 3.7).

Drugs causing serotonin syndrome
Serotonin is produced in presynaptic neurons from L-tryptophan and remains within vesicles until released into the synaptic space following axonal stimulation and acts at postsynaptic serotonin receptors. Reuptake mechanisms, degradation by monoamine oxidase type A, and feedback loops exist to keep its effects tightly controlled under normal circumstances.

A wide variety of drugs, including over-the-counter medications, drugs of abuse, and herbal products, either interfere with these homeostatic mechanisms or act as agonists at serotonin receptors (Box 3.2).

Serotonin syndrome may result from drug interactions with two or more serotonergic drugs during normal therapeutic use. The most severe cases occur with the combination of monoamine oxidase inhibitors (which inhibit the breakdown of serotonin) with selective serotonin re-uptake inhibitors (SSRIs), tricyclic antidepressants, or venlafaxine.

In the context of acute overdose, the serotonin syndrome generally occurs following overdose of antidepressants or drugs of abuse mainly.

Antidepressants
Around 15% of patients taking an overdose of SSRIs develop features of serotonin syndrome. This occurs more frequently following overdose of venlafaxine, a selective norepinephrine and serotonin inhibitor (SNRI), affecting around 30% of cases.

Drugs of abuse
Central nervous system stimulant drugs of abuse, such as amfetamines and 'ecstasy' (MDMA, 3,4-methylenedioxymethamfetamine), directly stimulate serotonin release from neuronal vesicles and frequently cause features of serotonin toxicity in overdose (see also Amfetamines and related compounds, pp. 182–183). This is seen much less commonly with overdose of methylphenidate, an amfetamine derivative used for the treatment of attention-deficit hyperactivity disorder, as it appears to be only a weak serotonin releaser.

Opioid drugs
Synthetic phenylpiperidine opioids (pethidine, tramadol, methadone, and fentanyl), dextromethorphan, and propoxyphene are weak serotonin re-uptake inhibitors and can unusually cause serotonin toxicity in overdose and when inadvertently taken with potent serotonergic drugs. Severe reactions and fatalities have been reported with pethidine, tramadol, and fentanyl.

Box 3.2 Drugs causing serotonin syndrome

- Increase in serotonin production:
  - L-tryptophan
- Inhibition of serotonin metabolism:
  - phenelzine
  - moclobemide
  - selegiline
  - methylthioninium chloride (high dose)
  - linezolid
- Increase in serotonin release:
  - amfetamines
  - methylphenidate
  - MDMA ('ecstasy')
- Inhibition of serotonin reuptake:
  - SSRI
  - tricyclic antidepressants
  - venlafaxine
  - trazodone
  - dextromethorphan
  - tramadol
  - pethidine
  - fentanyl
  - duloxetine
  - bupropion
  - sibutramine
  - St John's wort
- Serotonin receptor agonism:
  - buspirone
  - sumatriptan
  - lithium
  - LSD.

Morphine analogues (morphine, codeine, dihydrocodeine, buprenorphine) do not inhibit serotonin reuptake and do not cause serotonin toxicity.

Management

All serotonergic drugs should be immediately discontinued and supportive care instituted. Agitation or convulsions may be controlled with diazepam or lorazepam. Physical restraint should be avoided.

Cooled intravenous fluids, tepid sponging and use of fans may help in reducing the temperature. Mild cases usually resolve spontaneously within 24 hours using these measures and regular benzodiazepines.

Administration of 5-HT$_{2A}$ receptor antagonists, e.g. cyproheptadine or chlorpromazine, have anecdotally proved beneficial in moderate to severe cases, although no controlled trial evidence is available.

- Cyproheptadine adult dose: 12 mg orally, then 4–8 mg 6-hourly.
- Chlorpromazine adult dose: 12.5–25 mg IV, then 25 mg orally 6-hourly
- Dantrolene may be given although there is no evidence that it is effective in serotonin syndrome.
- Dantrolene adult dose: 1mg/kg IV over 15 minutes. Repeat doses may be given every 15 minutes to a maximum of 10 mg/kg.

If these measures fail, sedation, neuromuscular paralysis and ventilation should be undertaken. As hyperthermia is the result of excessive muscle activity, antipyretics are not useful.

Further reading

Boyer EW, Shannon M (2005). Current concepts: the serotonin syndrome. *N Engl J Med*, 352:1112–20.

Dunkley EJ, Isbister GK, Sibbritt D, et al. (2003). The Hunter Serotonin toxicity criteria: simple and accurate diagnostic decision rules for serotonin toxicity. *QJM*, 96:635–42.

Isbister GK, Bowe SJ, Dawson A, et al. (2004). Relative toxicity of selective serotonin reuptake inhibitors (SSRIs) in overdose. *J Toxicol Clin Toxicol*, 42:277–85.

Sternbach H (1991). The serotonin syndrome. *Am J Psych*, 148:705–13.

Whyte IM, Dawson AH, Buckley NA (2003). Relative toxicity of venlafaxine and selective serotonin reuptake inhibitors in overdose compared to tricyclic antidepressants. *QJM*, 96:369–74.

Malignant hyperpyrexia

Background
Malignant hyperpyrexia (hyperthermia) is a rare potentially fatal reaction occurring in susceptible patients exposed to some trigger agents such as volatile general anaesthetics or the neuromuscular blocking drug suxamethonium (succinylcholine).

It is a genetic disorder caused most commonly by mutations in the skeletal muscle ryanodine receptor type1 (RYR-1, chromosome 19q13.1) in up to 80% of affected individuals. In some patients, mutations in the *CACNA1S* gene encoding L-type voltage-gated calcium channel α-subunit have been identified. The disorder is inherited as an autosomal dominant trait with variable penetrance and the incidence of malignant hyperpyrexia is 1/10,000 to 1/50,000.

The defect results in excessive Ca^{2+} release in the sarcoplasmic reticulum and adenosine triphosphate (ATP) consumption leading to heat generation and cellular damage.

Onset of symptoms occurs within minutes to a few hours of administration of a general anaesthetic but may occur up to 12 hours postoperatively with recurrent episodes up to 24–36 hours postoperatively.

Malignant hyperpyrexia may occur despite a previous uneventful exposure to a trigger agent.

Clinical features
The systemic manifestations of malignant hyperpyrexia result from skeletal muscle hyper-metabolism.

Early signs
- *Metabolic*: elevated CO_2 production (raised end-tidal CO_2 on capnography, tachypnoea if breathing spontaneously), increased O_2 consumption (mixed venous oxygen saturation <75%), mixed metabolic and respiratory acidosis, profuse sweating, skin mottling.
- *Cardiovascular*: tachycardia, arrhythmias (especially ectopic ventricular beats and ventricular bigeminy), labile blood pressure.
- *Neurological*: masseter spasm (with succinylcholine), generalized muscle rigidity.

Later signs
- *Metabolic*: rapid increase in core body temperature, rhabdomyolysis
- *Cardiovascular*: cardiovascular collapse, cardiac arrhythmias and cardiac arrest
- *Haematological*: disseminated intravascular coagulation
- *Laboratory*: hyperkalaemia, elevated creatine kinase, myoglobinuria.

Diagnosis
The diagnosis should be considered *early* in any patient undergoing general anaesthesia who has *all* of the following features:
- unexplained, unexpected increase in end-tidal CO_2
- unexplained, unexpected tachycardia
- unexplained, unexpected increase in oxygen consumption.

Masseter muscle spasm and more generalized muscle rigidity after suxamethonium are usually self-limiting but indicate a high risk of susceptibility to malignant hyperpyrexia.

Differential diagnosis
- Malignant neuroleptic syndrome
- Serotonin syndrome
- Phaeochromocytoma
- Thyroid crisis
- Heat stroke
- Anaphylactic reaction
- Transfusion reactions
- Poisoning by amfetamines and other related drugs of abuse
- Exposure to dinitrophenol
- Baclofen withdrawal
- Infection/sepsis (e.g. meningitis, tetanus).

Management
Immediately
- Declare an emergency and call for help.
- Stop all trigger agents.
- Disconnect the vaporizer.
- Use high fresh gas flows (oxygen).
- Use a new, clean non-rebreathing circuit.
- Hyperventilate (use a minute volume 2–3 times normal) with 100% O_2 at high flow.
- Maintain anaesthesia with intravenous agents such as propofol until surgery completed.

Administer dantrolene. Give IV dantrolene 2–3 mg/kg initially (ampoules of 20 mg are mixed with 60 mL sterile water) and then 1 mg/kg. Dantrolene infusions should be repeated until the cardiac and respiratory systems stabilize. 36–50 ampoules may be needed for an adult patient. The maximum dose (10 mg/kg) may need to be exceeded.

Use active body cooling but avoid vasoconstriction. Convert active warming devices to active cooling, give cold intravenous infusions, cold peritoneal lavage, extracorporeal heat exchange

Monitoring
- Continue routine anaesthetic monitoring.
- Establish intravenous access with wide-bore cannulas.
- Consider inserting an arterial and central venous line and a urinary catheter.
- Monitor the patient for a minimum of 24 hours (ICU, HDU, or in a recovery unit) as recrudescence may occur.

The following should be monitored:
1 oxygen saturation, SpO_2
2 end-tidal CO_2
3 core and peripheral temperature
4 cardiac rhythm
5 invasive arterial BP, CVP
6 urine output
7 pH, arterial blood gases
8 potassium, creatinine
9 haematocrit, platelets, clotting
10 creatine kinase (peaks at 12–24 hours).

Check for signs of compartment syndrome.

Symptomatic treatment

Hypoxia
100% oxygen.

Hyperthermia
- 2–3 L of chilled IV 0.9% saline at 4° C.
- Surface cooling: wet, cold sheets, fans, and ice packs placed in the axillae and groin.
- Other cooling devices if available.
- Stop cooling once temperature lower than 38.5° C.

Hyperkalaemia
- Adults: 50 mL 50% dextrose with 50 IU insulin.
- Consider IV calcium chloride (if in extremis).
- Adult dose: 10 ml 10% calcium chloride.
- Dialysis may be required.
- Acidosis: Hyperventilate to normocapnoea.
- Give IV sodium bicarbonate if pH less than 7.2.

Arrhythmias
- Amiodarone: 300 mg IV for an adult (3 mg/kg).
- β-blockers (e.g. metoprolol/esmolol) if tachycardia persists.
- Calcium channel blockers should be *avoided* due to interaction with dantrolene.

Rhabdomyolysis/myoglobinuria
- Maintain urinary output >2–3 mL/kg/hour and urine pH greater than 7.0
- Fluids: IV crystalloids (e.g. 0.9% saline or lactated Ringer's solution).

Disseminated intravascular coagulation
Liaise with haematologist early. Consider administration of fresh frozen plasma, cryoprecipitate, and platelet concentrates.

Late management

- Patients should be counselled about the implications of hyperpyrexia.
- Patients with malignant hyperpyrexia (MH) or suspected of being MH-susceptible should be referred to a regional Malignant Hyperthermia Investigation Unit.

In the UK, advice can be obtained from:
The UK MH Investigation Unit
Academic Unit of Anaesthesia
Clinical Sciences Building
St James's University Hospital Trust
Leeds, LS9 7TF.
Direct line: 0113 206 5270. Fax: 0113 206 4140. Emergency Hotline: 07947 609601.

Further reading

Association of Anaesthetists of Great Britain and Ireland. *Guidelines for the management of a malignant hyperthermia crisis.* <http://www.aagbi.org/sites/default/files/MH%20guideline%20for%20web%20v2.pdf>.

Glahn KPE, Ellis FR, Halsall PJ, *et al.* (2010). Recognizing and managing a malignant hyperthermia crisis: guidelines from the european malignant hyperthermia group. *Br J Anaesth,* 105:417–20.

The anticholinergic syndrome

Background
The anticholinergic syndrome results from inhibition of muscarinic cholinergic transmission—it is perhaps more accurately described as the antimuscarinic syndrome.

Muscarinic receptors occur in the brain, on organs innervated by postganglionic parasympathetic nerves, and on sweat glands innervated by postganglionic sympathetic nerves. The anticholinergic syndrome may be predominantly peripheral, if a drug has poor CNS penetrance, or both peripheral and central, if the drug penetrates well into the CNS.

Epidemiology
Hundreds of compounds cause anticholinergic features, particularly in overdose. Many therapeutics medicines, such as antihistamines, tricyclic antidepressants, antipsychotics, and phenothiazines have 'off-target' anticholinergic effects.

The syndrome can result from overdoses of antimuscarinic antagonists such as atropine, benzatropine (not licensed for use in the UK), glycopyrronium bromide, hyoscine (scopolamine) hydrobromide, hyoscine butylbromide, and propantheline, as well as the antiparkinsonian medicines procyclidine, orphenadrine, and trihexyphenidyl (benzhexol). Glycopyrronium bromide has few central effects due to poor CNS penetration, while hyoscine hydrobromide can have severe central effects. Atropine has intermediate CNS penetration and mixed central/peripheral effects. Nefopam, a benzoxazocine often used as an analgesic in those with renal injury is an anticholinergic that may cause central anticholinergic effects at normal doses and in overdose.

Intentional ingestion of plant parts or mushrooms for hallucinogenic effects is a common cause in some localities. Plants include *Datura stramonium* (jimsonweed) and *Brugmansia* spp. (angel's trumpet) which contain tropical alkaloids such as atropine, hyoscine (scopolamine), and hyoscyamine. Mushrooms include *Amanita muscaria* which contains muscimol. Unintentional poisoning with plants of the *Mandragora* (mandrake) and *Belladonna* (deadly nightshade) genera will also cause anticholinergic features.

Anticholinergic eyedrops can cause systemic poisoning. Anti-travel sickness patches, containing hyoscine and placed behind the ear, or rubbing of eyes with hands contaminated by contact with plants, can cause ipsilateral mydriasis.

Clinical features
Peripheral effects
These include: nausea, vomiting, mydriasis, dry mouth, lack of sweating, flushing, tachycardia, paralytic ileus, and urinary retention.

Central effects
These include: agitation, confusion, tremor, ataxia, myoclonic jerking, hallucinations, psychosis, seizures, and coma.

Cardiac effects
Cardiac dysrhythmias and cardiovascular collapse occur in severe poisoning.

The combination of confusion, agitation, seizures, and lack of sweating can produce dangerous hyperthermia.

Confused patients can become highly distressed by urinary retention; their confusion often prevents them being able to localize the suprapubic pain.

Management
Ensure a clear airway, adequate ventilation, and removal of bronchial secretions.
- The benefit of gastric decontamination is uncertain. Consider activated charcoal (charcoal dose: 50 g for adults; 1 g/kg for children) only if the patient presents within 1 hour of ingestion of a potentially toxic amount.
- Administration of activated charcoal later than 1 hour post ingestion may be beneficial for sustained release (slow-/modified release) preparations; however, there is no clinical trial evidence to support this hypothesis.
- Monitor pulse, blood pressure, temperature, respiratory rate, and cardiac rhythm in symptomatic patients. Perform a 12-lead ECG.
- Observation for 6 hours after ingestion, without other specific treatments, will be sufficient for asymptomatic patients.

In more seriously poisoned patients the following measures may be required
- Consider arterial blood gas analysis in patients who have reduced conscious level (e.g. GCS <8; AVPU scale P or U) or have reduced oxygen saturations on pulse oximetry. Hypercapnia indicates the need for assisted ventilation.
- Correct hypoxia.
- Agitated adults can be sedated with oral or IV diazepam (0.1–0.3 mg/kg body weight). If ineffective, consider oral (5–10 mg) or parenteral (2–10 mg) haloperidol, 0.5–2 mg (oral or IV) initially in the elderly.

Management in children
In children, it is better to manage agitation without sedation and to carefully exclude other causes (e.g. hypoxia, infection, hypoglycaemia, and raised intracranial pressure). Consider nursing in a dark and quiet environment with a close relative present; seek expert paediatric advice. If required, for children over 3 years, buccal (3–5 years 5 mg; 5–10 years 7.5 mg; 10–16 years 10 mg) or IV (50–100 microgram/kg body weight) midazolam is generally the most appropriate drug for managing agitation and requires specialist paediatric care.
- Physostigmine can be used as an antidote for anticholinergic delirium. Retrospective studies have reported good efficacy compared to benzodiazepines but also cardiovascular complications and seizures when used in patients without severe anticholinergic features. The precise role of physostigmine is not clear. Most UK experts do not recommend use by those inexperienced in this syndrome.
- Mild hyperthermia should be treated with conventional cooling measures.
- In patients with pyrexia, monitor renal function and creatine kinase (CK) activity. Ensure adequate hydration and monitor urine output carefully.
- However, when body temperature exceeds 39.5° C, urgent cooling measures such as ice-baths and sedation (IV diazepam 10–20 mg IV in adults; 0.25 mg/kg body weight in children) should be used.

- Consider other causes as hyperthermia may be caused by conditions other than poisoning.
- Correct hypotension by raising the foot of the bed and by giving an appropriate fluid challenge. Treat brady- and tachyarrhythmias appropriately.

Children failing to respond to an appropriate intravenous fluid bolus require early discussion with the local paediatric intensive care unit (PICU).

Management in adults

- If severe hypotension persists despite the described measures, then central venous pressure monitoring should be considered. Manage in a critical care area or involve the critical care outreach team.
- When hypotension is mainly due to decreased systemic vascular resistance, vasopressors such as norepinephrine or high-dose dopamine (10–30 micrograms/kg/min) may be beneficial. The dose of vasopressor should be titrated against blood pressure. When hypotension is believed to be due to reduced cardiac output (e.g. where global hypokinesia is demonstrated on echocardiography) inotropic drugs such as dobutamine, or in severe cases epinephrine, may be beneficial.
- Single brief seizures do not require treatment. Give oxygen, check blood glucose, U&Es, and arterial blood gases. Correct acid–base and metabolic disturbances as required. If seizures are frequent or prolonged, control with intravenous diazepam (10–20 mg in adults; 0.25 mg/kg body weight in children) or lorazepam (4 mg in an adult and 0.1 mg/kg in a child).
- If unresponsive to these measures, consider phenobarbital sodium (10 mg/kg at maximum rate of 100 mg/minute; maximum dose 1 g). An alternative is phenytoin (loading dose 18 mg/kg IV infusion in adults and children, given via slow IV infusion (maximum rate 50 mg/minute) over 20–30 minutes with blood pressure and ECG monitoring). However, the use of phenytoin may worsen cardiotoxicity in the presence of sodium channel blocking agents.
- If convulsions persist, consider the need for referral to intensive care, general anaesthesia, intubation, and ventilation. There may continue to be epileptiform activity and measures to monitor and control this are necessary. Use of cerebral monitoring is therefore recommended. Thiopental is the preferred antiepileptic for status epilepticus not responding to the described measures. The role of newer agents such as propofol and levetiracetam in toxicological seizures is currently unclear because of a lack of clinical or animal studies.

If metabolic acidosis persists despite correction of hypoxia and adequate fluid resuscitation consider correction with intravenous sodium bicarbonate:

- In *adults*: an initial dose of 50 mmol (50 mL of 8.4%) sodium bicarbonate may be given and repeated as necessary, guided by arterial blood gas monitoring (aim for a pH of 7.44).
- In *children*: use 8.4% sodium bicarbonate diluted in an equal volume of 5% glucose and give a 'calculated' dose: dose (in mmol) = desired change in base deficit (current–target) × 0.3 × weight of child up to a maximum of 50 mmol. Caution is required if the solution is to be given by a peripheral venous line as it is irritant to veins and can cause local necrosis after extravasation. Administer at a rate of 1 mmol/minute.
- In both *adults* and *children*, recheck the acid–base status after administration of sodium bicarbonate. Large amounts of bicarbonate (several hundred mL) with repeated pH checking may ultimately be required to correct the metabolic acidosis. Monitor electrolytes since there is a risk of hypokalaemia and possibly hypernatraemia if substantial amounts of bicarbonate are administered.

Resist the temptation to treat arrhythmias with drugs. Arrhythmias are best treated by correction of hypoxia and acidosis.

Haemodialysis and haemoperfusion are of no value in primary therapy, but may be indicated for metabolic or renal complications.

Treat skin blisters as burns.

Further reading

Burns MJ, Linden CH, Graudins A, et al. (2000). A comparison of physostigmine and benzodiazepines for the treatment of anticholinergic poisoning. Ann Emerg Med, 35:374–81.

Krenzelok EP (2010). Aspects of Datura poisoning and treatment. Clin Toxicol, 48:104–10.

Patel RJ, Saylor T, Williams SR, et al. (2004). Prevalence of autonomic signs and symptoms in antimuscarinic drug poisonings. J Emerg Med, 26:89–94.

Vallersnes OM, Lund C, Duns AK, et al. (2009). Epidemic of poisoning caused by scopolamine disguised as Rohypnol tablets. Clin Toxicol, 47:889–93.

The opioid syndrome

Background

Opioids act on specific opioid receptors which can be classified into three main sub-types (μ, δ, κ). There is a natural endorphin system that acts via this receptor system.

In cases of poisoning, details of these sub-classifications are generally irrelevant, since toxicity depends on dose, and the μ receptor subtype is the common site of action of analgesic opioids currently in use.

Although the toxicity of opioids relates primarily to their effects on opioid receptors, some compounds, and/or their metabolites, have other pharmacological properties that may be important in poisoning.

Examples include: methadone (actions on potassium channels), dextropropoxyphene (actions on sodium channels), dextromethorphan (actions on NMDA receptors), and tramadol (actions on 5-HT receptors).

Mechanisms of toxicity

The key toxic effects of opioids are mediated by their actions on opioid receptors, centrally and peripherally. The principal risk is respiratory depression, coma, and airway obstruction leading to death from hypoxia. Other adverse effects include hypotension, delayed motility of the GI tract, in particular manifesting as delayed gastric emptying. Constipation is generally irrelevant in acute poisoning, although it may be a feature seen in opioid addicts. Delayed gastric motility may affect the speed at which opioids are absorbed from the GI tract, since absorption is minimal from the stomach. The formulation of the drug may also affect this, particularly for modified-release products. Nausea and vomiting are common adverse effects, and are more frequent in patients who are not receiving opioids regularly since tolerance develops to this adverse effect. Nausea and vomiting are due primarily to the effects of opioids on the chemotherapy receptor trigger zone, which lies outside the blood–brain barrier, and often rapidly follow intravenous doses of opioids.

A number of opioid compounds act as partial agonists (see Basic mechanisms of poisoning, pp. 4–7): buprenorphine, used primarily in management of opioid addicts in a sublingual formulation, and dihydrocodeine widely used as an analgesic, are the best examples (see Opioid analgesics, pp. 128–129).

Toxicokinetics

The route of administration of opioids is key to the speed and magnitude of their effects: opioid addicts tend to use the drugs by inhalation or intravenously to get rapid onset of effects. Nausea and vomiting, and delayed gastric emptying slow absorption in oral overdose.

Most opioids have relatively short half-lives (Table 3.8). Many opioid pharmaceutical preparations therefore modify the absorption of the opioid they contain.

In contrast, the onset of action of oral methadone is far slower than other opioids, in part because of slower systemic absorption, with a peak effect around 6 hours after administration. Codeine and dihydrocodeine are metabolized to more potent active metabolites (morphine and dihydromorphine respectively). This metabolism is polymorphic (CYP2D6), and 8% of a UK population will form little active metabolite from the parent. A smaller proportion over-expresses the enzyme and produce excess active metabolite with excess drug effect.

The duration of action of opioids relates to their rate of elimination (Table 3.8). Most are metabolized in the liver. The metabolite of morphine, morphine-6-glucuronide, is active and renally excreted, causing toxicity in renal impairment.

Opioid antagonists

Naloxone and naltrexone are pure opioid antagonists. They cause no effects given on their own in opioid-naïve individuals, but may produce withdrawal symptoms in addicts. Naltrexone is longer acting and generally used orally in the management of opioid dependency syndromes. Naloxone is used intravenously but is of much shorter action, the half-life in most individuals being between 45 and 90 minutes. This is much shorter than the half-life of opioids (Table 3.8).

Risk factors for toxicity

Drug interactions may unexpectedly increase opioid toxicity in patients on regular therapy. Drugs that inhibit the hepatic enzymes are particularly likely to produce such effects. Plasma concentration and toxicity of fentanyl is increased by erythromycin, ritonavir, and diltiazem; of methadone by ketoconazole, itraconazole, and voriconazole. The absorption of fentanyl from patches is increased by local or systemic temperature increase, producing potential

Table 3.8 Common opioid therapeutic half-lives (standard release formulations unless otherwise stated) and their important properties

Opioid	Approximate t½	Key features
Morphine	3 hours	Active metabolite morphine-6-glucuronide
Diamorphine	3 hours [morphine]	Rapidly metabolized to morphine
Codeine	3.5 hours	5–15% converted to active metabolite morphine. Polymorphic metabolism
Dihydrocodeine	3.5–4.5 hours	Partial agonist. Active metabolites, e.g. dihydromorphine. Polymorphic metabolism
Methadone	12–18 hours	Slow onset, long action
Fentanyl	2.5 minutes	Very potent, usually used transdermally
Tramadol	6 hours	Central 5-HT and noradrenergic effects; causes convulsions
Dextropropoxyphene	15 hours	Sodium channel blocker. This and active metabolite norproxyphene (t½ 27 hours) causes arrhythmias
Buprenorphine	6–40 hours	Partial agonist. slow absorption by buccal route: peak 3–4 hours after dosing

toxicity. Gradual accumulation of morphine-6-glucuronide in patients with renal impairment and the elderly may be unexpected. Co-ingestion of opioids with other CNS depressants, particularly ethanol and benzodiazepines, increases the risk of respiratory arrest and death.

Etorphine (Immobilon) is a parenteral veterinary opioid product with high potency. Its use may result in accidental or deliberate injection. The antidote diprenorphine (Revivon) is carried by vets, but high-dose naloxone is effective.

Clinical features

Pinpoint pupils, vomiting, delayed GI motility (in particular, delayed gastric emptying), respiratory depression, depression of consciousness, coma, and decreases in blood pressure and pulse rate. The principal differences in the effect of the drugs relates to the speed of onset. Route of administration determines speed of onset, the highest risk therefore being in IV drug users. Modified-release preparations, agents that undergo slow absorption, particularly methadone, and those with additional pharmacological properties (e.g. methadone, tramadol and dextropropoxyphene) require particularly careful monitoring. IV preparations act almost instantly, normal oral preparations usually have effects within 4 hours but slow-release formulations may take significantly longer, particularly if there is nausea or vomiting impairing gastric motility.

Methadone acts slowly with a peak effect at around 6–8 hours after oral dosing. It causes prolongation of the QT interval and the risk of torsade de pointes (see Opioids, pp. 194–195). Tramadol is converted to a more active opioid metabolite but also has effects on 5-HT systems and may cause convulsions (see Opioid analgesics, pp. 128–129). Dextropropoxyphene and its active metabolite norpropoxyphene are sodium channel blockers and cause QRS prolongation with risk of ventricular arrhythmia or sudden death.

Toxicity assessment

While blood and urine samples may be taken to confirm opioid ingestion, assessment is essentially clinical and based on route of administration, symptoms at presentation, and close monitoring of changes in the period after admission. History of multiple drug ingestion increases the risk of toxicity and such patients need particularly careful monitoring. Blood gas analysis may be useful to rapidly identify patients with CO_2 retention, an early marker of respiratory depression. Development of respiratory acidosis indicates the necessity for use of an antidote.

Investigations

Ensure that there is a clear airway and adequate respiration using an oximeter or blood gas analysis as necessary. Measure blood pressure, pulse rate, and respiration initially at least every 15 minutes in patients with any depression of consciousness, and perform 12-lead ECG and blood gases. Consider the risk of other medical illnesses, particularly in drug addicts, and perform appropriate screening tests, including biochemical, bacteriological, viral, and radiological.

Management

Management focuses on maintaining adequate ventilation, and in patients with significant respiratory depression use of naloxone intravenously as the antidote. If fentanyl patches are in place these should be removed. Consider activated charcoal in patients who have recently ingested a potentially toxic dose.

Observe all patients until they are fully recovered. In asymptomatic patients at least 4 hours after ingestion of standard release, and 8 hours after slow-release products or methadone. Observe 6 hours after the last administration of naloxone in intravenous or oral ingestion of normal release product, but at least 8 hours, and until asymptomatic, in those ingesting slow-release products and methadone. Observe all symptomatic patients who do not require naloxone until they are asymptomatic.

Treat hypotension with an intravenous fluid challenge after checking 12-lead ECG for arrhythmia (methadone). Hypotension will also often respond to naloxone. The management of opioid poisoning with naloxone is therefore based on the use of an appropriate dose to reverse the effect of the opioid ingested.

The initial dose of naloxone should be titrated to the patient's response, a starting dose of 400 micrograms slowly intravenously, followed by subsequent further doses usually initially to a maximum of 2 mg, at which point the diagnosis should be reviewed. Unusually large doses may be required for very significant opioid overdose, or for partial agonists and some patients may receive several milligrams of naloxone. In patients who have taken long-acting opioids repeat doses or a naloxone infusion may be required. An infusion of approximately 60% of the dose required to wake the patient per hour is sufficient to maintain most patients physiologically stable. Large volume dilution is not required (naloxone may be given in a pump with low volume dilution). As the patient recovers the dose should be reduced. Intramuscular naloxone is less rapidly absorbed and has a less predictable action.

It is important to monitor patients carefully since naloxone reverses the effect of opioids on the gut and there may be an increase in absorption of orally ingested agent with unexpected increases in opioid effects. For modified-release agents and methadone careful monitoring for several hours after the start of the infusion is needed to ensure that appropriate levels of reversal are achieved.

Do not use excess naloxone, as this will precipitate opioid withdrawal in addicts. If patients become agitated or distressed following naloxone this may be managed by a small dose of diazepam, but beware of precipitating respiratory depression.

Use of naloxone in patients who wish to self-discharge following opioid overdose in an attempt to protect them from sudden collapse is very unlikely to protect in slow-release products, mixed drug, or methadone ingestion.

Remember in drug addicts to check injection sites and provide general health warnings following recovery (see Introduction to problems of the drug abuser, pp. 180–181 and Opioids, pp. 194–195). Some agencies offer 'take-home' naloxone.

Further reading

Goldfrank L, Weisman RS, Errick JK, et al. (1986). A dosing nomogram for continuous infusion of intravenous naloxone. Ann Emerg Med, 15:566–70.

Melandri R, Re G, Lanzarini C, et al. (1996). Myocardial damage and rhabdomyolysis associated with prolonged hypoxic coma following opiate overdose. J Toxicol Clin Toxicol, 34:199–203.

Webster LR, Cochella S, Dasgupta N, et al. (2011). An analysis of the root causes for opioid-related overdose deaths in the United States. Pain Med, 12(Suppl 2):S26–35.

The stimulant syndrome

Background

The stimulant toxidrome is also sometimes referred to as the sympathomimetic toxidrome. It comprises a series of symptoms and signs—commonly dilated pupils, psychomotor agitation, tachycardia, and hypertension—related to increased activity of sympathetic neurotransmitters, in particular norepinephrine but also dopamine and serotonin.

Substances leading to the stimulant toxidrome

Recreational drugs

- Amfetamines including substituted amfetamines (amfetamine analogues) such as 3,4-methlyene-dioxymethamfetmaine (MDMA, 'ecstasy'), 3,4-methylenedioxy-N-ethylamfetamine (MDEA), (N-methyl-1-(3,4-methylenedioxyphenyl)-2-aminobutane (MBDB), paramethoxyamfetamine (PMA), para-metoxymethamfetamine (PMMA), 2,5-dimethoxy-4-chloroamfetamine (DOC) and methamfetamine
- Cocaine and synthetic cocaines such as fluorotropcaine and dimethocaine
- Synthetic piperazines such as 1-benzylpiperazine and meta-chlorophenylpiperazine
- Synthetic cathinones such as mephedrone (4-methylmethcathinone), methedrone, methylone, butylone, felphedrone, fluoromethcathinone and methylenedioxypyrovlaerone
- Other stimulant recreational drugs such as the pipradrols (e.g. diphenylprolinol (D2PM), desoxypirpradrol (2DPMP), the benzodifurans (e.g. bromo-DragonFLY) and the susbstiued pyrovalerones (e.g. naphthylpyrovalerone).

Pharmaceutical drugs

- Ephedrine, psudoephedrine
- Epinephrine, norepinephrine
- Dextroamfetamine
- Methylphenidate and ethylphenidate
- Phentermine
- Salbutamol and other β_2 agonists
- Theophylline, caffeine.

Clinical features

The common symptoms and signs that are seen in the stimulant toxidrome are:

- Central nervous system excitation: anxiety, psychomotor agitation, anxiety, delusions, paranoia, hallucinations and delusions
- Sweating
- Dilated pupils
- Tachycardia, palpitations
- Hypertension
- Bruxism (grinding of the jaws and teeth)
- Hypertonia, hyper-reflexia, tremor.

Hypokalaemia, hyperglycaemia, and a metabolic acidosis may also be seen in patients with a stimulant toxidrome (see Amfetamines and related recreational drugs, pp. 182–183 and Psychedelic agents, pp. 192–193).

Complications

The severe features and complications seen and the likelihood of these developing depend on the substance causing the stimulant toxidrome. As an example chest pain, acute coronary syndrome, and broad complex (ventricular) tachyarrhythmias are more commonly seen in individuals with acute cocaine toxicity; hyperpyrexia and serotonin toxicity (sometimes referred to as serotonin syndrome) are more common in individuals with acute MDMA (ecstasy) toxicity. Potential complications include:

- seizures
- chest pain (angina), acute coronary syndrome, and myocardial infarction
- arrhythmias: narrow complex tachycardias and more rarely ventricular tachycardia
- aortic dissection
- stroke—related to intracerebral haemorrhage and/or infarction
- mesenteric ischaemia
- hyperthermia: severe hyperthermia can be associated with significant secondary complications including rhabdomyolysis, disseminated intravascular coagulation, acute kidney injury and acute liver dysfunction.

Differential diagnosis

Toxicological

The anticholinergic toxidrome can present with clinical features that are similar to the stimulant toxidrome. However, features that are seen in the anticholinergic toxidrome that are not seen in the stimulant toxidrome include dry skin, urinary retention, and decreased bowel sounds; also the psychomotor agitation, tachycardia, and hypertension that are seen in patients with an anticholinergic toxidrome are usually less severe than that in the stimulant toxidrome (see The anticholinergic syndrome, pp. 83–84).

Other toxicological differential diagnoses for the stimulant toxidrome include neuroleptic malignant syndrome, (see Malignant hyperpyrexia, pp. 81–82) serotonin toxicity (see The serotonin syndrome, pp. 79–80) strychnine poisoning, and monoamine oxidase inhibitor poisoning (see Antidepressants, pp. 100–103).

Drug and/or alcohol withdrawal

The clinical features of drug and alcohol withdrawal can be difficult to differentiate from a stimulant toxidrome because many of the features seen in withdrawal are due to adrenergic excess. However, patients with drug and alcohol withdrawal generally have a more marked tremor and the psychomotor agitation is usually less severe. Management of drug and alcohol withdrawal is discussed in Drug and alcohol withdrawal, pp. 46–47.

Medical

Phaeochromocytoma and thyrotoxicosis can present with clinical features similar to those seen in the stimulant toxidrome.

Management

For specific management related to each of the substances that can cause the stimulant toxidrome and management of severe complications of the stimulant toxidrome readers should refer to the section covering each substance or group of substances.

Key management points

- Reduce central nervous stimulation by non-specific treatment; usually benzodiazepines titrated to response.
- Manage fluid balance, acidosis, and systemic complications, e.g. tachycardia, hypertension, rhabdomyolysis, hyperpyrexia, and convulsions.

The mainstay of management of the stimulant toxidrome is to decrease the significant central nervous system and psychomotor agitation associated with the toxidrome. The fever this excess muscle activity causes is associated with inadequate cooling and results in hyperpyrexia, muscle injury with rhabdomyolysis, seizures, metabolic acidosis and severe cardiovascular disturbance.

It is important that patients are managed in a quiet environment with minimal stimulation. Sedatives such as benzodiazepines are often required. In mild cases these should be given in small doses (e.g. oral diazepam (0.1–0.3 mg/kg body weight)) titrated against the patient's agitation. Patients with significant psychomotor agitation may require parenteral benzodiazepines in the first instance, and large doses (e.g. 1–2 mg/kg diazepam slowly in severe cases). Neuroleptics such as haloperidol should generally only be used as second-line agents as they can lower the seizure threshold.

In patients with seizures it is important to ensure adequate oxygenation, check the blood glucose, and correct acid–base abnormalities. Seizures should initially be treated with benzodiazepines, intravenous diazepam (10–20 mg in adults; 0.25 mg/kg body weight in children), or lorazepam (4 mg in an adult and 0.1 mg/kg in a child). Seizures that are resistant to treatment with benzodiazepines should be managed with intravenous phenobarbital sodium (10 mg/kg at maximum rate of 100 mg/minute; maximum dose 1 g).

Common cardiovascular features such as tachycardia and hypertension often settle with benzodiazepines. Beta-blockers have been controversial as they can theoretically result in unopposed alpha-stimulation and worsening hypertension and coronary artery vasoconstriction. Recent case series suggest that drugs labetalol are, however, relatively safe. Patients with ongoing severe hypertension (e.g. systolic BP > 200 mmHg, diastolic BP > 120–140 mmHg) despite sedation with benzodiazepines may require treatment with vasodilators such as nitrates (e.g. intravenous glyceryl trinitrate, starting at 1–2 mg/hour) or alpha-blockers (e.g. phentolamine, phenoxybenzamine), or labetalol (50 mg by slow IV injection)

Hyperthermia should be treated aggressively as persistent hyperpyrexia (temperature greater than 39–40° C) is associated with a poor prognosis and a high incidence of secondary complications. The management of recreational drug related hyperpyrexia is detailed within the sections detailing with individual drugs/drug classes. However, general management initially involves simple, conventional cooling methods (e.g. cold intravenous fluids, ice packs), together with benzodiazepine sedation. Patients with persistent pyrexia greater than 39–40° C should be discussed with a clinical toxicologist or poisons centre and further measures such as invasive cooling, dantrolene, or serotonin-specific agents such as cyproheptadine may be considered. Case reports also suggest benefit from chlorpromazine or atypical antipsychotics that act as antagonists on 5-HT receptors.

Further reading

Cregler LL, Mark H (1986). Medical complications of cocaine abuse. *N Engl J Med*, 315:1495–500.

Knuepfer MM (2003). Cardiovascular disorders associated with cocaine use: myths and truths. *Pharmacol Ther*, 97:181–222.

McCord J, Jneid H, Hollander JE, et al. (2008). Management of cocaine-associated chest pain and myocardial infarction: a scientific statement from the American Heart Association Acute Cardiac Care Committee of the Council on Clinical Cardiology. *Circulation*, 117:1897–907.

Schep LJ, Slaughter RJ, Beasley DM (2010). The clinical toxicology of metamfetamine. *Clin Toxicol*, 48:675–94.

Wood DM, Greene SL, Dargan PI (2011). Clinical pattern of toxicity associated with the novel synthetic cathinone mephedrone. *Emerg Med J*, 28:280–2.

Delirium (acute confusional state)

Background
ICD-10 defines delirium as:

An etiologically nonspecific organic cerebral syndrome characterized by concurrent disturbances of consciousness and attention, perception, thinking, memory, psychomotor behaviour, emotion, and the sleep-wake schedule. The duration is variable and the degree of severity ranges from mild to very severe.

The syndrome of delirium is characterized by:
1 Disorder of attention. This is the hallmark of the disorder. The presence of inattention may be variable and may be accompanied by disturbance in arousal, although arousal may also be normal. Commonly this is referred to as 'clouding of consciousness' (see later in section). Attention is commonly measured as forward (7±2) or reverse digit span. Other examples of tests of attention are simply WORLD backwards, serial sevens, or months of the year backwards, the latter has the advantage that is unlikely to be affected by educational level.
2 Acute or subacute (gradual over a period of days) onset.
3 Fluctuating course. This is not usually volunteered by the patient and is, along with the first two features, an important differentiating factor. It must therefore be actively enquired about when taking the third-party history (e.g. from nurse or relative) Patients present with intermittent lucid periods or with sleep–wake cycle reversal (being more somnolent during the day, with agitated, often hallucinated and wakeful periods overnight).
4 Other impairments of cognitive function tend to accompany the disorder of attention. Usually the patient is disorientated, more so for time than place (may be normal in a lucid phase). It is important to also ask about passage of time, the patient who suffers even from moderate levels of dementia, usually retains the innate awareness of passage of time. However, the patient who has been delirious will often volunteer a vastly abnormal account of same. There may also be cognitive perceptual deficits present.

Clouding of consciousness
This state reflects a change in alertness and arousal that is qualitatively different to that one would normally expect. Commonly this is taken to mean decreased arousal and awareness of one's environment, on a continuum from barely perceptible dulling of awareness to coma. A substantial minority of patients present with hyper-arousal and hyper-alertness. In both cases the defining characteristic is a disorder of attention (be that phasic, directed, divided, or modulated). In practice this reflects the inability to respond in a planned and appropriate manner to changes in the environment. In the former group of patients there is reduced attention with a somewhat drowsy state. In the latter group, there is a hyper alertness but loss of the ability to direct, divide, or modulate attention in an appropriate manner.

Other terms used to describe the disorder are: acute or subacute:-
• brain syndrome
• confusional state (non-alcoholic)
• infective psychosis

• organic reaction
• psycho-organic syndrome.

Delirium types
Dependent on the predominant state of arousal patients can be defined as suffering from *hypoactive* (decreased arousal), *hyperactive* (increased arousal), or *mixed* delirium (alternating states of hypo- and hyper-arousal), the latter being the commoner.

Along with any of these types the patient may experience hallucinations (commonly visual or tactile) or illusions which commonly are frightening. Alternatively the quiescent delirious patient may actually find these amusing! There may be secondary delusions of persecution.

Delirium in the context of the toxicology patient
This may be precipitated by acute intoxication or withdrawal from substances.

These patients fall broadly speaking into three groups
1 Substance-induced delirium, due to recreational use or intentional overdose. Recreational drugs commonly used include any combination of amfetamines, cocaine, heroin, gamma-hydroxybutyric acid (GHB), benzodiazepines or drugs commonly referred to as 'legal highs' (see relevant sections in Chapter 8, p. 181).

The patient may present with a cluster of psychotic phenomena characterized by hallucinations (typically visual, but often in more than one sensory modality), perceptual distortions, delusions (often of a paranoid or persecutory nature), psychomotor disturbances (excitement or stupor), and an abnormal affect, which may range from intense fear to ecstasy. Where there is significant impairment of attention, consciousness, and disorientation this presentation takes on the form of a delirium. Without this the presentation may be classified as a drug-induced psychosis. Usually the delirium resolves as the intoxication ends or within hours to days thereafter.

2 Substance withdrawal delirium, commonly due to alcohol withdrawal (delirium tremens) or increasingly, withdrawal from GBL/GHB, features of which may not differ qualitatively from substance-induced delirium. Other drugs associated with this include benzodiazepine withdrawal. Commonly this is preceded by a dependence syndrome. This is treated by prescription of adequate amounts of initially benzodiazepine (typically those with a medium length half-life such as diazepam or chlordiazepoxide) but also an antipsychotic such as haloperidol (chosen for its low anticholinergic side effects) if an adjuvant is needed.

In the case of GHB withdrawal clinical experience has shown regular prescription of baclofen (a GABA_B agonist) significantly reduces the severity of the delirium and the need for high doses of benzodiazepine/antipsychotic (see also Gamma-hydroxybutyrate and related compounds, pp. 188–189).

3 Delirium secondary to accidental or intentional overdose in a patient with pre-existing cognitive impairment. In the presence of pre-existing cognitive impairment the degree of insult (i.e. the amount of substance ingested in these individuals) can be quite small and still result in delirium. Psychotropic medications, (particularly with sedative properties), opioids,

or drugs with anticholinergic side effects (e.g. nefopam) are particularly implicated.

In the delirious patient it is impossible to accurately assess premorbid cognitive ability which is particularly important in an elderly patient in predicting prognosis.

A well-validated and useful tool used to diagnose delirium is a diagnostic algorithm such as the Confusion Assessment Method (sensitivity: 94–100%; specificity 90–95%). It uses four changes. The first change is an acute onset and fluctuating course with evidence of an acute change in mental status from the patient's baseline. Fluctuating (abnormal) behaviour often fluctuates during the day (tending to come and go, or increase and decrease in severity). The second change is when the patient has difficulty in focusing attention (e.g. being easily distractible) or having difficulty keeping track of what was being said. The third change is when the patient's thinking becomes disorganized or incoherent: such as rambling or irrelevant conversation, unclear or illogical flow of ideas, or unpredictable switching from subject to subject. The fourth change is an altered level of consciousness in the patient: score positive for any answer other than 'alert'. The diagnosis of delirium should be considered if the first and second change, and either the third or fourth change are present.

Dementia

In practice, the commoner differential diagnosis may be that of dementia (Table 3.9).

The IQCODE is an instrument that that has high reliability, sensitivity and specificity in diagnosing pre-existing cognitive decline, performs at least as well at screening as conventional cognitive screening tests.

Depression

A common problem is in determining whether patients presenting with a hypoactive delirium are, in fact, depressed. There may in fact be an underlying depressive illness, but this may be difficult to diagnose in the delirious patient. Again, third-party history is invaluable in this regard. Key features of depression are: insidious onset (commonly over a period of weeks to months); Normal consciousness; normal sleep onset sleep but early morning wakening (>2 hours before normal); pervasive low mood;

Table 3.9 Features differentiating delirium and dementia

Delirium	Dementia
Acute onset	Gradual onset
Altered consciousness	Normal alertness
Altered sleep–wake cycle	Normal sleep pattern ('sundowning')
Variability in presentation	Stable through day or worse in evening
Emotional lability and distress	Settled apart from aimless wandering or searching
Visual hallucinations	Hallucinations less common
	Poverty of mood commoner

emotional lability and distress; auditory hallucinations. This can be compared with features of delirium in Table 3.8.

Psychosis

Patients present with an acute, or insidious onset of a cluster of psychotic phenomena, typically including auditory hallucinations, illusions, delusions, psychomotor disturbances (excitement or stupor), and an abnormal affect, which may range from intense fear to ecstasy or indeed may be inappropriate to the situation. Consciousness is usually clear and orientation normal.

Risk factors

The greatest risk factor for delirium is pre-existing cognitive impairment, thereafter age along with multiple medical co-morbidities, multiple medications, and serious illness all contribute to increasing a patient's vulnerability whereby the addition of certain medications may precipitate delirium. Further, where cognitive impairment is less overt, identification of executive dysfunction or depression appears to be more predictive then memory tests per say. Substances which may cause delirium through intoxication or withdrawal can also be any of detailed in Delirium types (previous page), although obviously in much greater doses then would be needed in someone already at risk.

Treatment and outcomes

If there is a known toxic precipitant, or delirium forms part of a withdrawal syndrome, then treatment should be directed at the primary cause. In persons without previous cognitive impairment or other risk factors for delirium, generally one finds that the delirium resolves once the causal factor has been treated or within days to 1–2 weeks of same at most. The prognosis for those with ongoing risk factors and/or pre-existing cognitive impairment varies following treatment of the causal agent. It is also worth noting that in a significant proportion of this group the causal agent may not be found. A recent systematic review of the literature concluded that there is likely a link between delirium and long-term cognitive impairment.

Further reading

Brown LJ, McGrory S, McLaren L, et al. (2009). Cognitive visual perceptual deficits in patients with delirium. *JNNP*, 80:594–9.

Greene NH, Attix DK, Weldon BC, et al. (2009). Measures of executive function and depression identify patients at risk for postoperative delirium. *Anesthesiology*, 110:788–95.

Hall JB, Schweickert W, Kress JP (2009). Role of analgesics, sedatives, neuromuscular blockers, and delirium. *Crit Care Med*, 37(Suppl): S416–21.

Inouye SK (2000). Prevention of delirium in hospitalised patients: risk factors and targeted intervention strategies. *Ann Med*, 32:257–63.

Jorm AF (2004). The Informant Questionnaire on cognitive decline in the elderly (IQCODE): a review. *Int Psychogeriatr*, 16:275–93.

MacLullich AM, Beaglehole A, Hall RJ, et al. (2009). Delirium and long term cognitive impairment. *Int Rev Psychiatry*, 21:30–42.

Smith PJ, Attix DK, Weldon BC, et al. (2009). Executive function and depression as independent risk factors for postoperative delirium. *Anesthesiology*, 110:781–7.

Convulsions

Definition

There are numerous definitions of a 'convulsion'. Put simply, a convulsion is where the body muscles contract and relax rapidly and repeatedly, resulting in an uncontrolled shaking of the body. It should be noted that a convulsion is not the same as an epileptic seizure, since not all epileptic seizures result in a similar clinical condition.

Convulsions may be single and self-limiting or may be prolonged or repetitive in nature. Status epilepticus is the term used to refer to convulsive activity that is defined as either: (1) ongoing for longer than 15 minutes; or (2) more than two convulsive episodes without the regaining of consciousness in between. True status epilepticus in toxicological exposure is uncommon; examples of where it is more likely to occur is in association with exposure to theophylline and water hemlock (*Cicuta maculata*).

Drugs, chemicals, and other toxins associated with convulsions

A wide range of drugs, chemicals, and plants can be associated with the development of convulsions (Table 3.10). It should be noted that the convulsion may be a result of direct toxicity or may be secondary to a metabolic complication of the exposure. A summary follows of some common agents that are associated with convulsions on exposure. It should be noted that this list is not exhaustive and complete, and there may be other agents not listed that are associated with convulsions. Where an agent is known to be associated with the potential to cause convulsions, this will be mentioned in the clinical features subsection of individual sections later in this text book.

Table 3.10 Agents that may cause convulsions

Classification	Examples
Metals	Lead, arsenic, manganese, copper, lithium
Plants and plant material	Water hemlock (*Cicuta maculata*), nicotine, jimson weed
Recreational drugs	Amfetamine, cocaine, cathinones, piperazines, pipradrols, MDMA (3,4-methylenedioxymethamfetamine), gamma-hydroxybutyrate (GHB) and related analogues, phencyclidine
Pharmaceuticals	NSAIDs (particularly mefenamic acid), bupropion, phenytoin, digoxin, theophylline, lidocaine (lignocaine), chloroquine, carbamazepine, anti-histamines, salicylates, tramadol, tricyclic antidepressants, isoniazid, phenothiazines, SSRIs and similar antidepressants (particularly venlafaxine), olanzapine, clozapine, haloperidol
Household and/or industrial products	Caffeine, camphor oil, methanol, ethylene glycol, phenol, strychnine, cyanide
Environmental and/or accidental agents	Carbon monoxide, cyanide, hydrogen sulphide, helium, nitrous oxide, hydrocarbons (e.g. toluene, butane)
Pesticides	Organophosphates, pyrethrins, carbamates

Complications of convulsions

There are a number of potential complications that can occur in relation to a convulsion.

- There is a risk that during a convulsion, an individual may cause significant and/or permanent injury to themselves (e.g. intracranial haemorrhage secondary to head trauma during the convulsion).
- Convulsion in a patient who is vomiting increases the risk of aspiration and associated pneumonitis.
- Prolonged convulsions, whether sustained or repetitive, can be associated with a reduction in oxygen supply to the brain and other organs. In particular, this could lead to significant cerebral ischaemia and long-term neurological complications. Additionally, the cerebral ischaemia may in its own right perpetuate the convulsions.
- Prolonged sustained convulsions can lead to significant muscle injury, rhabdomyolysis, and associated acute kidney injury. The increased muscular activity associated with convulsions can lead to hyperthermia as a result of increased muscular heat production.
- Finally, metabolic acidosis is a common feature of convulsions, whether one-off or sustained, and is a result not only of the convulsion itself, but also the resultant tissue hypoxia that occurs during convulsion.

Differential diagnosis for the cause of convulsions

It is important that when assessing an individual who has had a convulsion which is thought to be drug related, that you also consider other reasons why the convulsion may have occurred. With drugs such as ethanol, gamma-hydroxybutyrate (GHB) and gamma-butyrolactone (GBL), which are associated with a physical dependency syndrome, cessation of use of the drug(s) involved may result in an individual suffering one or more convulsions as part of the withdrawal syndrome.

Other underlying medical conditions, such as meningitis and encephalitis, may not only cause convulsions but also may have other clinical features that may be misinterpreted as being drug related (e.g. pyrexia, tachycardia, confusion). There is also the possibility that an individual may have suffered either a head injury (secondary to a collapse or an intracranial event) that may be the precipitant for the convulsion.

Finally, the agent or agents that an individual has been exposed to may not in their own right be associated with convulsions, but they may cause metabolic disturbances that could lead to a convulsion. An example of this would be an insulin overdose causing profound hypoglycaemia and resultant convulsions.

Management of toxicity-related convulsions

Where convulsions occur or where there is the suspicion that they may occur, it is important that the potential for harm to the individual during the convulsion is minimized. If appropriate, the individual should be removed from ongoing exposure to the agent or agents that are thought to have precipitated the convulsion.

During a convulsion, where possible, supplemental oxygen should be administered to the patient. The use of airway adjuncts should not be used, as there is a risk of trauma to the patient and/or the healthcare professional during their insertion (but can be considered when the convulsion has ceased if appropriate).

Following a short, self-terminating seizure, there is no indication for the routine administration of an anti-convulsant. It is important that other non-toxicological causes for the convulsion are excluded and/or treated (see earlier in section). For example, where the convulsion is thought to be secondary to opioid toxicity and associated hypoxia, it would be appropriate to administer naloxone to reverse the opioid toxicity.

For those individuals with repetitive or ongoing convulsions, it is appropriate to consider the use of an anticonvulsant to control to convulsion. First-line treatment is with the use of a benzodiazepine.

These can be administered intravenously (route of choice if access available) intramuscularly, or rectally (slowest onset of effect), depending on the availability of an appropriate route. While there is probably no difference between the different benzodiazepines in management of poisoning-induced convulsions if equivalent doses are used, their stocking and availability is usually based on their use for non-drug-related convulsions. There is some logic to using a longer-acting benzodiazepine in this situation in an attempt to reduce the risk of further convulsions. For this reason diazepam (initially 10 mg intravenously in an adult) or lorazepam tends to be the drug of choice. There is a risk of respiratory depression and the patient's airway needs to be protected once the seizure has ceased.

Whilst phenytoin is often used as a second-line agent in the management of convulsions, it should be used with caution when it is suspected that the reason for the convulsion is drug related. It has sodium channel antagonist activity, which means that potentially it can increase the risk of cardiac toxicity if an individual is having a convulsion secondary to a drug known to block cardiac sodium channels (the resultant risk is potential worsening of QRS prolongation and the precipitation of a broad-complex tachycardia). An example of this would be an individual who presents with a cocaine-related convulsion, where both phenytoin and cocaine block cardiac sodium channels.

Therefore, in the situation of toxicity-related convulsions, often second-line treatment is with a barbiturate. In those who fail to respond to both benzodiazepines and barbiturates, then paralysis and ventilation should be considered. However, it is important to note that whilst this may treat the external features of the convulsion, there is the potential that there is ongoing 'cerebral convulsive activity'. Therefore where an individual is paralysed, continuous EEG monitoring should be undertaken and any underlying convulsive activity should be treated appropriately.

In some exposures there may be specific treatment warranted to reduce the toxicity related to the exposure and therefore treat the convulsion or prevent their recurrence. Examples of this would be pyridoxine for isoniazid toxicity, and pralidoxime for organophosphate exposure.

It is important that once the convulsive activity is controlled, that the individual's core body temperature is measured. Where this is elevated, either secondary to drug toxicity that precipitated the convulsion or as a result of prolonged convulsive activity, this should be managed accordingly (the management of hyperpyrexia is discussed in Malignant hyperpyrexia, pp. 81–82).

Finally, it is important that once the convulsion is controlled, that an appropriate history and examination is undertaken. This should look for evidence of other harm related to the agent or agents that an individual has been exposed to, as well as looking for complications related to the convulsion itself.

Further reading

Brust JC (2008). Seizures, illicit drugs, and ethanol. *Curr Neurol Neurosci Rep*, 8:333–8.

Ruffmann C, Bogliun G, Beghi E (2006). Epileptogenic drugs: a systematic review. *Expert Rev Neurother*, 6:575–89.

Shah AS, Eddleston M (2010). Should phenytoin or barbiturates be used as second-line anticonvulsant therapy for toxicological seizures? *Clin Toxicol*, 48:800–5.

Bleeding disorders

Background

Control of bleeding is complex and involves both clotting factors, platelets, and clot breakdown. Clotting disorders therefore involve excess haemorrhage, or increased clotting. Clinical toxicologists normally encounter excess bleeding, due to clotting factor deficiency, low platelet count, consumptive coagulopathy, or increased clot breakdown. Drugs may also cause a lesion, e.g. peptic ulceration, from which bleeding is a complication. Consultations regarding bleeding possibly related to poisoning therefore require a diagnostic approach and management based on an understanding of the potential mechanisms involved (Table 3.11). The detailed approach to specific agents is dealt with in Antithrombotic drugs, pp. 154–157; Coumarin rodenticides, pp. 311–312; and Common venomous snakes, pp. 332–333. This section will concentrate on the principles guiding initial diagnosis, assessment, and management.

Clotting dysfunction occurs in patients with impaired clotting factor synthesis in acute hepatic dysfunction, as in paracetamol or amanita toxicity, or in chronic severe liver disease.

Drugs reducing clotting for therapeutic purposes normally interfere with the clotting cascades or with platelet function (see Antithrombotic drugs, pp. 154–155). Prescription drugs that have anticoagulant properties include:

- heparins: synthetic and low molecular weight
- inhibitors of vitamin K, coumarins, and phenindiones
- derivatives of snake venoms, such as hirudin
- drugs targeted at specific clotting factors: e.g. dabigatran etexilate, a direct thrombin inhibitor, and apixaban and rivaroxaban, direct inhibitors of activated factor X (factor Xa).

All anticoagulants may cause devastating effects if there is uncontrolled bleeding into the CNS or gut.

Anticoagulants, particularly coumarins, are also used as rodenticides, and very long-acting agents are available; anticoagulant effects may last many months.

Table 3.11 Toxic causes of coagulation disorder

Physiological change	Potential toxins
Clotting factor synthesis deficiency	Coumarins, rodenticides, toxin-induced hepatic failure (e.g. paracetamol, amanita toxin)
Clotting factor function impairment	Heparins, specific factor inhibitors, hirudin.
Thrombocytopenia	Cytotoxics, antifolate drugs (e.g. methotrexate, co-trimoxazole), radiation, drug-induced immune thrombocytopenia (e.g. quinine)
Platelet function impairment	Anti-platelet drugs (NB this very rarely causes active bleeding unless there is another cause, e.g. peptic ulcer, varices, etc.)
Consumption coagulopathy	Snake bite, sepsis
Excess thrombolysis	Thrombolytics

Mechanisms of toxicity

Drugs that cause bleeding acutely affect some aspect of the coagulation system, and this will depend on their mode of action. Readers are referred to individual sections (see Antithrombotic drugs, pp. 154–157; Coumarin rodenticides, pp. 311–312) for more details.

Coumarins

These interfere with the action of vitamin K in synthesizing clotting factors II, VII, IX, and X by acting as inhibitors of vitamin K 2,3-epoxide-reductase in the liver. Effects are generally maximal 48–72 hours after a single overdose. Bleeding is more commonly seen during therapeutic use, where it may be a problem in as many as 10% of patients on therapy a year. Warfarin is very susceptible to drug metabolism interactions, and enzyme inhibitors increase the risk of bleeding within 24–48 hours of commencement.

Heparins

Heparins are given IV or, in the case of low-molecular-weight compounds, subcutaneously. Medication error is the commonest cause of bleeding, either by acute overdose or failure to monitor during IV dosing (see Antithrombotic drugs, pp. 154–155).

Snake peptides

Snake peptides such as hirudin irreversibly block thrombin, and have no natural inhibitors. Derivatives of hirudin have been developed and used therapeutically. This is rarely seen as a clinical cause as it is rarely used. Bleeding following snake bites are much commoner worldwide, and there will be a history or evidence of bite puncture in such cases (see Common venomous snakes, pp. 332–333).

Platelet inhibitors

These rarely cause spontaneous bleeding, although aspirin and NSAIDs (see Salicylates, pp. 124–127; Non-steroidal anti-inflammatory drugs, pp. 122–123) may cause upper GI ulceration. At therapeutic dose other clotting mechanisms are relatively unaffected.

Bleeding may occur in patients with *reduced platelet count*, a complication of drugs that inhibit folate metabolism and cytotoxics. Thrombocytopenia may also occur as a drug-induced autoimmune disorder, e.g. quinine. This can be a very dramatic presentation and follow very small amounts of quinine in a soft drink such as tonic water.

Thrombolytic products

Thrombolytic products are given parenterally, are generally relatively short-acting but medication errors may cause devastating effects if there is bleeding into the CNS or gut.

Toxicokinetics

Readers are referred to Antithrombotic drugs, pp. 154–157, for full details of the kinetics of warfarin and heparin. Warfarin undergoes hepatic metabolism. Unfractionated heparin is renally cleared after metabolism, but small heparin molecules are active, and contribute to therapeutic effects in not excreted.

Warfarin is used orally and most commonly presents due to excess effect during therapy. A single ingestion may also occur. In the former case precipitants include medication interactions due to effects on drug metabolism, either prescription of an inhibitor of warfarin metabolism, or stopping prescription of a long-term inducing agent. Maximal effect from such changes normally takes 2 or 3 days. Dietary change may also precipitate bleeding if vitamin K is lacking in the diet.

Heparin normally has a short half-life and action, if given in single excess dose IV due to medication error, only lasts a few hours. The anticoagulant hirudin is also a clotting factor antagonist.

Thrombolytic enzymes such as streptokinase are metabolized in the liver and have short half-lives of hours.

Risk factors for toxicity

Risk of bleeding is increased in the elderly and in patients with underlying clotting abnormalities, either hereditary or acquired, most commonly liver disease, and by presence of potential bleeding sites, e.g. peptic ulcer, oesophageal varices. Drug interactions are common with oral anticoagulants, and caution is required whenever new therapies are given to patients on these agents. As vitamin K is present in food, dietary change, starvation, or illness also affect warfarin sensitivity. Failure to attend routine monitoring, and risk of falls in the elderly, are reasons to reconsider use of warfarin.

Heparin is renally excreted, and accumulates in renal failure. This can be monitored by measuring the activated partial thromboplastin time (APTT). Low-molecular-weight heparins (LMWHs) do not affect this measurement at therapeutic doses and are normally dosed weight-related, adjusted for renal function. Renal impairment is a risk factor for bleeding with unfractionated and LMWH.

Renal impairment is also a major risk factor for bleeding with dabigatran etexilate, apixaban, and rivaroxaban. These drugs should also be avoided in liver disease.

Clinical features

The clinical features of bleeding depend on the site and extent of blood loss. Loss in the gastrointestinal tract may initially be occult, with patients presenting with collapse due to acute hypotension from unsuspected blood loss. Rectal, renal tract, and nasal bleeds are more obvious. Bleeding may present as catastrophic haemorrhage, but may also be fatal if intracerebral. Clues that indicate a toxic cause include drug history, or skin features of purpura, or bleeding following minor trauma.

Toxicity assessment

Assessment includes measurement of the effects of blood loss, including blood pressure, conscious level, and pulse rate, together with tests of coagulation. These need to be performed serially. National guidelines exist for managing prolongation of INR due to warfarin overdose in patients receiving the drug therapeutically, because of the difficulties in re-establishing warfarin in patients who have had large doses of vitamin K. In those not normally on warfarin, results will indicate a need for therapy but not precisely guide it (see Antithrombotic drugs, pp. 154–157).

Investigations

Assess blood loss by measuring blood pressure and pulse rate. Establish degree of anticoagulation by use of appropriate laboratory tests, INR for warfarin, APTT for heparin, platelet count, and platelet function tests if an anti-platelet drug is suspected. Measure full blood count, U&Es, and LFTs, the latter to exclude hepatic injury. If there is no clear history blood samples should be obtained for further laboratory analysis, for example, for specific anticoagulants (e.g. warfarin, rodenticides) or clotting factor assays (discuss with a haematologist prior to sampling for advice).

Management

Management depends on the extent of bleeding. Many patients on warfarin present to emergency departments from primary care only with abnormal blood tests. In this situation monitor pulse, blood pressure, and urine output and observe for features suggesting overt or occult bleeding. Transfusion and resuscitation is only needed in active bleeding while reversing anticoagulation is invoked. Readers are referred to the relevant sections for details (see Antithrombotic drugs, pp. 154–157; Coumarin rodenticides, pp. 311–312; and Common venomous snakes, pp. 332–333). Brief details of principles follow:

Warfarin and other vitamin K antagonists

Management depends on whether patients are receiving warfarin therapeutically. In all cases measure the INR at presentation, and monitor further as necessary (see Antithrombotic drugs, pp. 154–157). Vitamin K_1 is the natural antidote to warfarin and other coumarins, but if given in large excess to patients on warfarin will cause problems with subsequent anticoagulation control. National guidelines on management have been drawn up to address this.

Heparin

Monitor pulse, blood pressure, and urine output and observe for features suggesting overt or occult bleeding. Measure APTT, full blood count, U&Es, and LFTs. If the APTT is prolonged and there is no sign of bleeding, no further treatment is required. Monitor APTT every 6 hours until it is within the therapeutic range. If there is evidence of haemorrhage or very large amounts of heparin have been injected, consider administration of protamine sulfate after discussion with local haematologists. Protamine is itself an anticoagulant so care is needed in dosage.

Thrombocytopenia

This should be treated conventionally, and if drug induced the offending agent stopped.

Excess thrombolysis

Excess thrombolysis is not readily amenable to therapy. The agent should be stopped and patients treated as indicated by clinical complications.

Specific factor antagonists are being developed as an alternative to warfarin. Effective antidotes for these agents are not yet available, but are in development. They do not appear to be reversed by administration of clotting factors.

Further reading

British Society of Haematology (2011). Guidelines on Oral Anticoagulation with Warfarin, 4th edition. *Br J Haematol*, 154:311–24.

Berny P, Velardo J, Pulce C, D'amico A, Kammerer M, Lasseur R (2010). Prevalence of anticoagulant rodenticide poisoning in humans and animals in France and substances involved. *Clinical Toxicology*, 48:935–41.

Cruickshank J, Ragg M, Eddey D (2001). Warfarin toxicity in the emergency department: recommendations for management. *Emerg Med*, 13:91–7.

Kandrotas RJ (1992). Heparin pharmacokinetics and pharmacodynamics. *Clin Pharmacokinet*, 22:359–74.

Scottish Intercollegiate Guidelines Network (SIGN) (2008). *Management of Upper and Lower GI Bleeding*. Edinburgh: SIGN. <http://www.sign.ac.uk/pdf/sign105.pdf>

Chapter 4

CNS drugs

Anticonvulsants

Background
Anticonvulsants are widely prescribed for treatment of epilepsy, but some are also increasingly used as mood stabilizers in patients with psychiatric disease or for treatment of neuropathic pain.

Toxicity may occur as a result of acute overdose or due to chronic accumulation resulting from excessive dosing or drug interactions.

Generally, phenytoin and carbamazepine have greater toxicity in overdose than sodium valproate and the newer anticonvulsants, though case reports confirm that severe toxicity can occur uncommonly with the newer agents.

Phenobarbital is discussed in Other hypnotics, pp. 110–111.

Carbamazepine
Carbamazepine is an anticonvulsant widely used to treat generalized tonic–clonic or partial seizures and neuropathic pain (e.g. trigeminal neuralgia) and for prophylaxis in bipolar disorder.

Toxicokinetics
Standard-release preparations may have delayed absorption, with peak concentrations occurring 6–24 hours after ingestion, although more rapid absorption occurs with syrups or chewable tablets. Modified-release preparations are associated with further delay in absorption. The primary route of elimination is via hepatic metabolism (CYP3A4) with carbamazepine-10,11-epoxide the principal metabolite, which is responsible for some of the adverse effects of carbamazepine during therapeutic dosing. Carbamazepine has a half-life of 30–40 hours in treatment naïve patients, but this is shortened to 16–24 hours in those receiving chronic therapy as a result of auto-induction of metabolism. The epoxide metabolite has a half-life of about 6 hours.

Clinical features
In overdose, carbamazepine causes dry mouth, sinus tachycardia, ileus, nystagmus, ataxia, incoordination, coma which may be cyclical, convulsions which may be refractory, severe hypotension, and less commonly respiratory depression and arrest. The pupils are often dilated, a divergent strabismus may be present, and complete external ophthalmoplegia has been reported. QRS and QTc prolongation are observed occasionally in severe cases. Hallucinations may occur, particularly during recovery.

The ingestion of a modified-release formulation may result in delay in the onset of features and peak plasma carbamazepine concentrations; in one case, some 96 hours from the time of ingestion.

Investigations
An ECG should be performed. Blood glucose, U&Es, and arterial blood gases should be considered in patients with clinical evidence of toxicity.

Urgent measurement of plasma carbamazepine concentration is not required in asymptomatic patients, but is indicated when oral multiple-dose activated charcoal (MDAC) is being considered or if there is doubt about the diagnosis in patients with coma, respiratory depression, or arrhythmias. There is a good correlation between plasma carbamazepine concentrations and severity of poisoning. The usual therapeutic range is 4–12 mg/L (17–50 micromol/L) and serious complications are unusual at concentrations less than 25 mg/L (105 micromol/L). Life-threatening toxicity is associated with concentrations greater than 40 mg/L (168 micromol/L). Non-urgent measurement of carbamazepine concentrations during the recovery phase helps to time the re-introduction of carbamazepine therapy.

Management
A single dose of activated charcoal 50–100 g within 1 hour of ingestion substantially reduces absorption and should be administered to adults or children ingesting an overdose greater than 20 mg/kg, provided the airway can be protected.

The BP, pulse, respiratory rate, conscious level, and cardiac rhythm should be monitored and hypoxia and hypotension corrected. Metabolic acidosis that persists in spite of correction of hypoxia and administration of intravenous fluids may require correction with sodium bicarbonate.

Single self-terminating convulsions do not require treatment but frequent or prolonged convulsions should be controlled using intravenous diazepam (10–20 mg (0.1–0.3 mg/kg body weight) in adults; 0.1–0.3 mg/kg body weight in children) or lorazepam (4 mg in an adult and 0.05 mg/kg in a child). Give oxygen and correct acid–base and metabolic disturbances as required. Phenytoin (20 mg/kg by IV infusion in adults and children) should be considered in refractory cases.

Asymptomatic patients should be observed for a minimum of 6 hours (non-sustained-release preparations) or 12 hours (sustained-release preparations). If CNS features have not developed by this time they are unlikely to do so subsequently.

Enhanced elimination techniques
MDAC increases the elimination of carbamazepine significantly. The mean (±SD) clearance using this method was 113±44 mL/min in one study. MDAC should therefore be given in severe cases of carbamazepine poisoning in an initial dose of 50–100 g for adults, with repeated doses of 12.5 g/hour (or the equivalent 2- or 4-hourly).

The overall clearance during charcoal haemoperfusion in one study was only 28.8 mL/min due to cartridge saturation.

High efficiency haemodialysis may be useful but there is limited clinical experience available.

Oxcarbazepine
Oxcarbazepine is a keto-analogue of carbamazepine. It is indicated for partial seizures with or without secondarily generalization, either as monotherapy or adjunctive therapy.

Toxicokinetics
It is a pro–drug which is metabolized to the active metabolite 10-hydroxycarbazepine with a half-life of 1–5 hours. This metabolite is responsible for the drugs therapeutic effects and has a half-life of 7–20 hours.

Clinical features and management
Experience of overdose is limited but effects appear similar to those of carbamazepine and include nausea, vomiting, dizziness, ataxia, nystagmus, diplopia, tinnitus, vertigo, drowsiness, hyponatraemia, convulsions, bradycardia, and hypotension.

Management is as for carbamazepine poisoning. Activated charcoal may be considered in those ingesting greater than 40 mg/kg or more than their total daily dose (whichever is the larger) within 1 hour. Oxcarbazepine elimination is enhanced by MDAC in healthy volunteers, but clinical value in overdose is uncertain.

Phenytoin

Phenytoin is an antiepileptic and class 1b anti-arrhythmic agent. Toxicity is common during normal therapeutic use because of its low therapeutic index and the complex pharmacokinetic properties of phenytoin, including inter-individual variability and susceptibility to drug interactions. Because of this, and the high rate of unacceptable adverse effects such as gum hypertrophy, hirsutism, and acne, use has been declining.

Parenteral phenytoin preparations contain propylene glycol as a diluent and this may be associated with cardiovascular effects after rapid intravenous administration.

Fosphenytoin is a soluble prodrug of phenytoin, administered by IV or IM injection. It is converted to phenytoin in vivo (half-life of phenytoin formation 15 minutes). Toxicity is as for phenytoin, but preparations do not contain propylene glycol and cardiovascular toxicity after parenteral use may therefore be less likely.

Toxicokinetics

After oral use, absorption is slow and variable, with delayed time to peak concentration associated with higher therapeutic doses. Phenytoin is hydroxylated in the liver by CYP2C9 and CYP2C19. These processes are saturable at higher phenytoin concentrations within the therapeutic range, resulting in zero-order elimination. As a result, half-life in therapeutic dose ranges from 7–42 hours, but absorption and elimination are often prolonged in overdose, with elimination half-life between 24 and 230 hours.

Clinical features

Toxicity may occur with doses greater than 20 mg/kg phenytoin and may include nystagmus, dysarthria, cerebellar ataxia (which may be persistent), drowsiness, coma and, rarely, hypoglycaemia. Hallucinations and facial dyskinesia have been reported. Chronic high concentrations of phenytoin may lead to cerebellar atrophy.

Cardiovascular toxicity, including bradycardia, hypotension, and arrhythmias, may occur after rapid intravenous administration but are rare after oral ingestion.

Investigations

General investigations should be performed as for carbamazepine poisoning. Measurement of plasma phenytoin concentration is not generally necessary but may be helpful to confirm the diagnosis if MDAC is being contemplated. The usual therapeutic range for phenytoin is 10–20 mg/L (40–79 micromol/L). Symptomatic toxicity is usually associated with concentrations greater than 20 mg/L (79 micromol/L), while concentrations greater than 40 mg/L (159 micromol/L) are associated with serious toxicity.

Management

Asymptomatic patients should be observed for at least 4 hours. Agitation may require treatment with a benzodiazepine.

A single dose of activated charcoal (50–100 g) reduces phenytoin absorption if administered within 1 hour of ingestion and there is some evidence that multiple doses of activated charcoal increase phenytoin elimination. Haemodialysis may also be of benefit.

Sodium valproate

Sodium valproate is used to treat generalized and partial epilepsy, as a mood stabilizing agent in bipolar disorder, and in the management of migraine and chronic pain syndromes.

Toxicokinetics

It is available in standard and modified-release preparations, with time to peak plasma concentrations 1–2 hours and 3–8 hours respectively. The major route of elimination is via hepatic metabolism. Valproate taken in therapeutic doses has an elimination half-life of 8–14 hours, but this may be increased to more than 20 hours in overdose. Active metabolites may also contribute to prolonged toxicity.

Clinical features

Clinical manifestations of poisoning may occur with doses greater than 200 mg/kg and vary in severity from gastrointestinal disturbances and drowsiness to coma and death. In a multicentre series involving 133 cases with valproate concentrations greater than 100 mg/L, coma was present in 19 (15%) cases; all had plasma concentrations above 850 mg/L. Apart from central nervous system depression, fever, sinus tachycardia, muscle spasms, hypothermia, seizures, cardiovascular instability, hepatotoxicity, and thrombocytopenia have been observed. Cerebral oedema is uncommon, but has been seen following both acute and chronic overdose. Hypernatraemia, hypocalcaemia, hyperammonaemia, hyperosmolarity, and high anion gap metabolic acidosis may complicate the clinical picture.

Investigations

U&Es, blood glucose, LFTs, and amylase should be arranged, together with arterial blood gases and ammonia in severely poisoned patients.

Urgent measurement of valproate concentration is only usually necessary if haemodialysis is being considered or when there is doubt about the diagnosis. Serum valproate concentrations generally correlate with clinical features of poisoning, with those greater than 850 mg/L more likely to be associated with coma, respiratory depression, hypotension or metabolic acidosis. Concentrations encountered in therapeutic use are usually in the range 50–100 mg/L (350–700 micromol/L).

Management

Supportive measures, including correction of electrolyte and metabolic abnormalities, are the mainstay. The value of gut decontamination is unproven. Hypotension and convulsions should be managed conventionally, as for carbamazepine.

Some experimental and clinical data suggest that early intravenous supplementation with L-carnitine could improve survival in severe valproate-induced hepatotoxicity. Carnitine administration has been shown to speed the decrease of ammonaemia in patients with valproate-induced encephalopathy, although a correlation between ammonia concentrations and clinical condition was not always observed. As it does not appear to be harmful, L-carnitine is commonly recommended in severe poisoning, especially in children, although the clinical benefit in terms of liver protection or hastening of recovery from unconsciousness has not been established. A suggested regimen is a loading dose of 100 mg/kg IV over 30 minutes (maximum 6 g) followed by maintenance doses of 15 mg/kg IV every 4 hours.

Extracorporeal methods of elimination should be considered in patients with features of severe poisoning (coma or haemodynamic compromise) and plasma valproate concentration greater than 850 mg/L, particularly if severe hyperammonaemia and electrolyte and acid–base disturbances are present. Case reports suggest that haemodialysis decreases the elimination half-life of valproate to around 2 hours from approximately 30 hours following overdose. Continuous veno-venous haemofiltration and continuous veno-venous haemodiafiltration do not appear to be as effective as haemodialysis.

Gabapentin

Gabapentin is an anticonvulsant used to treat focal seizures with or without secondary generalization. It is also used for the management of chronic neuropathic pain and occasionally for migraine prophylaxis.

Toxicokinetics

After a therapeutic dose taken orally, maximum concentrations occur in 2–3 hours. The half-life is 5–7 hours.

Clinical features and management

Only a small number of cases of poisoning have been reported and most patients have developed few features even though they have often ingested other drugs. Ingestion of up to 90 g caused only gastrointestinal symptoms (vomiting and mild diarrhoea), transient drowsiness, dizziness, slurred speech, and ataxia. Many of the more severe cases involved patients with renal impairment, which is not surprising given that the kidney is the major route of gabapentin elimination.

Management is supportive, including observation for at least 6 hours after ingestion, with monitoring of conscious level, pulse, BP, and oxygen saturation. Haemodialysis is unlikely to be helpful.

Pregabalin

Pregabalin is a GABA analogue structurally related to gabapentin. It is used as adjunctive therapy in adults with partial seizures with or without secondary generalization, as a treatment for neuropathic pain and for generalized anxiety disorder.

Toxicokinetics

After ingestion, peak plasma concentrations occur within 1 hour (fasted) or 2.5 hours (with food). The drug is almost entirely excreted unchanged in the urine with a half-life of about 6 hours, which is prolonged in people with renal impairment. Development of renal failure may precipitate toxicity in patients taking chronic pregabalin therapy.

Clinical features and management

Experience of overdose is limited. CNS depression and myoclonus have been reported.

Management is primarily supportive. Activated charcoal (50 g for adults, 1 g/kg for children) may be considered for those presenting within 1 hour of ingesting doses greater than 25 mg/kg. Asymptomatic patients should be observed for at least 6 hours after overdose, monitoring conscious level. For symptomatic patients the pulse, blood pressure and oxygen saturation should be monitored and U&Es, creatinine, LFTs, and CK checked.

Haemodialysis may be effective in enhancing pregabalin elimination, but is unlikely to be required unless there is renal failure.

Lamotrigine

Lamotrigine is used for focal or generalized tonic–clonic seizures, occasionally for typical absence seizures in children and in the treatment of bipolar disorder.

Toxicokinetics

After ingestion of a therapeutic dose, peak concentrations occur in about 2.5 hours. The half-life in therapeutic use is 22–36 hours and has been reported to range between 10 hours and 19.5 hours after overdose.

Clinical features

Lethargy, ataxia, nystagmus, coma, seizures, cardiac conduction abnormalities (QRS prolongation and complete heart block), respiratory arrest and multi-organ failure have been reported.

A 32-year-old woman ingested lamotrigine 4.5 g and developed ataxia and rotational nystagmus but recovered over 48 hours. A 2-year-old developed generalized tonic–clonic seizure activity, tremor of limbs, muscle weakness, ataxia, and hypertonia after ingestion of 16 × 50 mg tablets. Symptoms resolved within 24 hours.

At least one patient has died after lamotrigine overdose.

Management

General management is supportive. Asymptomatic patients should be observed for at least 4 hours. Pulse, blood pressure, U&Es, and cardiac rhythm should be monitored in symptomatic patients.

Multiple doses of activated charcoal have been shown in volunteers to increase the elimination of lamotrigine in therapeutic doses. Clinical utility for overdose is uncertain.

Levetiracetam

Levetiracetam is used as adjunctive treatment for partial onset seizures with or without secondary generalization.

Toxicokinetics

Absorption is rapid with peak plasma concentration occurring 1.3 hours after ingestion. The elimination half-life of levetiracetam is about 7 hours and 95% is excreted unchanged in the urine.

Clinical features and management

Lethargy, vomiting, blurred vision, ataxia, coma, and respiratory depression have been observed. A 38-year-old woman who ingested 60 × 500 mg tablets presented with a GCS of 8 and recovered over 24–48 hours.

Management is supportive. Asymptomatic patients should be observed for at least 4 hours after overdose.

Tiagabine

Tiagabine is used as second-line adjunctive therapy for partial-onset seizures with or without secondary generalization.

Toxicokinetics

During therapeutic use peak plasma concentrations occur about 2.5 hours after ingestion. Elimination is via hepatic metabolism, with a half-life of 7–9 hours.

Clinical features and management

Lethargy, facial grimacing, nystagmus, posturing, agitation, confusion, coma, hallucinations, and seizures have been reported. Patients may be mute and withdrawn. The minimum dose reported to cause seizures is 96 mg.

After ingesting tiagabine 1500 mg, a 44-year-old woman suffered vomiting, hypersalivation, generalized rigidity, myoclonus, bradycardia, hypertension, and coma within 2 hours. Coma lasted until 10 hours. Recovery was complete by 26 hours. A 2-year-old girl weighing 13 kg suffered two generalized tonic–clonic seizures about 1.5 and 3.5 hours after ingesting 90 mg. A 14-year-old girl with no previous history of epilepsy developed status epilepticus following ingestion of up to 180 mg tiagabine. Management is supportive.

Topiramate

Topiramate is used as monotherapy or adjunctive treatment for partial seizures, with or without secondary generalization, primary generalized tonic–clonic seizures, and sometimes for migraine prophylaxis.

Toxicokinetics

It is rapidly absorbed, with peak concentrations occurring 2–3 hours after ingestion. Although subject to some hepatic metabolism, the major route of elimination is renal. The mean elimination half-life is approximately 21 hours.

Clinical features and management

Lethargy, ataxia, nystagmus, myoclonus, coma, seizures, and a non-anion gap metabolic acidosis have been observed; the latter may be due to inhibition of renal cortical carbonic anhydrase. Metabolic acidosis can appear within hours of ingestion and persist for days. A 33-month-old girl who ingested an unknown quantity of topiramate suffered visual hallucinations, slurred speech and severe ataxia; features resolved after 6 days.

Management is supportive. Activated charcoal (50 g for adults, 1 g/kg for children) may be considered if a patient presents within 1 hour of ingesting more than 20 mg/kg topiramate. Asymptomatic patients should be observed for at least 4 hours after overdose. Although topiramate is effectively removed by haemodialysis, this is unlikely to be required.

Zonisamide

Zonisamide is indicated as monotherapy or adjunctive treatment for adults with partial seizures, with or without secondary generalization.

Toxicokinetics

Peak plasma concentrations occur 2–5 hours after ingestion. It is metabolized in the liver but some parent drug is also excreted in the urine. Elimination is prolonged, with a mean half-life of about 60 hours.

Clinical features and management

There is very limited experience of zonisamide in overdose. The manufacturer reports features as somnolence, nausea, gastritis, nystagmus, myoclonus, bradycardia, hypotension, impaired renal function, and respiratory depression. Status epilepticus, cerebral oedema, and death have been reported.

Activated charcoal (50 g for adults, 1 g/kg for children) may be considered for patients presenting within 1 hour of ingesting more than 25 mg/kg zonisamide. Asymptomatic patients should be observed for at least 8 hours after overdose, monitoring conscious level, BP, pulse, temperature and cardiac rhythm. Management is otherwise supportive,

Further reading

Barrueto Jr F, Williams K, Howland MA, et al. (2002). A case of levetiracetam (Keppra) poisoning with clinical and toxicokinetic data. J Toxicol Clin Toxicol, 40:881–4.

Boldy DAR, Heath A, Ruddock S, et al. (1987). Activated charcoal for carbamazepine poisoning. Lancet, 1:1027.

Brandt C, Elsner H, Furatsch N, et al. (2010). Topiramate overdose: a case report of a patient with extremely high topiramate serum concentrations and nonconvulsive status epilepticus. Epilepsia, 51:1090–3.

Briassoulis G, Kalabalikis P, Tamiolaki M, et al. (1998). Lamotrigine childhood overdose. Pediatr Neurol, 19:239–42.

Buckley NA, Whyte IM, Dawson AH (1993). Self-poisoning with lamotrigine. Lancet, 342:1552–3.

Fakhoury T, Murray L, Seger D, McLean M, Abou-Khalil B. (2002). Topiramate overdose: clinical and laboratory features. Epilepsy Behav, 3:185–9.

Farrar HC, Herold DA, Reed MD (1993). Acute valproic acid intoxication: enhanced drug clearance with oral-activated charcoal. Crit Care Med, 21:299–301.

Fischer JH, Barr AN, Rogers SL, et al. (1994). Lack of serious toxicity following gabapentin overdose. Neurology, 44:982–3.

French LK, Mckeown NJ, Hendrickson RG (2011). Complete heart block and death following lamotrigine overdose. Clin Toxicol, 49:330–3.

Graudins A, Peden G, Dowsett RP (2002). Massive overdose with controlled release carbamazepine resulting in delayed peak serum concentrations and life-threatening toxicity. Emerg Med, 14:89–94.

Hojer J, Malmlund H-O, Berg A (1993). Clinical features in 28 consecutive cases of laboratory confirmed massive poisoning with carbamazepine alone. J Toxicol Clin Toxicol, 31:449–58.

Isbister GK, Balit CR, Whyte IM, et al. (2003). Valproate overdose: a comparative cohort study of self poisonings. Br J Clin Pharmacol, 55:398–404.

Kazzi ZN, Jones CC, Morgan BW (2006). Seizures in a paediatric patient with a tiagabine overdose. J Med Toxicol, 2:160–2.

Keranen T, Sorri A, Moilanen E, et al. (2010). Effects of charcoal on the absorption and elimination of the antiepileptic drugs lamotrigine and oxcarbazepine. Arzneimittelforschung, 60:421–6.

Khoo SH, Leyland MJ (1992). Cerebral edema following acute sodium valproate overdose. J Toxicol Clin Toxicol, 30: 209–14.

Klein-Schwartz W, Shepherd JG, Gorman S, et al. (2003). Characterization of gabapentin overdose using a poison center case series. J Toxicol Clin Toxicol, 41:11–5.

Larsen JR, Larsen LS (1989). Clinical features and management of poisoning due to phenytoin. Med Toxicol Adverse Drug Exp, 4:229–45.

Lee CH, Li JY (2008). Phenytoin intoxication and upper facial dyskinesia: an unusual presentation. Mov Disord 2008; 23:1188–9.

Lheureux PER, Hantson P (2009). Carnitine in the treatment of valproic acid induced toxicity. Clin Toxicol, 47: 101–11.

Lin G, Lawrence R (2006). Pediatric case report of topiramate toxicity. Clin Toxicol, 44:67–9.

Lofton AL, Klein-Schwartz W (2005). Evaluation of toxicity of topiramate exposures reported to poison centers. Hum Exp Toxicol, 24:591–5.

Lynch MJ, Pizon AF, Siam MG, et al. (2010). Clinical effects and toxicokinetic evaluation following massive topiramate ingestion. J Med Toxicol, 6:135–8.

O'Donnell J, Bateman DN (2000). Lamotrigine overdose in an adult. J Toxicol Clin Toxicol, 38:659–60.

Spiller HA, Krenzelok EP, Klein-Schwartz W, et al. (2000). Multicenter case series of valproic acid ingestion: serum concentrations and toxicity. J Toxicol Clin Toxicol, 38:755–60.

Spiller HA, Winter ML, Ryan M, et al. (2005). Retrospective evaluation of tiagabine overdose. Clin Toxicol, 43:855–9.

Sztajnkrycer MD (2002). Valproic acid toxicity: overview and management. J Toxicol Clin Toxicol, 40:789–801.

Thanacoody RHK (2009). Extracorporeal elimination in acute valproic acid poisoning. Clin Toxicol, 47:609–16.

Thundiyil JG, Anderson IB, Stewart PJ, et al. (2007). Lamotrigine-induced seizures in a child: case report and literature review. Clin Toxicol, 45:169–72.

Traub SJ, Howland MA, Hoffman RS (2003). Acute topiramate toxicity. J Toxicol Clin Toxicol, 41:987–90.

Verma A, St Clair EW, Radtke RA (1999). A case of sustained massive gabapentin overdose without serious side effects. Ther Drug Monit, 21:615–17.

Antidepressants

Background

Antidepressants are commonly taken in overdose, in part because of the disorders they are used to treat. They may be classified into four principal groups, all of which affect amine function in central neurons: tricyclic (and related) antidepressants and selective reuptake inhibitors increase postsynaptic quantities of monoamines (norepinephrine, serotonin, and dopamine) by preventing the normal reuptake of the amines, which terminates their biological activity. Presynaptic alpha-blockers affect the presynaptic autoreceptor which normally terminates amine release. Monoamine oxidase inhibitors (MAOIs) prevent breakdown of monoamines in the presynaptic terminal, increasing the quantities being released following a nerve impulse. The toxicity of these drugs depends in part on these actions, but also on the other pharmacological properties the individual compounds possess.

Antidepressant drugs differ in their relative toxicities. The most hazardous are MAOIs and tricyclics. Citalopram and venlafaxine are the most toxic of the more specific re-uptake inhibitors. Mirtazapine is the least toxic.

Tricyclic and related compounds

Although usually superseded by selective serotonin reuptake inhibitors (SSRIs) as first choice therapies for depression, tricyclic antidepressants (TCAs) are commonly prescribed as second-line agents and for other indications, e.g. chronic pain. Examples include amitriptyline, amoxapine (not licensed for use in the UK), clomipramine, dosulepin (dothiepin), doxepin, imipramine, lofepramine, nortriptyline, protriptyline, and trimipramine.

Mechanisms of toxicity

TCAs produce their therapeutic effects by blocking the uptake of monoamines in adrenergic or serotonergic nerve endings in the brain. Many first-generation TCAs also have other pharmacological properties which cause major effects in overdose. Antihistaminergic and anticholinergic effects cause sedation which may be severe enough to cause respiratory depression and acidosis.

Blockade of sodium influx channels in the myocardial membrane delays conduction velocity resulting in QRS prolongation and arrhythmias and possibly convulsions. The binding of TCAs to the sodium channel is pH dependent, and acidosis increases the degree of blockade. This explains why arrhythmias become more frequent in the presence of acidosis, and complications such as convulsions that cause acidosis result in arrhythmias, particularly ventricular tachycardias and fibrillation. Alpha-adrenoceptor antagonism causes vasodilation and secondary hypotension.

Cardiac arrhythmias and convulsions are the usual cause of death, but reduced conscious level and hypoxaemia with acidosis also contributes to arrhythmia and convulsion risk.

Within the tricyclics, dosulepin appears to have the greatest incidence of fits and arrhythmias, while lofepramine, which is converted to the active metabolite imipramine, is the least hazardous.

Toxicokinetics

TCAs may have delayed absorption after overdose. Most achieve peak concentrations within 6 hours of ingestion at therapeutic doses. The majority are very lipid-soluble and are metabolized in the liver, some to active metabolites which contribute to therapeutic effects or toxicity (Table 4.1).

There is little evidence of a close relationship between individual plasma concentration measurements of TCAs and their clinical effects in overdose and no clinical value in measuring these.

Clinical features

Features of TCA poisoning usually appear within 4 hours of overdose and initially comprise anticholinergic (dry mouth, blurred vision, sinus tachycardia, and drowsiness) and antihistaminergic effects (drowsiness). Depending on the dose ingested and speed of absorption, CNS and cardiovascular features may evolve at different rates and in different ways. Effects in more severe cases include:

CNS: pyramidal signs (brisk reflexes and extensor plantar responses, coma, convulsions, respiratory depression.

Cardiovascular: hypotension, ECG abnormalities (prolongation of the QRS interval and other intraventricular conduction disturbances), ventricular tachycardia, and ventricular fibrillation.

A cycle of clinical complications may develop in severe poisoning. Hypoxia and acidosis from respiratory depression increases the risk of sodium channel blockade induced arrhythmias. Arrhythmias may worsen acidosis (respiratory and metabolic) and hypotension may provoke reduced cerebral perfusion, increasing further the risk of convulsions. Hypokalaemia and renal and/or hepatic impairment may also occur.

During the recovery phase, agitation and psychosis may occur, probably due to prolonged anticholinergic effects, especially after substantial overdoses. Typical features include incoherent speech and plucking at the bedclothes. Urinary retention may also occur.

Table 4.1 Half-lives ($t\frac{1}{2}$) and potentially toxic doses of common antidepressants in various groups, and their active metabolites ([ ]) where applicable

Drug	Approximate $t\frac{1}{2}$ (hours)	Potentially toxic dose (mg/kg)
Amitriptyline	10–50	3
Dosulepin	11–40	3
Imipramine	9–20	4
Lofepramine	5	15
Citalopram	36	3
Escitalopram	27–33	1.5
Fluoxetine	24–96	6
[Norfluoxetine]	>150	
Paroxetine	12–18	3
Sertraline	26	7
Duloxetine	18	5
Venlafaxine	5–15	7
[Desmethylvenlafaxine]	[11–15]	
Mirtazapine	20–40	5
Mianserin	44	4
Trazodone	5–9	20

Toxicity assessment

The dose ingested is a key indicator of likely toxicity and the level of consciousness is in excellent marker of severity of poisoning. Convulsions and arrhythmias are unlikely in patients who are fully conscious, or have a GCS above 8. QRS intervals are a very useful marker of the degree of sodium channel blockade and correlate with the risk of arrhythmia and convulsions. QRS durations of greater than 160 ms are extremely dangerous, and those above 120 ms should be monitored very carefully. A Brugada syndrome pattern (seen in leads V1–3) is also sometimes seen. ECG monitors are not appropriate for measuring or monitoring cardiac conduction abnormalities and 12-lead ECGs must be performed if there is deterioration in the physiological or clinical status of the patient. Automated ECG machines automatically correct QT duration for heart rate change as QT is affected by heart rate under normal physiological circumstances. The machine nomograms are dependent on the shape of the T-wave and may be inaccurate in patients with poisoning. Automated measurements are a useful alerting signal for the clinician, but should not replace manual measurement. Nomograms have been published from case series of patients with torsade, which may be useful for comparison in this situation (see Cardiovascular toxicity, pp. 64–67).

Investigations

Blood pressure, pulse, temperature, conscious level, and cardiac rhythm, including a 12-lead ECG, should be assessed in all patients, together with U&Es, creatinine, and liver function tests. Urine output and renal function should be monitored carefully. Pulse oximetry may be useful in patients with any depression of consciousness. Blood gas analysis should be used to assess degree of acidosis in those with suspected respiratory depression or ECG abnormalities and to guide treatment with sodium bicarbonate.

The frequency of repeat physiological monitoring is dependent upon the degree of sedation as this is a marker of overall toxicity. Rapid reduction in consciousness within a few hours of overdose indicates severe poisoning.

Management

Management is determined by the clinical features; its objectives are to pre-empt potential toxicity by interventions to reduce the risk of cardiac arrhythmia predicted by ECG changes. Active treatment of complications such as arrhythmia and convulsions is mandatory.

The anticholinergic effects of TCAs delay gastric emptying and hence the opportunity for use of activated charcoal to reduce absorption may be longer; this should be considered in patients presenting within 1 to 2 hours of a potentially serious overdose (see Table 4.1). It is vital that the patient is able to protect their own airway and in comatose patients intubation is necessary if this procedure is being contemplated. Gastric lavage is potentially hazardous and may wash the tricyclic into the duodenum, leading to more rapid drug absorption and increased toxicity.

Patients with severe tricyclic poisoning require careful supportive management. Acid–base balance should be monitored and acidosis (which increases the risk of cardiac arrhythmias) should be corrected.

Arrhythmias

Arrhythmias are uncommon in patients who are conscious, and risk decreases with time; arrhythmias are unlikely to arise *de novo* more than 12 hours after overdose.

Prolongation of the QRS interval (e.g. >120 ms) is an indication for prophylactic sodium bicarbonate, aiming to achieve a pH of 7.5. An initial bolus dose of 50 mmol sodium bicarbonate is indicated, with repeat monitoring of 12-lead ECG, plasma potassium, and arterial pH and the dose titrated as required. Use of an 8.4% solution is generally recommended to achieve the rapid change in pH required, but extravasation may produce local tissue damage. If arrhythmias occur they should also be managed with bolus doses of 8.4% sodium bicarbonate, which may abolish arrhythmias, even in those without acidosis. Unless cardiac output is significantly compromised in spite of pH correction, anti-arrhythmic drugs are not used because they have negative inotropic and membrane effects, which may aggravate toxic myocardial effects.

TCAs may prolong the QT interval, a risk factor for torsade de pointes. Specific treatment includes intravenous magnesium sulfate (e.g. 8 mmol over 30–120 seconds), which may be repeated. Hypoxaemia, electrolyte disturbance, and acidosis should also be corrected. If these measures fail the arrhythmia may respond to atrial or ventricular pacing to increase the heart rate to 90 to 110 beats per minute. Isoproterenol by infusion may also be used if pacing is not possible. Classical antiarrhythmic drugs do not normally reduce risk of torsade, and some further prolong the QT interval.

Hypotension

Hypotension may be due to direct myocardial toxicity, for example sodium channel blockade, or to peripheral vasodilation, a particular feature of TCAs due to their alpha-adrenoceptor blocking actions. Patients with hypotension who do not respond to a fluid challenge should be managed in a high dependency area. The predominant cause should be identified and rectified if possible. Thus inotropes are used in myocardial depression and vasoconstrictors such as the alpha agonist phenylephrine may be used for vasodilation.

In patients who have suffered a cardiac arrest secondary to antidepressant poisoning, prolonged cardiopulmonary resuscitation is indicated and full recoveries have been documented after resuscitation over several hours.

CNS complications

Depression of consciousness may result in hypoxaemia. Protection of the airway is extremely important; serious poisoning is a common reason for intubation and ventilation.

Convulsions should be controlled with intravenous diazepam or lorazepam, although there is a risk of respiratory depression and patients may require subsequent ventilation. Acidosis and hypoxia should be corrected after a seizure to reduce the risk of arrhythmia. If patients are paralysed, appropriate EEG cerebral monitoring should be instituted to detect continuing electrical activity as left untreated this may cause brain damage.

Hyperthermia is also reported and may require cooling measures.

In the recovery phase, many patients become acutely disturbed, probably due to anticholinergic delirium and may need sedation; a long-acting benzodiazepine (e.g. diazepam) is normally effective.

Antidotes

Since a primary action of tricyclic antidepressants is that of an anticholinergic, the anticholinesterase physostigmine is used by some for the management of the CNS depression caused by tricyclic poisoning. CNS depression is generally short-lived in mild poisoning, and is a useful marker of more severe poisoning. European clinical toxicologists do not therefore advocate this antidote.

Sodium bicarbonate is a specific antidote for tricyclic antidepressant effects on sodium channels in the myocardium (as mentioned earlier).

Intravenous lipid emulsion® therapy may have a role in managing patients with resistant arrhythmia or hypotension where it sometimes appears to rapidly reduce toxic drug effects on the myocardium, possibly by redistribution of active compound or by intracellular actions including on the mitochondria. Its role is yet to be fully determined.

Selective reuptake inhibitors

SSRIs include citalopram, escitalopram, fluoxetine, fluvoxamine, paroxetine, and sertraline. Their toxicity following overdose is considerably less than that of TCAs.

Selective serotonin and norepinephrine reuptake inhibitors, (SNRIs) such as venlafaxine and duloxetine, appear intermediate in toxicity between SSRIs and TCAs.

Mechanisms of toxicity

These drugs are potent inhibitors of neuronal serotonin reuptake and toxicity arises from serotoninergic effects such as agitation and increased muscle activity, which may progress to a full-blown serotonin syndrome (see Serotonin syndrome, pp. 79–80). At high doses some SSRIs, e.g. citalopram and escitalopram, also have direct effects on myocardial and central ion channels causing ventricular intraconduction abnormalities prolongation of both QRS and QT intervals, convulsions, and arrhythmias.

Venlafaxine and its major active metabolite desmethylvenlafaxine are potent inhibitors of uptake of serotonin and norepinephrine into neurons and also have dose-dependent sodium channel blocking effects. Less is known about the toxicity of duloxetine, but effects are likely to be similar.

Toxicokinetics

Most SSRIs achieve peak concentrations within 6 hours of ingestion at therapeutic doses, but their nauseating effects may delay absorption in overdose.

There is little evidence of a close relationship between individual plasma concentration measurements of SSRIs and their clinical effects in overdose. More recent complex Bayesian statistical analysis has, however, shown a relationship between the concentrations of citalopram and some other antidepressants on clinical features such as QT prolongation on the ECG. At present this is a research tool and there is no place for routine monitoring of the plasma concentrations of these compounds.

The majority of SSRIs are very lipid-soluble compounds and are metabolized in the liver. Half-lives and doses associated with toxic effects are shown in Table 4.1.

Venlafaxine and duloxetine are both available as modified-release preparations and this may delay the onset of features in overdose.

Risk factors for toxicity

Ingestion of other drugs that are potentially pro-convulsive is likely to increase toxicity and patients with epilepsy or cardiac disease are at a greater risk of fits or arrhythmias. Co-ingestion of more than one agent acting on the serotonin system increases the risk of serotonin syndrome. Examples of serotonin active compounds include: SSRIs, SNRIs, MAOIs, TCAs, tramadol, triptans, linezolid, St John's wort, and the drugs of abuse MDMA (ecstasy), amfetamines, cocaine, and cathinone derivatives (see Serotonin syndrome, pp. 79–80). Clinicians should be aware that drug users may be aware of these interactions and use prescribed medications and illicit drugs together to prolong or intensify the effect of illicit compounds.

Clinical features

The timing of onset of clinical features may be delayed, especially in patients ingesting modified-release preparations.

Most patients will have only mild serotoninergic features including nausea, vomiting, agitation, and tachycardia. Sedation, convulsions, and coma may develop after large overdoses (>1.5 g). More severe cardiac effects include hypertension and changes to the ECG reflect disturbance of ion channel function. In particular, QT prolongation may occur with some SSRIs, e.g. citalopram. Although associated with a risk of torsade de pointes, this arrhythmia seems rare after SSRI overdose.

In large single overdoses or if SSRIs are taken in combination or with other serotoninergic drugs there is a risk of serotonin syndrome (restlessness, hyperpyrexia, rhabdomyolysis, and renal failure).

Venlafaxine (and probably duloxetine) cause clinical features similar to those of SSRIs, although cardiovascular symptoms including sinus tachycardia, hypotension, or hypertension may be more prominent. Agitation and seizures are common and there is risk of cardiotoxicity, with both QRS and QT prolongation reported, although interpretation of the ECG is difficult due to the marked sinus tachycardia that is often present following overdose. Hypoglycaemia may also occur.

Investigations

As for TCAs, initial blood tests include U&Es, creatinine, and liver function tests. In patients with elevation of temperature, creatine kinase should be checked, urine output carefully monitored, and renal function tests repeated. Blood gas analysis should be used to exclude acidosis in those with suspected ECG abnormalities.

Management

Appropriate management of airway and ventilation is essential for patients with a reduced level of consciousness.

Oral activated charcoal may be valuable if administered within 1–2 hours of ingestion.

Intravenous fluids may be necessary for patients with vomiting, pyrexia, or serotonin syndrome.

Convulsions may be treated with intravenous diazepam (10–20 mg in adults; 0.1–0.3 mg/kg body weight in children) or lorazepam (4 mg in adults and 0.1 mg/kg in children) if prolonged or recurrent.

Prolongation of QRS or QT intervals on the ECG should be managed as described for TCA poisoning.

Most cases of serotonin syndrome resolve within 24 hours without specific therapy. Benzodiazepines may be helpful for severe myoclonic jerking. Cyproheptadine and chlorpromazine, both 5-HT$_{2A}$ antagonists, may be used for severe serotonin syndrome although clinical evidence of benefit is lacking. Dantrolene may also be considered. Urinary alkalinization and, in more severe cases, haemodiafiltration may be useful for rhabdomyolysis.

Presynaptic alpha-blockers

Mirtazapine acts as a presynaptic alpha$_2$-antagonist, increasing central noradrenergic and serotoninergic neurotransmission. It also has H$_1$ antihistamine effects which are responsible for the sedative effects that are prominent in overdose. The half-life during therapeutic use and the dose associated with potential toxicity are shown in Table 4.1.

Clinical features

Mirtazapine causes sedation associated with reductions in blood pressure and pulse. Arrhythmias and toxicity seen with other antidepressant groups appear rare after overdose, although supraventricular tachycardias and QRS prolongation have been reported.

Investigations

As for SSRI overdose.

Management

Patients should be observed for at least 4 hours and activated charcoal administered if the patient presents soon after ingestion of a substantial dose. The ECG should be monitored if there are ECG abnormalities. Otherwise management is supportive.

Monoamine oxidase inhibitors

Non-specific MAOIs inhibit MAO types A and B and include isocarboxazid (not licensed for use in the UK), phenelzine, and tranylcypromine. Currently they are used infrequently in the management of depression and overdose is now uncommon. Moclobemide is a specific MAO type A inhibitor.

Mechanisms of toxicity

Non-selective MAOIs block intracellular monoamine oxidase and increase intracellular monoamine (nor-epinephrine, 5-hydroxytryptamine) concentrations. In overdose, the clinical features reflect this action; there is a prominent increase in noradrenergic outflow and major toxicity may result, with central agitation, convulsions, cardiac arrhythmias, hypotension, and in severe cases death. During (or up to 2 weeks after) therapeutic MAOI use, a hypertensive crisis may result from interactions with other antidepressants and tyramine-containing foods (e.g. cheese, alcohol, meat, and yeast extracts). Serotonin syndrome is also prominent after overdose.

Moclobemide is much less toxic in overdose but may also be associated with serotonin syndrome.

Toxicokinetics

Onset of features after overdose with non-selective MAOIs may be delayed for at least 12 hours, and maximum toxicity may not occur until 24–36 hours after ingestion.

Risk factors for toxicity

Serotonin syndrome is more likely in patients also exposed to other serotoninergic agents (see SSRIs).

Clinical features

The principal features of toxicity are CNS and autonomic dysfunction including agitation, abnormal movements, hyper-reflexia, muscular rigidity, convulsions, sweating, hyperpyrexia, hyperventilation, tachycardia hypotension or hypertension, urinary retention, and coma. Rhabdomyolysis, acute kidney injury, intractable seizures, coagulopathy, and haemolysis are recognized in severe cases. Occasionally, thrombocytopenia, hypotension, and cardiac failure have been reported.

Moclobemide is less toxic, but overdose may be associated with nausea, vomiting, hypotension or hypertension, tachycardia, agitation, dysarthria, drowsiness, and serotonin syndrome.

Investigations

The ECG, U&Es, and full blood count should be checked, together with the creatine kinase if the patient is symptomatic.

Management

Following non-selective MAOI overdose activated charcoal should be administered if the patient present sufficiently early and asymptomatic patients observed for at least 12 hours. Heart rate, blood pressure, temperature, respiratory rate, and conscious level should be monitored frequently. Hyperthermia may require use of cooling measures and sedation, e.g. with diazepam. Dantrolene may be required in severe cases. Diazepam may also be required for treating convulsions or severe hypertension, for which intravenous nitrates may also be necessary. Tyramine-containing foods should be avoided during the recovery phase.

Observation for at least 4 hours is recommended after moclobemide overdose, with activated charcoal administered if the patient presents soon after a large ingestion. Serotonin syndrome may require specific management, otherwise treatment is supportive.

Other antidepressants

Mianserin and maprotiline are tetracyclic antidepressants, while trazodone and viloxazine (neither is licensed for use in the UK) are structurally unrelated to TCAs. These drugs have anticholinergic and cardiotoxic effects that are less marked than those of TCAs, but they may cause serotonin syndrome in overdose.

In overdose, all may cause vomiting, reduced level of consciousness, ataxia, tachycardia or bradycardia, hypotension or hypertension, convulsions, and serotonin syndrome.

Hyponatraemia, ST elevation, heart block, and ventricular fibrillation can be features of mianserin overdose while trazodone may cause QT prolongation and torsade de pointes.

Management of specific toxic effects is as described for TCAs and SSRIs.

Further reading

Bateman DN (2005). Tricyclic antidepressant poisoning: central nervous system effects and management. *Toxicol Rev*, 24:181–6.

Buckley NA, McManus PR (2002). Fatal toxicity of serotoninergic and other antidepressant drugs: analysis of United Kingdom mortality data. *Br Med J*, 325:1332–3.

Isbister GK, Friberg LE, Stokes B, et al. (2007). Activated charcoal decreases the risk of QT prolongation after citalopram overdose. *Ann Emerg Med*, 50:593–600,

Kelly CK, Dhaun N, Laing WJ, et al. (2004). Comparative toxicity of citalopram and the newer antidepressants after overdose. *J Toxicol Clin Toxicol*, 42:67–71.

Liebelt EL, Francis PD, Woolf AD (1995). ECG lead aVR versus QRS interval in predicting seizures and arrhythmias in acute tricyclic antidepressant toxicity. *Ann Emerg Med*, 26:195–201.

Shannon M, Liebelt EL (1998). Toxicology reviews: targeted management strategies for cardiovascular toxicity from tricyclic antidepressant overdose: the pivotal role for alkalinization and sodium loading. *Pediatric Emerg Care*, 14:293–8.

Thanacoody HK, Thomas SH (2005). Tricyclic antidepressant poisoning: cardiovascular toxicity. *Toxicol Rev*, 24:205–14.

van Gorp F, Duffull S, Hackett LP, et al. (2012). Population pharmacokinetics and pharmacodynamics of escitalopram in overdose and the effect of activated charcoal. *Br J Clin Pharmacol*, 73:402–10.

Waring WS, Good AM, Bateman DN (2007). Lack of significant toxicity after mirtazapine overdose: a five-year review of cases admitted to a regional toxicology unit. *Clin Toxicol*, 45:45–50.

Antihistamines

Background

Antihistamines act as reversible competitive histamine receptor antagonists. The term generally refers to drugs which block the H_1 histamine receptor (Table 4.2), but may also encompass H_2 receptor antagonists (see later in this section).

H_1 antihistamines are used to treat allergic disorders such as seasonal allergic rhinitis and urticaria. They may also be prescribed for bites or stings, vestibular disorders including motion sickness and vomiting, including in palliative care. As a result of their widespread availability, including over-the-counter for some drugs, overdose is commonly encountered.

Sedating antihistamines

Sedating antihistamines are lipid-soluble drugs with large volumes of distribution that penetrate the CNS rapidly. They have non-specific actions which include anticholinergic effects and in some cases alpha$_1$ adrenergic and serotonergic actions.

In therapeutic use, anticholinergic effects and sedation are most pronounced with promethazine, alimemazine, and diphenhydramine, with effects less marked for chlorphenamine and cyclizine. Anticholinergic properties are useful in the treatment of motion sickness and other causes of vomiting but also contribute to the clinical features of overdose.

Blockade of fast sodium channels may also occur with toxic doses. Seizures may be provoked by sodium channel blockade in the brain, while in the myocardium this effect may result in delayed conduction and ventricular arrhythmias.

After therapeutic dosing peak plasma concentrations usually occur within 2–6 hours. Plasma half-lives vary between agents (Table 4.2).

Clinical features

Features encountered in overdose include the following:

Common

- Gastrointestinal disturbances, e.g. nausea and vomiting.
- Anticholinergic effects—these include sedation, which is exacerbated by other sedative co-ingestants including alcohol, as well as dry mouth, hot dry skin, dilated pupils, hyperthermia, tachycardia, ataxia, nystagmus, drowsiness, and agitation. Paralytic ileus and urinary retention may occasionally occur. Delayed gastric emptying is probably common.
- Hypotension may occur due to dehydration, vasodilatation, or (rarely) impaired myocardial function.

Uncommon

- Seizure threshold is reduced and convulsions occasionally occur. Diphenhydramine and hydroxyzine have been most commonly implicated. Seizures may result in acidosis which may in turn precipitate cardiac arrhythmias.
- Myoclonus, rigidity, hyperthermia, hyperkalaemia, metabolic acidosis, and rhabdomyolysis occur uncommonly.
- Electrocardiographic effects have been reported for some agents, e.g. diphenhydramine. These include prolongation of the QRS interval, reflecting impaired conduction velocity and of the QT interval, reflecting delayed cardiac repolarization. Ventricular arrhythmias including torsade de pointes have been reported, although these seem uncommon.
- Pulmonary oedema has been observed in severe poisoning and may be found at autopsy in fatal cases.

Non-sedating antihistamines

Non-sedating antihistamines are increasingly replacing sedating agents for treating allergic disorders. Their non-sedating properties result in part from more specific actions on the H_1 antihistamine receptor, with little or no anticholinergic actions. In addition, many are lipid-soluble pro-drugs that are converted to less lipophilic active metabolites during first-pass metabolism. These metabolites are active on peripheral H_1 receptors but penetrate the CNS poorly, limiting central effects. Some have long half-lives, prolonging their clinical effects, or are converted to active metabolites e.g. loratadine metabolized to desloratadine. Examples of non-sedating antihistamines are shown in Table 4.2.

Table 4.2 Pharmacokinetic properties and potentially toxic doses of sedating and non-sedating antihistamines

Antihistamine	Approximate t½ (therapeutic doses, hours)	Minimum potentially toxic dose (mg/kg)
Sedating		
Alimemazine[1]	5	4
Buclizine	15	7
Chlorphenamine[2]	28	2
Cinnarizine	3	15
Clemastine	3–4*	0.3
Cyclizine	20	14
Cyproheptadine	1–4	2
Diphenhydramine	2–9	5
Hydroxyzine	20	10
Ketotifen	18	0.3
Promethazine	7–14	5
Triprolidine	2–6	1
Non-sedating		
Acrivastine	1.5	4
Cetirizine	7–10	2
Desloratadine	27	1
Fexofenadine	11–15	20
Levocetirizine	8	1
Loratadine	11**	2
Mizolastine	7–17	2
Rupatadine	6–9	n/k

Previously termed
[1] trimeprazine and
[2] chlorpheniramine.
*Extended terminal half-life.
**Metabolized to desloratidine.

Clinical features

There is less experience with these drugs in overdose; clinical features are non-specific and include:

- Tachycardia.
- Drowsiness or agitation.
- Gastrointestinal disturbances.
- Dizziness and headache.
- QT interval prolongation and torsade de pointes occurred rarely with the older non-sedating antihistamines agents terfenadine and astemizole. These drugs have now been withdrawn from clinical practice as a result. There have been occasional reports of QT prolongation or arrhythmia with therapeutic doses of newer agents (e.g. loratadine) but a cause–effect relationship has not been proven.

Management of H₁ antihistamine overdose

- It is reasonable to administer activated charcoal to patients who have ingested potentially toxic amounts within approximately 1 hour, although there is no specific evidence of clinical benefit. Potentially toxic amounts are defined in Table 4.2.
- Monitor conscious level and respiration, especially following overdose of sedating agents. Provide supportive care for complications such as loss of airway or respiratory depression.
- A 12-lead ECG should be performed for determination of QRS and QT intervals.
- Asymptomatic patients should be observed for at least 6 hours after ingestion before discharge.
- Hypotension generally responds to intravenous fluids, which are also indicated in patients with dehydration as a result of fever.
- Convulsions should be treated with a benzodiazepine in the first instance, e.g. lorazepam
- Drug treatment of delirium or agitation should be avoided if possible. When necessary, cautious use of benzodiazepines may be useful. There are reports of successful treatment of delirium with anticholinesterases such as physostigmine (1–2 mg IV), although this drug is not available in the United Kingdom.
- Torsade de pointes and other ventricular arrhythmias should be managed by correction of hypoxia, acidosis, and electrolyte abnormalities. Intravenous bicarbonate may be beneficial even in the absence of acidosis. Torsade de pointes type ventricular tachycardia should be treated with intravenous magnesium sulfate in the first instance (see pp. 64–65).
- Active elimination methods are unlikely to be effective due to the large volumes of distribution of these agents.

Patients who have not developed clinical features within 6 hours are unlikely to do so and can be considered for discharge from hospital.

H₂ antihistamines

These drugs act on gastric mucosa, suppressing acid secretion. They have previously been used commonly to treat or prevent peptic ulceration and gastro-oesophageal reflux, although they are now largely superseded by newer agents, e.g. proton pump inhibitors. Examples of H₂ blockers are cimetidine, famotidine, nizatidine, and ranitidine. Overdose with these agents is not usually associated with significant toxicity.

Cimetidine is an inhibitor of several cytochrome P450 isoforms including CYP1A2, CYP2C9, CYP2C19, CYP2D6, CYP2E1, and CYP3A4. As a result it may precipitate drug interactions if co-administered with narrow therapeutic index drugs metabolized via these enzymes. Examples are warfarin, methadone, theophylline, lidocaine, and phenytoin.

Clinical features

Features occasionally encountered in overdose include dry mouth, nausea and vomiting, dizziness, drowsiness, disorientation, and bradycardia.

Serious complications of poisoning have not been reported. However, rapid intravenous administration of cimetidine has been reported to cause bradycardia and hypotension; cardiac arrest has been reported but is rare.

Management of overdose

Specific treatment is unlikely to be needed if these drugs are ingested alone.

Further reading

Cowen PJ (1979). Toxic psychosis with antihistamines reversed by physostigmine. *Postgrad Med J*, 55:556–7.

Mullins ME, Pinnick RV, Terhes, JM (1999). Life-threatening diphenhydramine overdose treated with charcoal hemoperfusion and hemodialysis. *Ann Emerg Med*, 33:104–7.

Köppel C, Ibe K, Tenczer J (1987). Clinical symptomatology of diphenhydramine overdose: an evaluation of 136 cases in 1982 to 1985. *J Toxicol Clin Toxicol*, 25:53–70.

Pragst F, Sieglinde H, Bakdash A (2006). Poisonings with diphenhydramine – A survey of 68 clinical and 55 death cases. *Forens Sci Int*, 161:189–97.

Scharman EJ, Erdman AR, Wax PM, *et al.* (2006). Diphenhydramine and dimenhydrinate poisoning: an evidence based consensus guideline for out-of-hospital management. *Clin Tox*, 44:205–23.

Zareba W, Moss AJ, Rosero SZ, *et al.* (1997). Electrocardiographic findings in patients with Diphenhydramine overdose. *Am J Cardiol*, 80:1168–73.

Antipsychotics

Background

Antipsychotic drugs can be classified by chemical structure or receptor specificity.

Older 'typical' or 'classical' antipsychotics (e.g. phenothiazines, thioxanthenes, butyrophenones) have dopamine D_1 and D_2 antagonist properties; as a result they are particularly associated with drug-induced extrapyramidal effects and hyperprolactinaemia in therapeutic use.

The newer 'atypical' antipsychotics (e.g. amisulpride, aripiprazole, clozapine, olanzapine, quetiapine, risperidone, zotepine [not licensed for use in the UK]) are weaker dopamine D_2 antagonists and have effects on serotonin (typically $5HT_{2A}$) and other CNS receptor systems that account for their lower risk of extrapyramidal effects.

Individual antipsychotic drugs may also antagonize other receptor systems including cholinergic, histaminergic and α-adrenergic receptors and may also affect myocardial ion channels. This spectrum of activity largely determines the pattern of toxicity seen in overdose.

Mechanisms of toxicity

Much of the toxicity of antipsychotics can be explained by their receptor interactions:

- Antidopaminergic effects (especially typical agents). Effects on the extrapyramidal system are primarily due to D_1 dopamine receptor blockade. This may cause increased muscle tone, movement disorder, particularly acute dystonia in overdose, or rarely thermogenesis (neuroleptic malignant syndrome).
- Anticholinergic effects (especially chlorpromazine, zuclopenthixol, clozapine, olanzapine) resulting in sedation, tachycardia, hypotension, dry mouth, urinary retention, etc.
- Antihistaminergic effects (especially chlorpromazine) contributing to sedation.
- Alpha-adrenoceptor antagonist activity (especially phenothiazines, clozapine, olanzapine, quetiapine) resulting in dose-related vasodilatation with hypotension and reflex tachycardia.
- Myocardial ion channel effects. Potassium channel inhibition (especially droperidol, amisulpride, sertindole, ziprasidone [last two not licensed for use in the UK]) results in QT prolongation with a risk of torsade de points. Risk was especially high with thioridazine, which has now been withdrawn from the market. Antipsychotics may also cause sodium channel blockade associated with QRS prolongation.

Toxicokinetics

The absorption profile of older antipsychotics is rather slow and erratic with peak concentrations often taking several hours. The onset of action of parenteral injections is more predictable. Depot injections release drug over days and weeks and may cause prolonged symptoms, especially if given accidentally to treatment naïve patients. Most antipsychotic drugs are lipid-soluble, have large volumes of distribution, are eliminated by hepatic metabolism, and have long half-lives (Table 4.3). Many also have active metabolites which may contribute to toxicity and duration of action.

Risk factors for toxicity

Age affects the risk of developing extrapyramidal features; dystonia is more common in young females,

Table 4.3 Commonly used antipsychotics from different classes, their half-life ($t\frac{1}{2}$) at therapeutic doses, and minimum potentially toxic doses (mg/kg body weight). Note. Toxic doses may be conservative in patients on long-term therapy, who may develop tolerance

Drug	$t\frac{1}{2}$ (therapeutic doses, hours)[a]	Minimum toxic dose (mg/kg)
Typical agents		
Chlorpromazine	8–35	5
Trifluoperazine	22	1
Haloperidol	13–35	0.5
Sulpiride	8–9	50
Atypical agents		
Olanzapine	30–38	1
Risperidone	24	1.5
Quetiapine	7	10
Aripiprazole	75–145	3
Amisulpride	12	25
Clozapine	17–19	10
Zotepine[b]	14–21	15

[a] NB $t\frac{1}{2}$ in overdose may be significantly longer, possibly because of delayed absorption or saturation of elimination pathways. Many also have active metabolites.

[b] Not licensed for use in the UK or USA

parkinsonian symptoms are much commoner in the elderly. Previous history of such reactions may indicate a higher incidence in repeat ingestion.

Patients with liver disease may have more severe effects due to delayed metabolism.

Co-ingestion of drugs that have cardiovascular actions will tend to exacerbate effects on the cardiovascular system, and co-ingestion of CNS depressants increase the risk of respiratory depression and obstruction of the upper airway.

Clinical features

The commonest features seen following acute ingestion of antipsychotics in overdose include:

- Depression of consciousness. This appears especially common after overdose of typical antipsychotics and the atypical agents clozapine, olanzapine, and quetiapine. If severe it may be associated with respiratory depression.
- Hypotension associated with tachycardia.
- Hypothermia and thermoregulation disturbance.
- Cardiac arrhythmias (conduction abnormalities and torsade de pointes).
- Acute dystonic reactions (e.g. oculogyric crisis).
- Convulsions may occur and may be more common with typical agents and with clozapine.

Rarely there may be rhabdomyolysis and renal failure.

Pulmonary oedema is also occasionally reported, perhaps due to ion channel effects in the lung.

Toxicity assessment

Assessment of toxicity is judged on history of dose ingested and clinical features, particularly CNS and cardiovascular effects. Hypothermia may occur due to peripheral vasodilatation and CNS depression. Concentration measurements are unhelpful.

Investigations

Blood should be taken for full blood count, U&Es, creatinine, and LFTs. A 12-lead ECG should be obtained. The QT interval should be measured carefully as it indicates the risk for torsade de pointes. Manual measurements should be made as many automated ECG machines are inaccurate in overdose. Automated rate correction may also be misleading but is an initial guide. The QRS duration should also be assessed (see Cardiovascular toxicity, pp. 64–67).

If there is CNS depression or the 12-lead ECG is abnormal, pulse oximetry and ECG monitoring is required and the 12-lead ECG should be repeated, ideally every 2–4 hours initially or if the clinical situation changes. Venous or arterial blood gases should also be taken.

In patients with ECG abnormalities or arrhythmias, serum magnesium should be checked. If there is increased muscle tone or hyperthermia creatine kinase should be monitored and fluids given to maintain adequate urine output.

Management

Pulse, BP, temperature, and respiration should be monitored, initially at 15-minute intervals; monitoring should be continued for at least 12 hours. Patients who have taken large overdoses and those exposed to agents with long half-lives (e.g. clozapine, olanzapine, haloperidol) should be monitored for longer periods.

Activated charcoal may be indicated in patients who present after significant overdose and may be considered up to 4 hours in patients who ingest large quantities of modified-release preparations with cardiotoxic potential, e.g. amisulpride.

Hypotension should be corrected conventionally initially by using intravenous fluids, but since many of these agents are alpha receptor antagonists and cardiac depressants, therapy with inotropes or an alpha-adrenergic pressor agent (e.g. norepinephrine) should be considered after adequate volume expansion.

Some patients may become agitated and this is best managed with a benzodiazepine (e.g. diazepam orally or IV 0.1–0.3 mg/kg).

Dystonic reactions should be managed by reassurance; an IV anticholinergic (e.g. procyclidine 5–10mg IV or IM in an adult) or a benzodiazepine (e.g. diazepam orally or IV 0.1–0.3 mg/kg) will often stop the reaction. Reactions may recur up to 24–36 hours after acute antipsychotic ingestion.

Convulsions should be managed conventionally with intravenous benzodiazepines if prolonged.

Torsade de pointes ventricular tachycardia caused by antipsychotic drugs is often delayed as absorption of drugs in this class is often slow and metabolites may also play a role in causation. It is managed by correcting hypoxia (oxygen) and acidosis (sodium bicarbonate) and by administration of intravenous magnesium sulfate. Overdrive cardiac pacing is occasionally needed. Lidocaine or phenytoin may be effective if multifocal ventricular arrhythmias occur.

Hyperthermia may indicate serotonin syndrome or rarely neuroleptic malignant syndrome. Monitoring of creatine kinase, active temperature lowering, and reducing agitation, initially with benzodiazepines, may be appropriate (see Serotonin syndrome, pp. 79–80). Rhabdomyolysis should be treated conventionally (see Rhabdomyolysis and compartment syndrome, pp. 77–78).

Pulmonary oedema or acute lung injury may require intubation and positive pressure ventilation. Mechanical ventilation may also be required for patients with marked impairment of consciousness.

Clozapine causes aplastic anaemia as an idiosyncratic reaction. It is important to check repeat blood counts, in patients exposed to this agent.

Other features of poisoning should be treated symptomatically.

Elimination techniques have no role because most antipsychotic drugs are very lipid-soluble and have high volumes of distribution.

Chronic exposure

Extrapyramidal effects may occur with therapeutic doses of antipsychotic drugs. They do not usually occur after overdose.

Acute dystonic reactions are more common in younger patients, particularly females. These present as prolonged muscle spasms in specific muscle groups. The most frequent is an oculogyric crisis. These reactions are extremely worrying for patients; the differential diagnosis includes tetanus. Acute dystonic reactions respond to intravenous diazepam or an anticholinergic agent (e.g. procyclidine—see under 'Management').

Akathisia is a sensation of acute restlessness and usually occurs more often in patients naïve to antipsychotics.

Parkinsonism is more common in the elderly, and normally requires several weeks of therapy. Specific drug therapy is usually not indicated for parkinsonian features, which often improve on withdrawal of the offending agent, although effects may become irreversible once established.

Tardive dyskinesia usually requires months or years of therapy and results from up-regulation of receptors in the context of chronic receptor blockade. It will usually diminish if an acute overdose is taken in a patient with this condition.

A more severe feature of chronic therapy with antipsychotics is the neuroleptic malignant syndrome (see Malignant hyperpyrexia, pp. 81–82). Key features of this are autonomic dysfunction, fluctuating consciousness, hyperthermia, and muscular rigidity. Rhabdomyolysis may occur with secondary renal failure. Management depends on the severity of the clinical features. Careful fluid balance is essential. Dantrolene and dopamine agonists may have a role in severe cases, though the latter may exacerbate psychosis. Their use should be discussed with an expert.

Further reading

Burns MJ (2001). The pharmacology and toxicology of atypical antipsychotic agents. *J Toxicol Clin Toxicol*, 39:1–14.

Glassman AH, Bigger Jr JT (2001). Antipsychotic drugs: prolonged QTc interval, torsade de pointes, and sudden death. *Am J Psychiatry*, 158:1774–82.

Isbister GK, Balit CR, Macleod D, et al. (2010). Amisulpiride overdose is frequently associated with QT prolongation and *torsade de pointes*. *J Clin Psychopharmacol*, 30:391–5.

James LP, Abel K, Wilkinson J, et al. (2005). Antipsychotic poisoning in young children. A systematic review. *Drug Saf*, 28:1029–44.

Li C, Gefter WB (1992). Acute pulmonary edema induced by overdosage of phenothiazines. *Chest*, 101:102–4.

Russell SA, Hennes HM, Herson KJ, et al. (1996). Upper airway compromise in acute chlorpromazine ingestion. *Am J Emerg Med*, 14:467–8.

Strachan EM, Kelly CA, Bateman DN (2004). Electrocardiogram and cardiovascular changes in thioridazine and chlorpromazine poisoning. *Eur J Clin Pharmacol*, 60:541–5.

Benzodiazepines

Background

Benzodiazepine compounds are prescribed for their sedative and anxiolytic effects and some have more specific uses. Clonazepam is used as a long-term therapy in the management of epilepsy, lorazepam and diazepam are used intravenously in the acute management of convulsions, and diazepam and chlordiazepoxide are used in the management of acute alcohol withdrawal. Midazolam is used as an intravenous sedative and as a buccal liquid for treatment of convulsions.

Benzodiazepines are also commonly abused by recreational drug users and occasionally also used illegally to sedate potential victims of theft or sexual assault.

Benzodiazepines are rarely fatal if ingested alone, but potentiate CNS depression caused by co-ingested agents, both drugs and ethanol. A number of drugs with similar profiles of action to benzodiazepines have been developed, the aim being to avoid the risk of dependency. Examples are zaleplon, zopiclone, and zolpidem. These agents have toxicity similar to shorter-acting benzodiazepines and are considered in Other hypnotics, pp. 110–111.

NB The benzodiazepine antagonist flumazenil has a half-life of only around 1 hour (range 45–90 minutes), far less than any of the commonly used drugs in Table 4.4.

Toxic doses

Establishing a toxic dose of a benzodiazepine in an individual patient is difficult, because tolerance develops within a few days in patients receiving the drugs regularly. As a general guide, an oral dose of 0.5 mg/kg of diazepam would be indication for close monitoring in hospital. For more potent agents such as lorazepam or flunitrazepam (not licensed for use in the UK) the equivalent dose would be 0.1 mg/kg and for a less potent drug such as chlordiazepoxide 1–1.5 mg/kg.

Table 4.4 Half-lives of benzodiazepines and similar drugs and their active metabolites ([ ]) where applicable

Benzodiazepines	t½ (hours)
Alprazolam	6–12
Bromazepam[a]	10–20
Chlordiazepoxide	5–30 [36–200]
Clobazam	12–60
Clonazepam	18–50
Clorazepate[a]	[36–200]
Diazepam	20–100 [36–200]
Flunitrazepam[a]	18–26 [36–200]
Flurazepam	[40–250]
Lorazepam	10–20
Lormetazepam	10–12
Midazolam	2–3 [1]
Nitrazepam	15–38
Oxazepam	4–15
Temazepam	8–22
Triazolam[a]	2

[a] Not licensed for use in the UK

For non-benzodiazepine sedatives doses of 0.5–1 mg per kilogram should be regarded as potentially serious.

Mechanisms of toxicity

Benzodiazepines bind to a specific benzodiazepine receptor on the gamma-aminobutyric acid (GABA) receptor complex, augmenting the actions of GABA, which increases permeability to chloride, resulting in reduced neuronal excitability.

Serious toxicity in children or adults is rare. In acute overdose the main complications are those of CNS depression. Obstruction to the upper respiratory tract may result in hypoxic brain injury. CNS depression is associated with hypotension and bradycardia.

Toxicokinetics

There is little evidence for dose dependency of kinetics, but these drugs are cleared by hepatic metabolism, and delayed elimination with increased risk of toxicity occurs in severe hepatic disease. Most benzodiazepines are very lipid-soluble and rapidly act on the CNS. Following oral dosing, peak effects normally occur within about 60–90 minutes, even for those drugs that require conversion to an active metabolite (e.g. clorazepate). Intravenous use results in rapid onset. Offset of effect depends to a large extent on redistribution into fat, particularly for the longer half-life agents (see Table 4.4). For some drugs in this class the action of metabolites is important in determining duration of effect in overdose. The diazepam metabolite nordiazepam has a half-life of approximately 100 hours and may contribute to delayed recovery of consciousness in severe overdose.

Risk factors for toxicity

The major risk factor for serious toxicity is co-ingestion of alcohol or other CNS depressants, with potential risk for obstruction of the upper respiratory tract, respiratory depression, and cerebral hypoxia. This is particularly important in patients who have ingested opiates where fatality rates appear much increased as compared to a single agent of either group alone.

Patients with severe liver disease may experience unexpected toxicity from small doses and patients with chronic lung diseases such as COPD, those with neuromuscular dysfunction, and the elderly are also at increased risk.

There is a risk of dependence, both physical and psychological, from all benzodiazepines; this seems more problematic with short-acting agents such as temazepam.

Clinical features

Benzodiazepines in overdose usually cause drowsiness, ataxia, dysarthria, and nystagmus. Coma, hypotension, bradycardia, and respiratory depression occasionally occur but clinical effects are seldom serious if benzodiazepines are taken alone. Coma usually lasts only a few hours but may be prolonged in elderly patients or those with liver failure.

Severe effects in overdose also include rhabdomyolysis and hypothermia.

Toxicity assessment

Toxicity assessment is based on clinical features and time from the ingestion. Key features are level of CNS depression, ability to maintain an airway and adequate oxygenation, and measurement of blood pressure and pulse, as indicators of central cardiovascular depression. It is important to observe the patient for sufficient time, and be particularly cautious in those patients with co-ingested CNS depressants. It is important to monitor oxygenation carefully using a pulse oximeter in patients with CNS depression, and routine observation should be done at least every 15 minutes initially in order to assess the stage of the clinical course.

Investigations

There are no specific investigations for benzodiazepine ingestion, however it is important to be certain that aspiration has not occurred in the patient with impaired CNS responses, i.e. GCS of 8 or less, or AVPU less than V. Routine pulse oximetry is appropriate in such patients and blood gas analysis may be necessary. Elevation in arterial carbon dioxide is an indication for further intervention, either using an antidote or mechanical respiratory support.

A 12-lead ECG should also be performed in anyone with CNS depression in order to ascertain there is no conduction abnormality (prolonged QRS or QT) that might indicate co-ingestion of an arrhythmogenic drug.

Management

Maintain a clear airway and adequate ventilation. If indicated consider respiratory support or antidote therapy with flumazenil (see 'Use of antidotes'). Consider activated charcoal (charcoal dose: 50 g for an adult, 1 g/kg for a child) in adults or children who have taken more than a potentially toxic amount within 1 hour, provided the airway can be protected. Patients who are asymptomatic at 4 hours are unlikely to develop severe toxicity.

Monitor level of consciousness, respiratory rate, pulse oximetry, and blood pressure in symptomatic patients.

Consider arterial blood gas analysis in patients who have a reduced level of consciousness (e.g. GCS <13, AVPU scale P or U) or have reduced oxygen saturations on pulse oximetry.

Correct hypotension by raising the foot of the bed and by giving an appropriate fluid challenge. If hypotension persists after fluid resuscitation seek expert advice to determine the mechanism of hypotension and appropriate management. Severe hypotension may be due to decreased systemic vascular resistance and/or reduced cardiac output.

There is no role for active elimination methods such as haemodialysis or haemoperfusion.

Use of antidotes

The specific benzodiazepine antagonist, flumazenil is available, but use in overdose is associated with potential hazards, particularly the risk of precipitating convulsions or acute withdrawal if given in the wrong situation. The antidote does have a role in patients for whom mechanical ventilation would otherwise be needed, particularly children who are naïve to benzodiazepines, or patients with COPD.

Flumazenil is contraindicated when patients have ingested multiple medicines, especially after co-ingestion with a tricyclic antidepressant or any other drug that causes seizures. This is because the benzodiazepine may be suppressing seizures induced by the second drug; its antagonism by flumazenil can reveal severe status epilepticus that can be very difficult to control. Contraindications to the use of flumazenil therefore include features suggestive of a tricyclic antidepressant ingestion including a wide QRS on ECG and large pupils. Flumazenil is also contraindicated in patients who have taken pro-convulsive drugs of abuse such as amfetamines or cocaine and also following cardiac arrest.

Flumazenil should be used with caution in patients with a history of seizures, head injury, or chronic benzodiazepine use. Flumazenil is not advised as a routine diagnostic test in patients with reduced conscious level because of the risk of precipitating convulsions.

When flumazenil is used to treat benzodiazepine overdose, is not necessary or appropriate to fully reverse benzodiazepine effects; all that is needed is to prevent the patient requiring ventilation. Most patients poisoned with benzodiazepines will respond to flumazenil (1 mg) but the antidote has a short half-life (about an hour). Because of this, patients with severe poisoning in whom flumazenil is indicated may need repeated doses (e.g. 0.5 mg intravenously over 1 minute, the same dose repeated if there is no response or only a partial response) or an intravenous infusion (e.g. 0.1–0.4 mg/hour).

Drug 'doping'

Management of patients who believe that they have been drugged, or their drink has been 'spiked' may be challenging. In reality the vast majority of such patients are suffering the effects of excess alcohol. Forensic tests for benzodiazepines are possible but must be done early after administration, and are rarely routinely available in hospital laboratories. If patients believe they have been subjected to drug-facilitated sexual assault they must be referred to an appropriate rape crisis team and the police.

Further reading

Gaudreault P, Guay J, Thivierge RL, et al. (1991). Benzodiazepinepoisoning. Clinical and pharmacological considerations and treatment. Drug Saf, 6:247–65.

Hojer J, Baechrendtz S, Gustafsson L (1989). Benzodiazepines poisoning: experience of 702 admissions to an intensive care unit during a 14-year period. J Intern Med, 226:117–22.

Kulka PJ, Lauven PM (1992). Benzodiazepine antagonists – an update of their role in the emergency care of overdose patients. Drug Saf, 7:381–6.

Weinbroum A, Rudick V, Sorkine P, et al. (1996). Use of flumazenil in the treatment of drug overdose: a double-blind and open clinical study in 110 patients. Crit Care Med, 24:199–206.

Mordel A, Winkler E, Almog S, et al. (1992). Seizures after flumazenil administration in a case of combined benzodiazepine and tricyclic anti-depressant overdose. Crit Care Med, 20:1733–4.

Veiraiah A, Dyas J, Cooper G, et al. (2012). Flumazenil use in benzodiazepine overdose in the UK: a retrospective survey of NPIS data. Emerg Med J, 29:565–9.

Wiley CC, Wiley JF 2nd (1998). Pediatric benzodiazepine ingestion resulting in hospitalization. J Toxicol Clin Toxicol, 36:227–31.

Other hypnotics

Background
The hypnotic potential of a drug refers to its ability to facilitate normal sleep through drowsiness. This property is distinct from sedation, which refers to the anxiolytic effects of a drug. Hypnotic toxicity may occur either as a result of deliberate self-harm or accidently, particularly in the elderly, as a result of accidental therapeutic excess.

Mechanism of toxicity
The majority of hypnotics exert their therapeutic and toxic effects by facilitating the action of the central inhibitory neurotransmitter gamma-amino butyric acid (GABA) binding to the chloride ion channel-gated $GABA_A$ receptor. $GABA_A$ receptors exist as pentamers of subunits and are highly heterogeneous. The different combinations of receptor subtypes appear to mediate different effects such as drowsiness, muscle relaxation and sedation.

The hypnotic property of a drug reflects its selectivity for the $alpha_1$ subunit of the $GABA_A$ receptor. Several classes of drugs are currently listed as hypnotics by the *British National Formulary* (Table 4.5), in addition to the benzodiazepines discussed elsewhere (see Benzodiazepines, pp. 108–109).

Toxicokinetics
The majority of hypnotics are highly lipid-soluble. They are rapidly absorbed from the gastrointestinal tract and often rapidly redistribute to fatty tissues. Hepatic metabolism is often required to increase water solubility to allow renal clearance. The metabolites of some hypnotics are active. The adverse effects of a hypnotic drug may therefore be prolonged, particularly following an overdose.

Risk factors for toxicity
The individual response to a particular dose of hypnotic is highly variable. Chronic users of hypnotics rapidly develop tolerance. The concurrent use of more than one hypnotic can have a marked synergistic effect. Ethanol also modulates $GABA_A$ receptor function and potentiates the actions of other hypnotics. Ethanol is not an effective hypnotic in clinical practice due to its diuretic action.

Toxicity may be enhanced in the frail elderly and in those with chronic lung, liver, or neuromuscular disease.

Clinical features
Clinical features of hypnotic toxicity are similar to ethanol intoxication and include dysarthria, ataxia, nystagmus decreased GCS, coma, hypotension, respiratory depression, and hypothermia.

Complications of hypnotic toxicity include aspiration pneumonia, rhabdomyolysis, pressure sores, renal failure, non-cardiogenic pulmonary oedema, and death.

Barbiturates are especially toxic and may cause hypotension and cardiac arrest.

Long-term users of some hypnotics may also experience a withdrawal reaction upon discontinuing the drug. These reactions can be severe and occasionally life threatening.

Investigations
Pulse oximetry and/or arterial blood gases should be considered in patients with a reduced level of consciousness. A chest X-ray should be arranged if aspiration pneumonia is suspected. Measurement of specific drug concentrations is generally not required.

Management
The majority of cases can be managed with good supportive care, including appropriate management of airway, breathing and circulation. A GCS of 9 or less and/or respiratory insufficiency should prompt an urgent review by an intensivist to ensure an adequate airway and ventilation.

Hypnotics that are agonists at the $alpha_1$ subunit of the $GABA_A$ receptor can be antagonized by flumazenil.

Dialysis has a limited role in enhancing the elimination of the majority of hypnotics due to their large volumes of distribution.

Specific clinical features and management issues for the different classes of hypnotics are detailed as follows:

Z-class hypnotics
These include zaleplon, zolpidem, and zopiclone (marketed as the isomer eszopiclone in the USA), which are all $GABA_A$ receptor agonists that are chemically distinct from the benzodiazepines. Initial expectations that the Z-class hypnotics might have a better side effect profile than conventional benzodiazepines have not been realized in clinical practice.

Several idiosyncratic features are associated with the Z-class hypnotics in overdose. Neuropsychiatric features, such as hallucinations and sleep-walking, have been described after zaleplon and zolpidem overdoses. Zaleplon poisoning can also turn urine blue/green. Haemolytic anaemia and methaemoglobinaemia have been reported following zopiclone poisoning.

Flumazenil can be used when there is coma or severe respiratory depression, in addition to supportive care. The half-life of flumazenil is approximately 1 hour. An intravenous infusion may therefore be required to maintain an adequate response. Flumazenil should not be used as a diagnostic challenge or in mixed overdoses, patients with a history of seizures, or those with head injuries, due to the risk of precipitating seizures.

Table 4.5 Examples of non-benzodiazepine hypnotic agents and their half-lives

Drug	Approximate t½ (hours)
Z-class hypnotics	
Zaleplon	1
Zolpidem	2.4
Zopiclone	3.5–6
Barbiturates	
Thiopental sodium	6–46[a]
Amobarbital (amylobarbitone sodium amytal)	8–42
Butobarbital	34–42
Secobarbital (quinalbarbitone)	15–40
Phenobarbital sodium	24–140
Sodium barbital[b]	27–33
Others	
Sodium oxybate	0.5
Chloral hydrate	See text
Clomethiazole (chlormethiazole)	4–8
Melatonin	3.5–4

[a] Action limited by redistribution

[b] Not licensed for use in the UK

Chloral hydrate

Chloral hydrate is rapidly converted to its active metabolite, trichloroethanol, by alcohol dehydrogenase. Trichloroethanol is inactivated by alcohol dehydrogenase and aldehyde dehydrogenase into trichloroacetic acid. There is a marked difference in the rate of metabolism between both adults and children, consequently the half-life is highly variable, but the half-life of trichloroacetic acid is several days.

A typical maximum therapeutic dose is 2 g, yet toxicity has been described at doses of 1.5 g. Fatal toxicity has been described following ingestion of 4 g in adults, yet individuals have survived following ingestion of 70 g.

In addition to the usually features of hypnotic toxicity, a sweet odour to the breath and constricted pupils have been reported, although these are not consistent findings, Chloral hydrate is a local irritant of the gastrointestinal tract and can cause ulceration or perforation following an overdose.

Chloral hydrate toxicity may be associated with ventricular arrhythmias, which are sometimes fatal. Chloral hydrate apparently sensitizes the myocardium to catecholamines. Consequently, beta-blockers appear effective in suppressing chloral hydrate-induced arrhythmias.

The may be a role for haemodialysis following severe poisoning. A single case report described a reduction in chloral hydrate half-life from 35 hours to 6 hours whilst on dialysis.

Clomethiazole (chlormethiazole)

Clomethiazole is a sedating hypnotic with anticonvulsant properties that is also licensed to treat acute alcohol withdrawal. The half-life is usually around 4 hours but this can increase to 8 hours in the elderly or in patients with hepatic impairment. In severe poisoning consciousness may be depressed for several days.

As with other hypnotics, there appears to be considerable individual susceptibility to the toxic effects of clomethiazole. Death has been described following blood concentrations of 1 mg/100 mL but survival following coma has been reported in individuals with concentrations of 3.6 mg/100 mL of blood. Treatment is supportive.

Sedative antihistamines

Antihistamines with sedative properties are sometimes used as hypnotics and promethazine is licensed for this purpose. A typical therapeutic dose is between 25 and 50 mg and toxicity has been reported at doses of 350 mg. Promethazine has an anticholinergic action. Delirium is frequently reported following promethazine poisoning. The risk of developing delirium correlates with the dose. There is also a risk of QT and QRS prolongation following promethazine overdose. Neuroleptic malignant syndrome has also been described in several cases of promethazine overdose. For further information on antihistamine toxicity see Antihistamines, pp. 104–105.

Sodium oxybate

Sodium oxybate is licensed for the treatment of narcolepsy with cataplexy. Sodium oxybate is better known as gamma-hydroxybutyrate (GHB) and is reviewed in Gamma-hydroxybutyrate and related compounds, pp. 188–189.

Melatonin

Melatonin is a naturally occurring hormone that is chemically similar to 5-hydroxytryptamine. It is synthesized in the pineal gland and has a regulatory function in controlling biological rhythms. It is licensed as a hypnotic for

adults aged over 55 years. There is limited experience with this drug in overdose, although it is not expected to produce severe toxicity. A single case report described a self-limiting period of increased lethargy and disorientation following use of four times the usual treatment dose.

Barbiturates

The barbiturates are derivatives of barbituric acid (Table 4.5). The addition of aliphatic side-chains to the central ring increases hypnotic potency whilst decreasing duration of action and accelerating metabolism. A classification of clinical uses of the barbiturates roughly corresponds to their duration of action.

(a) Short acting: the short-acting barbiturate thiopental sodium is licensed as an anaesthetic induction agent in humans. Although it has a prolonged elimination half-life, its duration of action is short as a result of rapid redistribution into fatty tissues. Thiopental has a profound depressive effect on the central nervous system and is consequently used for euthanasia in veterinary medicine.

(b) Intermediate acting; these include amobarbital, butobarbital, and secobarbital. They are now only available as hypnotics on a named-patient basis in the UK due to their narrow therapeutic range and the risk of serious toxicity following overdose.

(c) Long acting: these are used in the treatment of epilepsy. Phenobarbital is a non-selective cytochrome P450 inducer capable of inducing its own metabolism. The half-life of phenobarbital can range from 24–140 hours. Primidone is partially converted to phenobarbital, which is primarily responsible for its antiepileptic properties.

Veterinary barbiturates are also highly caustic and can cause alkaline burns if they come into contact with the skin or eyes.

Taken in overdose barbiturates cause similar features to other hypnotics, but the degree of respiratory depression is often much more marked. In addition, hypotension and cardiovascular collapse are common. Renal failure may occur as a result of hypotension or rhabdomyolysis. Cerebral oedema and aspiration pneumonia are complications. Bullous skin eruptions have been traditionally attributed to barbiturate toxicity. This finding is not unique to barbiturates and is seen in other agents that produce coma, such as carbon monoxide poisoning, other hypnotics, and opiates.

Multiple-dose activated charcoal may enhance the elimination of long-acting barbiturates and is recommended for severe poisoning with phenobarbital or with the phenobarbital precursors primidone or methylphenobarbitone.

Haemoperfusion or high efficiency haemodialysis may have a role in severe barbiturate poisoning.

Further reading

Holliman BJ, Chyka PA (1997). Problems in assessment of acute melatonin overdose. *South Med J*, 90:451–3.

Donovan KL, Fisher DJ (1989). Reversal of chloral hydrate overdose with flumazenil. *Br Med J*, 298:1253.

Illingworth RN, Stewart MJ, Jarvie DR (1979). Severe poisoning with chlormethiazole. *Br Med J*, 2:902–3.

Page CB, Duffull SB, Whyte IM, Isbister GK (2009). Promethazine overdose: clinical effects, predicting delirium and the effect of charcoal. *Quart J Med*, 102:123–31.

Stalker NE, Gambertoglio JG, Fukumitsu CJ, et al. (1978). Acute massive chloral hydrate intoxication treated with hemodialysis: a clinical pharmacokinetic analysis. *J Clin Pharmacol*, 18:136–42.

Lithium

Background
Lithium salts, including lithium carbonate and lithium citrate, have mood stabilizing properties and are used to treat patients with bipolar disorder and related conditions.

Mechanisms of toxicity
The pharmacological mechanisms of lithium toxicity are not fully understood. The drug interacts with various neurotransmitters and signalling pathways, including phosphoinositide hydrolysis, adenylate cyclase, glycogen synthase kinase-3 beta, and protein kinase C.

Lithium has a narrow therapeutic index, and adverse effects are dose-dependent; therapeutic drug monitoring aims to maintain serum concentrations between 0.5 and 0.8 mmol/L.

Toxicity may be:
- *acute*: acute ingestion in patients not previously receiving lithium
- *acute-on-therapeutic*: acute ingestion in patients receiving chronic lithium therapy
- *chronic accumulation*: this is the most common form of lithium toxicity and is more likely if there has been inadequate therapeutic drug monitoring. Precipitants include:
  - excessive dosing
  - renal impairment; chronic lithium therapy is associated with renal impairment in about 20% of patients
  - drug interactions that impair lithium clearance, e.g. thiazide diuretics, ACE inhibitors, angiotensin II antagonists, and NSAIDs
  - intercurrent illness, e.g. dehydration.

Toxicokinetics
Most lithium preparations used in clinical practice are modified-release formulations. Peak effects after therapeutic doses depend on the formulation, e.g. 30 minutes after elixir, whereas 4–5 hours after a modified-release preparation. In overdose, large quantities of lithium salt form concretions within the gut that significantly prolong absorption so that peak serum concentrations occur as late as 48–72 hours after ingestion.

Volume of distribution corresponds closely with the total body water compartment and clearance is almost exclusively by renal excretion. Intracellular lithium transport is complex and distribution to the brain and other organs is typically delayed by at least several hours after peak serum concentrations.

After therapeutic doses, the serum half-life is around 8–45 hours, but this may be considerably prolonged after lithium overdose.

Risk factors for toxicity
Toxic effects are greatest after acute-on-therapeutic ingestion or chronic accumulation. Other predictors of severe toxicity include:
- age greater than 50 years
- impaired renal function
- dehydration
- hyponatraemia.

Clinical features
Clinical features are often delayed, sometimes by up to 24 hours, due to time taken for lithium to distribute to the tissues. Features of toxicity are summarized in Table 4.6 and include gastrointestinal disturbances, cardiovascular effects, neurological dysfunction, and nephrogenic diabetes insipidus.

Investigations
The clinical severity of poisoning should be assessed by:
- Measurement of U&Es and creatinine to assess renal function. Hypernatraemia may result from lithium-induced nephrogenic diabetes insipidus.
- An ECG should be performed and ECG monitoring instituted in patients at high risk of toxicity. Non-specific ST segment and T-wave changes have been reported, as have QTc prolongation, sinus node dysfunction, and asystole.
- Measurement of a plasma or serum lithium concentration (ensure collection bottle does not contain lithium heparin). Collect sample:
  - *immediately* in patents with suspected chronic accumulation, and in patients with moderate or severe features after acute-on-therapeutic overdose.
  - *at 6 hours* in patients after acute or acute-on-therapeutic overdose when clinical features are absent or mild.
  - *repeat every 6–12 hours* until it is evident that the lithium concentration is not continuing to increase.

Interpretation of lithium concentrations
Note that lithium concentrations may be very high in the absence of serious clinical features after acute overdose, until ingested lithium is redistributed from the blood. Conversely, serious features of intoxication may occur with concentrations raised modestly above the therapeutic range in the context of chronic toxicity. Therefore, assessment of toxicity relies heavily on clinical judgement in addition to drug concentrations.

Repeating the plasma concentrations during recovery from poisoning helps in timing the restarting of chronic lithium therapy, if this is deemed appropriate. Lithium treatment should normally be confined to less than 5 years, unless the severity of underlying psychiatric illness and/or risk of relapse indicate a more prolonged course. The decision to discontinue lithium should be considered with an appropriate psychiatry specialist.

Table 4.6 Clinical features of lithium poisoning

Mild	Moderate	Severe
Nausea	Confusion	Cardiac arrhythmia: sinoatrial block, sinus and junctional bradycardia, conduction defects
Diarrhoea	Blackouts	
Blurred vision	Fasciculation	
Dizziness	Hyper-reflexia	
Tremor	Myoclonus	Hypotension
Weakness	Restlessness	Renal failure
Drowsiness	Choreoathetosis	Ataxia
Polyuria	Stupor	Coma
	Hypernatraemia	Convulsions

Management

Forced emesis and forced diuresis are of no benefit. Lithium is not bound to activated charcoal and this method of decontamination is also therefore of no value. Gastric lavage, WBI, and sodium polystyrene sulfonate, a cation exchange resin, may reduce lithium absorption, and in the latter case increase lithium clearance, but data demonstrating improved clinical outcomes are lacking.

Patients should be rehydrated with intravenous fluids and electrolyte imbalances should be corrected. An adequate airway and ventilation should be ensured in patients with a reduced conscious level. Hypotension that is unresponsive to volume re-expansion may require treatment with inotropic agents.

Isolated convulsions may be treated with diazepam but paralysis and mechanical ventilation may be needed if convulsions are recurrent or refractory (see also Convulsions, pp. 91–92).

Enhanced elimination techniques

Haemodialysis is highly efficient at removing circulating lithium, but redistribution of lithium from the tissues causes blood concentrations to 'rebound' when haemodialysis is stopped. Prolonged haemodialysis (>18 hours) or repeated sessions are needed for adequate tissue clearance.

Other elimination techniques are increasingly accessible and might impose fewer delays than implementation of haemodialysis, for example, continuous arterio-venous haemodiafiltration (CAVHDF) and continuous veno-venous haemodiafiltration (CVVHDF). These allow an increased rate of lithium clearance and can normally be implemented over a sufficiently long period as might allow effective lithium clearance, for example, over 24 hours. The rate of overall lithium clearance is limited by diffusion between the intracellular and extracellular compartments so that both haemodialysis and haemofiltration techniques require prolonged treatment. Haemodialysis may be preferred in patients with very high serum lithium concentrations and severe toxicity that require prompt reversal. However, hypotension leading to myocardial infarction has been reported during haemodialysis treatment for lithium toxicity. In patients with haemodynamic instability, continuous haemofiltration might cause less perturbation and be better tolerated.

Indications for dialysis

Dialysis should be considered if:
- severe clinical features of toxicity are present, regardless of lithium concentration, e.g. seizures, severe arrhythmia, features of extrapyramidal toxicity

- severe toxicity is likely to develop, based on the pattern of ingestion, timing, and quantity ingested
- high serum lithium concentrations even if clinical features of toxicity have not yet developed (e.g. >7.5 mmol/L after acute, or >4 mmol/L after acute-on-therapeutic or chronic accumulation).

Monitoring lithium concentrations

Lithium concentrations need to be monitored after dialysis to detect a rebound increase in circulating concentrations, which is particularly common if haemodialysis has been instituted for an insufficient duration. The end-point of dialysis is reduced tissue lithium concentrations. If this has been achieved by dialysis of sufficient duration, then rebound of serum concentration does not occur and there is effective resolution of toxicity, e.g. resolution of neurological features.

Further reading

Amdisen A (1988). Clinical features and management of lithium poisoning. *Med Toxicol Adverse Drug Exp*, 3:18–32.

Dunne FJ (2010). Lithium toxicity: the importance of clinical signs. *Br J Hosp Med*, 71:206–210.

El Balkhi S, Megarbane B, Poupon J, et al. (2009). Lithium poisoning: is determination of the red blood cell lithium concentration useful? *Clin Toxicol*, 47:8–13.

Eyer F, Pfab R, Felgenhauer N, et al. (2006). Lithium poisoning: pharmacokinetics and clearance during different therapeutic measures. *J Clin Psychopharmacol*, 26:325–30.

Ghannoum M, Lavergne V, Yue CS, et al. (2010). Successful treatment of lithium toxicity with sodium polystyrene sulfonate: a retrospective cohort study. *Clin Toxicol*, 48:34–41.

Offerman SR, Alsop JA, Lee J, et al. (2010). Hospitalized lithium overdose cases reported to the California poison control system. *Clin Toxicol*, 48:443–8.

Waring WS (2006). Management of lithium toxicity. *Toxicol Rev*, 25:221–30.

Waring WS (2007). Delayed cardiotoxicity in chronic lithium poisoning: discrepancy between serum lithium concentrations and clinical status. *Basic Clin Pharmacol Toxicol*, 100:353–5.

Waring WS, Laing WJ, Good AM, et al. (2007). Pattern of lithium toxicity predicts poisoning severity: evaluation of referrals to a regional poisons unit. *Quart J Med*, 100:271–6.

Wilting I, Heerdink ER, Mersch PP, et al. (2009). Association between lithium serum level, mood state, and patient-reported adverse drug reactions during long-term lithium treatment: a naturalistic follow-up study. *Bipolar Disord*, 11:434–40.

Chapter 5

Analgesics

Paracetamol

Background

Paracetamol (acetaminophen, 4-hydroxyacetanilide, N-acetyl para-aminophenol, 4-acetamidophenol) is commonly used as an analgesic and antipyretic. Its widespread availability as an over-the-counter product contributes to its frequent use in overdose. In the United Kingdom, for example, paracetamol is involved in more than 40% of all overdose episodes.

Although paracetamol has an excellent safety profile when used in recommended doses, excessive doses can be associated with severe and potentially fatal toxic effects, especially fulminant hepatic failure (FHF). Paracetamol remains one of the most common agents involved in fatal poisoning, in spite of the availability of antidotes that are highly effective provided these are used soon after poisoning.

Mechanisms of toxicity

Taken in therapeutic doses, most paracetamol is conjugated in the liver with glucuronide or sulfate to form non-toxic metabolites, but a small amount is converted by to the reactive intermediate alkylating metabolite N-acetyl-para-benzo-quinone imine (NAPQI), principally by the hepatic cytochrome P450 isoenzyme CYP2E1, with a smaller contribution from CYP3A4 and CYP1A2. This is rapidly metabolized in glutathione-dependent reactions to non-toxic cysteine and mercapturic acid conjugates that are subsequently excreted in the urine and (to a lesser extent) the bile. After administration of toxic paracetamol doses, hepatic glutathione becomes depleted and NAPQI accumulates, binding to key cell constituents and setting in progress a sequence of events resulting in hepatocellular death.

Toxicokinetics

Paracetamol is rapidly absorbed after ingestion with peak blood concentrations occurring within an hour of a therapeutic dose and almost always within 4 hours following overdose.

The elimination t½ of paracetamol is approximately 2 hours after a therapeutic dose. This is increased to about 3 hours following overdose without liver damage because of saturation of the usual sulphation and glucuronidation pathways and to over 7 hours in patients who subsequently developed liver damage, with the prolongation in t½ correlated with the extent of subsequent liver damage.

Risk factors for toxicity

In animal studies paracetamol hepatotoxicity is enhanced by factors associated with hepatic glutathione depletion, increased formation of NAPQI, and/or pre-existing liver disease. Observational evidence suggests that these factors are also relevant to human poisoning, although in the UK and elsewhere these are no longer considered when deciding if patients with paracetamol poisoning should be treated with an antidote.

Glutathione depletion

This occurs with impaired recent (over several days) food intake, for example, in depression, chronic alcoholism, active HIV infection, or anorexia nervosa. Clinical clues to recent starvation include a low plasma urea, ketonuria, or abnormal liver function. Because glutathione is related to acute starvation, it may be present in patients who are overweight but who have not eaten properly in the days prior to overdose.

Enhanced NAPQI formation

Formation of NAPQI is increased by hepatic enzyme induction, especially when affecting CYP2E1. Causes include the following:

- Chronic excess alcohol ingestion. Enzyme induction is usually associated with very substantial chronic alcohol intake, but because a threshold for induction is not well defined. To further complicate the issue, there is evidence that acute ingestion of alcohol, which is common in patients with overdose in the context of self-harm, is protective against hepatotoxicity. As a result patients who regularly ingest large amounts of alcohol but who are sober when ingesting paracetamol may be at particular risk.

- Treatment with enzyme-inducing drugs including antiepileptic agents (e.g. carbamazepine, phenytoin, phenobarbital, primidone), antituberculous chemotherapy (rifampicin, rifabutin), and antiviral drugs (e.g. efavirenz, nevirapine). St John's wort, a herbal preparation sometimes used to treat depression, is a CYP3A4 inducer and in theory may also enhance toxicity of paracetamol.

Clinical clues of hepatic enzyme induction include the history of alcohol or medication use and the presence of a raised gamma-glutamyl transferase (GGT).

Pre-existing liver disease

There is epidemiological evidence to suggest an increased risk of hepatotoxicity after paracetamol overdose in patients with pre-existing liver disease including vital hepatitis, non-alcoholic liver disease, and Gilbert's syndrome.

Other possible factors affecting risk of toxicity

Other factors that may affect risk of paracetamol-induced hepatotoxicity have been suggested by animal research or human observational studies, although evidence is weaker and these are not generally taken into account when deciding on use of antidotes.

Young children may be more resistant to paracetamol hepatotoxicity than adults at equivalent weight-adjusted doses. Conversely, risks may be higher in elderly adults, although firm conclusions cannot be drawn from currently available information.

People of Caucasian origin appear to have on average increased metabolic activation of paracetamol compared with people of African racial origin and some epidemiological studies provide limited evidence supporting and increase in risk. The clinical implications of this have not been studies in detail.

Cigarette smoking is associated with induction of CYP1A2 and observational studies have shown a small apparent increased in risk of hepatotoxicity in smokers. It is difficult, however, to exclude a contribution from confounders such as diet, health state, alcohol use, etc.

Some epidemiological studies have suggested an increase in risk for females compared with males. Also, use of oestrogen-containing oral contraceptives appears to be associated with small increases in oxidative metabolism; the effects of this on risk of hepatotoxicity have not been studies in detail.

As already discussed, acute ingestion of alcohol appears to provide some protection against paracetamol-induced hepatotoxicity.

Clinical features

Early features of paracetamol poisoning are usually non-specific, e.g. nausea and vomiting. Consciousness is not directly affected and impairment usually indicates co-ingestion of sedative drugs or alcohol. Paracetamol may be ingested in combination analgesics containing opioids (e.g. codeine, dihydrocodeine) and features of poisoning with these agents may also be present.

Patients with significant paracetamol poisoning progress to develop features of hepatotoxicity and, less commonly, renal impairment in the days after ingestion, with these features developing more rapidly in those with severe poisoning.

Hepatotoxicity

The most prominent toxic effect after severe poisoning is hepatic necrosis. Hepatic tenderness may appear after about 12 hours. Subsequently abnormal liver function associated with derangement of clotting may develop with maximum effects seen 3–6 days after ingestion in patients who recover spontaneously.

Severely poisoned patients develop progressively clinical features of liver dysfunction, culminating in FHF with associated jaundice, confusion, encephalopathy, spontaneous bruising, ascites, acidosis, and hypoglycaemia. Raised intracranial pressure may ensue as a result of cerebral oedema, resulting in headache, reduced level of consciousness, papilloedema, and brainstem coning marked by pupillary dilatation and cardiac dysrhythmias. Disseminated intravascular coagulation (DIC) may complicate FHF.

The speed of progression of liver failure is related to the severity of poisoning, with jaundice developing within 24 hours in some patients with very severe poisoning.

Nephrotoxicity

A minority of patients (~2%) with paracetamol toxicity may develop renal failure, thought to be due to metabolic activation of paracetamol in the kidney. This is sometimes accompanied by loin pain, haematuria, and proteinuria. The plasma creatinine increases, starting on day 2 after overdose and usually peaking between days 3 and 6 with recovery to normal by day 9, although occasionally renal impairment may progress over 2 weeks or more. Plasma urea is unreliable as a marker of renal function due to impaired hepatic urea production as a result of hepatotoxicity.

Renal failure usually occurs in patients with severe hepatic necrosis but renal failure can occasionally occur in isolation.

Other features

Hypoglycaemia

Hypoglycaemia may occur 12–72 hours after overdose due to impairment of hepatic gluconeogenesis.

Lactic acidosis

Lactic acidosis may be an early feature of poisoning or may complicate later FHF. Lactic acidosis usually indicates a poor clinical outcome.

Uncommon effects

Uncommon effects reported with paracetamol poisoning include acute pancreatitis sometimes associated with paralytic ileus; neutrophilia and thrombocytopenia; ECG changes, including non-specific ST segment or T wave changes, or prominent U waves which may relate to hypokalaemia. Arrhythmias including ventricular fibrillation have also been reported but appear very rare and may have been due to other coingestants, especially dextropropoxyphene,

Diagnosis

The diagnosis of paracetamol poisoning is usually obvious, but some patients may not volunteer a history of paracetamol ingestion.

Establishing the severity of poisoning is important as this determines the need for use of an antidote such as acetylcysteine; this is not always straightforward.

Severity of poisoning is gauged from the history of ingestion, the plasma paracetamol concentration related to the time since ingestion and, in later presenters, the presence of liver function abnormalities. However, the history is often an unreliable indicator of the severity of poisoning, with limited correlation between reported doses and subsequently measured plasma paracetamol concentrations. The interval between ingestion and blood concentration measurement may be unknown or reported inaccurately by patients who may be distressed or intoxicated.

When there is doubt about the need for antidotal treatment, the clinician should err on the side of caution and the patient should always be treated.

Investigations

Measurement of plasma paracetamol concentration

Samples should be taken from all patients reporting acute paracetamol overdose at 4 hours after ingestion in patients presenting within that period. Samples taken less than 4 hours after overdose cannot be used for risk assessment because concentrations may still be increasing. For patients presenting more than 4 hours after overdose the sample should be taken as soon as possible.

Risk of severe paracetamol toxicity after acute overdose, and therefore the need for antidotal therapy, is assessed by plotting the plasma paracetamol concentration against the time since ingestion on a nomogram. The nomogram currently used in the UK classifies patients as requiring an antidote if the concentration is above a 'treatment' line starting at 100 mg/L (0.66 mmol/L) at 4 hours, with the concentration falling exponentially with a $t\frac{1}{2}$ of 4 hours to 50 mg at 8 hours, 25 mg at 12 hours, etc. (Figure 5.1). This is sometimes called the '100 line'. When assessing the time since ingestion, the treating clinician should use the earliest time that paracetamol might have be taken in overdose.

Paracetamol treatment nomograms were developed by relating patient outcomes to paracetamol concentrations in the pre-antidote era, when about 60% of patients whose paracetamol concentration was above line starting at 200 mg/L and falling exponentially with a $t\frac{1}{2}$ of 4 hours to 100 mg at 8 hours, 50 mg at 12 hours, etc. subsequently developed hepatic necrosis without specific treatment. In the UK, this higher, '200' line, was used for most patients, with the '100' line used only for patients with risk factors for enhanced hepatoxicity. However, following reports of fatal hepatotoxicity after lower paracetamol concentrations had been observed in patients without apparent risk factors present, the single '100' treatment line has been used since 2012.

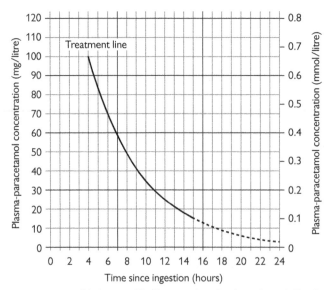

Fig 5.1 Paracetamol treatment nomogram (Medicines and Healthcare products Regulatory Agency). This Crown copyright material is reproduced by permission of the Medicines and Healthcare products Regulatory Agency (MHRA) under delegated authority from the Controller of HMSO. Available at: <http://www.mhra.gov.uk/home/groups/pl-p/documents/drugsafetymessage/con184396.pdf> (accessed 30 September 2013).

There are variations in management guidelines for paracetamol poisoning around the world. In North America and Australasia the threshold for treatment is based on a treatment line starting at 150 mg/L at 4 hours (the '150 line'), while in Denmark all patients with confirmed paracetamol overdose are treated with an antidote; paracetamol concentrations are measured but only to confirm that the drug has been ingested.

It is important to emphasize that there is a progressive increase in risk of hepatotoxicity with increasing paracetamol concentrations at any time point after ingestion with no absolute cut-off point identifying patients with a zero risk. As a result no nomogram has perfect sensitivity and specificity for detecting patients at risk of severe hepatotoxicity, as evidenced by the occasional reports of patients apparently below conventional treatment lines who develop unexpected hepatic failure that is sometimes fatal. While some of these may have been misclassified because the history may have been inaccurate or risk factors may not have been identified, it is clear that some patients develop severe hepatotoxicity at unexpectedly low paracetamol concentrations, although this seems very rare. There is a need to balance the risks of this with those of adverse reactions associated with more widespread antidote use in patients at lower risk. The benefits and risks of acetylcysteine for patients presenting with paracetamol concentrations between the '100' and '150' lines seem finely balanced, which underlies the differences in thresholds used in different countries.

Assessment of renal and liver function
Samples should be sent for U&Es, creatinine, LFTs including GGT, and clotting. These should be repeated at least daily in patients with clinically important paracetamol overdose and more frequently if values are changing rapidly.

Hepatic necrosis is indicated by increases in aspartate and alanine transaminase (AST and ALT) which can peak at values as high as 500× normal, usually 3–6 days after overdose. Impairment of synthetic hepatic function, specifically reduced production of clotting factors, especially factors II, V, and VII, results in an increase in prothrombin time (PT) or its international normalized ratio (INR). There are also increases in bilirubin, although the latter is less sensitive.

Liver function and clotting are usually only deranged 24 hours or longer after overdose, but early measurement is useful as abnormalities may indicate pre-existing liver disease, which is thought to predispose to a worse outcome, or point to evolving liver damage relating to paracetamol ingestion earlier than has been reported by the patient.

An elevated gamma GGT may indicate that the patient ids at high risk due to hepatic enzyme induction, e.g. by chronic ethanol intake or enzyme-inducing drugs.

Hypokalaemia due to kaliuresis is a common dose-dependent effect in early paracetamol poisoning and appears to be independent of vomiting and use of acetylcysteine. Hypophosphataemia due to renal phosphate loss is also seen at this stage.

In early paracetamol poisoning fibrinogen concentrations are increased while reduced levels may occur in patients with severe liver dysfunction due to DIC.

In patients who develop FHF, levels of factor V are reduced and those of factor VIII increased in those who subsequently die and the VIII/V ratio is sometimes used as a prognostic indicator in this group.

Management

The most important management step at initial presentation is to assess the severity of poisoning as this determines the need for an antidote, which can be life-saving. Antidotes are not used in all patients because of the significant associated risk of adverse effects.

Assessment of ingested dose

An accurate history of the preparation taken and the amount involved is essential for appropriate early management and for deciding on use of antidotes after staggered overdose, when the timing of overdose is uncertain and after repeated supratherapeutic dosing, but the history of the timing of overdose and/or the amount involved may be unreliable.

An overdose of 150 mg/kg paracetamol or more (i.e. >12 g in an 80 kg patient) carries a significant risk of hepatotoxicity, although lower doses (e.g. 75–150 mg) may also be associated with hepatic necrosis in particularly susceptible individuals. For obese patients, a maximum weight of 110 kg should be used.

A reduced level of consciousness should alert the clinician to the possibility of other sedative drugs being involved as these may require specific therapy.

Prevention of paracetamol absorption

Administration of activated charcoal may be of some value for preventing paracetamol absorption if administered soon after a significant overdose and should be considered for patients reporting ingestions greater than 150 mg/kg within 1 hour.

Gastric aspiration or lavage has also been used for very large ingestions in patients who present early as activated charcoal has limited capacity for drug binding. These methods, however, carry risks, including that of aspiration. They are therefore not generally recommended for paracetamol poisoning, as effective antidotes are available for those absorbing potentially toxic amounts.

Supportive care

Fluid and electrolyte therapy may be required for patients who are vomiting.

Antidotes

Antidotes for paracetamol poisoning act by replenishing hepatic glutathione to increase the amount available for detoxification of NAPQI. Two antidotes have been used in routine clinical practice, methionine and n-acetylcysteine, although methionine is currently used very rarely.

Acetylcysteine

Acetylcysteine and its metabolite cysteine replenish glutathione and benefits may also occur as a result of direct antioxidant effects. The drug can be administered orally or by intravenous infusion. It has a t½ of 2–6 hours, although a prolonged terminal t½ of 15 hours has been reported.

Acetylcysteine is effective for preventing liver dysfunction in patients with substantial paracetamol overdose when used by the intravenous or oral routes. It is almost universally effective at preventing severe liver dysfunction if administered within 8 hours of overdose, but efficacy subsequently declines. It is therefore critically important that administration is commenced within 8 hours, or as soon as possible after that for patients who present later. There is a lack of evidence for efficacy of acetylcysteine when used more than 15 hours after overdose, but current management guidelines recommend use in patients with severe paracetamol poisoning at any time after ingestion. One reason for this is that acetylcysteine

has been shown to be effective for preventing mortality in patients with established paracetamol-induced FHF, although this may be a non-specific action as the antidote has also appears to have benefit in patients with liver failure from other causes.

Intravenous acetylcysteine

The usual intravenous infusion regimen for acetylcysteine in the UK is 150 mg/kg in 200 mL infusion fluid over 1 hour, followed by 50 mg/kg in 500 mL infusion fluid over 4 hours, followed by 100 mg/kg in 1000 mL infusion fluid over 16 hours, giving a total dose of 300 mg/kg acetylcysteine infused over 21 hours. The same dose is used in children as in adults, but the volume of diluent needs to be reduced (Table 5.1). A ceiling weight of 110 kg should be used for obese patients.

The initial infusion, which delivers half the total dose of acetylcysteine, was previously administered over 15 minutes rather than 1 hour. It is therefore not surprising that dose-related adverse effects (see following 'Adverse effects' subsection) were very common during or soon after this first infusion had been given. Administration over the longer 1-hour period, as currently recommended in the UK and elsewhere, is a logical modification, although there is currently no direct evidence that this reduces the risk of adverse effects.

Following completion of acetylcysteine infusion, U&Es, LFTs, and clotting should be checked. If these are normal or improving, no further antidote is required and the patient can be considered for discharge, although they should be warned to return in the very unlikely event that they develop abdominal pain or vomiting. An elevated INR of 1.3 or less may result from acetylcysteine therapy and, in the absence of a raised ALT, should not be considered to indicate liver damage. Some clinicians also measure paracetamol concentration after acetylcysteine as persisting detectable concentrations, e.g. from massive overdose, prolonged paracetamol t½ or delayed absorption, are a further reason to continue acetylcysteine infusion. It is unusual, however, for paracetamol to be detected at this time after overdose.

If values are deteriorating, further 16-hour infusions (100 mg/kg) should be administered until improvement is documented, although there is no direct evidence that this improves clinical outcomes.

Adverse effects

The most common adverse effects of intravenous acetylcysteine are nausea and vomiting, affecting about half of all recipients. So-called 'anaphylactoid' reactions usually occur during or soon after the first infusion and are characterized by flushing, itching, and urticaria and are experienced by about a quarter of recipients. More severe anaphylactoid effects such as angio-oedema, bronchospasm, tachycardia, and/or hypotension, are much less common. Anaphylactoid reactions are not a true allergic phenomenon but caused by dose-related histamine-release from mast cells. People with a history of atopy or asthma appear at higher risk, while high paracetamol concentrations associated with severe overdoses appear to be protective.

Anaphylactoid reactions are sometimes severe and fatalities have been reported, although this is very rare and often associated with inadvertent acetylcysteine overdose.

Anaphylactoid reactions are managed by suspending the infusion and, in more severe cases, administering an

Table 5.1 Adult dose table for acetylcysteine (Medicines and Healthcare products Regulatory Agency)

	Adult acetylcysteine prescription (each ampoule = 200mg/mL acetylcysteine)				Please circle appropriate weight and volume	
Regimen	First Infusion		Second Infusion		Third Infusion	
Infusion fluid	200 mLs 5% glucose or sodium chloride 0.9%		500 mLs 5% glucose or sodium chloride 0.9%		1000 mLs 5%. glucose or sodium chloride 0.9%	
Duration of infusion	1 hour		1 hour		16 hours	
Drug dose	150 mg/kg acetylcysteine		50 mg/kg acetylcysteine		100 mg/kg acetylcysteine	
Patient Weight[1]	Ampoule volume[2]	Infusion Rate	Ampoule volume[2]	Infusion Rate	Ampoule volume[2]	Infusion Rate
Kg	mL	mL/h	mL	mL/h	mL	mL/h
40–49	34	234	12	128	23	64
50–59	42	242	14	129	28	64
60–69	49	249	17	129	33	65
70–79	57	257	19	130	38	65
80–89	64	264	22	131	43	65
90–99	72	272	24	131	48	66
100–109	79	279	27	132	53	66
≥110	83	283	28	132	55	66

[1] Dose calculations are based on the weight in the middle of each band. if the patient weighs less than 40kg use the paediatric dosage table.

[2].Ampoule volume has been rounded up to the nearest whole number

antihistamine such as chlorphenamine (50 mg IV). Once the reaction has settled the infusion can be restarted at a lower rate. The rare very severe reactions may require administration of corticosteroids and epinephrine and critical care management of the airway, respiration, and circulation.

Acetylcysteine has a direct effect on clotting, prolonging the prothrombin time by up to 1–3 seconds. This is important because it can be misinterpreted as the development of hepatic impairment.

Oral acetylcysteine

In the United States intravenous acetylcysteine was not licensed until 2004 and paracetamol overdose was usually treated with oral acetylcysteine using a loading dose of 140 mg/kg, followed by further doses of 70 mg/kg given every 4 hours to a total of 17 doses. This appears about as effective for preventing hepatotoxicity as the intravenous regimen; there is indirect evidence that it may be slightly less effective for patients presenting early but slightly more effective for late presenters.

The most common adverse effects of oral acetylcysteine are vomiting and diarrhoea but serious adverse effects including anaphylactoid reactions are very rare. The unpleasant smell of the medication and the prolonged course required are disadvantages of this route of administration and may discourage adherence.

Methionine

Studies comparing treated patients with untreated historical controls demonstrated that oral methionine in a dose of 2.5 g every 4 hours for a total of four doses was effective at reducing the frequency of hepatotoxicity.

Adverse effects include nausea, vomiting, and irritability and hepatic encephalopathy may be precipitated in susceptible individuals. For this reason late use of methionine, e.g. more than 10 hours after overdose, has been discouraged. The evidence for efficacy of methionine is

more limited than that for acetylcysteine (oral or intravenous). For this reason acetylcysteine has remained the antidote of choice for paracetamol poisoning.

Addition of methionine to paracetamol tablets has been suggested as a means of preventing severe toxicity. Although suitable preparations have been developed, these have not been widely used.

Enhanced elimination techniques

Haemodialysis and charcoal haemoperfusion, while effective for enhancing paracetamol elimination, have no role in the early management of paracetamol poisoning, although haemodialysis is sometimes needed for acute renal failure.

Management of liver failure

Early transfer of patients developing severe hepatic dysfunction is important for maximizing probability of survival. Discussion with a liver unit if recommended for patients with any of the following features:

• PT over 25–30 seconds and rising
• early encephalopathy
• creatinine over 200 micromol/L and rising
• pH less than 7.3
• systolic blood pressure less than 80 mmHg.

A detailed account of the management of hepatic failure caused by paracetamol poisoning is outside the scope of this book. Briefly, rigorous management of fluid balance, prevention of hypoglycaemia, administration of intravenous acetylcysteine and aggressive treatment of acidosis (sodium bicarbonate), renal failure (haemodialysis), circulatory failure (inotropes), infections (antibiotics), active haemorrhage (vitamin K, clotting factors, blood), and cerebral oedema (mannitol, ultrafiltration) are essential. Intracranial pressure monitoring assists with early diagnosis of cerebral oedema (see also Hepatic failure, pp. 73–74).

Liver transplantation is a valuable treatment option for patients who otherwise have a very high risk of mortality, with a 5-year survival of more than 50%. In one recent series 58% of recipients were surviving an average of 9 years post transplantation. The challenge is to identify patients who would not otherwise survive. The modified King's College Criteria is one of several scoring systems advocated:

- arterial pH less than 7.3 or lactate greater than 3.0 mmol/L in spite of adequate fluid resuscitation
- concurrent findings of:
  - encephalopathy grade III or IV
  - creatinine greater than 300 micromol/L, and
  - INR higher than 6.5 or PT longer than 100 seconds.

Hyperphosphataemia also appears to be associated with a worse prognosis in patients with liver failure.

Chronic paracetamol poisoning

There is increasing evidence of harm from chronic paracetamol use, especially following use of excessive doses.

Staggered overdoses involve intentional consumption of excess paracetamol over a prolonged duration (e.g. >1 hour) or in several single episodes. These may often involve large total doses of paracetamol carrying a substantial risk of hepatoxicity. The treatment nomogram is of no value in assessing risk of subsequent toxicity following staggered overdose and all patients who may have ingested potentially toxic amounts should be treated with acetylcysteine.

Excess therapeutic paracetamol can also result in FHF. Excess ingestion may occur because the patient is unaware of the hazards or they may have inadvertently used more than one paracetamol-containing preparation.

Clinical trials have also demonstrated that increases in hepatic transaminases in patients treated with regular therapeutic doses of paracetamol are common, although often transient in spite of continuing therapy. There are, however, occasional anecdotal reports of liver failure with usual therapeutic doses of paracetamol, often in patients with other risk factors for hepatotoxicity.

Clinical features, investigation and management
Clinical features, investigation, and management of chronic excess paracetamol ingestion are as for acute overdose, except that the paracetamol concentration is not of value in assessing the risk of liver dysfunction, although it may confirm ingestion. As a result risk assessment has to rely on the history of ingestion and there is a lack of high-quality evidence of the value of this approach. Current UK guidelines suggest that patients reporting ingestions of more than 150 mg/kg in any 24-hour period should be considered for intravenous acetylcysteine, unless they have normal LFTs and clotting more than 24 hours after the last paracetamol intake. Some susceptible patients ingesting smaller amounts, e.g. greater than 75 mg/kg/24 hours, may also be at risk, but there is currently no agreed method of identifying those who may be susceptible to these lower doses and current UK guidance suggests that clinical judgement should be used, taking into account the dose reported to be ingested and the apparent reliability of the history. The presence of an abnormal ALT or INR result at any time, or a detectable paracetamol concentration more than 24 hours after the last dose may indicate developing paracetamol hepatotoxicity and patients with these features should be treated with acetylcysteine

In patients treated with an antidote, plasma creatinine, LFTs and clotting should be repeated after the full 21-hour treatment course and the patient managed subsequently as for patients with acute paracetamol overdose.

Intravenous paracetamol overdose

The increasing popularity of intravenous paracetamol as an analgesic and antipyretic for hospital in-patients has been accompanied by many reports of inadvertent overdose. Management is as for oral paracetamol overdose except that the lower threshold of 60 mg/kg has been proposed for antidotal treatment for adults and children in the UK. If the dose is uncertain but the interval is known, the paracetamol nomogram can be used, except that acetylcysteine treatment is recommended at half the concentration of the usual treatment line (e.g. 50 mg/L at 4 hours). This is a very conservative approach, pending the availability of more evidence, taking into account the complete ands rapid bioavailability of paracetamol after intravenous infusion and the probable high risk status of many patients because of starvation associated with acute illness or surgical procedures.

Paracetamol overdose in pregnancy

The limited information available suggests that severe fetal hepatotoxicity and intrauterine death can occur after maternal paracetamol overdose, but are unlikely to be encountered in the absence of severe maternal toxicity. There is no evidence that pregnant women are at increased risk for paracetamol hepatotoxicity.

Data on the safety of use of acetylcysteine are limited but do not point to a risk of teratogenesis. Current experience suggests that benefits of acetylcysteine use for severe paracetamol poisoning during pregnancy outweigh any unknown risks to the fetus and that early treatment offers mother and fetus the best chance of a successful outcome.

For calculation of acetylcysteine doses, it may be advisable to use the patient's current rather than pre-pregnancy weight, up to a maximum of 110 kg.

Further reading

Bateman DN, Dear J (2010). Medicine, poison, and mystic potion: a personal perspective on paracetamol Louis Roche lecture, Stockholm, 2009. *Clin Toxicol*, 48:97–103.

Bridger S, Henderson K, Glucksman E, et al. (1998). *Deaths from low dose paracetamol poisoning BMJ*, 316:1724–5.

Buckley N, Eddleston M (2007). Paracetamol (acetaminophen) poisoning. *Clin Evid*, 12:2101.

Ferner RE, Dear JW, Bateman DN (2011). Management of paracetamol poisoning. *BMJ*, 342:d2218.

McElhatton PR, Sullivan FM, Volans GN (1997). Paracetamol overdose in pregnancy analysis of the outcomes of 300 cases referred to the Teratology Information Service. *Reprod Toxicol*, 11:85–94.

Mitchell JR, Jollow DJ, Potter WZ, et al. (1973). Acetaminophen-induced hepatic necrosis. IV. Protective role of glutathione *J Pharmacol Exp Ther*, 187:211–17.

Prescott LF, Illingworth RN, Critchley JA, et al. (1979). Intravenous N-acetylcystine: the treatment of choice for paracetamol poisoning *BMJ*, 2:1097–100.

Sandilands EA, Bateman DN (2009). Adverse reactions associated with acetylcysteine. *Clin Toxicol*, 47:81–8.

Smilkstein MJ, Knapp GL, Kulig KW, et al. (1988). Efficacy of oral N-acetylcysteine in the treatment of acetaminophen overdose. Analysis of the national multicenter study (1976 to 1985). *N Engl J Med*, 319:1557–62.

Thomas SHL (1993). Paracetamol (acetaminophen) poisoning. *Pharmacol Ther*, 60:91–120.

Non-steroidal anti-inflammatory drugs

Background

Non-steroidal anti-inflammatory drugs (NSAIDs) are widely prescribed and several are also available for over-the-counter sale.

NSAIDs come in different chemical groupings:

- propionic (arylpropionic) acid derivatives: fenbufen, ibuprofen, ketoprofen, naproxen, tiaprofenic acid
- oxicams (enolic acid derivatives): meloxicam, piroxicam, tenoxicam
- acetic acid derivatives; indometacin, sulindac, etodolac, diclofenac, nabumetone
- fenamates; mefenamic acid
- selective cyclo-oxygenase (COX)-2 inhibitors: celecoxib, etoricoxib.

To a very large extent these chemical differences make little difference to toxicity in overdose, but are more relevant to the toxicity in long-term therapeutic use. Key differences in toxicity in long-term use relate to adverse cardiovascular risk profile and rates of GI ulcer formation.

The main toxicity of NSAIDs seen in overdose is on the kidney. In very large doses CNS or hepatic effects may be seen, but these are uncommon, except following overdose with mefenamic acid.

Toxicity is generally low, and, for example, ingestion of less than 100 mg/kg of ibuprofen, the widest used NSAID, is unlikely to cause features. Patients ingesting more than this require careful assessment and in those ingesting more than 400 mg/kg of ibuprofen toxicity is extremely likely.

Mefenamic acid is unique in that it causes convulsions more commonly than other NSAIDs. In a study of 29 cases of mefenamic acid poisoning, convulsions were recorded in 38% of patients, although these were rarely persistent. Bloody diarrhoea may also be a feature of mefenamic acid overdose, and diarrhoea is also a relatively common adverse effect in therapeutic use.

Mechanisms of toxicity

NSAIDs cause their principal effects in overdose because of their actions on COX enzymes, particularly in the kidney. Prostaglandins are important in maintaining renal circulation and in the control of electrolyte handling in the kidney. In overdose NSAIDs inhibit prostaglandin metabolism, initially causing a relative increase in potassium loss which may be sufficient to cause hypokalaemia. Subsequently renal shutdown occurs because of secondary vascular changes and acute kidney injury develops. In very large doses CNS depression has been reported; this may be due to effects on central prostaglandin production. Hepatic damage with acute hepatitis is rarely reported, and the mechanisms are not well understood.

Topical preparations are non-toxic unless swallowed. Suppositories may cause local toxicity to the rectum with ulceration, but this is not a normal presentation in overdose. Parenteral administration of excess doses of these drugs is normally only a hazard in patients at increased risk of toxicity (see later in section).

Toxicokinetics

NSAIDs are rapidly absorbed, as would be expected from their use as analgesics. They have a small volume of distribution as a result of plasma protein binding. They are eliminated via hepatic metabolism or via the kidneys. Most NSAIDs have short $t\frac{1}{2}$ (Table 5.2), for example the half-life of ibuprofen in overdose is 1.5–3 hours. Some, however, are available as modified-release preparations which may the delay onset of maximum effects and prolong toxicity.

Risk factors for toxicity

The key determinants of toxicity are the dose ingested and presence or absence of risk factors, and, in the case of therapeutic use, length of elimination, with long-$t\frac{1}{2}$ drugs being potentially more toxic.

NSAIDs are the commonest cause of acute kidney injury seen in UK renal units. In the vast majority of these patients overdose is not a factor, but there is often a pre-existing risk factor.

Key risk factors at the time of ingestion are as follows:

- increased age
- pre-existing renal disease
- hypovolaemia
- hypotension
- co-ingestion of nephrotoxic agents.

Thus co-ingestion of drugs that may cause hypotension, or NSAID overdoses associated with vomiting and secondary dehydration or electrolyte disturbance will be at increased risk of renal damage.

The toxic effects of NSAIDs are thought to be more severe in children, although, it is difficult to confirm this objectively.

Some patients with asthma are sensitive to the effects of aspirin and NSAIDs, which increase their risk of exacerbations of bronchospasm.

Pregnancy

There is no evidence that exposure to these agents in pregnancy caries any increased risk to the mother. Exposure in the first weeks of pregnancy is also not hazardous to the fetus. Because of the importance of prostaglandins in later development, however, exposure

Table 5.2 Common NSAIDs and their half-life ($t\frac{1}{2}$) at therapeutic dose and estimated minimum potentially toxic doses (mg/kg body weight)

Drug	Approximate $t\frac{1}{2}$ (hours)	Potentially toxic dose (mg/kg)
Short half-life		
Diclofenac	1.1	15
Ketoprofen	1.8	10
Mefenamic acid	2.0	40
Ibuprofen	2.1	100
Etodolac	3.0	50
Indometacin	4.6	7.5
Long half-life		
Naproxen	14	35
Nabumetone	26	100
(active metabolite)	(22)	
Piroxicam	57	5

to NSAIDs after 30 weeks of pregnancy increases the risk of premature closure of the ductus arteriosus and oligohydramnios. The incidence and severity of premature closure of the ductus arteriosus beyond 30 weeks appears to be dose related.

In circumstances where exposure to NSAIDs has occurred during the third-trimester, it is sensible to monitor the fetus regularly for oligohydramnios. Fetal circulation should be monitored via fetal echocardiogram following any NSAID exposure in late pregnancy. Oligohydramnios may be detected through serial scans measuring amniotic fluid volume and growth. Detection of an abnormality following third-trimester exposure to an NSAID warrants referral to a fetal medicine unit for further investigation.

Clinical features

Gastrointestinal

Vomiting is often seen and NSAIDs may cause acute GI irritation after overdose but this is unusual. Liver damage is possible, but is not to be expected without other features of significant poisoning.

Renal

Alterations in renal blood flow due to inhibition of prostaglandin synthesis causes disturbance of electrolyte excretion, with initial kaliuresis, followed by acute tubular damage and renal failure at higher doses.

Risk of renal damage is likely to be increased by co-ingestion of other potentially nephrotoxic agents, particularly those also associated with renal damage, such as ACE inhibitors, as well as in the elderly or those with renal disease.

CNS

Tinnitus and headache may occur. In more serious poisoning, there may be drowsiness (occasionally excitation), disorientation, or coma. Rarely (apart from mefenamic acid, see below) patients develop convulsions.

Laboratory

In serious poisoning acidosis may occur and an increase in INR may be observed, probably due to interference with the actions of clotting factors in the circulation.

Other

Asthmatics with aspirin sensitivity may suffer bronchospasm, which is treated conventionally.

Mefenamic acid

Produces nausea, vomiting, and, occasionally, bloody diarrhoea. Drowsiness, dizziness, and headaches are common and hyper-reflexia, muscle twitching, and dose-dependent convulsions occur. Hypoprothrombinaemia and acute kidney injury have been reported.

Toxicity assessment

Assessment of toxicity following ingestion is based on dose and clinical features. Toxicity is unlikely to occur at low doses (see Table 5.2), will be made more likely by co-ingestion of nephrotoxic drugs, and is more likely in those who are hypovolaemic, the elderly, or who have existing renal disease. These patients should be monitored more carefully. Monitoring is primarily therefore aimed at assessing renal function over time.

Investigations

Blood should be taken for creatinine, U&Es, and LFTs at baseline and repeated at intervals in patients with suspected severe poisoning. A full blood count is necessary if there is any evidence of haematemesis or melaena.

Evidence confirming the extent of renal impairment may take several days to develop.

Monitoring of acid–base status by blood gas analysis and assessment of clotting is necessary in patients with suspected severe poisoning.

Management

The key features in managing patients with non-steroidal ingestion are firstly administration of activated charcoal in those who present soon (e.g. within an hour) after a potentially toxic overdose. In practice, prompt attendance is unusual and this approach is rarely used.

Careful physiological monitoring of BP, pulse rate, respiration, and conscious level at regular intervals over the first few hours after ingestion is necessary in all but the mildest cases. In symptomatic patients regular (15-minute) nursing observations are appropriate. Urine output and fluid balance should also be monitored. Depending on the agent and dose ingested and the anticipated duration of effects, patients may require monitoring in hospital for between 4 and 12 hours after ingestion.

Appropriate replacement of fluid in those who are vomiting, adequate hydration, and maintenance of an appropriate blood pressure is necessary, particularly in patients who ingest hypotensive agents or other nephrotoxic drugs.

In patients who have brief convulsions, treatment is generally not required. In those with persistent seizures an intravenous benzodiazepine (e.g. diazepam 10–20 mg, or lorazepam 4 mg in adults) can be used.

In the case of metabolic derangement, careful monitoring of acid–base balance is important, using arterial or venous bicarbonate and pH as appropriate to the clinical situation. Appropriate fluid and bicarbonate replacement should be implemented in the management of metabolic acidosis. An initial dose of 50 mmol sodium bicarbonate should be administered, and the response monitored with the target pH of 7.4.

Renal replacement therapy is appropriate in those with severe renal injury; recovery of renal function is to be expected if the cause is acute tubular necrosis. Haemodialysis is ineffective for enhancing NSAID elimination.

Other clinical supportive measures should be applied as necessary.

Further reading

Balali-Mood M, Critchley JA, Proudfoot AT, et al. (1981) Mefenamic acid overdosage. Lancet, 1:1354–6.

Goddard J, Strachan FE, Bateman DN (2003). Urinary sodium and potassium excretion as measures of ibuprofen nephrotoxicity. J Toxicol Clin Toxicol, 41:747.

Kim J, Gazarian M, Verjee Z, Johnson D (1995). Acute renal insufficiency in ibuprofen overdose. Pediatr Emerg Care, 11:107–8.

Kulling PE, Backman EA, Skagius AS, et al. (1995). Renal impairment after acute diclofenac, naproxen, and sulindac overdoses. J Toxicol Clin Toxicol, 33:173–7.

Mattana J, Perinbasekar S, Brod-Miller C (1997). Near-fatal but reversible acute renal failure after massive ibuprofen ingestion. Am J Med Sci, 313:117–19.

Oker EE, Hermann L, Baum CR, et al. (2000). Serious toxicity in a young child due to ibuprofen. Acad Emerg Med, 7:821–3.

Turnbull AJ, Campbell P, Hughes JA (1988). Mefenamic acid nephropathy – acute renal failure in overdose. BMJ, 296:646.

Zuckerman GB, Uy CC (1995). Shock, metabolic acidosis, and coma following ibuprofen overdose in a child. Ann Pharmacother, 29:869–71.

Salicylates

Background

Aspirin (acetylsalicylic acid) is a non-steroidal anti-inflammatory analgesic with anti-inflammatory and antiplatelet actions that is widely used for cardiovascular risk reduction. Ingestion of aspirin is the most common form of salicylate poisoning. This may occur in the context of self-harm, but toxicity may also arise from accidental overdose, including use of more than one aspirin-containing preparation.

Salicylate toxicity may also result from percutaneous absorption of salicylic acid (used in keratolytic agents) and ingestion of methyl salicylate (oil of wintergreen). As a result of the high concentration of methylsalicylate, oil of wintergreen preparations are highly toxic, especially if ingested, but systemic toxicity may also occur after dermal use, especially if the skin is damaged or broken.

Between 1950 and 1970, salicylate poisoning was a common cause of severe and fatal poisoning, especially in children; the incidence of salicylate poisoning has fallen substantially since then. Use of aspirin as analgesia is contraindicated in children because of the link to Reye's syndrome and this has also reduced use, while the introduction of child-resistant containers has also reduced the incidence of childhood salicylate poisoning.

Toxicokinetics

Aspirin is usually absorbed rapidly via the stomach, duodenum, and jejunum, although this may be delayed if enteric-coated preparations have been used or large tablet masses are formed as a result of delayed tablet dissolution.

Once absorbed, aspirin is hydrolysed rapidly to salicylic acid by non-specific esterases in the intestinal wall and other tissues. As much as 35% of a therapeutic dose may be hydrolysed during the course of absorption. While some salicylic acid is then eliminated unchanged, variable amounts are conjugated with glycine to produce salicyluric acid and with glucuronic acid to form salicyl phenolic glucuronide, the major urine metabolites of acetylsalicylic acid after a therapeutic dose. In addition, salicyl acyl glucuronide and the ring hydroxylation products of salicylic acid, namely gentisic acid, and its glycine conjugation product, gentisuric acid, are all formed in minor amounts and excreted into the urine. The relative proportions of unchanged salicylic acid and salicyl phenolic glucuronide in the urine depend on the body load of salicylate to be eliminated because the formation of salicyluric acid and salicyl phenolic glucuronide is capacity-limited, resulting in zero-order metabolism.

After a therapeutic dose (acetylsalicylic acid 600 mg), unchanged salicylic acid, salicyluric acid, and salicyl phenolic glucuronide accounted for 9%, 75%, and 11% of urine salicylate respectively. In contrast, when plasma salicylate concentrations were very high (>700 mg/L), salicylic acid accounted for 65% while salicyluric acid and the phenolic glucuronide accounted for 22% and 15% respectively. Thus, after salicylate overdose, the major metabolic pathways become saturated and renal excretion of salicylic acid becomes increasingly important. This pathway is extremely sensitive to changes in urine pH (see 'Urinary alkalinization' subsection).

Thus, the time needed to eliminate a given fraction of a dose of salicylic acid increases with increasing dose. As a result, in usual therapeutic doses, aspirin has an elimination $t\frac{1}{2}$ of 2–4.5 hours but this may increase to an apparent $t\frac{1}{2}$ as long as 36 hours in overdose.

Mechanisms of toxicity

The mechanisms of toxicity of salicylates are shown in Figure 5.2. Salicylate enters the brain, where it stimulates the respiratory centre directly. An increase in the rate and depth of respiration occurs and respiratory alkalosis develops. The mechanism by which salicylate stimulates the respiratory centre is uncertain; it is most likely to be due to uncoupling of oxidative phosphorylation within the brainstem itself.

Salicylate causes a marked and progressive increase in oxygen consumption. Uncoupling of oxidative phosphorylation is thought to be responsible and is manifest clinically as hyperpyrexia, particularly in children. At very high salicylate concentrations, tissue oxygen uptake becomes progressively impaired, probably due to inhibition by salicylate of a wide variety of NAD^+-dependent dehydrogenases. The consequent impairment of the oxidation of fuel substrates leads to accumulation of acid intermediates and the development of metabolic acidosis.

Both hyperglycaemia and hypoglycaemia have been described. Although hypoglycaemia is less common in children than in adults, it is often more severe when it does occur. Uncoupling of oxidative phosphorylation increases tissue demand for glucose oxidation. The brain seems especially sensitive to this effect, and CNS glucose depletion (neuroglycopenia) can occur in the presence of normal blood glucose concentrations. If hepatic glycogen stores are adequate, catecholamine production stimulates glycogenolysis, leading to hyperglycaemia, which may persist for several days.

Although rarely a clinical problem, salicylate poisoning is often accompanied by hypoprothrombinaemia due to a warfarin-like action of salicylates on the physiologically important vitamin K-epoxide cycle.

Risk factors for toxicity

Toxicity is related to the dose ingested, with doses less than 125 mg/kg likely to be associated with mild or no toxic effects. Doses greater than 250 mg/kg are usually associate with moderate toxicity and those greater than 500 mg/kg with severe toxicity.

Clinical features

Recognition of salicylate poisoning is commonly delayed and the prognosis is poor, particularly in young children and the elderly, who are more likely to develop serious complications such as hypoglycaemia and metabolic acidosis.

The features of salicylate poisoning are summarized in Table 5.3. Nausea and vomiting, tinnitus and

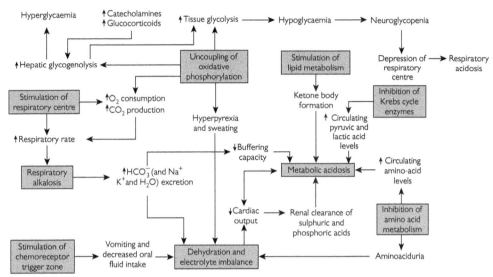

Fig 5.2 Mechanisms of aspirin toxicity. Reproduced from David A. Warrell, Timothy M. Cox, and John D. Firth, *Oxford Textbook of Medicine*, 5th edition, Figure 9.1.4, 2010, with permission from Oxford University Press.

deafness, sweating, hyperventilation, and fluid loss are common features in moderate poisoning. Features in severe poisoning include irritability, confusion, delirium, fever, hypokalaemia, non-cardiogenic pulmonary oedema, increased INR, and coma. Less common complications include tremor, convulsions, hypoglycaemia and hyperglycaemia, cerebral oedema, fluid retention, renal failure, haematemesis, thrombocytopaenia and DIC.

Disturbances of fluid, acid–base and electrolyte balance are common. Dehydration may develop rapidly as a result of vomiting, sweating, and hyperventilation.

Respiratory alkalosis is usually the dominant initial acid–base disturbance in adults and older children (e.g. >4 years). This is often accompanied by some degree of metabolic acidosis. Arterial pH is often normal or high (normal or reduced hydrogen ion concentration). Alkalosis is advantageous because salicylic acid (a weak acid) is maintained in its ionized state, which prevents it from entering cells. In contrast, when metabolic acidosis dominates, acidaemia develops (arterial pH decreases) and more salicylate becomes un-ionized and crosses cell membranes, particularly in the brain, to cause the neurological features that characterize severe poisoning.

In children less than 4 years of age, respiratory alkalosis is less common and metabolic acidosis predominates, with a low arterial pH (raised hydrogen ion concentration) being common. This acidosis may increase salicylate transfer across the blood–brain barrier.

Table 5.3 Clinical features of salicylate poisoning in adults

Mild-to-moderate poisoning (<700 mg/L; <5.1 mmol/L)	Severe poisoning (>700 mg/L; >5.1 mmol/L)	Less common complications of severe poisoning
Deafness	All features occurring in less severe poisoning	Tremor
Tinnitus	Confusion	Convulsions
Nausea and vomiting	Irritability	Cerebral oedema
Hyperventilation	Delirium	Renal failure
Sweating	Fever	Haematemesis
Fluid loss	Coma	Hypoglycaemia or hyperglycaemia
Respiratory alkalosis	Non-cardiogenic pulmonary oedema	Thrombocytopenia
Metabolic acidosis	Acidaemia	Disseminated intravascular coagulation
	Hypokalaemia	
	Increased INR	

Hypokalaemia occasionally complicates salicylate poisoning, even before treatment is begun, but it is exacerbated by the administration of sodium bicarbonate for the purpose of urine alkalinization.

Non-cardiogenic pulmonary oedema is a complication of salicylate poisoning and is associated with greater age, smoking, chronic intoxication, acidosis, and neurological complications. It may also be precipitated or aggravated by fluid overload.

Investigations

Check U&Es (including chloride and bicarbonate), creatinine, INR, and blood glucose. A chest X-ray is indicated if there are cardiorespiratory features.

The plasma salicylate concentration should be measured urgently in patients who have ingested more than 125 mg/kg of aspirin and in patients who have taken methyl salicylate or salicylamide. The sample should be taken at least 2 hours (symptomatic patients) or 4 hours (asymptomatic patients) after ingestion, since it may take several hours for peak plasma concentrations to occur and up to 12 hours for enteric-coated preparations. Repeat samples should be taken every 2 hours until concentrations are falling.

Arterial blood gases should be taken in all patients with the features of poisoning. Capillary gases or venous blood gases are a suitable alternative for use in children.

Assessment of severity

The severity of poisoning is assessed on the basis of clinical and biochemical features together with the plasma salicylate concentrations.

Plasma salicylate concentrations of 250–500 mg/L (1.8–3.6 mmol/L) suggest mild poisoning, though the presence of metabolic acidosis will increase severity.

Plasma salicylate concentrations of 500–700 mg/L (3.6–5.1 mmol/L) suggest moderate poisoning.

Severe salicylate poisoning is usually associated with plasma salicylate concentrations of 700 mg/L (5.1 mmol/L) or more, but the severity of intoxication should not be assessed on this basis alone. Clinical features (particularly coma, fever, and non-cardiogenic pulmonary oedema), age (>70 years) and acidaemia are also important and are associated with high mortality.

Management

Activated charcoal may be given (50–100 g in an adult, 1 g/kg for a child), although its efficacy is unproven. Current NPIS recommendations suggest use for adults or children who have ingested more than 125 mg/kg salicylate, or any amount of methyl salicylate, within the previous hour.

High-quality supportive care is essential in patients with moderate to severe poisoning, including appropriate general management of complications such as hypoglycaemia and hyperglycaemia, seizures, non-cardiogenic pulmonary oedema, and hyperthermia.

Dehydration, electrolyte imbalance, and, most importantly, metabolic acidosis should be corrected. If the serum potassium concentration is within the normal range, metabolic acidosis can be corrected by the intravenous infusion of sodium bicarbonate 50–100 mmoL (e.g. 50–100 mL 8.4%, alternatively 333–667 mL of 1.26% sodium bicarbonate) given over 30 minutes; the administration of bicarbonate may need to be repeated.

Use of elimination techniques

Increased salicylate elimination can be achieved by urine alkalinization and by haemodialysis. Forced alkaline diuresis is no longer used as it does not increase salicylate excretion and may precipitate pulmonary oedema. Salicylate t½ is reduced by multiple-dose activated charcoal but this method is not generally recommended as it is less effective than urine alkalinization and haemodialysis.

Urinary alkalinization

As the relationship between the renal clearance of salicylates and urine pH is logarithmic, urine alkalinization should be undertaken in patients with a plasma salicylate concentration higher than 500 mg/L, particularly if acidosis is present. The therapeutic aim is to make the urine alkaline (ideally pH 7.5–8.5), and in adults this may be achieved by administration of sodium bicarbonate, 225 mmol (225 mL of 8.4%); further doses of bicarbonate are given as required. Plasma potassium should be checked 1–2-hourly and hypokalaemia should be corrected before administration of sodium bicarbonate, as this will lower the serum potassium concentration further. Urinary alkalinization need not be delayed whilst awaiting haemodialysis.

Haemodialysis/haemodiafiltration

In patients with severe poisoning, haemodialysis or haemodiafiltration should be considered, particularly when severe acid–base abnormalities are present. Specific indications include salicylate concentration greater than 900 mg/L (6.4 mmol/L), especially when the patient is unresponsive to urine alkalinization, persisting severe metabolic acidosis (e.g. pH <7.2 H^+ 63 nmol/L), renal failure, non-cardiogenic pulmonary oedema, coma, convulsions, or other CNS effects not resolved by correction of acidosis

Children and older adults (>70 years) have increased morbidity from salicylate poisoning and may require haemodialysis or haemodiafiltration at an earlier stage.

Haemofiltration

Haemofiltration is much less efficient than haemodialysis or haemodiafiltration, but is an alternative in hospitals without these facilities, particularly if transfer is likely to be delayed.

Further reading

Broderick TW, Reinke RT, Goldman E (1976). Salicylate-induced pulmonary edema. Am J Roentgenol, 127:865–6.

Brubacher JR, Hoffman RS (1996). Salicylism from topical salicylates: review of the literature. J Toxicol Clin Toxicol, 34:431–6.

Chan TYK (1996). The risk of severe salicylate poisoning following the ingestion of topical medicaments or aspirin. Postgrad Med J, 72:109–12.

Chapman BJ, Proudfoot AT (1989). Adult salicylate poisoning: deaths and outcome in patients with high plasma salicylate concentrations. *QJM*, 72:699–707.

Heffner J, Starkey T, Anthony P (1979). Salicylate-induced non-cardiogenic pulmonary edema. *West J Med*, 130:263–6.

Jacobsen D, Wiik-Larsen E, Bredesen JE (1988). Haemodialysis or haemoperfusion in severe salicylate poisoning? *Hum Toxicol*, 7:161–3.

Patel DK, Hesse A, Ogunbona A, *et al.* (1990). Metabolism of aspirin after therapeutic and toxic doses. *Hum Exp Toxicol*, 9:131–6.

Proudfoot AT, Brown SS (1969). Acidaemia and salicylate poisoning in adults. *Br Med J*, 2:547–50.

Proudfoot AT, Krenzelok EP, Brent J, *et al.* (2003). Does urine alkalinization increase salicylate elimination? If so, why? *Toxicol Rev*, 22:129–36.

Opioid analgesics

Background

The management of chronic pain remains a major therapeutic challenge. Although opioid compounds have pain-relieving properties, this has invariably been associated with a risk of drug dependence and the development of tolerance to pharmacological effects. Clinical studies suggest that in chronic pain syndromes opioids are not particularly effective as analgesics, nevertheless very large quantities are prescribed for this purpose and these drugs are therefore commonly seen as components of an overdose. Details of the pharmacology and toxicology of opioid drugs are provided in The opioid syndrome, pp. 85–86.

Accidental poisoning is a particular risk for more potent agents such as fentanyl. Morphine is also used as a long-term analgesic, being available in modified-release preparations (Table 5.4). Potential hazards arise from the following factors:

- Codeine, dihydrocodeine, and, more recently, tramadol are available as combination tablets with paracetamol. The sedative effects of the opioid may mask the history and particular care is required to recognize the possibility of co-ingested paracetamol.
- Some drugs are available as modified-release formulations and their absorption can be unpredictable in overdose. Delayed onset of major sedative effect can be missed without appropriate monitoring.
- Many of these drugs have active metabolites which may contribute to their therapeutic action and their effects in overdose (e.g. tramadol).
- Several opioid analgesics are metabolized by the hepatic P450 isoform CYP2D6, which is subject to a genetic polymorphism. About 8% of the population do not express this enzyme, while a small number of individuals have multiple gene copies resulting in increased rates of metabolism. For codeine (metabolized to morphine) and tramadol (metabolized to o-desmethyltramadol), the consequences can either be lack of efficacy or unexpected toxicity, depending on individual genetic profile. These enzyme systems are also subject to drug interactions causing induction or inhibition of metabolism, further complicating clinical effects in overdose.

- Some drugs in this group, e.g. tramadol and dextropropoxyphene, have other important pharmacological effects. Tramadol has actions on both opioid receptors and 5-HT and norepinephrine reuptake systems, the latter being a factor in its potential to cause convulsions and serotonin syndrome. Dextropropoxyphene ($t\frac{1}{2}$=15 hours) was removed from the European market because both it, and its active metabolite norproxyphene ($t\frac{1}{2}$=27 hours) are sodium channel blockers and caused arrhythmias in overdose.

Mechanisms of toxicity

These drugs are competitive agonists for opioid receptors. Their principal analgesic and respiratory depressant effects result from agonism at the MOP (or μ) receptor (see The opioid syndrome, pp. 85–86).

The principal differences in the effect of opioids relates to their speed of onset, which for oral preparations depend on gastric emptying rate and metabolism and is more gradual for opioids converted to more active metabolites (e.g. codeine), than a pure agonist such as morphine. Opioids slow gut motility and this may affect rates of absorption in overdose, with both delayed and prolonged effects resulting from retention of tablets within the stomach.

Toxicokinetics

Most drugs in this group have relatively short $t\frac{1}{2}$ (Table 5.4). Some are formulated in modified-release preparations to prolong clinical effects. Peak onset in overdose may therefore be difficult to predict, and patients should be monitored for an appropriate period depending on the preparation and formulation.

Opioid metabolism interactions are possible, resulting in increased toxicity (see The opioid syndrome, pp. 85–86) or decreased efficacy.

Risk factors for toxicity

The effects of opioids may be enhanced in the following circumstances:

- Opioid naïve patients, particularly children, who are therefore at greater risk.

Table 5.4 Commonly prescribed opioids

Opioid	Approximate $t\frac{1}{2}$ (hours)	Key features
Codeine	3.5	5–15% converted to active metabolite morphine. Polymorphic metabolism via CYP2D6
Buprenorphine	6–40	Partial agonist. Slow absorption by buccal route—peak probably 3–4 hours after dosing. Transdermal preparation available
Dextropropoxyphene (propoxyphene)	15	Sodium channel blocker. This and its active metabolite norproxyphene ($t\frac{1}{2}$ 27 hours) causes arrhythmias
Dihydrocodeine	3.5–4.5	Partial agonist. Active metabolites, e.g. dihydromorphine. Polymorphic metabolism via CYP2D6
Fentanyl	3–4	Very potent. Short $t\frac{1}{2}$
		Used via buccal and transdermal (e.g. 72 hours patch) routes
Oxycodone	3–3.5	Active metabolites. Polymorphic metabolism. Modified-release preparations commonly used
Tramadol	6	Potent active metabolites: parent drug and metabolite have SSRI and SNRI effects
Methadone	13–47	Prolonged action. Potassium channel blocker causing QT interval prolongation and torsade de pointes
Morphine	3	Modified-release preparations commonly used. Active metabolite morphine 6 glucuronide may accumulate in renal impairment

- Co-ingestion of sedative drugs or alcohol; mixed ingestions are therefore hazardous.
- Drug interactions, especially those involving inhibition of hepatic drug metabolizing enzymes.
- Renal impairment, which may exacerbate toxicity of opioids with active metabolites subject to renal elimination, e.g. morphine, diamorphine (heroin), pethidine, and codeine.

Risk of toxicity is high with fentanyl patches. Drug release is temperature dependent, and toxicity may occur by heating. Transfer to another person sleeping in the same bed may also occur causing severe poisoning in someone not tolerant to opioid effects. Buccal fentanyl preparations are also potentially hazardous for opioid naive individuals, particularly children. See also The opioid syndrome, pp. 85–86.

Clinical features

Depending on the preparation ingested, peak effects may occur within 4–6 hours for normal formulations and up to 8–10 hours for modified-release agents, although the presence of nausea and vomiting may delay absorption and maximum effects for longer.

All analgesic opioids

Nausea and vomiting, reduced conscious level, respiratory depression, and coma with small pupils are the classical features of opioid ingestion. Opioids also cause veno-dilation and may, by their central depressant effect, lower blood pressure and pulse rate. In severe poisoning rhabdomyolysis has been reported. Reduced gut motility may prolong the onset and duration of the effects of slow-release preparations above those normally expected.

In some patients, opioids, particularly codeine, cause significant histamine release with flushing, urticaria, and itch. Rarely bronchospasm may also ensue.

Tramadol

In addition to the features already mentioned, tramadol may cause convulsions, sweating, increased muscle tone, and Serotonin syndrome, pp. 79–80.

Dextropropoxyphene

Sodium channel blockade with QRS prolongation on the ECG and risk of arrhythmia, exacerbated by hypoxia and/or acidosis secondary to opioid induced respiratory depression.

For details of methadone, heroin, and buprenorphine, see Opioids pp. 194–195.

Toxicity assessment

Opioid effects are usually easily identified. Careful monitoring of conscious level, oxygenation, pulse, and blood pressure is essential, initially every 15 minutes for 4 hours after ingestion, but longer periods of monitoring are required for slow-release preparations (8 hours).

Understanding expected timeframes of onset and offset of the effects is necessary. The differential diagnosis includes toxicity of other sedatives including gamma-hydroxybutyrate. Pin-point pupils may also occur in cholinergic poisoning, e.g. with organophosphorus compounds.

Investigations

U&Es, creatinine, and creatine kinase should be checked, the latter especially in patients with severe hypotension or who have been unconscious for a period. Arterial blood gases should be performed in patients with suspected respiratory depression or circulatory failure. If there is uncertainty of the preparation ingested, paracetamol concentrations should be checked and appropriate treatment given. An ECG should be performed if dextropropoxyphene or methadone may have been involved. Specific drug concentrations are not clinically useful.

Management

Establish that the patient is conscious and can maintain their airway. If opioid ingestion has been recent (1–2 hours), and the patients can protect their own airway consider use of activated charcoal (50 g in an adult, 1 g/kg in a child). Opioid skin patches should be removed.

In patients with features of severe opioid intoxication, particularly depressed consciousness and respiration, naloxone is indicated. Naloxone is a pure opioid antagonist and dose should be titrated to the clinical response of the patient. Its duration of action is shorter than all opioid drugs, and repeated doses are likely to be required. An initial intravenous starting dose of 400 micrograms is given and titrated to achieve the required clinical response (maximum initial dose 2 mg). It may be appropriate to consider use of a naloxone infusion in patients whose conscious level subsequently declines., An hourly dose of approximately 60% of the initial dose required to awake the patient adequately is a good starting point; however, as naloxone may increase gut motility resulting in more rapid absorption of opioid, a paradoxical initial increase in toxicity may occasionally occur. For opioids with active metabolites, continued metabolism may result in increasing toxicity, requiring larger doses of naloxone. Further information about naloxone dosing and adverse effects is provided in The opioid syndrome, pp. 85–86.

On discontinuing naloxone it is necessary to monitor the patient for a further period of at least 6 hours to ensure that no recurrence of opioid effect is seen.

In patients who have hypotension or hypoperfusion, ensure adequate hydration. Rhabdomyolysis should be treated conventionally (see Rhabdomyolysis and compartment syndrome, pp. 77–78). Treat opioid-induced urticaria with a sedative antihistamine and wheeze with bronchodilators.

Tramadol

Monitor temperature and perform a 12-lead ECG. Ensure QRS and QT intervals are normal; consider further ECGs if conscious level deteriorates. Brief convulsions do not require treatment, but prolonged or recurrent episodes should be managed conventionally with intravenous benzodiazepines (diazepam (10–20 mg in adults; 0.1–0.3 mg/kg body weight in children) or lorazepam (4 mg in adults; 0.1 mg/kg in children): beware additional respiratory depression.

Other treatments may be required, depending on co-ingestants and individual response to the opioid overdose.

Further reading

Goldfrank L, Weisman RS, Errick JK, et al. (1986). A dosing nomogram for continuous infusion of intravenous naloxone. Ann Emerg Med, 15:566–70.

Hawton K, Bergen H, Simkin S, Brock A, et al. (2009). Effect of withdrawal of co-proxamol on prescribing and deaths from drug poisoning in England and Wales: time series analysis. BMJ, 338:b2270.

Jovanovic-Cupic V, Martinovic Z, Nesic N (2006). Seizures associated with intoxication and abuse of tramadol. Clin Toxicol, 44:143–6.

Stamer UM, Stuber F, Muders T, et al. (2008). Respiratory depression with tramadol in a patient with renal impairment and CYP2D6 gene duplication. Anesth Analg, 107:926–9.

Cardiovascular acting agents

Beta-adrenoceptor antagonists

Background

Beta-adrenoceptor antagonists (beta-blockers) are widely used for the treatment of ischaemic heart disease, hypertension, thyrotoxicosis, migraine prophylaxis, arrhythmias, and anxiety.

Mechanisms of toxicity

These are competitive antagonists at the beta-adrenergic receptor; cardio-selective agents bind preferentially to $beta_1$ receptors in cardiac tissue with less binding affinity to $beta_2$ receptors, e.g. in respiratory tissue. The extent of $beta_1$ selectivity is normally derived from *in vitro* tests involving isolated tissue from a variety of animal species, and applicability to human pharmacology is questionable. Moreover, the clinical relevance is made even less certain by functional crossover between receptor subtypes so that the clinical effects may vary only slightly between so-called highly $beta_1$ selective agents (e.g. bisoprolol, atenolol) and non-selective ones (e.g. propranolol). Some beta-adrenoceptor antagonists have sodium channel blocking effects (sometimes termed 'quinidine-like effects' or 'membrane stabilizing activity' (MSA)) and partial agonist activity at adrenoceptors, ('intrinsic sympathomimetic activity' (ISA)).

Toxicological effects are related to beta-adrenoceptor blockade:

- $Beta_1$ receptor blockade (predominant effects):
  - bradycardia
  - hypotension
  - reduced cardiac output and cool peripheries
- $Beta_2$ receptor blockade:
  - bronchospasm
- $Beta_3$ receptor blockade:
  - negatively inotropic.

Exposure to very high drug concentrations may result in effectively irreversible receptor blockade, in contrast to the reversible competitive antagonism observed after therapeutic doses. Toxicity may be prolonged and resistant to conventional treatment for bradycardia and hypotension.

Toxicokinetics

Beta-adrenoceptor antagonists vary substantially in their pharmacokinetics. Hydrophobic (lipid soluble) agents such as propranolol, metoprolol, and labetalol have large volumes of distribution, distribute widely, including to the CNS, and are metabolized by the liver. In some cases metabolites may be active (e.g. propranolol). Propranolol has substantial first-pass metabolism and limiting bioavailability after oral ingestion. Hydrophilic agents such as atenolol, nadolol, and sotalol have small volumes of distribution and are eliminated in the urine. Half-lives of beta-blockers in normal doses vary from less than 10 minutes (esmolol) to about 12 hours (sotalol). There is limited information available on toxicokinetics after overdose.

Risk factors for toxicity

Cardiac features of toxicity are more likely if co-ingested with other drugs acting on the cardiovascular system, e.g. greater likelihood of heart block if co-ingested with calcium channel blocker, more profound hypotension if co-ingested with an antihypertensive agent. Those at highest risk of significant cardiovascular toxicity are elderly patients and those with established ischaemic heart disease or renovascular disease.

Clinical features

Features of toxicity are evident within 6 hours of ingesting a non-sustained release preparation, 8 hours after a sustained release preparation, and within 12 hours after sotalol ingestion.

Cardiovascular features

Cardiac features are prominent, with bradycardia and hypotension being common. Cardiac conduction defects, e.g. first- or second-degree AV block, may occur, as may peripheral cyanosis. Pulmonary oedema, cardiogenic shock and asystole are features of severe poisoning. Sotalol, which is also a potassium channel antagonist, may cause QT prolongation and torsade de pointes ventricular tachycardia.

Central nervous system features

CNS effects include reduced consciousness, seizures, hallucinations, absent pupillary reflexes, and coma; these are more common after ingestion of agents with high lipid solubility (Table 6.1).

Other features

Bronchospasm may occur, particularly in patients with pre-existing pulmonary disease. Hypoglycaemia and hypocalcaemia have also been reported but appear uncommon.

Investigations

U&E, creatinine and glucose should be measured and a 12-lead ECG performed to assess for features of heart

Table 6.1 Properties of some beta-adrenoceptor antagonists

	Cardio-selective	Lipid solubility	Comments
Acebutolol	Yes	Low	ISA
Atenolol	Yes	Low	
Betaxolol	Yes	Low	MSA
Bisoprolol	Yes	Moderate	
Carvedilol	No	Moderate	Also α-blocker
Celiprolol	Yes	Low	
Esmolol	Yes	Low	Parenteral, short-acting
Labetalol	No	Moderate	Also α-blocker
Metoprolol	Yes	Moderate	
Nadolol,	No	Low	
Nebivolol,	Yes	High	Vasodilating via nitric oxide
Oxprenolol	No	Moderate	ISA
Pindolol	No	Moderate	ISA, MSA
Propranolol	No	High	MSA
Sotalol	No	Low	Potassium channel blocker
Timolol	No	Low	

block and, in the case of sotalol, QT interval prolongation. Significant sodium channel blockade may cause prolongation of the QRS duration.

Detection of cardiovascular effects requires frequent haemodynamic and electrocardiographic monitoring.

Management

Oral activated charcoal should be considered for patients presenting within 1 hour of a significant ingestion, provided that no contraindications exist. Later administration may be beneficial for overdose involving delayed-release preparations, but there is no direct evidence of clinical benefit.

Intravenous fluids should be used to ensure adequate hydration.

Bradycardia may respond to atropine; large doses are sometimes required (e.g. 3 mg in an adult or 0.04 mg/kg in a child. An isoproterenol (isoprenaline) infusion may allow restoration of haemodynamic stability, and high rates of administration may be required: an initial infusion rate of 5–10 micrograms/minute can be used in an adult, titrating the dose as required. Very large doses (e.g. 800 micrograms/minute) have sometimes been effective. Other inotropic agents, e.g. dobutamine, epinephrine, or norepinephrine, may also be required.

Glucagon appears capable of restoring the beta-adrenoceptor-linked intracellular cascade and should be considered if there are features of severe toxicity including severe hypotension, heart failure, or cardiogenic shock. Glucagon is normally administered as an intravenous bolus (e.g. of 5–10 mg over 10 minutes in an adult), followed by an infusion (1–5 mg per hour titrated to clinical response). It may be necessary to discuss with the duty pharmacist to ensure adequate glucagon can be made available. Vomiting is a common adverse effect, and might necessitate reducing the rate of administration. Hyperglycaemia, hypokalaemia, and hypocalcaemia may also occur.

Limited data suggest that hyper-insulinaemia euglycaemic therapy (HIET) might also be effective for poisoning with beta-adrenoceptor antagonists, perhaps by stimulating glucagon secretion and should be considered where other measures have failed. Further details of the method can be found in Cardiovascular toxicity, pp. 64–67.

Internal or external cardiac pacing may correct bradycardia, but may not restore blood pressure and can be ineffective due to electromechanical dissociation. In severe poisoning, mechanical support using intra-aortic balloon counter-pulsation or cardiopulmonary bypass (if available) may be considered for use until drug toxicity has resolved.

Certain beta-blockers (e.g. propranolol) have quinidine-like effects, prolonging the QRS duration and causing arrhythmia; in theory, intravenous bicarbonate might help but clinical data to support this are lacking.

Nebulized salbutamol may be an effective treatment for bronchospasm.

Intravenous lipid emulsion administration and haemodialysis have been reported after beta-blocker overdose, but insufficient data exist to support their role in clinical practice. Lipid-soluble beta-adrenoceptor antagonists would not be expected to be cleared effectively by haemodialysis or haemoperfusion due to their large volumes of distribution.

Further reading

Bailey B (2003). Glucagon in beta-blocker and calcium channel blocker overdoses: a systematic review. *J Toxicol Clin Toxicol*, 41:595–602.

Cave G, Harvey M (2009). Lipid emulsion may augment early blood pressure recovery in a rabbit model of atenolol toxicity. *J Med Toxicol*, 5:50–1.

DeWitt CR, Waksman JC (2004). Pharmacology, pathophysiology and management of calcium channel blocker and beta-blocker toxicity. *Toxicol Rev*, 23:223–38.

Kolcz J, Pietrzyk J, Januszewska K, et al. (2007). Extracorporeal life support in severe propranolol and verapamil intoxication. *J Intensive Care Med*, 22:381–5.

Mégarbane B, Karyo S, Baud FJ (2004). The role of insulin and glucose (hyperinsulinaemia/euglycaemia) therapy in acute calcium channel antagonist and beta-blocker poisoning. *Toxicol Rev*, 23:215–22.

Page C, Hacket LP, Isbister GK (2009). The use of high-dose insulin-glucose euglycemia in beta-blocker overdose: a case report. *J Med Toxicol*, 5:139–43.

Salhanick SD, Wax PM (2000). Treatment of atenolol overdose in a patient with renal failure using serial hemodialysis and hemoperfusion and associated echocardiographic findings. *Vet Hum Toxicol*, 42:224–5.

Stellpflug SJ, Harris CR, Engebretsen KM, et al. (2010). Intentional overdose with cardiac arrest treated with intravenous fat emulsion and high-dose insulin. *Clin Toxicol*, 48: 227–9.

Thanacoody HK, Waring WS (2008). Toxins that affect the cardiovascular system. *Clin Med*, 8:92–95.

Wax PM, Erdman AR, Chyka PA, et al. (2005). Beta-blocker ingestion: an evidence-based consensus guideline for out-of-hospital management. *Clin Toxicol*, 43:131–46.

Calcium channel blockers

Background

Calcium channel blockers are widely used in the management of a range of cardiovascular (e.g. hypertension, ischaemic heart disease, and arrhythmias) and non-cardiovascular (migraine, Raynaud's phenomenon) conditions. Calcium channel blocker toxicity can result in severe and life-threatening clinical effects. There is increasing use of modified-release preparations; overdose of these preparations can be particularly problematic as it results in delayed onset and prolonged toxicity.

Mechanisms of toxicity

Calcium channel blockers bind to L-type calcium channels in cardiac and vascular smooth muscle cells. This leads to decreased calcium availability within myocardial and vascular smooth muscle cells resulting in decreased myocardial contractility, impaired myocardial conduction, and peripheral arterial vasodilatation. Calcium channel blockers also bind to L-type calcium channels in beta-islet cells in the pancreas resulting in decreased pancreatic insulin release; they also cause peripheral insulin resistance. The combination of hypo-insulinaemia and insulin resistance results in poor cellular glucose supply and hyperglycaemia. This is important because glucose is the preferred energy substrate for the ischaemic myocardium and therefore this poor cellular glucose availability worsens myocardial performance and adds to the direct negative inotropic effects of calcium channel blockers.

Calcium channel blockers have limited or no binding to other L-type calcium channels in skeletal muscle or neurological tissues.

There are three classes of calcium channel blockers in clinical use:

1 dihydropyridines (e.g. nifedipine, nimodipine, amlodipine, felodipine); greater peripheral vascular activity (vasodilatation)
2 benzothiazepines (e.g. diltiazem); mixed cardiac and peripheral effects
3 phenylalkylamines (e.g. verapamil); greater cardiac effects (negative inotropic and chronotropic actions).

This relative selectivity remains, but is less prominent, in overdose.

Toxicokinetics

The calcium channel blockers all have good oral bioavailability and peak concentrations of standard-release preparations occur within 1–2 hours. They are metabolized by various hepatic pathways, these can become saturated in overdose, decreasing hepatic first-pass metabolism and prolonging half-life, and thereby increasing drug concentrations. The calcium channel blockers are all highly protein bound with a large volume of distribution and therefore extracorporeal techniques are of no value in managing toxicity.

Many calcium channel blockers are available in sustained-release preparations. These are absorbed slowly, the onset of clinical features may be delayed for more than 12–18 hours after ingestion, and drug concentrations may not peak until over 24–36 hours after ingestion.

Risk factors for toxicity

Cardiac features of toxicity are more likely if co-ingested with other drugs acting on the cardiovascular system,

e.g. risk of heart block increased if co-ingested with a beta-adrenoceptor blocker or more profound hypotension if co-ingested with an antihypertensive agent. Those at highest risk of significant cardiovascular toxicity are elderly patients and those with established ischaemic heart disease or renovascular disease. Significant toxicity can occur with ingestion of just one or two tablets of a calcium channel blocker in toddlers.

Clinical features

Features of toxicity are usually evident within 6–8 hours of ingestion of a standard, non-sustained-release preparation and within 12–18 hours after ingestion of a sustained-release preparation. Clinical features are largely confined to the cardiovascular system.

Cardiovascular features

Cardiovascular effects predominate with myocardial depression and peripheral vasodilatation leading to hypotension. Severe hypotension can occur and patients can deteriorate rapidly due to a variable combination of direct myocardial suppression and peripheral vasodilatation. It is therefore important to assess cardiovascular status carefully in patients with hypotension related to calcium channel blockers to determine which of these mechanisms is predominating. Myocardial conduction delay can lead to bradycardia, AV conduction abnormalities, and heart block. Patients with dihydropyridine (e.g. nifedipine) toxicity may initially have a reflex tachycardia related to marked peripheral vasodilatation in the context of minimal effects on cardiac conduction; however, bradycardia is more common in patients with severe calcium channel blocker toxicity. Patients with severe toxicity can develop cardiogenic shock with resultant pulmonary oedema, complete heart block, and asystole.

Metabolic effects

Lactic acidosis can occur in patients with significant hypotension and can worsen toxicity due to a decrease in ionized calcium concentrations. Calcium channel blockers cause hyperglycaemia and there is a strong negative correlation between both presentation and peak blood glucose concentrations and outcome. Hyperkalaemia and hypocalcaemia may occur.

Other features

Patients with severe toxicity may develop central nervous system toxicity secondary to severe hypotension including agitation, confusion, seizures and occasionally coma, but if significant drowsiness is present in the absence of cardiovascular effects co-ingestants or an alternative cause of neurological depression should be considered. Ileus can occur as a secondary effect in patients with marked cardiovascular toxicity but other gastrointestinal effects are uncommon. Acute pancreatitis, hepatotoxicity, and mesenteric infarction have also been reported.

Investigations

Electrolytes, renal function, and glucose should be measured and in patients with significant toxicity an arterial blood gas should be taken to assess acid–base status. A 12-lead ECG should be performed to assess for features of heart block.

Management

Oral activated charcoal should be considered for patients presenting within 1 hour of a significant ingestion, provided that no contraindications exist. Multiple-dose activated charcoal and/or WBI should be considered in patients with significant sustained-release calcium channel blocker ingestions and this may be beneficial even in later presenters.

Patients with standard-release preparation ingestions should be observed for at least 12 hours after ingestion and those with sustained-release ingestions should be observed for up to 24 hours after ingestion. All patients should be placed on a cardiac monitor and have regular observations of heart rate and blood pressure.

Bradyarrhythmias

Patients with bradycardia associated with cardiovascular compromise should be treated initially with atropine (initial dose 0.5–1.2 mg in an adult, 0.02 mg/kg in a child, maximum dose 3 mg in an adult 0.04 mg/kg in a child). Patients with significant heart block not responding to atropine may require temporary pacing. External pacing can be attempted but is rarely successful and patients will generally require internal pacing with a high pacing threshold. If available, isoproterenol (isoprenaline) may be useful for patients with significant bradyarrhythmias.

Hypotension

Initial management of hypotension should be with a standard fluid challenge. Hypotension not responding to a fluid challenge should be managed initially with intravenous calcium, although this is generally only successful in those with mild–moderate hypotension and not in those with severe or persistent hypotension. Calcium should be used in caution in patients who may have concomitant digoxin toxicity. Calcium chloride has a greater ionized calcium content and so is preferred to calcium gluconate, but either agent can be used. An initial dose of 5–10 mL 10% calcium chloride (or 20–30 mL calcium gluconate) given over 5 minutes can be repeated up to three or four times. If patients respond to this, a calcium infusion (up to 10 mL/hour of 10% calcium chloride) can be used with monitoring of serum calcium concentrations.

Patients with severe hypotension not responding to a fluid challenge and calcium should be managed with hyper-insulinaemia euglycaemia therapy (HIET). This facilitates myocardial glucose supply, improves calcium signalling, and also at the doses used, insulin is a positive inotrope. If the serum potassium concentration is less than 2.5 mmol/L prior to starting HIET, give 20 mmol of potassium over 30 minutes and recheck electrolytes. Patients should be treated with a loading bolus dose of 1 unit/kg of short-acting insulin (Humulin-S® or Actrapid®) with 50 mL of 50% or 100 mL of 20% dextrose. This should be followed with a maintenance infusion of 0.5–2.0 units/kg/hour of insulin titrated to blood pressure/cardiac output, which may be increased further to a maximum of 10 units/kg/hour if required. Sufficient 10% dextrose should be given to maintain euglycaemia, checking capillary glucose every 15–20 minutes initially and after an insulin dose change and every 30–60 minutes when on a stable insulin dose. Serum potassium concentration should be checked every 2–4 hours and supplementary potassium given as required.

Whilst it is important to monitor closely for hypoglycaemia and hypokalaemia, despite the large doses of insulin used, HIET is well tolerated and significant hypoglycaemia and hypokalaemia are rarely a problem because of the insulin resistance associated with calcium channel blocker toxicity. A good marker of clinical improvement is increasing glucose and potassium requirements which are an indication of decreasing insulin resistance associated with amelioration of calcium channel blocker toxicity.

Conventional inotropes and vasopressors are generally less effective as they require effective intracellular calcium signalling and should generally only be used alongside or after HIET and guided by bedside or invasive monitoring. If hypotension is predominantly due to peripheral vasodilatation, a vasopressor such as norepinephrine is preferred. If predominantly due to myocardial depression, an inotrope such as epinephrine or dobutamine is preferred. Some patients may have a mixed picture requiring a combination of agents. Alternative inotropes such as phosphodiesterase inhibitors are generally limited in their efficacy due to peripheral vasodilatation associated with their use. There are case reports of the use of metaraminol in patients with resistant hypotension in calcium channel blocker toxicity.

Whilst glucagon is an antidote of choice in beta-adrenoceptor blocker toxicity, it is less effective in calcium channel blocker toxicity as, to be effective, it requires effective intracellular calcium signalling. It can be considered in patients with resistant hypotension at an initial dose of 5–10 mg IV over 1–2 min.

In severe poisoning, mechanical support using intra-aortic balloon counter-pulsation, cardiopulmonary bypass, or extracorporeal membrane oxygenation (if available) may be considered.

Preliminary data from animal studies suggests that intravenous lipid emulsion (e.g. 1.5 mL/kg 20% Intralipid® as an intravenous bolus followed by 0.25–0.5 mL/kg/minute for 30–60 minutes to a maximum of 500 mL, repeated once or twice if necessary) may have a role in the management of severe hypotension resistant to other therapy, but it has not been compared with other options and there is limited clinical experience.

Further reading

DeWitt CR, Waksman JC (2004). Pharmacology, pathophysiology and management of calcium channel blocker and beta-blocker toxicity. *Toxicol Rev*, 23:223–38.

Engebretsen KM, Kaczmarek KM, Morgan J, et al. (2011). High-dose insulin therapy in beta-blocker and calcium channel-blocker poisoning. *Clin Toxicol*, 49:277–83.

Greene SL, Gawaramman I, Wood DM, et al. (2007). Relative safety of hyperinsulinaemia/euglycaemia therapy in the management of calcium channel blocker overdose: a prospective observational study. *Intensive Care Med*, 33:2019–24.

Kolcz J, Pietrzyk J, Januszewska K, et al. (2007). Extracorporeal life support in severe propranolol and verapamil intoxication. *J Intensive Care Med*, 22:381–5.

Mégarbane B, Karyo S, Baud FJ (2004). The role of insulin and glucose (hyperinsulinaemia/euglycaemia) therapy in acute calcium channel antagonist and beta-blocker poisoning. *Toxicol Rev*, 23:215–22.

Salhanick SD, Shannon MW (2003). Management of calcium channel blocker overdose. *Drug Saf*, 26:65–79.

Thanacoody HK, Waring WS (2008). Toxins that affect the cardiovascular system. *Clin Med*, 8:92–5.

ACE inhibitors and angiotensin receptor antagonists

Mechanisms of toxicity

Angiotensin-converting enzyme (ACE) inhibitors prevent cleavage of angiotensin I to angiotensin II, thereby substantially reducing circulating angiotensin II concentrations. In contrast, angiotensin receptor antagonists competitively inhibit angiotensin II receptor binding, with high affinity for the AT_1 receptor subtype. Both block the renin–angiotensin–aldosterone cascade, which is the mechanism responsible for therapeutic and adverse effects. The predominant toxic effects are attributable to hypotension, particularly when co-ingested with other antihypertensive agents. ACE inhibitors but not angiotensin receptor antagonists, are capable of preventing enzymatic degradation of bradykinin. Elevated bradykinin concentrations may provoke endothelium-dependent nitric oxide release, which is capable of causing vasodilatation and hypotension independent of effects on angiotensin II or aldosterone. Key features of the presently available drugs are shown in Table 6.2.

Clinical features

The onset of hypotension is usually within 1–2 hours of drug ingestion, and reaches a maximum 4–6 hours later. Hypotension may persist for more than 1–2 days after ingestion.

When determining the extent of any hypotensive effect it is important to consider that the baseline blood pressure might have been high, particularly if prescribed for hypertension. Therefore, an apparently 'normal' blood pressure might still represent a significant fall from usual values. There is a commonly held perception that the dose–response relationship is comparatively flat beyond the normal therapeutic dose range so that overdose

might cause only a modest blood pressure effect in most patients. However, severe hypotension and acute lidney injury have been reported after overdose involving ACE inhibitors or angiotensin receptor blockers. Clinical features are due to vasodilatation and hypotension, including postural dizziness, reduced conscious level, flushing and erythema, myocardial ischaemia, metabolic acidosis and, rarely, acute pancreatitis.

Risk factors for toxicity

Severe hypotension is most likely to occur when co-ingested with other antihypertensive agents including diuretics and calcium channel blockers. Hypotension may cause tissue hypoperfusion, particularly in patients with pre-existing cardiovascular or renovascular disease who are less able to compensate for large changes in systemic blood pressure. Hyperkalaemia is a recognized feature and appears to be a consequence of impaired renal function and a direct effect of ACE inhibition or angiotensin receptor blockade on renal electrolyte transport.

Management

Oral activated charcoal should be considered for patients presenting within 1 hour of a significant ingestion, provided that no contraindications exist. Detection of cardiovascular effects requires frequent haemodynamic and electrocardiographic monitoring, up to at least 4 hours after ingestion.

If there is haemodynamic disturbance, then intravenous fluids should considered to ensure adequate hydration. Cognitive state, urine output, and vital signs should be monitored frequently to allow detection of organ hypoperfusion. Most patients will recover with only minimal supportive care. However, a fall of more than 30 mmHg systolic blood pressure or evidence of organ hypoperfusion indicate severe toxicity, and the use of intravenous pressor agents to increase systemic blood pressure should be considered.

Pressor agents, particularly noradrenaline (norepinephrine), exert a direct vasoconstrictor effect and may increase systemic blood pressure in ACE inhibitor or angiotensin receptor antagonist toxicity. High doses may be required to establish satisfactory blood pressure, and caution is needed to avoid worsening organ hypoperfusion. This should normally be undertaken in a critical care environment to allow close monitoring. Where needed, pressor agents can be discontinued within 12 hours in most cases.

Table 6.2 Pharmacokinetic characteristics associated with therapeutic use of selected ACE inhibitors (upper panel) and angiotensin receptor antagonists (lower panel)

Name	Half-life (hours)	Toxic dose (mg/kg)	Renal excretion
Captopril	2	4	>90%
Enalapril	11	1	>90%
Fosinopril	4	1	40%
Lisinopril	13	1	>90%
Perindopril	9	0.5	70%
Quinapril	3	1	>90%
Ramipril	17	0.2	70%
Trandolapril	22	0.1	70%
Zofenopril[a]	6	2	>90%
Azilsartan	11	6	50%
Candesartan	9	0.6	60%
Eprosartan	5	40	30%
Irbesartan	13	20	<5%
Losartan	2	2	10%
Olmesartan	15	1.5	40%
Telmisartan	24	3	<5%
Valsartan	6	6	30%

[a] Not licensed for use in the UK

Angiotensin II administration

Infusion of angiotensin II allows restoration of blood pressure after ACE inhibitor overdose, but existing reports are confined to a research setting and pharmaceutical preparations of this agent are not readily available.

Further reading

Baffoni L, Durante V, Grossi M (2004). Acute pancreatitis induced by telmisartan overdose. *Ann Pharmacother*, 38:1088.

Christie GA, Lucas C, Bateman DN, et al. (2006). Redefining the ACE-inhibitor dose-response relationship: substantial blood pressure lowering after massive doses. *Eur J Clin Pharmacol*, 62:989–93.

Cohen V, Jellinek SP, Fancher L, *et al.* (2011). Tarka (trandolapril/ verapamil hydrochloride extended-release) overdose. *J Emerg Med*, 40:291–5.

Forrester MB (2007). Adult lisinopril ingestions reported to Texas poison control centers, 1998–2005. *Hum Exp Toxicol*, 26:483–9.

Galea M, Jelacin N, Bramham K, *et al.* (2007). Severe lactic acidosis and rhabdomyolysis following metformin and ramipril overdose. *Br J Anaesth*, 98:213–15.

Ghatak A, Farrer M (2009). Refractory hypotension and ECG changes in a case of nicorandil and lisinopril overdose and role of vasopressor in management. *J Cardiovasc Med*, 10:649–53.

Lip GY, Ferner RE (1995). Poisoning with anti-hypertensive drugs: angiotensin converting enzyme inhibitors. *J Hum Hypertens*, 9:711–15.

Lucas C, Christie GA, Waring WS (2006). Rapid onset of haemodynamic effects after angiotensin converting enzyme-inhibitor overdose: implications for initial patient triage. *Emerg Med J*, 23:854–7.

Newby DE, Lee MR, Gray AJ, *et al.* (1995). Enalapril overdose and the corrective effect of intravenous angiotensin II. *Br J Clin Pharmacol*, 40:103–4.

Thanacoody HK, Waring WS (2008). Toxins that affect the cardiovascular system. *Clin Med*, 8:92–5.

Antidysrhythmic drugs

Background

Antidysrhythmic drugs are not commonly involved in drug overdose, but are important because most have a low therapeutic index and are highly toxic when taken in overdose. In addition, toxicity may develop as a result of therapeutic use.

There are several ways of classifying antidysrhythmic drugs, e.g. on the basis of cellular electrophysiological effects, sites of action, or chemistry. The Singh Vaughan Williams method classifies antidysrhythmics into four major classes based on electrophysiological characteristics and is commonly used.

Class I antidysrhythmics

These block fast sodium channels in the heart and neuronal tissues, slowing the Phase 0 depolarization that results from fast sodium entry. In neuronal tissue this effect gives rise to local anaesthetic properties. Within the central nervous system severe sodium channel blockade may result in confusion, agitation, and convulsions. In the heart, sodium channel blockade slows conduction velocity, especially in specialist conducting tissues and this may terminate re-entry circuits. However, arrhythmias can also be precipitated ('pro-arrhythmia') and sodium channel blockade may be associated with reduced myocardial contractility and excitability.

Class I antidysrhythmics can be further subdivided according to additional properties as follows:

Class Ia

This group includes quinidine, procainamide, and disopyramide. In addition to sodium channel blockade, Class Ia agents are characterized by delayed cardiac repolarization as a result of blockade of potassium channels (e.g. I_{kr}). This ancillary class III effect (see later in this section), increases action potential duration (APD) and the effective refractory period (ERP) and is reflected by QT prolongation on the ECG. Class Ia drugs, especially disopyramide, also have anticholinergic properties, quinidine has alpha-adrenergic blocking actions and procainamide has neuromuscular and ganglion blocking effects. These properties contribute to adverse effects and to the clinical features observed in poisoning.

Severe and potentially fatal poisoning may occur with doses in an adult as low as 1 g (quinidine, disopyramide) or 5 g (procainamide). Clinical features of poisoning with class Ia drugs include:

- Nausea, vomiting, abdominal pain, and diarrhoea.
- Anticholinergic features (especially with disopyramide). These may include sedation (exacerbated by other sedative co-ingestants including alcohol), dry mouth, hot dry skin, dilated pupils, hyperthermia, tachycardia, ataxia, nystagmus, drowsiness, and agitation. Paralytic ileus and urinary retention may occasionally occur. Delayed gastric emptying is probably common.
- Drowsiness, lethargy, confusion, with convulsions occurring in severe poisoning.
- Metabolic acidosis and hypokalaemia may occur in severe poisoning
- 'Cinchonism' is a feature of poisoning with quinidine. It is characterized by flushing, tremor, dizziness, tinnitus, deafness, and visual disturbances.

- ECG effects include PR, QRS, and QT interval prolongation. Sinus tachycardia or bradycardia, heart block, and torsade de pointes may occur. Torsade de pointes may also occur with therapeutic dosing (e.g. 'quinidine syncope') but is more common with higher plasma concentrations, e.g. after overdose or drug interaction.
- Reduced myocardial contractility may result in hypotension and pulmonary oedema.

Class Ib

Examples are lidocaine (previously termed lignocaine), phenytoin, mexiletine, and tocainide. These drugs shorten APD and ERP. Actions are more pronounced in rapidly depolarizing or ischaemic tissue.

Lidocaine is available as parenteral and topical products. It has a short half-life of 10–20 minutes but action is prolonged by active metabolites. Elimination is also delayed in patients with hepatic impairment or poor cardiac output, who are at increased risk of toxicity, generally as a result of inadvertent therapeutic overdose. Ingestion of topical preparations can also occasionally result in systemic toxicity, although oral bioavailability is low. Toxicity may also occur after extensive topical use involving damaged skin or mucous membranes, through which it is readily absorbed. Toxicity has also occurred after urethral and rectal instillation.

Mexiletine and tocainide are orally active class Ib agents that are now used rarely if ever. Phenytoin is considered further in Anticonvulsants, p. 99.

Features of poisoning with class Ib drugs include:

- Numbness of the mouth, which is usually present after significant ingestions.
- Nausea and vomiting.
- Restlessness, dizziness, agitation confusion, visual disturbances, hallucinations, tinnitus.
- Muscle twitching and shivering, paraesthesia.
- Depressed myocardial contractility, peripheral vasodilatation, hypotension.
- Convulsions, coma, and apnoea.
- Sinus bradycardia, asystole, conduction defects, heart block, and nodal and ventricular tachyarrhythmias. NB the QRS and QT intervals are not prolonged.

Class Ic

Drugs in this group, including flecainide, lorcainide (not licensed for use in the UK), encainide (not licensed for use in the UK), and propafenone, are potent sodium channel blockers but do not affect APD or ERP. They have a narrow therapeutic index and doses twice or more than the usual daily dose may cause significant toxicity.

Features of poisoning include:

- Nausea, vomiting, mydriasis, blurred vision.
- Depressed myocardial contractility, hypotension, and pulmonary oedema.
- ECG abnormalities including marked QRS and QT interval prolongation and giant inverted T-waves. Cardiac conduction disturbances with bradycardia, nodal or ventricular tachycardia (including torsade de pointes) may occur.
- Hypoxia, metabolic acidosis, hypokalaemia, hyperglycaemia, leucocytosis.
- Coma, convulsions, and respiratory depression.

Class II

These are antisympathetic agents and include beta-blockers and bretylium. Poisoning with beta-blockers is dealt with in Beta-adrenoceptor antagonists, pp. 132–133.

Class III

Amiodarone, dronedarone, and dofetilide (not licensed for use in the UK) block cardiac potassium channels including I_{kr} to inhibit the outward movement of potassium, delaying repolarization with consequent increase in APD and ERP. The beta-blocker sotalol also has class III properties, while amiodarone also has weak beta-blocking and calcium channel blocking effects.

Unlike other antidysrhythmic drugs, amiodarone does not usually cause serious toxicity if taken in a single overdose, due to its widespread distribution. Toxicity may, however, occur due to accumulation of therapeutic doses.

Dronedarone is an orally active agent used to prevent recurrence in non-permanent atrial fibrillation. Unlike amiodarone, it does not contain iodine and is therefore less likely to disturb thyroid function. It has, however, been associated with abnormal liver function and in some cases acute liver failure.

Bretylium is an anti-fibrillatory drug that initially stimulates and then inhibits noradrenaline (norepinephrine) release. It has occasionally been used intravenously in the context of cardiac arrest. Transient hypertension and exacerbation of arrhythmias associated with catecholamine release may occur after use, with subsequent sustained hypotension due to vasodilatation.

Features of poisoning with class III drugs include:

- Nausea, vomiting, and sweating
- Hypotension, tachycardia
- Bradycardia and AV block may occur and have been reported with therapeutic loading doses of amiodarone
- QT interval prolongation and torsade de pointes.

Class IV

Non-dihydropyridine calcium channel antagonists such as diltiazem and verapamil block slow calcium channels and, as a result, have actions that are most pronounced in nodal tissue. Poisoning with calcium channel blockers is described in Calcium channel blockers, pp. 134–135.

Other antidysrhythmic drugs

Drugs falling outside the Singh Vaughan Williams classification, sometimes referred to as 'Class V' agents, include:

- Digoxin and other cardiac glycosides (discussed in Digoxin, pp. 142–145).
- Adenosine, a purine nucleotide that slows atrioventricular conduction via blockade of the A1 adenosine receptor. It is administered as an intravenous bolus for diagnosing or terminating supraventricular arrhythmias. It has a very short half-life and poisoning is unlikely.
- Magnesium sulfate is used intravenously to treat torsade de pointes ventricular tachycardia. Adverse effects include flushing, nausea, drowsiness, slurred speech, loss of deep tendon reflexes and even paralysis, hypotension, and coma. Bradycardia,

prolongation of the PR QRS intervals, conduction defects, heart block, and asystole have also been reported.

Management of overdose with class I and III drugs

- Prevent further administration of suspect drug (e.g. when poisoning from therapeutic use).
- Give activated charcoal to patients who have ingested potentially toxic doses within approximately 1 hour.
- Monitor pulse, blood pressure, conscious level, and respiration for up to 12 hours in asymptomatic patients (longer for modified-release preparations).
- Perform a 12-lead ECG for determination of QRS and QT intervals and analysis of arrhythmias (see also Cardiovascular toxicity, pp. 64–67).
- Assess for acidosis (arterial blood gases or venous bicarbonate) correcting with sodium bicarbonate as required. Bicarbonate may reverse QRS widening and prevent arrhythmias associated with sodium channel blockade (e.g. with flecainide).
- Measure electrolytes and correct abnormalities as appropriate.
- Provide airway and respiratory support as appropriate. Consider managing patients with significant poisoning in a critical care environment.
- Treat hypotension with intravenous fluids, watching for features of developing pulmonary oedema. Inotropic agents may be needed in some patients.
- Treat convulsions with a benzodiazepine, e.g. lorazepam.
- Treat bradycardias associated with impaired cardiac output with atropine and, if necessary, temporary pacing.
- Treatment of tachyarrhythmias is complex and specialist advice should be sought. Hypoxia, acidosis, and electrolyte abnormalities should be corrected. Torsade de pointes associated with class Ia and III agents is treated using magnesium sulfate. For other ventricular arrhythmias, intravenous bicarbonate may be beneficial even in the absence of acidosis. Lidocaine has been used successfully for ventricular tachycardia associated with class Ia drugs.
- Intravenous lipid emulsion therapy may be considered for severe poisoning with class I and III drugs, especially if severe clinical effects have been unresponsive to conventional therapy (See Cardiovascular Toxicity, p. 67).
- Enhanced elimination methods are unlikely to be useful because of the large volumes of distribution of these drugs

Further reading

Denaro CP, Benowitz NL (1989). Poisoning due to class 1B antiarrhythmic drugs. Lignocaine, mexiletine and tocainide. Med Toxicol Adverse Drug Exp, 4:412–28.

Kim SY, Benowitz NL (1990). Poisoning due to class 1A antiarrhythmic drugs, Quinidine, procainamide and disopyramide. Drug Saf, 3:394–420.

Köppel C, Oberdisse U, Heinemeyer G (1990). Clinical course and outcome in class IC antiarrhythmic overdose. Clin Toxicol, 28:433–44.

Leatham EW, Holt DW, McKenna WJ (1993). Class III antiarrhythmics in overdose. Presenting features and management principles. Drug Saf, 9:450–62.

Nitrates

Background and therapeutic use

Organic nitrates have been used in clinical medicine since the 19th century. The nitrates currently available are glyceryl trinitrate (GTN, nitroglycerin), isosorbide dinitrate, and isosorbide mononitrate. They are available in a variety of preparations designed for use via several different routes (Table 6.3).

Nitrates are predominately used for the management of coronary ischaemia and left ventricular failure. Additionally, GTN ointment can be used in the management of anal fissures (due to the smooth muscle relaxant effects of nitrates).

Mechanism of toxicity

Nitrates are metabolized to release nitric oxide (NO), which is normally produced from blood vessel endothelial cells and is a potent vasodilator. NO stimulates guanylate cyclase in the vascular smooth muscle cells leading to an increase in intracellular cGMP concentration. This results in relaxation of the blood vessel smooth muscle with consequent vasodilatation. This affects arterioles, including coronary arterioles, but is particularly predominant in venules, especially at lower concentrations. This dilatation of the venous system leads to a reduction in the left ventricular filling pressure, while arteriolar dilatation reduces systemic vascular resistance and reduced blood pressure. Cardiac output is maintained as a result of the reduced afterload and the reflex tachycardia that occurs as a result in the fall in blood pressure.

Toxicokinetics

Following oral ingestion, nitrates are rapidly absorbed from the gastrointestinal tract.

Glyceryl trinitrate

GTN is subject to extensive pre-systemic metabolism to di- and mononitrates which are of much lower potency. As a result, GTN has limited effects after oral ingestion and acute overdose by ingestion is unlikely to have important clinical consequences unless the doses involved are very large. GTN is absorbed via the mucous membrane of the mouth and across the skin and these routes avoids first-pass metabolism, allowing clinically useful plasma concentrations of GTN to be achieved. Sublingual GTN achieves peak blood concentrations after about 3 minutes, while buccal and transdermal preparations are designed to release GTN over several hours. GTN has a plasma half-life of approximately 1–3 minutes.

Table 6.3 Available nitrate preparations

Drug	Routes	Preparations
Glyceryl trinitrate	Sublingual	Tablet, aerosol spray
	Buccal	Long-acting tablets
	Parenteral	
	Transdermal	Patches, ointment
Isosorbide dinitrate	Oral	Standard or modified-release tablets
	Parenteral	
Isosorbide mononitrate	Oral	Standard or modified-release tablets

Isosorbide dinitrate

Isosorbide dinitrate is also rapidly absorbed after oral ingestion and undergoes rapid first-pass metabolism to the biologically active isosorbide mononitrate. The half-life in plasma is 0.5–2 hours. Modified-release preparations are available.

Isosorbide mononitrate

Isosorbide mononitrate is well absorbed with peak blood concentrations achieved within an hour of ingestion of a standard preparation. It has a half-life of 4–5 hours. Modified-release preparations are available to extend its duration of action.

Risk factors for toxicity

The toxic dose of oral nitrates varies between individuals, with some individuals being able to tolerate higher does than others. Regular prolonged use of nitrate preparations is associated with tolerance and this affects therapeutic and adverse effects. These individuals may be resistant to some of the clinical features of nitrate poisoning.

Concurrent use of nitrates with phosphodiesterase type 5 inhibitors such as sildenafil, tadalafil, and vardenafil is contraindicated because of the increased risk of severe hypotension.

Toxicity is also likely to be more severe in patients receiving treatment with other vasodilators, in those with heart disease, and in the elderly.

Anyone who has ingested more than 3–4 mg/kg of isosorbide mononitrate/dinitrate respectively should have a medical assessment. Sublingual absorption of more than two or three tablets or transdermal exposure to more than one patch of GTN is potentially associated with toxicity. As noted earlier, swallowing of sublingual GTN tablets is associated with a lower risk of toxicity.

Clinical features of nitrate poisoning

Clinical effects develop rapidly after oral ingestion of isosorbide mononitrate or dinitrate and may persist for many hours especially after use of modified-release preparations.

The pattern of clinical features of nitrate poisoning do not appear to differ between the type and/or preparation of nitrate involved.

Commonly reported features of nitrate poisoning are similar to the adverse effects reported by users of these products in therapeutic doses. These include flushing, sweating, restlessness, headache, nausea and vomiting, hypotension (which may be postural and associated with syncope), tachycardia, and palpitations. Less commonly, there are reports of raised intracranial pressure and associated confusion and/or other neurological deficits. There are also reports of retinal toxicity from excess recreational use of nitrates.

Methaemoglobinaemia has been reported after therapeutic use of massive doses of sublingual GTN.

Toxicity assessment

Severity of poisoning is assessed on the basis of the extent of hypotension and tachycardia.

Investigations

There are no specific investigations required and measurement of plasma nitrate concentrations is not clinically useful. It may be appropriate to perform an ECG, especially in patients with underlying heart disease, although nitrate overdose is not associated with specific features. Measurement of methaemoglobin is only needed following massive overdose if there is a clinical suspicion of methaemoglobinaemia.

Management

Patients should be observed for at least 4 hours after ingestion of an oral or a sublingual preparation (12 hours if a modified/sustained-release preparation has been ingested). Patients who are asymptomatic after this time can be discharged and advised that it is unlikely that they will develop symptoms. Individuals with suspected nitrate toxicity related to transdermal absorption should be observed for at least 4 hours after removal of the patches.

Patients who present within an hour of ingestion of a potentially toxic amount of a nitrate should be given activated charcoal (50 g in adults, 1 g/kg in children).

Where toxicity is thought to be related to a transdermal nitrate patch, this should be removed and the area washed thoroughly to prevent any ongoing absorption from nitrates remaining on the skin after removal of the patch.

Management of toxicity associated with nitrates is largely supportive. Analgesia may be required for headache. Hypotension should be treated initially with conservative measures, such as elevation of the foot of the bed and/or legs, and the use of intravenous fluids. In those individuals with severe hypotension unresponsive to these measures, then the use of inotropes may be indicated, based on the individual clinical situation. If the cause is predominantly decreased systemic vascular resistance, vasoconstrictor agents such as norepinephrine may be most appropriate, titrating the dose of against blood pressure. If hypotension is thought to result from reduced cardiac output, inotropic drugs (e.g. dobutamine, epinephrine) may be more appropriate.

Use of elimination techniques

Haemodialysis and haemoperfusion are not clinically useful because of the large volumes of distribution of these agents.

Further reading

Sobrino JM, Fernández N, Martinez A, et al. (1992). Massive ingestion of isosorbide-5-mononitrate and nitroglycerin: suicide attempt by an adolescent girl without previous heart disease. Eur Heart J, 13:145.

Vignal-Clermont C, Audo I, Sahel J, et al. (2010). Poppers-associated retinal toxicity. N Engl J Med, 363:1583–5.

Digoxin

Background

Digoxin is a cardiac glycoside (cardenolide) used in the treatment of supra-ventricular arrhythmias, especially atrial fibrillation, and also occasionally in the treatment of heart failure.

Other cardiac glycoside-based medications, e.g. digitoxin and ouabain, are no longer in clinical use and are unlikely to be encountered in overdose. Cardiac glycosides are, however, present in some plants and ingestion of these can precipitate toxicity. The foxglove (*Digitalis purpurea*) contains digitoxin and gitoxin in its leaves and digitalin in its seeds. Yellow (*Thevetia peruviana*) and Pink (*Nerium oleander*) oleander also contain cardiac glycosides, especially in the seeds. Yellow oleander is commonly used as a method of self harm in South Asia. Lilly of the valley (*Convallaria majalis*) contains cardiac glycosides in all part of the plant. Cardiac glycosides are also found in red squill (*Drimia maritime*) (see also Common plant poisonings, pp. 320–323).

Mode of toxicity

The pharmacological receptor target of this class of compounds is the Na^+/K^+-ATPase transporter on the membrane of myocardial cells and cardiac conducting tissue. Blockade of this transporter by cardiac glycosides prevents inward potassium transport and results in increasing concentrations of intracellular Na^+ and Ca^{2+} ions. In toxicity this is associated with a rise in extracellular K+.

The clinical outcome of digoxin toxicity is usually atrio-ventricular (AV) block and bradycardia, with reduced conduction velocity through the cardiac conducting system as a result of enhanced vagal tone. The myocardium becomes more excitable and electrical automaticity is increased, resulting in extrasystoles and arrhythmias. The binding of digoxin to the Na^+/K^+-ATPase is increased in hypokalaemia and hypomagnesaemia, thus increasing digoxin toxicity.

Digoxin poisoning presents in three different scenarios:
1 Acute overdose in patients not taking digoxin therapeutically.
2 Acute overdose in patients taking regular digoxin.
3 Following chronic accumulation in patients on therapy. This may be associated with:
   • deterioration in renal function
   • drug interactions which:
     • increase serum digoxin concentrations: numerous drugs inhibit P-glycoprotein; these increase systemic bioavailability and inhibit renal tubular and biliary secretion of digoxin resulting in increases in serum digoxin concentration that can be substantial. Examples include amiodarone, erythromycin, clarithromycin, diltiazem, verapamil, felodipine, itraconazole, ketoconazole, quinidine, tacrolimus, indinavir, and ritonavir
     • reduce plasma potassium: examples include potassium-losing diuretics (e.g. furosemide, bendroflumethiazide), and corticosteroids.

Risk factors for toxicity

Risk of severe toxicity (all presentations) is increased for the following groups:
• age greater than 55 years
• renal and/or cardiac disease
• males.

Toxicokinetics

Digoxin is incompletely absorbed after ingestion with a systemic bioavailability of about 70%. Peak blood concentrations occur at around 6 hours after a therapeutic dose.

The volume of distribution of digoxin is large, about 7–8 L/kg in an adult, as a result of binding of the drug to the Na^+/K^+-ATPase transporter in peripheral tissues, especially heart and skeletal muscle. As a result, enhanced elimination methods such as haemodialysis are of limited value for removing digoxin.

The elimination of digoxin is predominantly renal. In patients with normal renal function taking therapeutic doses, digoxin half-life ranges from 20–50 hours, but half-life is longer (e.g. up to 5 days) in patients with renal impairment.

Concentrations in normal therapeutic use are usually in the range of 1–2 ng/mL (1.3–2.6 nmol/L).

Clinical features

Cardiac

Digoxin toxicity may be associated with a wide range of arrhythmias which may result from excessive degrees of heart block or ventricular excitability of a combination of these. Specific cardiac features include bradycardia with marked PR and QRS prolongation on the ECG. Various degrees of AV block with associated escape rhythms may be evident. Sinus arrest may occur. Serious tachyarrhythmias are less common but may be supra-ventricular or ventricular in origin. Ventricular ectopics are common with bigeminy or trigeminy characteristic. Ventricular tachycardia and fibrillation can also occur. Atrial tachycardia with variable degrees of AV block is highly characteristic of digoxin toxicity but is not common. Arrhythmias are more common in patients with pre-existing cardiac disease.

Impairment of cardiac output with hypotension may occur in severe digoxin toxicity.

Cardiac features may be aggravated by co-ingested drugs which increase AV block, e.g. beta blockers, diltiazem, or verapamil.

Gastrointestinal

Nausea and vomiting are common features of digoxin toxicity. Diarrhoea may occur but is less characteristic.

Nervous system

Visual disturbances described as a yellow tinge to vision (xanthopsia) are characteristic but very uncommon. Confusion and occasionally psychosis can occur. Convulsions have been reported but are rare.

Laboratory

To assess the clinical severity of poisoning the following should be performed:
• The serum electrolytes and serum magnesium should be measured. In acute poisoning a serum potassium higher than 5 mmol/L usually indicates significant toxicity.
• Plasma creatinine should be measured to assess renal function.
• A 12-lead ECG should be performed. This should be repeated at regular intervals over the first 4–24 hours in acute or acute-on-chronic poisoning.

- Measurement of the plasma digoxin concentration should normally be delayed until at least 6 hours after ingestion, except in symptomatic patients. A measurement made at least 6 hours after ingestion is necessary for determining doses of digoxin antibody. Earlier measurements may confirm ingestion, but because of the time taken for digoxin to distribute, are less useful in calculating antidote doses. Plasma digoxin concentrations greater than 4 ng/mL (5.2 nmol/L) are suggestive of severe poisoning, especially after chronic accumulation.
- Arterial blood gases should be measured in patients with hyperkalaemia or other features of severe toxicity. Hyperkalaemia is commonly associated with metabolic acidosis.

Toxicity assessment

In digoxin poisoning assessment of toxicity is based on the presence of clinical features, particularly nausea and vomiting and bradycardia, as well as the results of investigations, with toxicity related to the degree of hyperkalaemia, the plasma concentrations of digoxin, and the presence of ECG changes (e.g. heart block). Poor prognostic factors are a high degree of AV block, hyperkalaemia, and episodes of ventricular tachycardia.

In acute poisoning plasma concentrations of digoxin do not correlate well with features of toxicity but are useful to confirm ingestion.

Acute changes in plasma concentration may assist in determining the extent of poisoning, but clinical management should be based on the features of poisoning, not plasma concentrations of digoxin in isolation.

Clinical course in acute poisoning

Clinical features develop within 1–2 hours of acute ingestion, but cardiac features usually take longer, with maximal effects usually not present for at least 6–12 hours.

Asymptomatic patients should be observed for at least 6 hours after an acute digoxin overdose.

Chronic accumulation of digoxin

The risk factors for chronic accumulation are pre-existing renal impairment and advanced age. GI features including nausea, vomiting, and diarrhoea tend to be more prominent, together with general symptoms including anorexia, general malaise, headache, weakness, blurred vision, and less commonly alterations in colour perception. Rarely confusion, hallucinations, and delirium may occur.

In these patients any type of cardiac arrhythmia may occur. Pre-existing cardiac disease and electrolyte disturbances caused by concomitant diuretic therapy increase the risk of toxicity, and also make serum potassium rise less easy to interpret as a marker of acute digoxin poisoning.

Management

The pulse and blood pressure should be measured frequently and the patient should be placed on an ECG monitor to detect disorders of cardiac rhythm.

Activated charcoal may reduce absorption of digoxin if administered soon (e.g. within 1 hour) after ingestion of a potentially toxic overdose, e.g. more than 3 mg in an adult or more than 50 micrograms/kg in a child for a single acute overdose. Lower amounts may be toxic in patients taking acute overdoses in the context of chronic therapy.

Hyperkalaemia, if present, is a marker of the urgent need to give digoxin antibody. Life-threatening hyperkalaemia should be treated with insulin and glucose while the antibody is being prepared. Hypokalaemia and hypomagnesaemia should be corrected as these increase the myocardial toxicity of digoxin. Calcium should not be used first line in the treatment of hyperkalaemia or hypocalcaemia as it increases ventricular automaticity and may precipitate arrhythmias (consult an expert if considering).

Metabolic acidosis should be treated with intravenous sodium bicarbonate.

In patients who have ingested glycosides other than digoxin (e.g. digitoxin, foxglove, or yellow oleander) the laboratory digoxin assay is less accurate but nevertheless helpful in confirming ingestion of active material.

Repeat digoxin concentrations may need to be measured before commencing therapy and serum potassium measurements, which are more easily obtained, may be of use in monitoring progress of digitalis effect on the myocardium.

Bradycardia should be treated with atropine (e.g. 1.2 mg initial dose in an adult, 0.02 mg/kg for a child). Repeat doses may be necessary.

If bradycardia does not respond to atropine and an appropriately calculated dose of digoxin antibody, a temporary pacing wire should be inserted and used.

Ventricular arrhythmias secondary to digoxin may respond to intravenous magnesium, even if the serum magnesium concentration is initially normal. As infusion of 4–8 mmol/hour may be required in cases of recurrent ventricular arrhythmia. Class 1a and 1C antiarrhythmics (e.g. quinidine, flecainide, disopyramide) may affect AV nodal conduction adversely and should not be used.

Digoxin-specific antibody fragments

Antigen binding fragments (Fab), derived from antidigoxin antibodies raised in sheep, are effective in the management of digoxin toxicity but use should be restricted to patients with severe poisoning. The affinity constant of digoxin antibody fragments for digoxin is higher than that of the Na^+/K^+-ATPase, so digoxin binds preferentially to the antibody fragments, becoming pharmacologically inactive. Digoxin antibody complexes are then eliminated in the urine (half-life 16–20 hours in patients with normal renal function). Features of severe poisoning are usually reversed within an hour of administration of antibodies, although complete reversal may take as long as 24 hours.

Indications

Treatment indications are based on the patient's clinical condition and serum potassium. Patients who have no impairment of cardiac output, and whose heart rate is reasonably well maintained, may not require antidotal therapy.

Indications for digoxin antibody include:
- life-threatening dysrhythmias
- severe heart block, marked bradycardia
- cardiac compromise in patients with underlying cardiac disease
- serum potassium higher than 6 mmol/L
- elevated serum digoxin in a symptomatic patient. An arbitrary cut-off of 7 ng/mL (9 nmol/L) in patients with acute overdose, or 4 ng/mL in chronic toxicity, may be considered a useful marker.

Dose calculation

Digoxin antibodies (Fab fraction) are specific and bind digoxin in a molar ratio. It is usually not necessary to completely bind all digoxin present. In patients on chronic therapy, although recommended by the manufacturers, complete neutralization of digoxin is inappropriate because the beneficial effects of the drug will be impaired. This would include those with chronic accumulation of digoxin and those who have taken an acute overdose who are also receiving the drug regularly.

In patients who have ingested an acute overdose all that is required is to prevent or reverse the acute toxic effects of digoxin; excess use of antibody is unnecessary and costly.

Approximately 50% of the dose calculated to completely neutralize digoxin should be administered initially and the response to this dose monitored. A clinical effect should be clearly seen within 1–2 hours. If this is inadequate, further doses can be administered.

In the event of a good response, patients still need to be monitored for at least 6–12 hours, but a second dose of antibody should only be given in the event of a recurrence of toxicity. This may occur due to tissue redistribution or continued absorption of digoxin from the GI tract.

Once digoxin antibody has been administered, further measurements of serum digoxin are not useful because the assay measures both free and bound digoxin, with redistribution of digoxin from tissues into the blood (bound to antibody) often resulting in very high plasma total digoxin concentrations in patients who are clinically improving.

Digoxin antibody complex is not removed by haemodialysis, but use of the method in patients with acute kidney injury will reduce acute effects of digoxin on the heart. Acute kidney injury is therefore not a contraindication to using the antibody, although digoxin antibodies may persist in the blood for many days and there is a theoretical risk of dissociation of digoxin with consequent recurrent toxicity.

The dose of digoxin antibodies required for full neutralization in digoxin poisoning can be calculated as shown in Box 6.1 (NB *normally use half the calculated dose*):

NB digoxin assay kits are *not* designed to measure levels greater than 5 ng/mL (6.4 nmol/L), so exercise caution when using high digoxin levels to calculate the dose (see Box 6.2).

The estimated number of vials required for full neutralization for adults and children heavier than 20 kg is shown in Table 6.4, which is for the product DigiFab®. This has replaced the previous market leader Digibind® which was

---

Box 6.1 Calculation of dose

Adults and children (>20 kg):

(a) Dose of digoxin ingested known
Full neutralization dose of DigiFab® is:
Number of vials = amount of digoxin ingested (mg) × 1.6
Round up to the nearest vial

(b) Serum digoxin concentration known:
Full neutralization dose of DigiFab® is:
Number of vials = serum digoxin concentration (ng/mL) × weight (kg)/100
Round up to the nearest vial

To calculate the number of milligrams to be prescribed multiply the number of vials by 40 (as there are 40 mg DigiFab®/vial).

Box 6.2 Converting units

micrograms/L(or ng/mL) × 1.28 = nmol/L
nmol/L × 0.781 = micrograms/L (or ng/mL)

---

withdrawn by the manufacturer in 2011. Doses in practice are similar.

The estimated dose of DigiFab® (in mg) required for full neutralization for infants and children less than 20 kg is shown in Table 6.5. The number of vials can be obtained by dividing the dose in mg by 40. For very small doses, a 40 mg vial can be diluted with 36 mL of sterile isotonic (0.9%) saline to achieve a concentration of 1 mg/mL.

Digoxin antibody fragments may also be used to treat cardiac glycoside poisoning arising from plant poisoning. Dosing is based on clinical severity, and monitoring of response to increments of antibody.

Adverse effects

Adverse effects of digoxin antibody fragments include:

• Allergy: anaphylactic, hypersensitive or febrile reactions have been reported but are not common because of the lower antigenicity of the Fab fragment compared to the intact antibody. Rash (sometimes purpuric), facial swelling, urticaria, and thrombocytopenia have occurred. Risk is likely to be increased in patients with asthma or antibiotic allergies. Patients

---

Table 6.4 Calculation of DigiFab® doses according to weight and serum digoxin concentration (adults and children >20 kg). As described previously, the normal starting dose should be 50% of this calculated dose

Weight	Serum digoxin concentration (ng/mL)				
(kg)	2	4	8	12	16
40	1 vial	2 vials	3 vials	5 vials	7 vials
60	1 vial	3 vials	5 vials	7 vials	10 vials
70	2 vials	3 vials	6 vials	9 vials	11 vials
80	2 vials	3 vials	7 vials	10 vials	13 vials
100	2 vials	4 vials	8 vials	12 vials	16 vials

Data from DigiFab®

Table 6.5 Calculation of Digifab® doses according to weight and serum digoxin concentration (children ≤20 kg). As described earlier, the normal starting dose should be 50% of this calculated dose

Weight (kg)	Serum digoxin concentration (ng/mL)				
	2	**4**	**8**	**12**	**16**
1	1 mg	1.5 mg	3 mg	5 mg	6.5 mg
3	2.5 mg	5 mg	10 mg	14 mg	19 mg
5	4 mg	8 mg	16 mg	24 mg	32 mg
10	8 mg	16 mg	32 mg	48 mg	64 mg
20	16 mg	32 mg	64 mg	96 mg	128 mg

Data from DigiFab®

with allergy to papain, chymopapain, or other papaya extracts are at increased risk as papain is used to cleave the antibody to derive the Fab fragments.

• Hypokalaemia may be precipitated by digoxin antibody fragments. Plasma potassium should therefore be monitored frequently during therapy.

• In patients on chronic therapy, use of digoxin antibody fragments may cause features of the underlying disease to recur, e.g. heart failure or arrhythmias.

Little information is available on the use of digoxin antibody fragments during pregnancy, however in the context of severe digoxin toxicity, pregnancy is not a contraindication since the risk of adverse maternal and fetal effects from poisoning are likely to outweigh any possible adverse effects of the antibody fragments.

Use of elimination techniques

Haemodialysis and haemoperfusion are unlikely to be effective for removing digoxin because of its large volume of distribution. Haemodialysis may be needed to treat hyperkalaemia and acidosis in the context of renal failure.

Multiple-dose activated charcoal can reduce the half-life of digoxin but the role of this in therapy in the management of digoxin poisoning is uncertain.

Further reading

Antman EM, Wenger TL, Butler VP, et al. (1990). Treatment of 150 cases of life-threatening digitalis intoxication with digoxin-specific Fab antibody fragments. *Circulation*, 81:1744–52.

Bateman DN (2004). Digoxin-specific antibody fragments: how much and when? *Toxicol Rev*, 23:135–43.

Bilbault P, Oubaassine R, Rahmani H, et al. (2009). Emergency step-by-step specific immunotherapy in severe digoxin poisoning: an observational cohort study. *Eur J Emerg Med*, 16:145–9.

Eddleston M, Rajapakse S, Rajakanthan K, et al. (2000). Anti-digoxin Fab fragments in cardiotoxicity induced by ingestion of yellow oleander: a randomised controlled trial. *Lancet*, 355:967–72.

Hickey AR, Wenger TL, Carpenter VP, et al. (1991). Digoxin immune Fab therapy in the management of digitalis intoxication: safety and efficacy results of an observational surveillance study. *J Am Coll Cardiol*, 17:590–8.

Lapostolle F, Borron SW, Verdier C, et al. (2008). Assessment of digoxin antibody use in patients with elevated serum digoxin following chronic or acute exposure. *Intensive Care Med*, 34:1448–53.

Lapostolle F, Borron SW, Verdier C, et al. (2008). Digoxin-specific Fab fragments as single first-line therapy in digitalis poisoning. *Crit Care Med*, 36:3014–18.

Rajapakse S (2009). Management of yellow oleander poisoning. *Clin Toxicol*, 47:206–12.

Smith TW, Haber E, Yeatman L, et al. (1976). Reversal of advanced digoxin intoxication with Fab fragments of digoxin-specific antibodies. *N Engl J Med*, 294:797–800.

Ujhelyi MR, Robert S (1995). Pharmacological aspects of digoxin-specific Fab therapy in the management of digitalis toxicity. *Clin Pharmacokinet*, 28:483–93.

Woolf AD, Wenger T, Smith TW, et al. (1992). The use of digoxin-specific Fab fragments for severe digitalis intoxication in children. *N Engl J Med*, 326:1739–44.

Theophylline

Background and therapeutic use

Theophylline (1,3 dimethylxanthine) is a prescription-only medication mainly used as a modified-release tablet or capsule preparations for the treatment of chronic obstructive pulmonary disease (COPD) and asthma. A combination product (Do-Do ChestEze®) containing theophylline, caffeine, and ephedrine is also available without prescription via pharmacies.

Theophylline is also available in the intravenous preparation aminophylline, which also contains ethylenediamine to improve solubility. This is used in the management of acute asthma exacerbations (but not COPD) and also in the management of neonatal apnoea. Toxicity may arise from administration of aminophylline to patients already taking oral theophylline preparations or as a result of dose calculation errors, which are especially common in neonates.

Mechanisms of toxicity

Theophylline and the other methylxanthines have their actions through increased adrenergic activity. This occurs by: (1) increased release of catecholamines and stimulation at β_1/β_2-receptors; (2) adenosine antagonism leading to increased noradrenaline (norepinephrine) and adrenaline (epinephrine) release and inhibition of histamine related bronchoconstriction; and (3) inhibition of intracellular phosphodiesterase which is responsible for the degradation of cAMP the post-synaptic second messenger involved in β-receptor activity.

Toxicokinetics

The oral bioavailability of theophylline is almost 100%, with maximal absorption occurring within 6–10 hours following ingestion of standard-release theophylline preparations. The majority of theophylline products available are modified-release preparations; maximal absorption with these occurs within 15–20 hours of ingestion. The time to peak theophylline concentrations is typically 1–3 hours and 8–16 hours with standard and modified-release preparations respectively, so the onset of theophylline toxicity may be delayed when modified-release preparations have been ingested.

The volume of distribution of theophylline is small (about 0.5 L/kg), making it amenable to extracorporeal removal.

The majority of theophylline (>90%) is metabolized by the hepatic cytochrome P450 isoenzyme system, particularly the CYP1A2 isoenzyme. Half-life is dependent on a number of factors, and is approximately 4–5 hours in healthy non-smoking adults. Factors that inhibit CYP activity can significantly alter theophylline clearance, increasing risk of chronic accumulation and associated toxicity. Elimination may be prolonged after overdose (apparent half-life up to 30 hours).

Acute toxic effects correlate well with serum theophylline concentrations; the usual therapeutic range is 10–20 mg/L (55–110 micromol/L). Life-threatening toxic features occur at serum concentrations of greater than 60 mg/L (330 micromol/L) and fatalities are associated with concentrations of greater than 80 mg/L (440 micromol/L). In chronic accumulation the severity of poisoning is less well correlated with concentration, more severe clinical features occurring at lower concentrations, with fatalities at concentrations of greater than 40 mg/L (220 micromol/L).

Acute overdose ingestions of more than 3 g in adults (>40 mg/kg in children) are potentially serious.

Risk factors for toxicity

Risk of toxicity is enhanced in neonates (especially when premature) and the elderly and those with underlying cardiac or respiratory disease. Toxicity may also be precipitated by drugs inhibiting theophylline metabolism, e.g. macrolide and quinolone antibiotics, cimetidine, verapamil, and allopurinol. Risk of toxicity is higher at any particular theophylline concentration with chronic rather than acute intoxication.

Clinical features

Vomiting is common, occurring in 75% of cases. It is often pronounced and resistant to anti-emetic treatment. In protracted vomiting, associated haematemesis can occur. Diarrhoea and abdominal pain may also accompany the vomiting.

Theophylline stimulates the respiratory centre leading to hyperventilation and respiratory alkalosis. In cases of severe theophylline toxicity, this respiratory centre stimulation can lead to respiratory failure and/or respiratory arrest.

Anxiety/agitation, insomnia, tremor, irritability, dilated pupils, hallucinations, and convulsions all occur. Convulsions can often be prolonged and/or recurrent, and resistant to treatment with conventional anti-epileptic medications. Rhabdomyolysis can be a complication. Cardiac arrhythmias associated with toxicity include sinus tachycardia or atrial or ventricular ectopy progressing to ventricular tachycardia or fibrillation in severe poisoning

Toxicity assessment

The clinical features of acute theophylline toxicity can be graded, as shown in Table 6.6. This grading system is useful in determining the need for enhancing elimination of theophylline.

Chronic theophylline toxicity

Chronic theophylline toxicity can occur due to excess dosing or the concurrent use of medications that inhibit the metabolism of theophylline.

The pattern of toxicity differs from that observed in acute overdose. There is an increased incidence of convulsions, which are typically more resistant to treatment. Tachycardias are also more common in chronic theophylline toxicity, occurring in approximately 35% of chronic

Table 6.6 Grading of severity of theophylline poisoning on clinical signs/symptoms

Grade	Clinical features
1	Vomiting, diarrhoea, anxiety, tremor, sinus tachycardia, potassium 2.6–3.4 mmol/L
2	GI bleeding, confusion, supra-ventricular tachycardia, potassium <2.6 mmol/L, arterial pH <7.2 or >7.6, rhabdomyolysis
3	Convulsions, mean arterial BP <60 mmHg, sustained ventricular tachycardia
4	Recurrent convulsions, ventricular fibrillation, cardiac arrest

poisonings (compared to 10% in acute poisonings). Conversely, vomiting and hypokalaemia are less frequent with chronic toxicity.

Investigations

All patients require an initial ECG to determine the underlying cardiac rhythm. Continuous cardiac monitoring should be undertaken where there is evidence of theophylline toxicity.

Urea and electrolytes should be measured, paying particular attention to the plasma potassium. Theophylline-associated β_2-receptor stimulation results in an intracellular shift of potassium, with resultant intracellular hyperkalaemia and systemic hypokalaemia, which is present in 85% of acute theophylline poisonings. Total body potassium burden is normal, despite the systemic hypokalaemia. Electrolytes should be monitored every 1–2 hours in the acute phase of severe poisoning. Other metabolic disturbances include hypomagnesaemia, hypocalcaemia, hypophosphataemia, and hyperglycaemia.

Arterial blood gases should be performed in patients with clinical features or substantial overdose. Metabolic acidosis or respiratory alkalosis may be demonstrated.

Plasma theophylline concentrations should be measured urgently in patients with clinical features of toxicity, including hypokalaemia. In patients with severe poisoning (e.g. theophylline concentration >60 mg/L) measurements should be repeated every 2–4 hours. The grading system in Table 6.6 is a better guide to severity than concentrations alone.

Management

A clear airway and adequate ventilation and oxygenation should be ensured. It is appropriate to monitor oxygen saturation, especially in patients with underlying respiratory disease.

Asymptomatic patients should be observed for at least 4 hours (standard-release preparations) or 12 hours (modified-release preparations) after overdose.

Activated charcoal (50 g in adults, 1 g/kg in children) should be considered in patients who present within an hour of ingestion of a potentially toxic amount of theophylline (>20 mg/kg). As the majority of theophylline preparations are modified-release, administration more than 1 hour after ingestion may be appropriate. This may not be possible in individuals with severe theophylline toxicity due to vomiting. Care should be taken not to induce vomiting with the activated charcoal in the setting of an unprotected airway. Whole bowel irrigation is also sometimes used to prevent further absorption of modified-release preparations, although efficacy is uncertain.

Theophylline-induced vomiting should be treated with anti-emetics; ondansetron (e.g. 8 mg by slow IV injection) appears most effective. Patients with severe neurotoxicity (coma and/or convulsions) are increased risk of aspiration if they have significant vomiting.

Sinus tachycardia and supra-ventricular tachycardias not associated with haemodynamic comprise do not need treatment routinely. Where there is evidence of haemodynamic compromise, first-line therapy is short-acting beta-blockers (e.g. esmolol or metoprolol). Caution is advised in individuals with underlying COPD and/or asthma, in whom it may be more appropriate to consider the use of calcium channel blockers such as verapamil. Ventricular tachycardia with cardiac output should be treated with IV magnesium by infusion initially and then DC cardioversion. There is some evidence that amiodarone may be safe in this group of patients, although other antiarrhythmmics, such as lidocaine (lignocaine) should be avoided due to the increased risk of convulsions. Ventricular tachycardia without cardiac output should be treated in accordance with current standard Advance Life Support (ALS) algorithms.

Theophylline-related agitation and/or anxiety is best treated with benzodiazepines, the dose titrated to the patient's clinical condition. Haloperidol should be avoided as it lowers seizure threshold.

Convulsions should be initially be treated with benzodiazepines (diazepam: 10–20 mg in adults or 0.1–0.3 mg/kg in children; lorazepam: 1–4 mg in adults or 0.05 mg/kg in children).

The replacement of potassium in patients with theophylline toxicity should be undertaken very cautiously. Although there is systemic hypokalaemia, the total body burden of potassium is normal. Over-treatment during the acute phase of theophylline toxicity may result in clinically significant rebound hyperkalaemia during recovery. Therefore, potassium supplementation should only occur if the serum potassium is less than 2.8 mmol/L; replace at a rate of no more than 10 mmol per hour in the majority of cases, with regular monitoring of the serum concentration, which should continue in the recovery phase because of the risk of rebound hyperkalaemia.

Hypomagnesaemia may accompany hypokalaemia and should be corrected with parenteral magnesium. Severe metabolic acidosis that persists in spite of fluid resuscitation and correction of hypoxia may be treated with sodium bicarbonate. Note that overcorrection of acidosis may exacerbate hypokalaemia.

The management of chronic theophylline toxicity is the same as that for acute theophylline toxicity. In asymptomatic patients with an incidental finding of an elevated theophylline concentration, management may be by withholding theophylline treatment or reducing the daily prescribed dose.

Use of elimination techniques

Multiple-dose activated charcoal (MDAC) enhances theophylline elimination by reducing entero-hepatic circulation and is almost as effective as charcoal haemoperfusion. Its use can be limited in acute theophylline poisoning by intractable vomiting and/or paralytic ileus. It should be considered for patients with features of significant toxicity, especially when associated with a plasma theophylline concentration greater than 40 mg/L.

Charcoal haemoperfusion should be considered in the setting of grade 3 or 4 acute theophylline toxicity or a theophylline concentration of greater than 100 mg/L. Where this is not readily available, or a patient is too unstable to transfer to a centre where this can be provided, then haemodialysis could be used instead. Charcoal haemoperfusion enhances theophylline clearance to a greater extent, but haemodialysis has comparable effects on reducing theophylline morbidity and is associated with fewer complications.

There is a case report of successful use of continuous veno-venous haemofiltration for enhancing elimination of theophylline after overdose.

Further reading

Sessler CN (1990). Theophylline toxicity: clinical features of 116 consecutive cases. *Am J Med*, 88: 567–76.

Shannon M (1993). Predictors of major toxicity after theophylline overdose. *Ann Intern Med*, 119:1161–7.

Shannon M (1999). Life-threatening events after theophylline overdose: a 10-year prospective analysis. *Arch Intern Med*, 159:989–94.

Shannon MW (1997). Comparative efficacy of hemodialysis and hemoperfusion in severe theophylline intoxication. *Acad Emerg Med*, 4:674–8.

Other common pharmaceutical toxins

Antibiotics and antituberculous drugs

Background and therapeutic use of antibiotics

Antibiotics are used in the management of bacterial infections and sepsis. Generally the adverse effects seen with antibiotics occur in therapeutic use rather than as a result of intentional overdose. Most antibiotics are well tolerated in overdose. This section will discuss the potential for toxicity associated with some of these drugs and in addition will discuss the significant toxicity that can be associated with overdose of the antituberculous agents.

Antibiotics can be divided into a number of different classes (e.g. penicillins, cephalosporins, aminoglycosides, fluoroquinolones, macrolides, etc.) based on their mechanism of action and their spectrum of antibacterial activity. A detailed review of the mechanisms of action is beyond the scope of this book and these are generally not important in the toxicity seen with these agents.

Antibiotics

Penicillins and cephalosporins

Penicillins (e.g. amoxicillin, co-amoxiclav, phenoxymethylpenicillin) and cephalosporins (e.g. cefuroxime, cefalexin, cefotaxime) are of very low toxicity and acute overdoses are usually well tolerated. Some patients may develop self-limiting nausea and vomiting. Patients who are allergic to penicillin may develop skin rashes and/or other allergic/anaphylactic reactions. Rare effects reported include crystalluria and haematuria after very large oral overdoses and convulsions and encephalopathy after high-dose intravenous cephalosporin administration in patients with renal impairment. Large intravenous doses of penicillin can be associated with convulsions.

Hospital assessment is unlikely to be required for lone-penicillin/cephalosporin ingestion.

Macrolides

Macrolides such as erythromycin, clarithromycin, and azithromycin are generally of low toxicity. Acute overdose may be associated with self-limiting gastrointestinal symptoms such as nausea, vomiting and diarrhoea. Intravenous erythromycin lactobionate causes dose-related QTc prolongation and increases the risk of torsade de pointes. High dose oral poisoning with macrolides could theoretically be associated with QTc prolongation, particularly in patients on chronic therapy with cytochrome P450 3A4 inhibitors such as ketoconazole or fluconazole. Liver function abnormalities, renal impairment, hypokalaemia, pancreatitis, ototoxicity and thrombophlebitis have been reported after therapeutic use.

Management is supportive. Patients with erythromycin ingestions greater than 150mg/kg should have a 12-lead ECG to exclude QTc prolongation and be observed for 6 hours post-ingestion. Renal and liver function should be assessed in symptomatic patients.

Fluoroquinolones

This group of antibiotics, including ciprofloxacin, levofloxacin, and moxifloxacin, are also generally of low toxicity and well tolerated in overdose. There are, however, reports of acute kidney injury in patients with very large (4–19 g) ingestions, with some patients developing an interstitial nephritis. Some fluoroquinolones, including moxifloxacin, can cause QTc interval prolongation with a theoretical risk of torsade de pointes. Adverse effects reported after therapeutic use include nausea, vomiting, diarrhoea, tachycardia, hypotension, hypoglycaemia, rhabdomyolysis, toxic epidermal necrolysis, tendonitis, hepatotoxicity, photosensitivity, and seizures.

Treatment of overdose is supportive. Patients should be observed for at least 4 hours after overdose with monitoring of pulse, blood pressure, and cardiac rhythm. A 12-lead ECG should be performed for assessment of QTc interval.

Aminoglycosides

These antibiotics (e.g. gentamicin, tobramycin, streptomycin, amikacin) are available as topical (eye and ear), nebulizer fluid, and parenteral preparations. Toxicity is unlikely to occur after oral ingestion because of the very low systemic bioavailability of these polar compounds and therefore only occurs when excessive doses are given to patients being given intravenous aminoglycosides for sepsis.

Aminoglycosides cause dose-related nephrotoxicity, ototoxicity, and vestibular toxicity due to inhibition of mitochondrial metabolic processes. Vestibular toxicity occurs due to destruction of hair cells in the cochlea and the sensory cells in the inner ear. The elderly, those with renal impairment, and neonates are at greater risk of toxicity. Cumulative toxicity may occur after prolonged courses of high-dose aminoglycoside therapy. Ototoxicity may be irreversible. Neuromuscular paralysis may occur rarely after rapid intravenous administration.

The mainstay of management is to stop administration of the drug and ensure that the patient is well hydrated; in patients with significant renal impairment, renal replacement therapy (e.g. haemofiltration) may be necessary to remove the aminoglycoside and to manage associated renal failure. Referral for specialist assessment of auditory and vestibular function is recommended in those with ototoxicity and vestibular toxicity.

Other antibiotics

Chloramphenicol, sulfonamides, and tetracyclines are of low toxicity after overdose. Management is symptomatic and supportive. Chloramphenicol is occasionally associated with bone marrow aplasia after therapeutic use.

Metronidazole overdose may cause anorexia, vomiting, diarrhoea, headache, dizziness, and occasionally insomnia and drowsiness. Green or black urinary discolouration has been reported. Liver function abnormalities, seizures, peripheral neuropathy, and blood dyscrasias have occurred with intensive or prolonged therapeutic use. Taken with alcohol, metronidazole may provoke a disulfiram-like reaction with sudden onset of excitement, nausea, headache, dizziness, flushing, and dyspnoea. Treatment of overdose is symptomatic and supportive. Disulfiram-like reactions are treated by discontinuing therapy and infusion of intravenous fluids.

Trimethoprim overdose can be associated with vomiting, dizziness, ataxia, drowsiness, dysuria, headache, and confusion and occasionally hyperkalaemia and hyponatraemia. Bone marrow depression has been reported after therapeutic use and after overdose. Treatment is symptomatic and supportive.

Background and therapeutic use of antituberculous drugs

Antituberculous drugs (e.g. rifampicin, ethambutol, isoniazid, and pyrazinamide) are used in combination for the treatment of *Mycobacterium tuberculosis* (TB) infection.

If patients present after an overdose of their own medication that has been prescribed for the treatment of TB, it is important that this is restarted once features of toxicity have settled.

Antituberculous drugs

Isoniazid

This is the most toxic of the antituberculous agents; significant toxicity is seen with ingestion greater than 20 mg/kg and severe toxicity with ingestions greater than 60–80 mg/kg.

Isoniazid metabolites complex with pyridoxine to form inactive complexes, resulting in a functional pyridoxine deficiency and inhibition of pyridoxine-dependent enzyme systems. In addition, isoniazid interferes with the synthesis and metabolism of the inhibitory neurotransmitter gamma-aminobutyric acid (GABA) resulting in agitation and seizures.

The most significant features seen in isoniazid poisoning are seizures, severe metabolic acidosis, and coma. Other features include nausea and vomiting, hypotension rhabdomyolysis, hyper-reflexia, hallucinations, and acute tubular necrosis. The seizures seen in isoniazid poisoning are often refractory to conventional anticonvulsant therapy and toxicity can be prolonged. The specific antidote in those not responding is pyridoxine.

All patients should be observed for at least 6 hours post ingestion; patients that are asymptomatic at this time can be discharged. Management of isoniazid toxicity involves general supportive care (rehydration, maintenance of the airway) and in those with severe toxicity treatment of seizures, correction of metabolic acidosis and use of the antidote pyridoxine.

Patients with a significant metabolic acidosis (pH <7.30) should be treated with 1–2 mL/kg intravenous 8.4% sodium bicarbonate to correct the acidosis. Intravenous high-dose pyridoxine therapy should be given to patients with seizures not responding to benzodiazepines. The dose of pyridoxine is 1 g for each gram of isoniazid ingested (to a maximum of an initial dose of 5 g). If the intravenous preparation is not available, pyridoxine tablets can be administered orally, or via a nasogastric tube after crushing. Benzodiazepines act synergistically with pyridoxine and further doses of benzodiazepines (e.g. diazepam 10–20 mg in adults, 0.1–0.3 mg/kg in children) should be used in circumstances where insufficient pyridoxine is available. Seizures resistant to benzodiazepines and pyridoxine should be managed with barbiturates. Phenytoin is ineffective for isoniazid-related seizures.

Rifampicin

Acute rifampicin overdose is generally well tolerated with only gastrointestinal effects such as nausea, vomiting, and diarrhoea and cutaneous effects such as flushing and itching in most patients. Red discolouration of skin, mucous membranes, skin, sweat, and urine may occur as a result of the presence of rifampicin and its metabolites. Other effects that can occur but that are more likely with larger ingestions include convulsions, metabolic acidosis, hepatic and renal toxicity, bleeding, dizziness, blurred vision, lethargy, confusion, ataxia, and peripheral neuritis. There are reports of facial and peri-orbital oedema in children with rifampicin overdose.

Symptomatic patients and/or those with an ingestion of more than 50 mg/kg should be observed for 6 hours post ingestion. Those with ongoing symptoms should have U&Es and LFTs checked to exclude hepatic and/or renal injury.

Treatment of toxicity is supportive. Acidosis and convulsions may require treatment with sodium bicarbonate and benzodiazepines respectively.

Pyrazinamide

There is little information on the toxicity associated with acute overdose of pyrazinamide. Toxicity seen with therapeutic use of pyrazinamide includes hepatotoxicity and hyperuricaemia sometimes associated with gout.

Ethambutol

Acute overdose of ethambutol is usually well tolerated with only gastrointestinal effects reported, such as nausea, vomiting, and abdominal pain. However, there are reports of fatalities associated with ethambutol overdose and more significant features such as confusion, pyrexia, hallucinations. Optic neuropathy may occur with larger ingestions, e.g. over 10 g. Patients should be observed for 6 hours post ingestion; management is supportive. Recovery from optic neuritis may take weeks or months and may be incomplete.

Further reading

Bredemann JA, Krechel SW, Eggers GW Jr (1990). Treatment of refractory seizures in massive isoniazid overdose. *Anesth Analg*, 71:554–7.

Dharnidharka VR, Nadeau K, Cannon CL, et al. (1998). Ciprofloxacin overdose: acute renal failure with prominent apoptotic changes. *Am J Kidney Dis*, 31(4):710–12.

Farrar HC, Walsh-Sukys MC, Kyllonen K, et al. (1993). Cardiac toxicity associated with intravenous erythromycin lactobionate: two case reports and a review of the literature. *Pediatr Infect Dis J*, 12:688–91.

Lheureux PP, Gris M (2005). Pyridoxine in clinical toxicology: a review. *Eur J Emerg Med*, 12:78–85.

Maw G, Aitken P (2003). Isoniazid overdose : a case series, literature review and survey of antidote availability. *Clin Drug Investig*, 23:479–85.

Rezkalla MA, Pochop C (1994). Erythromycin induced torsades de pointes: case report and review of the literature. *S D J Med*, 47:161–4.

Antidiabetic drugs

Background
A wide range of antihyperglycaemic agents exist with different pharmacological mechanisms of action and toxicological profiles. Some of these are capable of causing severe toxicity, and patients normally require urgent medical assessment and treatment. For example, poisoning by sulphonylureas, biguanides and insulin are associated with moderate to severe poisoning in 5%, 12%, and 15% of cases respectively; fatal poisoning occurs in 1%, 6% and 4% of cases respectively

Insulin
Insulin, an endogenous hormone secreted by the pancreatic beta cells, acts via its tyrosine kinase-linked receptor to alter glucose and electrolyte transport, enhancing glucose and potassium uptake into cells, especially skeletal muscle, myocardium and adipose tissue. Pharmaceutical preparations of insulin and analogues differ in their onset and duration of action, and range from those with very rapid onset of effect (e.g. Humalog ®) to those with a very prolonged duration of action (e.g. Glargine ®). Data concerning the pharmacokinetic properties of typical therapeutic dosages gives some indication of the likely onset and duration of hypoglycaemia, however, in the context of overdose hypoglycaemia is usually more severe and more prolonged than anticipated from therapeutic kinetics (see Table 7.1). Ingestion of insulin does

Table 7.1 Pharmacokinetic characteristics of selected insulins during therapeutic use

Type	Onset (minutes)	Peak (hours)	Duration (hours)
Humalog®	15	0.5–1	2–5
Humalog Mix®	15	0.5–1	15
Actrapid®	30	1.5–3.5	7–8
Insulatard®	90	4–12	24
Insulatard ge®a	60–90	4–12	24
Mixtard 10–50®a	30	2–8	24
Monotard®a	60–120	7–14	16–22
Ultratard®a	120–240	8–24	28
Velosulin®a	30	1–3	8
Humulin I®	120	4–12	24
Humulin Lente®	60–120	10–12	22–26
Humulin M2®a	30	3–4	15–22
Humulin M3®	<120	4–12	24
Humulin M4®a	30	4–6	15–22
Humulin M5®a	30	3–4	15–22
Humulin MI®	30–60	4–6	15–22
Humulin S®	30–60	2–5	6–8
Humulin Zn®a	60–120	10–14	24–36
Lantus®	240	10–16	24
Lentard MC®a	60–120	6–14	15–24
Levemir®	180–240	14	24
Glargine®	240	10–16	24
NovoMix 30®	10–20	1–4	24

a Not licensed for use in the UK

not result in systemic effects because insulin is degraded in the gastrointestinal tract.

Iatrogenic toxicity may arise as a drug administration error or when changing between insulin types or formulations. Patients with dementia and poor eyesight may be at increased risk of insulin toxicity due to inadvertent administration errors.

Clinical features
Parenteral administration of insulin may cause profound hypoglycaemia and activation of neurohormonal counter-regulatory mechanisms. Clinical features are arising from hypoglycaemia and the associated neurohormonal features include agitation, altered behaviour, excess sweating, slurred speech, tachycardia, seizures, reduced conscious level, and coma. Insulin overdose may also be associated with hypokalaemia.

Management
Hypoglycaemia should be reversed by administration of intravenous dextrose or glucose, with a target plasma glucose concentration of ≥4 mmol/L. Higher target concentrations may be needed to avoid symptoms in diabetes patients with poor glucose control that normally have much higher concentrations. Prolonged intravenous infusion may be required after substantial overdose, and there is a risk of hepatocellular glycogen accumulation resulting in reversible liver dysfunction. Lactate provides an alternative substrate for brain metabolism, and lessens the risk of neuroglycopenia. Glucagon and octreotide antagonize the effects of insulin and may reduce the quantity of carbohydrate administration needed to maintain euglycaemia.

The principal goal is to prevent hypoglycaemic episodes, but monitoring of fluid balance and electrolytes is also important, and hypokalaemia should be corrected if needed.

Surgical excision may be considered in cases where a large subcutaneous insulin depot is identified and there is ongoing hypoglycaemia.

Profound or prolonged hypoglycaemia may lead to persisting neurological deficits, for example, cognitive impairment and delayed reaction times have been described. This emphasizes the importance of rapid correction and maintenance of normal glucose concentrations during the acute episode to minimize the risks of long-term sequelae.

Metformin
Metformin, a biguanide, enhances tissue sensitivity to insulin and inhibits lactate dehydrogenase, the enzyme responsible for conversion of lactate to pyruvate. As a result gluconeogenesis is inhibited because pyruvate is the main substrate for this pathway. Toxicity is mainly due to inhibition of lactate dehydrogenase and development of severe lactic acidosis. Metformin ingestion alone does not cause significant hypoglycaemia.

Clinical features
Metformin overdose may cause abdominal pain, vomiting, diarrhoea, and metabolic disturbance. Severe lactic acidosis is associated with agitation, tachypnoea, hypotension, reduced conscious level, and seizures.

Management
Urea, electrolytes, creatinine, and lactate should be measured, together with arterial blood gases in patients with clinical features of toxicity.

Hypoxia should be corrected and adequate fluid replacement provided. Metabolic acidosis should be corrected using sodium bicarbonate, monitoring plasma potassium and sodium.

Patients who develop severe lactic acidosis require close observation of haemodynamic status, urinary output, serum electrolytes, and acid–base balance, and, where appropriate, correction of fluid or electrolyte disturbance. Haemodialysis or haemodiafiltration using a bicarbonate buffer should be considered in patients with severe toxicity, or where electrolyte and acid–base disturbance cannot be corrected by conventional measures.

Sulphonylureas
These include glibenclamide, gliclazide, glimepiride, glipizide, and tolbutamide. These bind to a specific islet cell receptor stimulating insulin secretion and provoking hypoglycaemia. They also enhance peripheral tissue sensitivity to insulin. Duration of action varies between agents, with t½ after therapeutic dosing ranging from 2–4 hours (glipizide) to 25–60 hours (chlorpropamide).

Clinical features
Onset of hypoglycaemia is normally within 8 hours of overdose, but may be delayed for up to 48 hours after ingestion of modified-release preparations or those with a long t½.

Management
Hypoglycaemia should be corrected as for insulin overdose.

Octreotide, a potent inhibitor of pancreatic insulin release, has been reported to lessen the duration of hypoglycaemia after sulphonylurea ingestion, and is effective in patients that fail to respond to dextrose administration alone.

Meglitinides
This group includes nateglinide and repaglinide. Like sulphonylureas, these stimulate insulin secretion via a specific receptor site on pancreatic beta cells and may cause significant hypoglycaemia. However, onset of hypoglycaemia is more rapid, for example within 30 minutes of overdose, and the duration of action is shorter. The clinical features and management are as for sulphonylureas.

Thiazolidinediones
Pioglitazone and rosiglitazone are thiazolidinediones and stimulate peroxisome proliferator-activated receptor gamma (PPAR-γ), thereby increasing peripheral insulin sensitivity. Abnormal liver biochemistry and congestive heart failure have been described occasionally after therapeutic use, but these have not been reported after acute ingestion. Rosiglitazone was withdrawn in Europe in 2010 after being associated with cardiovascular events including myocardial infarction and heart failure. Pioglitazone remains widely prescribed. In usual therapeutic doses it has a t½ of 5–6 hours but is converted to active metabolites with t½ of up to 23 hours.

There is limited information available on the clinical features of thiazolidinedione overdose, but serious clinical effects are not anticipated. Hypoglycaemia would not be expected.

Incretin mimetics
Glucagon-like peptide-1 (GLP-1) is a naturally occurring peptide that increases post-prandial insulin secretion; GLP-1 is subject to degradation by dipeptidyl peptidase-IV (DPP-IV). Exenatide and liraglutide are GLP-1 analogues normally administered by subcutaneous injection. Saxagliptin, sitagliptin, and vildagliptin are DPP-IV inhibitors available as oral formulations.

There is limited experience of overdose involving incretin mimetics. Their pharmacological actions are insulin-dependent so significant hypoglycaemia is not be expected.

Acarbose
Acarbose is an alpha-glucosidase inhibitor that prevents hydrolysis of complex carbohydrates within the small intestine and thereby reduces or delays their systemic absorption. Gastrointestinal effects are common, including diarrhoea and abdominal pain and these might also be anticipated after overdose. Bioavailability is 1–2% so systemic effects of overdose are unlikely, and hypoglycaemia is not a recognized feature. The duration of effect is around 4–6 hours after therapeutic doses, but may be longer after overdose.

Further reading
Flatt PR, Bailey CJ, Green BD (2009). Recent advances in antidiabetic drug therapies targeting the enteroinsular axis. *Curr Drug Metab*, 10:125–37.

Forrester MB (2006). Pattern of thiazolidinedione exposures reported to Texas poison centers during 1998–2004. *J Toxicol Environ Health A*, 69:2083–93.

Glatstein M, Garcia-Bournissen F, Scolnik D, et al. (2010). Sulfonylurea intoxication at a tertiary care paediatric hospital. *Can J Clin Pharmacol*, 17:e51–e56.

Graveling AJ, Frier BM (2009). Hypoglycaemia: an overview. *Prim Care Diabetes*, 3:131–9.

Pelavin PI, Abramson E, Pon S, et al. (2009). Ex-tended-release glipizide overdose presenting with delayed hypoglycemia and treated with subcutaneous octreotide. *J Pediatr Endocrinol Metab*, 22:171–5.

Rath S, Bar-Zeev N, Anderson K, et al. (2008). Octreotide in children with hypoglycaemia due to sulfonylurea ingestion. *J Paediatr Child Health*, 44:383–4.

Tsujimoto T, Takano M, Nishiofuku M, et al. (2006). Rapid onset of glycogen storage hepatomegaly in a type-2 diabetic patient after a massive dose of long-acting insulin and large doses of glucose. *Intern Med*, 45:469–73.

von Mach MA, Gauer M, Meyer S, et al. (2006). Antidiabetic medications in overdose: a comparison of the inquiries made to a regional poisons unit regarding original sulfonylureas, biguanides and insulin. *Int J Clin Pharmacol Ther*, 44:51–6.

Waring WS, Alexander WD (2004). Emergency presentation of an elderly female patient with profound hypoglycaemia. *Scott Med J*, 49:105–7.

Wiernsperger NF, Bailey CJ (1999). The antihyperglycaemic effect of metformin: therapeutic and cellular mechanisms. *Drugs*, 58(Suppl 1):31–9.

Antithrombotic drugs

Background

Control of bleeding is complex and involves clotting factor synthesis and function, platelets, and clot breakdown mechanisms (thrombolysis). The differential diagnosis of bleeding from a toxicological perspective is discussed in Bleeding disorders, pp. 93–94.

Drugs reducing clotting normally interfere with clotting factor synthesis, individual components of the clotting cascades, or with platelet function. Clotting cascades are classically described as the *extrinsic* (tissue factor) and *intrinsic* (contact activation) pathways, depending on the triggers and clotting factors involved. The two pathways join to a common pathway, in which factor X activation results in prothrombin conversion to thrombin, activation of fibrinogen, and clot formation by fibrin (Figure 7.1). The extrinsic cascade is thought to be the primary pathway for the initiation of blood coagulation, and the intrinsic pathway is now believed to have less importance *in vivo*, since hereditary deficiencies in this pathway do not normally cause bleeding.

Bleeding disorders

Therapeutic agents that can precipitate bleeding disorders include:

- Vitamin K antagonists: coumarins (e.g. warfarin, phenindione)
- Specific clotting factor inhibitors: e.g. dabigatran etexilate, a direct thrombin inhibitor, and apixaban and rivaroxaban, direct inhibitors of activated factor X (factor Xa)
- Heparins: unfractionated or low molecular weight
- Derivatives of snake venoms: hirudin analogues (e.g. lepirudin, bivalirudin)
- Thrombolytics: agents that promote clot breakdown. There are two types, non-specific agents, including the enzymes streptokinase and urokinase, and specific tissue plasminogen activators such as alteplase which only act to increase fibrin breakdown in the presence of a clot.
- Antiplatelet drugs: aspirin, adenosine diphosphate receptor inhibitors (clopidogrel, ticlodipine), glycoprotein IIB/IIIA inhibitors (abciximab, eptifibatide—IV use only), adenosine reuptake inhibitors (dipyridamole).

Bleeding disorders may also be caused by toxins that affect liver or bone marrow function, and hence impair synthesis of clotting factors or platelets, have immunological action causing platelet destruction (drug-induced immune thrombocytopenia) or cause clot formation by triggering the clotting cascade, typically snake venoms (see Common venomous snakes, pp. 332–333).

Both clotting factors and platelets have relatively short half-lives (t½) and drugs that impair their production cause bleeding in a short time frame. Recovery requires re-synthesis of the relevant component.

Anticoagulants, particularly coumarins, are also used as rodenticides, and very long-acting agents are available; anticoagulant effects from these agents may last many months (see Coumarin rodenticides, pp. 311–312).

Coumarins

Mechanisms of toxicity

Warfarin and other classical coumarin anticoagulants such as phenindione all interfere with the action of vitamin K in synthesizing clotting factors II, VII, IX, and X by acting as inhibitors of vitamin K 2,3 epoxide-reductase (VKORC1), a key pathway in the activation of vitamin K in the liver, and for the synthesis of these clotting factors. Polymorphisms of the gene encoding VKORC1 reduce enzyme expression and render affected individuals very sensitive to the anticoagulant effects of warfarin.

The onset of anticoagulant effects is dependent on the t½ of the clotting factors affected, and commences within about 7–10 hours of dosing (factor VII t½ is about 5 hours), but is generally maximal 48–72 hours after initiation. Warfarin may also inhibit other enzyme pathways, including vitamin K quinone-reductase, which activates clotting factors. The effects of warfarin are monitored using the prothrombin time, expressed as a ratio, reported as the international normalized ratio (INR) to standardize readings of prothrombin time between laboratories.

Warfarin is metabolized in the liver and is very susceptible to drug interactions. Enzyme inhibitors of the hepatic microsomal enzyme families CYP1A2, CYP2C9, and CYP3A4 increase the risk of bleeding, an effect usually seen within 48–72 hours of commencement. Commonly prescribed enzyme inhibitors include: the

---

The intrinsic and extrinsic pathways both lead to the common step of conversion of factor X to Xa.

The intrinsic pathway
Initial stimulus (surface contact) causes the cascade
XII → XIIa
↓
XI → XIa
↓
IX → IXa + VIII, platelet membrane
phospholipid and calcium ⟶

The extrinsic pathway
Tissue damage
↓
VII → tissue factor on cells
↓
VIIa
↙
X → Xa
↓
Prothrombin → thrombin
↓
Fibrinogen → fibrin → fibrin clot

Fig 7.1 Clotting cascade pathways.

konazole antifungals (e.g. fluconazole and ketoconazole); antibiotics (e.g. ciprofloxacin and other quinolones), macrolides (e.g. clarithromycin and erythromycin), metronidazole, amiodarone, cimetidine, and some statins (e.g. fluvastatin and simvastatin). Some foodstuffs may also contain compounds that inhibit warfarin clearance, for example cranberry juice has been reported to do this. In practice, large quantities of foodstuffs are normally needed for a clinically important effect.

Recent studies have indicated a very strong genetic basis for the variability in warfarin dosing between patients, but while this may assist in preventing the risk of therapeutic over-anticoagulation, it has little relevance to managing overdose.

Toxicokinetics

Warfarin is mixture of two isomers, R- and S-warfarin. The S isomer is up to five times more potent than the R isomer in man. The metabolism of S- and R-warfarin is by different enzyme pathways: The more potent S-warfarin is predominantly metabolized to 7-hydroxywarfarin by CYP2C9, while R-warfarin is metabolized by CYP1A2 to 6- and 8-hydroxywarfarin and by CYP3A4 to 10-hydroxywarfarin. This is important in the aetiology of drug interactions and also explains why CYP2C9 poor metabolizers have reduced warfarin dose requirements.

The t½ of racemic warfarin is around 35 hours; the onset of action depends upon inhibition of clotting factor synthesis. Most commonly excess anticoagulation occurs during therapeutic dosing, and thus maximal anticoagulant effect is observed at presentation. In acute overdose, however, onset of maximal effect is delayed, usually by 48–72 hours, and offset of toxic effects on coagulation will depend on rates of warfarin elimination and dose.

Vitamin K can be used to overcome the action of warfarin by competitive reactivation of vitamin K epoxide-reductase. The speed of recovery depends on the dose of vitamin K administered and the rates of clotting factor re-synthesis.

Phenindione is an alternative vitamin K antagonist which is occasionally used in patients sensitive to warfarin. It has more likelihood of causing adverse reactions than warfarin, such as leucopenia, rashes, agranulocytosis, renal dysfunction, and liver damage. Management of overdose is similar to warfarin.

Long-acting anticoagulants are designed to overcome warfarin resistance in rodents. The 4-hydroxy derivatives difenacoum and brodifacoum are the most commonly used. These are more potent than warfarin and appear to have zero-order elimination, accounting for their very long duration of action. The implication for management of overdose in man is the need for prolonged therapy and monitoring over several months (see Coumarin rodenticides, pp. 311–312).

Risk factors for toxicity

Risk of bleeding is higher in the elderly and in patients with underlying clotting abnormalities, either hereditary or acquired, most commonly liver disease, and by presence of potential bleeding sites, e.g. peptic ulcer, varices, recent surgery, stroke, etc. Drug interactions are common with oral anticoagulants, and caution is required whenever new therapies are given to patients on these agents. As vitamin K is present in food, dietary change, starvation, or illness, also affect warfarin sensitivity, which is also increased in CYP2C9 slow hydroxylators and in those with specific VKORC1 polymorphisms. Failure to attend routine monitoring and risk of falls in the elderly are risk factors for bleeding and reasons to reconsider use of warfarin. Oral anticoagulant drugs should also be used with great caution in liver disease.

Clinical features

The most important clinical effect of anticoagulant excess is bleeding, the clinical importance of which depends on the site and extent of blood loss. Blood loss in the gastrointestinal tract may be covert, while rectal and nasal bleeding is more obvious. Bleeding may present as catastrophic haemorrhage, but may cause major neurological deficit, or even be fatal if intracerebral. It may be difficult to diagnose if retroperitoneal.

Toxicity assessment

Assessment includes assessment of acute blood loss, including blood pressure, conscious level, and pulse rate, together with tests of coagulation. National guidelines exist for managing prolongation of INR due to warfarin excess in patients receiving therapeutic anticoagulation. Because of the difficulties in re-establishing warfarin in patients who have been given large doses of vitamin K to treat therapeutic warfarin excess, these are stratified against INR. In those not normally on warfarin, INR results indicate the need for therapy but do not precisely guide it, as there is no hazard to such patients from excess vitamin K.

Investigations

Assess blood loss by clinical examination including measuring blood pressure and pulse rate. Establish degree of anticoagulation by use of INR. Measure the full blood count, U&Es, and LFTs.

Management of warfarin excess

Management depends on the extent of bleeding; many patients present only with abnormal blood tests. In this situation monitor pulse, blood pressure, and urine output and observe for features suggesting overt or occult bleeding. Transfusion and resuscitation is needed in active bleeding while anticoagulation is being reversed.

Patients taking chronic warfarin therapy

Measure the INR at presentation and monitor at least 12-hourly for a minimum of 48 hours following acute overdose.

If there is *active bleeding*, give vitamin K_1 (phytomenadione) by slow IV injection: 5–10 mg for adults (100 micrograms/kg for children) and prothrombin complex concentrate (25–50 units/kg), or if unavailable fresh frozen plasma (15 mL/kg). Further management depends on clinical response. Discuss when to repeat INR measurements, when to stop vitamin K_1, and the role of recombinant activated factor VII with a local haematologist.

If there is no active bleeding but the INR is dangerously prolonged (INR ≥8.0), give vitamin K_1 by slow IV injection: 1–3 mg for adults, 0.015–0.030 mg/kg (15–30 micrograms/kg) for children. A paediatric preparation containing 2 mg/0.2 mL is available. Further doses may be given as necessary, titrated to INR. Excess vitamin K_1 may make it difficult to re-establish anticoagulation. Warfarin should be normally restarted when the INR is less than 5.

Patients who are not prescribed warfarin

Take a careful history and measure the INR at presentation. Give vitamin K_1 if there is no active bleeding *and* more than 0.25 mg/kg warfarin has been ingested, or the INR is higher than 4.0. In these patients the adult dose of vitamin K_1 is 10–20 mg orally (250 micrograms/kg for a child). Delay oral vitamin K_1 until at least 4 hours after use of activated charcoal, as charcoal absorbs vitamin K. Repeat INR at 24 hours and consider need for further vitamin K_1. If there is active bleeding, or life-threatening haemorrhage, give prothrombin complex concentrate (30–50 units/kg) or, if unavailable, fresh frozen plasma (15 mL/kg). Give vitamin K_1 by slow IV injection: 10–20 mg for an adult (250 micrograms/kg for a child).

If the history is uncertain or less than 0.25 mg/kg warfarin has been ingested, repeat the INR every 24–48 hours after ingestion, depending on the initial dose and initial INR. If the INR remains normal for 24–48 hours and there is no evidence of bleeding, no further monitoring is necessary (see Coumarin rodenticides, pp. 311–312).

Specific clotting factor antagonists

Dabigatran

Dabigatran etexilate is a direct thrombin inhibitor, Standard coagulation tests do not reflect the effect of this drug due to its mode of action.

Dabigatran has a peak plasma concentration that occurs within 0.5–2 hours of a therapeutic dose in healthy volunteers. The terminal $t\frac{1}{2}$ in therapeutic use is 12–14 hours, but may be prolonged in renal impairment. Because of its mode of action there are no specific antidotes. Recombinant activated factor VII or prothrombin complex concentrates may have some efficacy based on animal studies, but at present there is no good evidence of an effective antidote in man.

Factor Xa inhibitors

Rivaroxaban and apixaban are direct inhibitors of activated factor X (factor Xa). As for dabigatran, standard coagulation tests do not reflect their effect. The peak plasma concentration of rivaroxaban is reached between 2 and 4 hours after a therapeutic dose. After oral administration of a 10 mg therapeutic dose, the elimination $t\frac{1}{2}$ is between 7 and 11 hours. The actions of rivaroxaban appear to be reversed effectively by prothrombin complex concentrates.

Risk factors for toxicity

Renal impairment is a major risk factor for bleeding with dabigatran etexilate, apixaban, and rivaroxaban. These drugs should also be avoided in liver disease.

Heparins

Mechanisms of toxicity

Heparin is a mucopolysaccharide, which acts by non-specific binding with clotting factor serine proteases, particularly antithrombin III, but also factors IX–XII, kallikrein, and thrombin. Unfractionated heparin, as the name suggests, is not a single molecule but a complex mixture. Heparin breakdown products are smaller heparin-like molecules and are also active anticoagulants. This explains why unfractionated heparin is dosed in units not mg. In repeat dosing anticoagulant action increases as smaller active heparin molecules accumulate. Low-molecular-weight heparins (LMWHs) avoid this problem and also have more activity against factor X, and less against activated factor II.

The effect of heparin is monitored by the activated partial thromboplastin time (APTT), but LMWHs do not affect this measurement at therapeutic doses. This explains why LMWHs are normally prescribed as a weight-related dose, adjusted for renal function.

Toxicokinetics

Intravenous heparins are rapidly broken down; effective $t\frac{1}{2}$ is of the order of 1–2.5 hours after single doses. Metabolism results in smaller molecular-weight compounds which are often biologically active, and contribute to anticoagulation. This is the reason that the required dose of heparin varies during regular therapy as the effective potency increases with time as smaller active molecules accumulate.

LMWHs do not share this problem and can be dosed by weight. They are given subcutaneously and route of administration is the primary factor affecting duration of action of low-molecular-weight agents.

Risk factors for toxicity

As with warfarin, risk of bleeding is increased in the elderly, in patients with underlying clotting abnormalities and liver disease, and by presence of potential bleeding sites. Heparin excretion, including that of LMWHs, is renal so renal failure is a further risk factor for bleeding.

Toxicity assessment

Assessment includes measurement of the effects of any acute blood loss, including blood pressure, conscious level, and pulse rate, together with the APTT.

Investigations

Assess blood loss by measuring blood pressure and pulse rate, lying and standing, and repeat as indicated by clinical status. Establish degree of anticoagulation by use of APTT. In the case of LMWHs discuss with haematologists. Measure full blood count, U&Es, and LFTs as a baseline.

Management

Monitor pulse, blood pressure, and urine output and observe for features suggesting overt or occult bleeding. Measure initially APTT full blood count, U&Es, and LFTs. If the APTT is prolonged but there is no sign of bleeding, no further acute treatment is required. Monitor physiological parameters to detect occult blood loss and repeat the APTT every 6 hours until it is within the therapeutic range.

If there is evidence of haemorrhage, or very large amounts of heparin have been injected, consider administration of protamine sulfate (e.g. 1 mg for every 100 units heparin, at a rate not exceeding 5 mg/minute, up to a maximum of 50 mg). The dose requirement for protamine varies with time from heparin injection, as the concentrations of heparin fall. Associated clinical risk factors may also influence use of this antidote. Protamine sulfate can cause severe hypotension and anaphylactoid reactions. In excess dosing protamine is itself an anticoagulant. It should only be given when facilities for resuscitation and treatment of anaphylactoid shock are available and after discussion with local haematologists. Repeat APTT after 4 hours. Treat hypovolaemia with fluids and blood transfusion as indicated.

If excess heparin has been given accidentally, stop heparin and observe for 6 hours if asymptomatic. Monitor APTT every 6 hours until it is within the therapeutic range. Heparin can then be restarted if clinically indicated. If there is haemorrhage, give protamine sulfate 25–50 mg IV at a rate not exceeding 5 mg/min. Repeat APTT after

4 h, noting cautions mentioned earlier regarding potential adverse effects of protamine.

Clotting factor inhibitors

Hirudin irreversibly blocks thrombin, and has no natural inhibitors. Lepirudin (not licensed for use in the UK) and bivalirudin are derivatives of hirudin, developed for therapeutic use. Lepirudin is used in patients with heparin-induced thrombocytopenia. Dose is titrated according to the APTT.

Bivalirudin is used in the management of acute ischaemic heart disease and as an anticoagulant. Both are used intravenously and overdose will cause bleeding, which can be reversed by clotting factor concentrates. These drugs have specialist haematological use and management of dose excess by the use of these as antidotes for excess IV dosing of the active should be discussed with a haematologist. Indications for intervention would include active bleeding or risk of this, e.g. recent surgery.

Thrombolytic products

There are two types: non-specific agents, including the enzymes streptokinase and urokinase, and specific tissue plasminogen activators such as alteplase which only act to increase fibrin breakdown in the presence of a clot. They are generally relatively short-acting. As with all anticoagulants these may cause devastating effects if there is bleeding into the CNS or gut. Manufacturers recommend the infusion of fresh frozen plasma or fresh blood as therapy. They also suggest that synthetic antifibrinolytics may be administered.

Platelet antagonists

Examples of platelet antagonists are shown in Table 7.2. All of these may cause bleeding. In the case of aspirin, however, the main toxicity is due to its metabolic effects (see Salicylates, pp. 124–127).

Bleeding seems unusual in acute overdose with the oral antiplatelet agents. Antiplatelet actions are longer for those agents that irreversibly bind to their target receptor (aspirin, prasugrel, and ticagrelor) and re-establishment of coagulation is dependent on synthesis of new platelets.

The action of the glycoprotein IIB/IIIA inhibitors is shorter as these drugs have short $t\frac{1}{2}$, generally of the order of 30 minutes (abciximab) to 2.5 hours (eptifibatide). Platelet function normally recovers within 48 hours after therapeutic dosing. Experience in overdose is limited.

Risk factors for toxicity

As for drugs affecting coagulation, risk of bleeding is increased in the elderly and in patients with underlying clotting abnormalities, either hereditary or acquired, most commonly liver disease, and by presence of potential bleeding sites, e.g. peptic ulcer or recent surgery.

Table 7.2 Platelet antagonists

Drug	Target site	Other comments
Aspirin	Cyclo-oxygenase	Irreversible effect, t½ of action about 3 days
Clopidogrel	Adenosine diphosphate receptor inhibitor	Active metabolite responsible for effects. t½ 8 hours
Dipyridamole	Adenosine uptake inhibitor. At larger doses phosphodiesterase inhibitor	May cause hypotension, ECG changes and coma in overdose
Prasugrel	Adenosine diphosphate receptor inhibitor	Active metabolite irreversibly binds to receptor. Duration of effect 5–9 days
Ticagrelor	Adenosine diphosphate receptor inhibitor	Parent and active metabolite irreversibly bind to receptor. Duration of effect 5–9 days
Abciximab	Glycoprotein IIB/IIIA inhibitor	Murine antibody used IV. Possibility of allergic reaction
Eptifibatide	Glycoprotein IIB/IIIA inhibitor	Synthetic peptide used IV. Potentially dialysable
Tirofiban	Glycoprotein IIB/IIIA inhibitor	Used IV. Potentially dialysable

Management

The management of bleeding is supportive and depends on the extent and severity of bleeding. Transfusion and resuscitation is needed in active bleeding. The benefit of platelet transfusion is unclear, particularly in the presence of excess antagonist as this will also act on donor platelets.

Further reading

Cruickshank J, Ragg M, Eddey D (2001). Warfarin toxicity in the emergency department: recommendations for management. *Emerg Med*, 13:91–7.

Eeerenberg ES, Kamphuisen PW, Sijpkens MK, *et al.* (2011). Reversal of new oral anticoagulants. *Circulation*, 124:1508–10.

Kandrotas RJ (1992). Heparin pharmacokinetics and pharmacodynamics. *Clin Pharmacokinet*, 22:359–74.

Keeling D, Baglin T, Tait C, *et al.* (2011). Guidelines on oral anticoagulation with warfarin – fourth edition. Br J *Haematol*, 154:311–24.

Johnson JA, Gong L, Whirl-Carrillo M, *et al.* (2011). Clinical Pharmacogenetics Implementation Consortium Guidelines for CYP2C9 and VKORC1 genotypes and warfarin dosing. *Clin Pharmacol Ther*, 90:625–9.

Lasseur R (2010). Prevalence of anticoagulant rodenticide poisoning in humans and animals in France and substances involved. *Clin Toxicol*, 48:935–41.

Antiviral drugs

Background

Antiviral drugs are used as treatment or to suppress a range of infections including those associated with the human immunodeficiency virus (HIV), influenza viruses, herpes simplex and zoster, cytomegalovirus (CMV), respiratory syncytial virus, and viral hepatitis.

Antiretroviral drugs

Background and therapeutic use

The majority of drugs inhibit the HIV enzymes reverse transcriptase or protease. Reverse transcriptase is required for the HIV virus, an RNA virus, to make complementary DNA for incorporation into the host DNA for subsequent transcription of viral proteins. Protease inhibitors block the HIV protease enzyme required for cleaving HIV protein precursors. Treatment strategies involve use of multiple drugs, often two nucleoside reverse transcriptase inhibitors with a nucleoside reverse transcriptase inhibitor or protease inhibitor.

Nucleoside reverse transcriptase inhibitors

Seven drugs are currently in clinical use: abacavir, didanosine, emtricitabine, lamivudine, stavudine, tenofovir, and zidovudine.

In therapeutic dose adverse effects include nausea, vomiting, abdominal pain, headache, itching, rash, and fever. Life-threatening lactic acidosis associated with hepatic steatosis has also been reported. Myopathy, bone marrow depression, and encephalopathy can also occur. Specific drugs are associated with hypersensitivity reactions (e.g. abacavir, strongly associated with HLA-B*5701 allele), pancreatitis (e.g. didanosine), and peripheral neuropathy (e.g. didanosine) in therapeutic use.

There is limited experience of significant toxicity following acute overdose, although GI disturbances, tiredness, fatigue, nystagmus, ataxia, transient bone marrow failure, and convulsions have been reported.

Non-nucleoside reverse transcriptase inhibitors

Three drugs are in clinical use: efavirenz, etravirine, and nevirapine. Their principal adverse effects in therapeutic use are skin hypersensitivity reactions.

Few cases of acute overdose have been reported and toxicity appears to be low. Toxic features have included nausea, headache, fever, fatigue, sleep disturbances, oedema, impaired concentration, disinhibition, and aggression. Elevated hepatic transaminases have also been recorded.

Protease inhibitors

Nine drugs (or combinations) are in clinical use: atazanavir, darunavir, fosamprenavir, indinavir, lopinavir with ritonavir, nelfinavir (not licensed for use in the UK), ritonavir, saquinavir, and tipranavir.

In therapeutic use, protease inhibitors cause lipodystrophy. Data on acute overdoses are limited. Nausea, vomiting, abdominal pain, and diarrhoea have been reported and nephrolithiasis has been documented after acute indinavir overdose.

Other antiretrovirals

Three drugs are in clinical use: enfuvirtide is a fusion inhibitor administered by subcutaneous injection used in HIV unresponsive to other agents; maraviroc is a CCR5 chemokine receptor antagonist used in patients infected exclusively with CCR5-trophic HIV. Raltegavir (not licensed for use in the UK) is an HIV integrase inhibitor used when non-nucleoside reverse transcriptase inhibitors cannot be used because of intolerance, drug interactions, or viral resistance.

No cases of acute overdose have been reported with these agents; toxicity in therapeutic use appears to be low. Dose-related postural hypotension has been observed with maraviroc so may be anticipated after overdose.

Anti-herpesvirus drugs

Most members of this class of compounds inhibit herpesvirus DNA polymerase, preventing viral replication. Inosine is an immunostimulant.

Five drugs are in clinical use for herpes simplex virus (HSV) and varicella zoster virus (VZV) infection. These are aciclovir, famciclovir, foscarnet sodium, inosine pranobex, and valaciclovir.

Few cases of acute overdose have been reported. Oral overdoses are unlikely to cause significant toxicity although large doses can cause acute renal injury due to drug precipitation in the kidney. Large IV overdoses of aciclovir and its pro-drugs can cause neurotoxic effects such as impaired consciousness, dysarthria, myoclonus, agitation, coma, hallucinations, and seizures.

Anti-cytomegalovirus drugs

Four drugs are primarily in clinical use for CMV infection: cidofovir, ganciclovir, foscarnet sodium, and valganciclovir.

Common adverse effects from therapeutic use of these drugs include myelosuppression and nephrotoxicity.

Few cases of acute overdose have been reported. All except valganciclovir are poorly absorbed orally and little toxicity is expected after oral overdose. GI disturbances, neutropenia, hyperkalaemia, and renal dysfunction have been reported after overdose with ganciclovir and renal dysfunction after overdose of aciclovir. Intravenous overdose of foscarnet can cause paraesthesia, seizures, coma, and electrolyte abnormalities especially Mg^{2+} and Ca^{2+}.

Antiviral hepatitis drugs

Most members of this class of compounds inhibit viral enzymes, preventing viral replication. Six drugs are in clinical use: adefovir dipivoxil, entecavir (not licensed for use in the UK), interferon-α, lamivudine, ribavirin, and telbivudine. Adefovir and lamivudine inhibit viral reverse transcriptase; the toxicity of lamivudine has already been considered under antiretroviral drugs. Telbivudine inhibits viral DNA polymerase; entecavir inhibits reverse transcription, DNA replication and transcription. Interferon α is an immunomodulator; ribavirin may interfere with RNA metabolism and/or enhance T cell immunity.

Few cases of acute overdose have been reported. Lamivudine (and potentially entecavir) can cause life-threatening lactic acidosis associated with hepatic steatosis in therapeutic use. Entecavir can cause severe skin reactions, telbivudine can cause rhabdomyolysis, and ribavirin can cause haemolysis. Adefovir may cause renal failure in overdose.

Anti-influenza drugs

Background and therapeutic use
Amantadine blocks an ion channel M2 in influenza A, preventing uncoating when the virus is taken up into a cell. Oseltamivir and zanamivir are neuraminidase inhibitors.

Amantadine
Amantadine is licensed for the prophylaxis and treatment of influenza A infection and also for treatment of Parkinson's disease, where it has complex actions as a monoamine oxidase A and NMDA inhibitor and alters effects of dopamine, noradrenaline, and serotonin substance, although clinical use is now very uncommon.

Overdose can cause severe cardiotoxicity with QRS and QT prolongation, hypokalaemia, anticholinergic-like delirium, and seizures. Torsade de pointes and cardiopulmonary arrest can occur. These features may be delayed for up to 36 hours after overdose. Adult respiratory distress syndrome has also been reported.

Neuraminidase inhibitors
No intentional overdoses with oseltamivir or zanamivir have been reported. Toxicity is expected to be low. Nausea, vomiting, and dizziness have been experienced after high doses of oseltamivir in clinical trials.

Zanamivir is administered as a dry powder for inhalation. Oral bioavailability is very low and toxic effects from ingestion are not anticipated.

Management of antiviral drug overdose

Management of overdose with antiviral agents is supportive. Use of oral activated charcoal could be considered if this can be administered soon after a large overdose.

Full blood count, U&Es, and liver function should be checked.

Convulsions associated with antiviral overdose (e.g. with aciclovir, foscarnet, or amantadine) should be treated with a benzodiazepine in the first instance.

In patients with amantadine overdose, treatment involves checking and replacing electrolytes, sodium bicarbonate for prolonged QRS duration, magnesium infusion for torsade de pointes with over-pacing if magnesium alone is unsuccessful. Benzodiazepines or barbiturates may be needed for agitation and seizures; otherwise supportive care should be administered as required.

Further reading
Ar MC, Ozbalak M, Tuzuner N, *et al.* (2009). Severe bone marrow failure due to valganciclovir overdose after renal transplantation from cadaveric donors: four consecutive cases. *Transplant Proc*, 41:1648–53.

Carr A, Cooper D (2000). Adverse effects of antiretroviral therapy. *Lancet*, 356:1423–30.

Claudet I, Maréchal C (2009). Status epilepticus in a pediatric patient with amantadine overdose. *Pediatr Neurol*, 40:120–2.

Haefeli WE, Schoenenberger RA, Weiss P, *et al.* (1993). Acyclovir-induced neurotoxicity: concentration-side effect relationship in acyclovir overdose. *Am J Med*, 94:212–15.

Hargreaves M, Fuller G, Costello C, *et al.* (1988). Zidovudine overdose. *Lancet*, 2:509.

Lafeuillade A, Poizot-Martin I, Dhiver C, *et al.* (1991). Zidovudine overdose: a case with bone-marrow toxicity. *AIDS*, 5:116–17.

Lehman HP, Benson JO, Beninger PR, *et al.* (2003). A five-year evaluation of reports of overdose with indinavir sulfate. *Pharmacoepidemiol Drug Saf*, 12(6):449–57

McNicholl I. Adverse effects of antiretroviral drugs. HIV InSite. <http://hivinsite.ucsf.edu/InSite?page=ar-05-01>.

Moore EC, Cohen F, Kauffman RE, *et al.* (1990). Zidovudine overdose in a child. *N Engl J Med*, 322:408–9.

Pickus OB (1988). Overdose of zidovudine. *N Engl J Med*, 318:1206.

Schwartz M, Patel M, Kazzi Z, *et al.* (2008). Cardiotoxicity after massive amantadine overdose. *J Med Toxicol*, 4:173–9.

Selwyn PA, Lezza A (1990). Zidovudine overdose in an intravenous drug user. *AIDS*, 4:822–4.

Caffeine

Background and therapeutic use

Caffeine (1,3,7-trimethylxanthine) is a methylxanthine closely related to theophylline which is present in drinks such as tea (typically 0.1–0.4 mg/mL), coffee (ground coffee 0.4–1.2 mg/mL, instant coffee (0.2–0.8 mg/mL), and cola (0.2–0.3 mg/mL). 'Energy drinks' such as Red Bull® also contain around 0.3 mg/mL of caffeine. Chocolate contains 1 mg/g of caffeine.

Caffeine is also present in some combination preparations with analgesics such as paracetamol and aspirin; typical amounts of caffeine found in these preparations are 30–65 mg per tablet. The addition of caffeine is claimed to enhance analgesic effects, but may also contribute to adverse effects, including headache with excessive doses or after withdrawal.

Caffeine is also available on prescription as an oral or intravenous preparation. Both of these preparations have been used in the management of spontaneous and post-lumbar puncture-related low-pressure headache; high-doses of caffeine may be required for these indications. Additionally, both oral and intravenous caffeine are also indicated to treat neonatal apnoea.

Mechanisms of toxicity

Caffeine and the other methylxanthines have their actions through increased adrenergic activity. This occurs by:

1 increased release of catecholamines and stimulation at ß1/ß2-receptors
2 adenosine antagonism leading to increased norepinephrine and epinephrine release;
3 inhibition of intracellular phosphodiesterase which is responsible for the degradation of cAMP the postsynaptic second messenger involved in ß-receptor activity.

Toxicokinetics

The bioavailability of caffeine following oral administration is almost 100%. Food taken at the same time as caffeine does not alter either the overall bioavailability or the peak plasma concentrations. However, the presence of food in the stomach delays the time from ingestion to the peak caffeine concentration. Peak concentrations occur within 30–60 minutes of ingestion when caffeine is taken without food.

The volume of distribution of caffeine is low (about 0.7 L/kg), meaning that potentially extra-corporeal removal of caffeine is possible.

The majority of caffeine (>95%) is metabolized by the hepatic cytochrome P450 isoenzyme system, especially CYP1A2. The half-life of caffeine is dependent on a number of factors and is reported to be 4–5 hours in healthy, non-smoking adults and shorter in smokers due to induction of CYP1A2. Other factors influencing CYP1A2 can also increase or decrease the clearance of caffeine; inhibition of this isoenzyme can lead to an increased risk of toxicity. A small proportion of caffeine is metabolized to other methylxanthines, particularly theophylline and theobromine. This metabolic pathway is of greater significance in neonates than in children or adults.

Toxicity associated with caffeine is dose-related. Data from published case reports and case series suggest that the potential fatal dose of caffeine is 150–200 mg/kg in adults. Reports also suggest that fatalities are associated with serum caffeine concentrations higher than 80 mg/L.

However, there have been reports of individuals surviving after much larger ingestions and/or higher serum concentrations. There is some suggestion that neonates and infants are more tolerant to the effects of caffeine, and therefore survive with higher serum caffeine concentrations. The usual therapeutic range for caffeine in the treatment of neonatal apnoea is 10–20 mg/L (50–100 micromol/L) but concentrations as high as 35 mg/L (180 micromol/L) are sometimes required.

Risk factors for toxicity

Risk of toxicity is likely to be enhanced in neonates (especially when premature) and infants, as caffeine clearance is reduced during the first 6 months of life. Increased risk is also likely in the elderly and those with underlying cardiac or respiratory disease, as is the case with the related methylxanthine theophylline. Inhibitors of CYP2A1 (e.g. macrolide and quinolone antibiotics, cimetidine, verapamil and allopurinol) delay caffeine elimination and enhance the risk of toxicity

Clinical features

Because caffeine is a methylxanthine, the clinical features of caffeine poisoning are similar to those seen with theophylline poisoning.

Vomiting is common and is often very pronounced and resistant to treatment with anti-emetics. In protracted vomiting, associated haematemesis can occur. Anorexia, diarrhoea, and abdominal pain may also be features.

Hypertension and sinus tachycardia are common but bradycardias have also been reported. Supraventricular and ventricular arrhythmias may occur and myocardial ischaemia or infarction has been reported.

Caffeine, similar to other methylxanthines, stimulates the respiratory centre leading to hyperventilation and associated respiratory alkalosis. In cases of severe caffeine toxicity, this respiratory centre stimulation can lead to respiratory failure and/or respiratory arrest.

Individuals consume caffeine containing products for their neurological stimulant effects at low doses (50–200 mg). However, larger ingestions are associated with anxiety and/or agitation, insomnia, tremor, irritability, dilated pupils, hallucinations, and convulsions. These convulsions often can be prolonged and/or recurrent, and resistant to treatment with conventional anti-epileptic medications. Fever, rhabdomyolysis and disseminated intravascular coagulation may also occur

Methylxanthines are associated with ß2-receptor stimulation, which results in a shift of potassium into the intracellular compartment, with a resultant intracellular hyperkalaemia and associated systemic hypokalaemia. It is important to note the total body potassium burden is normal, despite this systemic hypokalaemia. Hypomagnesaemia, hypocalcaemia, hypophosphataemia, and hyperglycaemia may also occur with caffeine toxicity.

Toxicity assessment

The severity of poisoning is established from the clinical features, with convulsions and ventricular arrhythmias signifying life-threatening poisoning. Unlike theophylline, there is no specific grading system for caffeine-related toxicity. However, despite this, since the clinical features are similar, the grading of severity could be compared to that for grading theophylline toxicity.

Chronic accumulation

Regular excessive dosing with caffeine may produce anxiety, agitation, restlessness, insomnia, tachycardia, tremors, and exaggerated tendon reflexes ('caffeinism').

Investigations

All patients require an initial ECG to determine the underlying cardiac rhythm. Continuous cardiac monitoring should be undertaken where there is evidence of caffeine toxicity.

Urea and electrolytes, particularly plasma potassium, should be measured. Caffeine-associated ß2-receptor stimulation results in an intracellular shift of potassium, with resultant intracellular hyperkalaemia and systemic hypokalaemia, but with a normal total body potassium burden. Electrolytes should be monitored every 1–2 hours in the acute phase of severe poisoning.

Concentrations of magnesium, calcium, phosphate, and glucose should be measured in patients with caffeine toxicity. Hypomagnesaemia, hypocalcaemia, hypophosphataemia, and hyperglycaemia may occur.

Arterial blood gases should be performed in patients with clinical features or substantial overdose. Metabolic acidosis or respiratory alkalosis may be demonstrated.

Creatine kinase should be measured in severe poisoning, especially in the context of convulsions.

Whilst caffeine concentrations can be measured, they are not routinely available in most hospitals and/or the results are not available in a time frame that will alter an individual patient's management. Additionally, although caffeine is in part metabolized to theophylline, there is no indication for routine measurement of theophylline concentrations in caffeine toxicity.

Management

Patients who have ingested less than 30 mg/kg of caffeine are likely to develop only mild features of toxicity.

Activated charcoal (50 g in adults, 1 g/kg in children) should be considered in patients who present within an hour of ingestion of a potentially toxic acute overdose of caffeine (>30 mg/kg in adults or >15 mg/kg in children). Due to the severe intractable vomiting, it may not be possible to administer the activated charcoal in individuals with severe caffeine toxicity. Additionally, in those with a reduced level of consciousness, care should be taken not to induce vomiting with the activated charcoal in the setting of an unprotected airway.

Tachycardias, particularly sinus tachycardia and supra-ventricular tachycardia, that are not associated with haemodynamic comprise should not be treated routinely. When there is evidence of haemodynamic compromise, first-line treatment is with short-acting beta-blockers (e.g. esmolol or metoprolol). Caution is advised in those individuals with underlying COPD and/or asthma, and it may be more appropriate to consider the use of calcium channel blockers such as verapamil in these patients. Ventricular tachycardia with cardiac output should be treated with IV magnesium infusion initially and then DC cardioversion. There is some evidence that amiodarone may be safe in this group of patients, but other antiarrhythmics, such as lidocaine (lignocaine) should be avoided due to the increased risk of convulsions. Ventricular tachycardia

without cardiac output should be treated in accordance with the current standard Advance Life Support (ALS) algorithms.

The management of caffeine-related agitation and/or anxiety is best treated with benzodiazepines. These can be given by any appropriate route, and the dose should be titrated to the patient's clinical condition. Haloperidol should be not used as a first-line drug in the management of agitation/anxiety, as it lowers the seizure threshold and therefore will increase the risk of convulsions.

Convulsions associated with caffeine toxicity should initially be treated with benzodiazepines (diazepam: 10–20 mg in adults or 0.1–0.3 mg/kg in children; lorazepam: 1–4 mg in adults or 0.05 mg/kg in children).

The replacement of potassium in patients with caffeine toxicity should be undertaken cautiously. Although there is systemic hypokalaemia, the total body burden of potassium is normal. Over-treatment during the acute phase of caffeine toxicity may result in a clinically significant rebound hyperkalaemia in the recovery phase. Therefore, consideration for potassium supplementation should only occur if the serum potassium is less than 2.8 mmol/L and replacement should be at a rate of no more than 10 mmol per hour in the majority of cases, with regular monitoring of the serum potassium concentration. Due to the risk of rebound hyperkalaemia, monitoring should continue in the recovery phase where potassium supplementation has been given.

Use of elimination techniques

There is a role for the use of multi-dose activated charcoal in the management of theophylline toxicity to enhance elimination by reducing its entero-hepatic circulation. Cases of neonatal caffeine toxicity have also been treated using this method with apparently accelerated resolution of toxicity. There is, however, little information available on the effects of this method on caffeine elimination or on clinical outcomes.

Caffeine withdrawal syndrome

Individuals who consume large amounts of drinks or pharmaceutical preparations containing caffeine can develop a withdrawal syndrome on discontinuation. Typically symptoms start within 24 hours of the last use of caffeine and can last for up to a week. Classical features of the caffeine withdrawal syndrome include tiredness, yawning, headache, lethargy, irritability, anxiety or nervousness, and low mood or depression.

Management is largely supportive, although some individuals may report that their symptoms are eased by re-introduction of small amounts of caffeine.

Further reading

Dietrich AM, Mortensen ME (1990). Presentation and management of an acute caffeine overdose. *Pediatr Emerg Care*, 6:296–8.

Leson CL, McGuigan MA, Bryson SM (1988). Caffeine overdose in an adolescent male. *J Toxicol Clin Toxicol*, 26:407–15.

Shum S, Seale C, Hathaway D, et al. (1997). Acute caffeine ingestion fatalities: management issues. *Vet Hum Toxicol*, 39:228–30.

Chloroquine

Background and therapeutic use
Chloroquine is an antimalarial drug, also used to treat various connective tissue diseases. Poisoning is rare but may be life threatening. It is more commonly encountered in malaria endemic countries, as well as in France, where chloroquine has featured in a popular guide to suicide.

In adults, doses higher than 5 g are likely to be fatal, although death may occur with lower doses.

Mechanisms of toxicity
The pronounced cardiovascular toxicity of chloroquine is related to its sodium channel blocking properties (membrane stabilizing activity). This reduces inward sodium flux (phase 0 of the action potential), outward potassium flux (phase 3), and inward voltage-dependent calcium flux (phase 2). As a result chloroquine inhibits spontaneous depolarization, slows conduction, lengthens the refractory period, and increases the electrical depolarization threshold. Toxicity results in depressed cardiac contractility, impaired conductivity, decreased excitability, and an increased risk of re-entrant arrhythmias. Cardiovascular collapse mainly occurs because of negative inotropic effects, but peripheral vasodilatation also occurs.

Hypokalaemia is not due to true potassium depletion, rather increased intracellular distribution of potassium due to HERG (human ether-a-go-go related gene) potassium channel blockade. Excessive blockade of HERG potassium channels may worsen other pro-arrhythmic effects in relation to intraventricular blockage, automaticity increase, and QT prolongation; however, it may also be protective, resulting in the inhibition of membrane Na^+/K^+-ATPase pumps that enhances cardiac inotropism.

Toxicokinetics
Gastrointestinal absorption of chloroquine is rapid and complete, with peak concentrations within 1–2 hours and about 90% bioavailability. The drug is concentrated in red cells. The apparent volume of distribution is large (150–800 L/kg for plasma and 200 L/kg for blood) with about 50–65% plasma protein binding.

Chloroquine is metabolized in the liver by de-alkylation (30–50% of chloroquine) by the cytochrome P450 isozymes CYP2C8, CYP3A4, and CYP2D6, producing pharmacologically active metabolites including desethylchloroquine and bis-desethylchloroquine. The terminal $t\frac{1}{2}$ is long (60 days) with clearance equally by kidneys and liver at 0.7–1 L/hour/kg (plasma) and 0.1 L/hour/kg (blood).

Risk factors for toxicity
Risk of toxicity is increased in:
• patients with pre-existing cardiovascular disease
• the elderly.

Clinical features
Clinical features usually develop 0.5–6 hours after ingestion; early features may be severe, with cardiac arrest occasionally the first clinical manifestation. Cardiovascular deterioration may, however, also occur up to 24 hours after ingestion; risk of death is greatest in the first 48 hours if cardiovascular failure occurs.

Typical features of chloroquine poisoning include the following:
• *Cardiovascular*: hypotension is common. Collapse and cardiovascular failure with impaired cardiac output or vasodilatation may result in organ failure. Cardiac features may be worsened by co-ingestion of other cardiotoxicants, including beta blockers, calcium channel blockers, and sodium channel blockers.
• *Gastrointestinal*: nausea and vomiting are frequent. Early vomiting may decrease gastrointestinal chloroquine absorption but may also precipitate aspiration pneumonia.
• *Central nervous system*: visual disturbances (blurred vision, diplopia, photophobia, and transient blindness) and audio-vestibular dysfunction (dizziness, buzzing, deafness) are common with an early onset. Anxiety, agitation, impairment of consciousness and seizures may occur. CNS features are generally correlated to the severity of cardiovascular failure, although direct CNS toxicity may also occur. Painless proximal myopathy, mild rhabdomyolysis and peripheral neuropathy are rarely encountered.
• *Respiratory system*: tachypnoea may occur; apnoea is rare, usually resulting from convulsions. Aspiration pneumonia may complicate impaired consciousness. Acute lung injury or respiratory distress syndrome (ARDS) with alveolar haemorrhage may develop late in severe cases. Pulmonary toxicity is directly related to membrane stabilizing activity.
• *Metabolic*: hypokalaemia, hyperlactataemia, and metabolic acidosis are common, with severity proportional to cardiovascular compromise. Hypokalaemia rarely results in ECG abnormalities. The lowest reported value (0.8 mmol/L) was associated with tetraparesis. Serum potassium is correlated with blood pressure reductions and QT or QRS prolongation.

Toxicity assessment
Factors suggesting a high risk of toxicity include the reported dose (e.g. >4 g in an adult) and rapid onset of clinical features, especially cardiovascular collapse. A BP lower than 100 mmHg and QRS prolongation of more than 100 ms also suggest severe toxicity. Blood or plasma chloroquine concentrations also correlate well with severity but are not generally available

Investigations
The following should be performed:
• Measurement of electrolytes, especially potassium, together with creatinine, lactate, coagulation, and liver function tests. These should be repeated frequently in patients with features of poisoning.
• A 12-lead ECG should be performed and repeated regularly during the acute phase of poisoning. Early abnormalities (best seen in standard lead II) include flattened or inverted T waves, ST segment depression, and prolongation of QTc and QRS intervals (see Figure 3.1, p. 64). Ventricular dysrhythmias including extrasystoles, torsade de pointes, ventricular tachycardia, and ventricular fibrillation, may occur. Right bundle branch block and Brugada syndrome (coved or 'saddle back' ST elevation with >2 mm J-point elevation

accompanied by gradually descending ST segment and negative T-wave) may be observed. Atrioventricular block and supraventricular tachycardia are less common.
- Arterial blood gases should be performed in patients with severe features.

Management
Pulse, blood pressure, cardiac rhythm, urine output, and O_2 saturation should be monitored continuously in patients with significant intoxication.

Oral activated charcoal should be administered in patients admitted less than 2 hours after ingestion of more than 15 mg/kg chloroquine, in the absence of contraindications. Gastric lavage is not indicated.

Early aggressive management improved survival in comparison to conventional supportive treatment in a randomized controlled trial. In the presence of at least one poor prognostic factor, the following three measures are mandatory:
1 Tracheal intubation and mechanical ventilation
2 High-dose diazepam (see 'Use of antidotes')
3 Epinephrine infusion (0.25 micrograms/kg/minute IV continuous infusion titrated to blood pressure with 0.25 micrograms/kg/minute increments)

In addition, 8.4% sodium bicarbonate is recommended in the event of hypotension with a widened QRS complex and repeated until QRS width narrows to a maximum dose of 1–2 meq/kg. Potassium administration should be considered in parallel, e.g. 2 g KCl for each 25 meq of bicarbonate.

Anti-arrhythmic medications should be avoided, including class I agents like lidocaine: there is a risk of precipitating further arrhythmias or seizures and worsening cardiovascular status due to negative inotropic and chronotropic effects.

In patients requiring increasing doses of epinephrine, haemodynamic monitoring is mandatory to monitor volume status, cardiac output, and systemic vascular resistance. Echocardiography or right heart catheterization should be used according to availability and experience.

Hypokalaemia may be protective and should not be corrected aggressively, especially in the early hours. The required high doses of potassium may lead to sudden rebound hyperkalaemia during the recovery phase, as chloroquine is cleared. However, in case of torsade de pointes or ventricular extrasystoles, cautious potassium administration is helpful. Doses of 80 mmol/day (K^+ >2 mmol/L) or 160 mmol/day (K^+ <2 mmol/L) are recommended.

Convulsions should be treated with diazepam. Phenytoin should be avoided as it may worsen sodium channel blockade.

Extracorporeal life support, when available, should be considered in case of refractory cardiac arrest or cardiovascular failure, e.g. in patients with an epinephrine infusion rate greater than 3 mg/hour in the presence of renal or respiratory failure. These recommendations are based on small patient series and case reports only.

Use of antidotes
There is increasing interest in the use of high-dose diazepam in chloroquine poisoning. The mechanism of action is unknown and indications for use are poorly defined.

Experimental animal models have been used to assess mortality reduction (rat), cardiac protection, and increased chloroquine renal elimination (pig) but in these studies diazepam was administered with or before chloroquine.

Research in human poisoning had suggested reduced clinical severity when chloroquine is co-ingested with diazepam and benefit has been reported with empirical administration of diazepam following chloroquine overdose. No significant ECG improvement was observed in comparison to placebo, however, in a randomized trial involving patients with moderate poisoning.

Administration of high doses of diazepam requires intubation and mechanical ventilation to avoid pulmonary aspiration. The recommended regimen is 2 mg/kg IV over 30 minutes followed by 2 mg/kg/hour.

Use of elimination techniques
There is no indication for haemofiltration, haemodialysis, or haemoperfusion for accelerating chloroquine elimination.

These methods are ineffective because of the large volume of distribution, high protein binding, and red cell uptake of chloroquine.

Further reading
Clemessy JL, Angel G, Borron SW, et al. (1996). Therapeutic trial of diazepam versus placebo in acute chloroquine intoxications of moderate gravity. *Intensive Care Med*, 22:1400–5.

Clemessy JL, Favier C, Borron SW, et al. (1995). Hypokalaemia related to acute chloroquine ingestion. *Lancet*, 346:877–80.

Clemessy JL, Taboulet P, Hoffman JR, et al. (1996). Treatment of acute chloroquine poisoning: a 5-year experience. *Crit Care Med*, 24:1189–95.

Ducharme J, Farinotti F (1996). Clinical Pharmacokinetics and metabolism of chloroquine. *Clin Pharmacokinet*, 31:257–74.

Jordan P, Brookes JG, Nikolic G, et al. (1999). Hydroxychloroquine overdose: toxicokinetics and management. *J Toxicol Clin Toxicol*, 37:861–4.

Ling Ngan Wong A, Tsz Fung Cheung I, Graham CA (2008). Hydroxychloroquine overdose: case report and recommendations for management. *Eur J Emerg Med*, 15:16–18.

Mégarbane B, Bloch V, Hirt D, et al. (2010). Blood concentrations are better predictors of chloroquine poisoning severity than plasma concentrations: a prospective study with modeling of the concentration/effect relationships. *Clin Toxicol* 2010; 48:904–15.

Riou B, Barriot P, Rimailho A, et al. (1988). Treatment of severe chloroquine poisoning. *N Engl J Med*, 318:1–6.

Colchicine

Background and therapeutic use

Colchicine is an antimitotic agent used in the treatment of gout and familial Mediterranean fever and occasionally pericarditis and Behçet's disease. For acute gout a dose of 500 micrograms is given 2–4 times daily until pain is relieved or diarrhoea or vomiting occurs, or when a cumulative dose of 6 mg is reached. For familial Mediterranean fever the usual dose is 0.5–2 mg daily.

Colchicine is also the toxic component of the bulbs and other parts of a number of plants including *Colchicum autumnale* (Autumn crocus or meadow saffron) and *Gloriosa superba* (glory lily).

Colchicine poisoning is uncommon, but is important because it can cause severe and life-threatening features.

Mechanism of action

Colchicine binds selectively to the intracellular protein tubulin in cells throughout the body. This prevents tubulin polymerization and interferes with cellular motility, intracellular transport mechanisms, and cellular mitosis. Colchicine also has effects within leucocytes and disrupts phagocytosis, chemotaxis, and cytokine production.

Toxicokinetics

Colchicine is rapidly but incompletely absorbed from the gut, reaching peak concentrations in the blood within 1–2 hours of ingestion. It has high first-pass metabolism resulting in systemic bioavailability of less than 50%. Colchicine has a large volume of distribution, particularly after overdose. Plasma protein binding is limited (10–50%). Colchicine is metabolized by deacetylation and demethylation, mainly via hepatic CYP3A4; the parent drug and its metabolites are mostly excreted in the bile, with about 10–20% excreted in the urine. Colchicine and its metabolites undergo enterohepatic recirculation. As a result the terminal half-life is prolonged (30–60 hours) and the drug can be detected in leucocytes for up to 9 days after an intravenous dose. As a consequence, toxicity can be delayed and prolonged.

Toxic dose

Toxicity with colchicine is dose-dependent but there is overlap between therapeutic and toxic doses making it difficult to establish a 'toxic dose' for colchicine. The fatality rate is high after acute ingestions greater than 0.5 mg/kg but doses lower than these can cause gastrointestinal and haematological effects and death has been reported. In case reports fatality has been associated with oral doses as low as 7 mg but survival has occurred after reported doses as high as 60 mg.

All colchicine overdoses should be taken seriously and be referred for medical assessment.

Clinical features of colchicine poisoning

The clinical features of colchicine appear in three phases:

Early phase (first 24 hours)

There can be delay of 6 hours before the initial irritant gastrointestinal features are seen. Patients develop nausea, vomiting, abdominal pain, and diarrhoea. The diarrhoea can be severe leading to dehydration, electrolyte disturbances, hypovolaemia, and hypovolaemic shock in severe cases. Bloody diarrhoea can also occur.

Intermediate phase (24 hours to 7 days)

This phase is characterized by widespread organ dysfunction. Patients develop effects as follows:

- Neurological: confusion, delirium, drowsiness convulsions and coma.
- Cardiac: hypotension, arrhythmias and cardiac arrest; arrhythmias typically occur 24–36 hours after ingestion.
- Renal: acute kidney injury, sometimes associated with haematuria
- Hepatic: tender hepatomegaly associated with raised blood transaminase concentrations.
- Metabolic: metabolic (including lactic) acidosis, hypokalaemia, hyponatraemia, hypocalcaemia, hypoglycaemia or hyperglycaemia, hypophosphatemia.
- Respiratory: pulmonary oedema and ARDS; this is multifactorial, relating to direct colchicine toxicity in the lungs, respiratory muscle weakness and cardiac failure.
- Haematological: leucocytosis is seen in the initial phase and is followed 48–72 hours after ingestion by bone marrow suppression with pancytopenia and an increased risk of sepsis. The nadir of the leucocyte count occurs up to 10 days after acute poisoning and patients remain susceptible to sepsis during this time period.
- Muscular: colchicine has direct toxic effects on both cardiac and skeletal muscle leading to shock and rhabdomyolysis respectively.

Patients with severe poisoning develop multi-organ failure often associated with bone marrow aplasia, sepsis, disseminated intravascular coagulation, cerebral oedema, and convulsions. Lactic acidosis may result from circulatory failure or inhibition of cellular metabolism. When poisoning is fatal, death typically occurs 8–72 hours after ingestion and is related to intractable hypotension, sepsis or cardiac arrest.

Late phase (>7 days after ingestion)

Patients who survive the intermediate phase develop a rebound leucocytosis with recovery of bone marrow activity. Alopecia is seen in this phase at 2–3 weeks. Patients may also develop a myopathy, neuropathy, or combined myoneuropathy with proximal limb weakness and distal sensory loss; this can persist for several weeks.

Management

All patients should be observed for at least 6–12 hours after ingestion. Patients who are asymptomatic at this stage can be discharged with advice to return if gastrointestinal symptoms occur.

Patients who present within an hour of a significant ingestion of colchicine (e.g. >0.1 mg/kg) should be given activated charcoal (50 g in adults, 1 g/kg in children). Multiple-dose activated charcoal (MDAC; 50 g every 4 hours in adults, 1 g/kg every 4 hours in children) potentially has a role, particularly in those with large ingestions (e.g. >0.3 mg/kg). There are no data to demonstrate a benefit from MDAC but it is theoretically of benefit because of the enterohepatic circulation of colchicine. MDAC administration may be limited by the significant vomiting seen in colchicine poisoning.

Supportive care is the mainstay of treatment. Patients with significant symptoms in the 'early phase' should be managed in a critical care environment with cardiac monitoring, adequate hydration, and management of organ dysfunction when it occurs. Shock may result from depressed myocardial function or intravascular hypovolaemia as a result of fluid loss and patients may require intravenous fluids, inotropes, or vasopressors for cardiovascular collapse. Other treatments that might be required include antibiotics for sepsis, renal replacement therapy for acute kidney injury, and respiratory support for acute respiratory distress syndrome. An intravenous benzodiazepine (e.g. diazepam 10–20 mg or 0.1–0.3 mg/kg in children) is appropriate first-line treatment for convulsions.

Patients with significant features in the early phase of poisoning should have frequent full blood counts (at least 12-hourly) together with monitoring of renal function, glucose, liver function, creatinine kinase, and clotting. Blood and urine colchicine concentrations are not widely available and are not useful as they do not correlate with the severity of poisoning.

Granulocyte colony stimulating factor (G-CSF) has been used in patients with colchicine-related leucopenia and thrombocytopenia. G-CSF should be considered in patients with leucopenia in consultation with a haematologist.

Colchicine-specific Fab fragments have shown to be effective at restoring tubulin function *in vitro* and there is a report of successful use of Fab fragments in a case of colchicine poisoning. However, colchicine Fab fragments are not widely available. Haemodialysis and other extracorporeal procedures are not useful because of the large volume of distribution and high protein binding of colchicine.

Enhanced elimination techniques
MDAC may increase elimination of colchicine by interrupting enterohepatic circulation. Haemodialysis and haemoperfusion, however, do not enhance drug removal because of its large volume of distribution associated with tissue binding; haemodialysis may, however, be needed in the management of renal failure.

Chronic colchicine toxicity
This may occur with use of excessive doses for therapy or as a result of factors that impair colchicine elimination. These include impairment of renal or liver function or drug interactions. Colchicine is a substrate for CYP3A4 and P-glycoprotein and co-prescription of inhibitors of these (e.g. erythromycin, clarithromycin, ketoconazole, grapefruit juice, tolbutamide, ciclosporin, HIV protease inhibitors) may precipitate toxicity and fatalities have been reported.

Features of chronic toxicity develop gradually and may include vomiting, diarrhoea, abdominal pain, gastrointestinal haemorrhage, muscular weakness, skin rashes, renal and hepatic impairment alopecia, peripheral neuropathy, and bone marrow depression.

Myopathy and rhabdomyolysis have been reported with the concomitant use of colchicine and statins, fibrates, ciclosporin, or digoxin

Further reading
Finkelstein Y, Aks SE, Hutson JR, et al. (2010). Colchicine poisoning: the dark side of an ancient drug. *Clin Toxicol*, 48: 407–14.

Harris R, Marx G, Gillett M, et al.(2000). Colchicine-induced bone marrow suppression: treatment with granulocyte colony-stimulating factor. *J Emerg Med*, 18:435–40.

Milne ST, Meek PD (1998). Fatal colchicine overdose: report of a case and review of the literature. *Am J Emerg Med*, 16:603–8.

Sauder P, Kopferschmitt J, Jaeger A, et al. (1983). Haemodynamic studies in eight cases of acute colchicine poisoning. *Human Toxicol*, 2:169–73.

Iron poisoning

Background

Iron is available in a variety of medicinal preparations and these are the commonest source of ingestion. Rarely exposure may occur in laboratory environments, for example, in schools where iron salts are available. Most multivitamin preparations contain insufficient iron to be toxicologically significant. Medicinal products may, however, be far more dangerous. Today the major risks from iron poisoning are from deliberate self-harm.

Iron toxicity also results from hepatic iron accumulation in patients who require repeat transfusion. In these patients clinical features are similar to haemochromatosis and therapy is needed to reduce total body iron content. The urgency of treatment and clinical features are very different in chronic iron overload to acute poisoning. However, principles of iron removal are similar, in that a chelating agent is used to reduce iron body load. The key difference between acute and chronic poisoning relates to the symptom pattern and the urgency for therapy.

Therapeutic iron salts are ferrous derivatives. Quantities of elemental iron available in each salt vary (Table 7.3). It is important to calculate the elemental iron from the quantity ingested. Thus 200 mg of ferrous sulfate contains 65 mg elemental iron, while 300 mg ferrous gluconate contains only 35 mg elemental iron. Clinicians should be wary of 'modified-release' preparations since the clinical profile of poisoning may differ in patients taking these products due to delayed absorption.

Mechanisms of toxicity

The precise mechanism by which iron causes toxicity is poorly understood. It acts as a cellular toxin, particularly on the liver, kidney, and brain. Locally it is corrosive and irritant in the GI tract causing vomiting and haematemesis. Its metabolic actions may result in metabolic acidosis. This process takes approximately 24 hours to complete.

Iron preparations damage and stain the mucosa of the upper GI tract, causing ulceration and haemorrhage. Circulating iron is initially bound to transferrin; in large overdoses, the capacity of transferrin is exceeded, leaving excessive circulating free iron. This is taken up by the reticuloendothelial system and transferred to hepatocytes, where it is concentrated in mitochondria, disrupting metabolism resulting in cell death, especially in the periportal regions.

Circulating free iron is a potent vasodilator, and this effect contributes to the development of hypotension and shock which are important clinical features in severe poisoning. In the severely affected patient, major iron toxicity appears to derive from intracellular hepatic actions. The time taken for iron absorption and the hepatic uptake that precede consequent hepatic damage allow a window of opportunity for treatment. Thus appreciation of the

Table 7.3 Elemental iron content of commonly used iron salts

Iron preparation	Elemental iron
Ferrous sulfate (dried)	32%
Ferrous gluconate	12%
Ferrous fumarate	32%
Ferrous chloride	28%

timescales, the various ways in which iron causes its toxicity, and the symptoms produced is essential to the prompt and appropriate management of iron ingestion.

Toxicokinetics

The precise kinetic profile of iron in overdose is poorly understood. Measurement of iron concentrations is key as it provides an index of the total body burden of iron. Normally iron is absorbed by active transport, but in overdose these processes may be overwhelmed, or the cells involved damaged by the acute GI effects of iron.

Following overdose peak concentrations of iron usually occur between 4 and 6 hours after ingestion. Estimating the body burden from a single concentration is often challenging as the precise time interval from ingestion may be unclear and nausea and vomiting induced by iron may perturb GI motility and hence delay absorption. It is therefore not unusual to see a potentially toxic concentration early in the course of management that rapidly falls to a less significant level. It is, however, extremely difficult to predict clinically which patients will, and will not follow this pattern. Management can be further complicated by haemolysis, which elevates serum iron but may also be secondary to a very high iron concentration in blood. Clinicians should be very wary of laboratory results which suggest an unsuitable sample and in such patients tend to a proactive management strategy.

Risk factors for toxicity

The clearest risk factor for toxicity is systemic dose. Ingested dose is a guide, but history can be unreliable and the actual absorbed dose is also affected by vomiting. Ingestion of a slow-release product may lead to inappropriate reassurance from initial iron concentration.

Acute iron overdose in pregnancy is occasionally fatal for mother and fetus. It must be managed as in the non-pregnant patient; there is no evidence of teratogenicity from desferrioxamine.

Clinical features

In the majority of patients with iron poisoning, only the features of gut irritation are present. Systemic toxicity is less common but can sometimes be fatal. Identifying higher-risk patients is a major challenge.

Iron poisoning is often said to have four phases, however this has uncertain clinical value.

- **Within 6 hours of ingestion:** nausea, vomiting, abdominal pain, and diarrhoea. Vomitus and stools may be grey or black.
- **6–12 hours after ingestion:** mild cases improve; in more serious cases hypoperfusion (cool peripheries and hypotension), reduced level of consciousness and metabolic acidosis may occur. High serum iron concentration may effect coagulation, typically prolonging APTT. If no liver injury, coagulation normalizes as iron concentrations fall
- **More than 12 hours after ingestion:** most patients improve and recover, but in serious cases there may be some initial improvement, followed by recurrence of vomiting and GI bleeding. Shock can result from hypovolaemia or direct cardiotoxicity. Evidence of hepatocellular necrosis with abnormal LFTs, jaundice, bleeding, hypoglycaemia, encephalopathy, and metabolic acidosis is evident. Renal failure may occur.

- **2–5 weeks after ingestion:** rarely, gastric scarring, stricture, or pyloric stenosis leading to bowel obstruction may occur.

It is crucial to understand that the initial GI symptoms (nausea, vomiting, abdominal pain, diarrhoea, and bleeding) are caused by direct effects of iron on the gut mucosa. Shock (normally not caused by blood loss), acidosis, impaired consciousness, convulsions, and subsequent features of hepatocellular necrosis and hepatic encephalopathy reflect systemic toxicity resulting from the effects of excessive absorbed elemental iron.

Investigations

- Full blood count, serum urea and electrolytes, liver function tests, and a clotting screen should be performed. In patients with suspected severe poisoning repeat regularly and measure arterial blood gases.
- Serum iron concentration should be measured immediately in suspected severe poisoning, or at 4–6 hours after ingestion in others. A second iron concentration taken 2 hours after the first is mandatory in all but mild cases. Measurement of total iron-binding capacity does not help differentiate episodes of severe poisoning and is therefore not recommended.

Abdominal radiography may confirm ingestion but is not accurate for determining dose and is potentially inappropriately reassuring.

Toxicity assessment

As the standard antidote desferrioxamine causes adverse effects (mainly hypotension), and prevents subsequent assessment of iron concentrations due to assay interference, it should not be given indiscriminately. It is critically important to identify patients who will benefit.

Severe poisoning is indicated by severe hypotension, coma, metabolic acidosis and/or severe GI bleeding. Patients with these features require immediate treatment with desferrioxamine, although the dose may need discussion with experts.

The majority of patients do not have these features, and are thus more challenging to assess. There is no one simple test to establish poisoning severity. The amount of elemental iron ingested gives an indication of likely severity; more than 20 mg/kg is likely to result in clinical features; more than 75 mg/kg expected to result in severe features with occasional fatalities; more than 150 mg/kg causes severe poisoning with a high risk of fatality.

The normal method for assessing severity of iron poisoning is to measure a serum iron concentration. Interpretation of the results is often difficult as there are few studies on kinetics in acute overdose. Some studies suggest peak concentrations occur about 4 hours after ingestion and in mild poisoning will decline rapidly thereafter. For these reasons it is difficult in the first few hours after ingestion to use the single measurement as a method of assessing severity. A second iron concentration taken 2 hours after the first is mandatory in all but mild cases. Even less is known about serum iron levels following overdose with slow release formulations.

When interpreting serum iron concentrations, values:

- **<55 micromol/L (<3 mg/L)** indicate mild or no toxicity. Desferrioxamine is not indicated.
- **55–90 micromol/L (3–5 mg/L)** suggest moderate toxicity. Concentrations should be re-measured after 2 hours; if rising and the patient is symptomatic desferrioxamine should be considered. If rising and the patient is asymptomatic, continue to monitor for at least 12 hours. If falling and the patient is asymptomatic, further intervention is unlikely to be required.
- **>90 micromol/L (>5 mg/L)** are consistent with severe poisoning and, if clinical features are present are an indication for antidote use and intensive monitoring. If the patient is asymptomatic concentrations can be repeated after a further 2 hours.

Other clinical features of more severe poisoning include haemolysis and a high anion gap. Leucocytosis and hyperglycaemia may also indicate more severe poisoning but their absence does not exclude it.

Management

Minor overdoses (<20 mg elemental iron/kg body weight) do not require admission to hospital or treatment. The main treatment for severe poisoning is desferrioxamine. Other therapies include replacement of fluid and blood losses, correction of hypoxia and/or metabolic acidosis using sodium bicarbonate and conventional measures for liver and renal failure.

Preventing absorption

Patients ingesting more than 20 mg elemental iron/kg body weight should be admitted to hospital. Activated charcoal adsorbs iron poorly and is not used. Gastric aspiration or lavage should be considered if a patient presents within 1 hour of ingestion of a very large quantity of iron, but most patients with severe poisoning will be vomiting, making this difficult and/or unnecessary. No intra-gastric therapies (e.g. chelation or bicarbonate) are of value. If a slow-release iron formulation has been ingested whole-bowel irrigation should be considered.

Desferrioxamine

Desferrioxamine chelates iron, and should be administered urgently in severe iron poisoning (defined by the presence of coma, shock, metabolic acidosis, or severe GI bleeding). Treatment should not be delayed pending the results of serum iron concentrations but a sample must be obtained before treatment. Desferrioxamine is given as an intravenous infusion, initially at a rate of 15 mg/kg/hour; the maximum dose advised is 80 mg/kg in 24 hours. This binds a relatively small quantity of iron and higher doses may be used in selected patients. There are case reports where much larger doses have been administered with apparent success, although hypotension, pulmonary oedema and ARDS have also been reported. Rare reported adverse effects include thrombocytopenia, hearing and visual disturbances, and allergy. Desferrioxamine may be stopped when clinical improvement occurs. The iron–desferrioxamine complex (ferrioxamine) is excreted in the urine, turning it orange-red in colour. It is dialysable if renal failure develops.

Further reading

Bosse GM (1995). Conservative management of patients with moderately elevated serum iron levels. *J Toxicol Clin Toxicol*, 33:135–40.

Chang TP, Rangan C (2011). Iron poisoning: a literature-based review of epidemiology, diagnosis and management. *Pediatr Emerg Care*, 27:978–85.

Chyka PA, Butler AY, Holley JE (1996). Serum iron concentrations and symptoms of acute iron poisoning in children. *Pharmacotherapy*, 16:1053–8.

Madiwale T, Liebelt E (2008). Iron: not a benign therapeutic drug. *Curr Opin Paediatr*, 18:174–9.

Robertson A, Tenenbein M (2005). Hepatotoxicity in acute iron poisoning. *Hum Exp Toxicol*, 24:559–62.

Tenenbein M (1996). Benefits of parenteral deferoxamine for acute iron poisoning. *J Toxicol Clin Toxicol*, 34:485–9.

Methotrexate and other chemotherapeutic agents

Chemotherapeutic agents

Chemotherapeutic agents (cytotoxic drugs) are used for the treatment of cancer and inhibit cell proliferation by various mechanisms. Those in common use include:
- alkylating drugs, e.g. cyclophosphamide
- anthracyclines, e.g. doxorubicin
- antimetabolites, e.g. methotrexate
- vinca alkaloids, e.g. vincristine
- platinum compounds, e.g. carboplatin
- protein kinase inhibitors, e.g. imatinib
- monoclonal antibodies, e.g. trastuzumab.

Overdose usually occurs as a result of accidental administration of a toxic dose during the course of treatment. Cases of intentional overdose or malicious administration with homicidal intent occur rarely.

Clinical features

Toxicity common to all chemotherapeutic agents generally results from damage to normal cells, especially those with rapid turnover, e.g. GI mucosa, bone marrow, hair follicles

GI: vomiting, diarrhoea, mucositis, oropharyngeal ulceration, haemorrhagic enteritis.

Skin: erythematous rashes, alopecia.

Haematological: bone marrow suppression leading to leucopenia, anaemia, and thrombocytopenia. The white cell count usually falls to its lowest level at around 6–12 days after acute overdose.

Investigations

After overdose with chemotherapeutic agents, check full blood count (FBC), serum urea, and electrolytes and liver function tests. The FBC may be normal initially but pancytopenia may develop over the next 7–12 days. Even if asymptomatic, the FBC should be repeated weekly for 4 weeks after overdose.

Management

Consider giving activated charcoal if ingestion of an orally active agent has occurred within 1 hour.

If pancytopenia occurs, consultation with a haematologist is advisable; isolation and reverse barrier nursing should be instituted and the patient closely monitored for signs of infection. Treat suspected neutropenic sepsis with broad-spectrum antibiotics as per local protocols. Blood or platelet transfusions or use of recombinant G-CSF may be necessary.

Methotrexate

Methotrexate is an antimetabolite which competitively inhibits the enzyme dihydrofolate reductase which is essential for the synthesis of purines and pyrimidines. Oral, intravenous, and intrathecal methotrexate is used in oncology. Once-weekly oral doses are also used for the treatment of inflammatory disorders such as rheumatoid arthritis and Crohn's disease.

Accidental overdoses commonly occur as a result of patients mistakenly taking oral methotrexate daily rather than weekly.

Toxicokinetics

Absorption of oral methotrexate depends on dose, with incomplete absorption associated with doses greater than 2–3 mg/kg. Peak concentrations occur 1–2 hours after an oral dose. The main route of excretion is renal. The $t\frac{1}{2}$ is dose-dependent with values of 3–10 hours after doses of less than 60 mg and 8–15 hours after high-dose parenteral therapy.

Risk factors for methotrexate toxicity

Methotrexate toxicity is more common after chronic excess oral dosing rather than after a single acute ingestion.

Hypoalbuminaemia, ascites, folate deficiency, renal impairment, and concomitant use of non-steroidal anti-inflammatory drugs predispose to methotrexate toxicity.

Clinical features

Following ingestion or parenteral use

Other than the usual GI, skin, and haematological manifestations associated with anticancer chemotherapy, recognized late complications of methotrexate overdose include hepatotoxicity, renal failure, and interstitial pneumonitis.

Following intrathecal use

Acute: headache, back or shoulder pain, nuchal rigidity and fever, resulting from chemical arachnoiditis.

Subacute: paresis, usually transient, paraplegia, nerve palsies, and cerebellar dysfunction.

Chronic: leucoencephalopathy manifested by irritability, confusion, ataxia, spasticity, occasionally convulsions, dementia, somnolence, coma, and rarely, death.

Systemic toxicity may occur following a large intrathecal overdose.

Investigations

Monitor FBC, serum U&Es, and liver function tests as for other chemotherapeutic agents.

Measure methotrexate concentration 4–6 hours after ingestion.

Management

- Consider giving activated charcoal if a potentially toxic dose (>1 mg/kg) has been ingested within 1 hour.
- Pancytopenia should be managed as for other chemotherapeutic agents (see earlier in section).
- Consider use of calcium folinate (leucovorin) or glucarpidase as antidotes for methotrexate toxicity (see later in section).
- If an antidote is not available, urinary alkalinization with sodium bicarbonate may be used to enhance elimination of methotrexate. Administer 1.5 L of 1.26% sodium bicarbonate over 3 hours.
- Following an intrathecal overdose, seek urgent neurosurgical advice. CSF drainage or ventriculolumbar perfusion should be performed.

Antidotes

Two antidotes are available for treatment of methotrexate toxicity:
- calcium folinate (folinic acid, leucovorin)
- glucarpidase.

Calcium folinate

This is given intravenously based on the dose ingested and methotrexate concentration. It should *not* be used intrathecally.

If the methotrexate dose is known, give an equal or greater dose of intravenous calcium folinate 6-hourly until the methotrexate concentration is known, then treat as shown in Table 7.4.

If the methotrexate dose is unknown, give intravenous calcium folinate 100 mg/m² body surface area until the methotrexate concentration is known, then treat as shown in Table 7.4.

Continue treatment until methotrexate concentration is $< 5 \times 10^{-8}$ M (<0.05 micromol/L).

Glucarpidase

Glucarpidase causes enzymatic degradation of methotrexate to glutamate and 4-deoxy-4-amino-N10-methylpteroic acid (DAMPA) which then undergo hepatic metabolism. It is not licensed for use in the UK and is only available on a named-patient basis. It is administered as an adjunct to calcium folinate in patients with methotrexate toxicity and renal impairment in a dose of 50 units/kg by slow intravenous infusion over 5 minutes. Glucarpidase has also been administered intrathecally for intrathecal methotrexate overdose.

Adverse effects reported include allergic reactions and occasionally hypertension or arrhythmias.

Cyclophosphamide and ifosfamide

Cyclophosphamide and ifosfamide are alkylating agents used in various cancer chemotherapy regimens. Cyclophosphamide is also used in the treatment of immunological disorders such as systemic lupus erythematosus and ANCA-associated vasculitis.

Toxicokinetics

Cyclophosphamide and ifosfamide are pro-drugs requiring metabolic activation in the liver. Metabolites are excreted in the urine and clearance is delayed if there is renal impairment.

Cyclophosphamide is metabolized to the active metabolites 4-hydroxycyclophosphamide and phosphoramide mustard. The parent drug is well absorbed orally and has a t½ of 4–10 hours, although active metabolites persist for longer.

Ifosfamide is metabolized to the active metabolite ifosforamide mustard. T½ of the parent drug is 4–15 h and varies with dose.

Acrolein is a metabolic product following administration of either drug in humans and is thought to be responsible for development of haemorrhagic cystitis.

Clinical features

Haematological: bone marrow suppression. A reduced white cell count is usually apparent by day 6 and may last 12–18 days.

Renal tract: haemorrhagic cystitis and renal failure.

CVS: left ventricular failure.

CNS: optic neuropathy may occur after high doses of cyclophosphamide. Ifosfamide can cause a dose-related encephalopathy causing symptoms ranging from somnolence or agitation to an acute confusional state, hallucinations, seizures, stupor, mutism, and reduced level of consciousness, possibly leading to coma and death.

Investigations

Monitor FBC, serum U&Es, and liver function tests as for other chemotherapeutic agents.

Urinalysis should be performed.

A chest X-ray should be carried out in patients with symptoms and signs of cardiac failure.

Management

- Consider giving activated charcoal if a potentially toxic dose has been ingested within 1 hour.
- Regular monitoring of pulse, blood pressure, oxygen saturation, and cardiac rhythm is essential.
- Ensure adequate hydration to maintain a urine output higher than 100 mL/hour.
- Pancytopenia should be managed as for other chemotherapeutic agents (see earlier in section).
- Mesna (Uromitexan®, sodium 2-mercaptoethane sulphonate) inactivates acrolein in the urine and is given to reduce the risk of haemorrhagic cystitis. Following overdose, mesna should be administered as soon as possible and doses repeated after 4 and 8 hours. In severe toxicity, further doses or more frequent administration should be considered. The total dose of intravenous mesna should be 60% of the dose of cyclophosphamide taken (weight for weight). For example, if 4 g of cyclophosphamide has been taken, give 800 mg mesna at 0, 4, and 8 hours (total 2.4 g). Frequent bladder emptying should be avoided once mesna has been given.
- In children or high-risk patients the dose of mesna should be up to 40% of the cyclophosphamide dose four times at 3-hourly intervals (i.e. 160% w/w total dose).
- Methylthioninium chloride (methylene blue) has been used to treat ifosfamide-induced encephalopathy. A suggested dosing regimen is: 50 mg (diluted in 50–100 mL normal saline and administered over 30 minutes) every 4 hours until the neurological status is improved.

Vincristine

Vincristine is a vinca alkaloid which acts by disrupting the microtubule assembly which is necessary for cell mitosis.

Overdose is usually iatrogenic, resulting from dose miscalculation or administration by the wrong route.

Toxicokinetics

Vincristine is poorly absorbed after oral ingestion and is only used via the intravenous route. It is excreted primarily in the bile with a terminal t½ ranging from 15–155 hours. Concomitant use of drugs which inhibit cytochrome 3A4 (e.g. itraconazole) may enhance toxicity.

Table 7.4 Calculation of calcium folinate dose

Methotrexate concentration	Calcium folinate dose
>50 micromol/L	1000 mg/m²
($>5\times10^{-5}$ M)	(6-hourly IV, or 3 hourly if renal impairment)
5–50 micromol/L	100 mg/m²
(5×10^{-5} M to 5×10^{-6} M)	(3-hourly IV)
0.5–5 micromol/L	30 mg/m²
(5×10^{-6} M to 5×10^{-7} M)	(6-hourly IV/PO)
<0.5 micromol/L	10 mg/m²
($<5\times10^{-7}$ M)	6-hourly PO/IV

Clinical features

Following intravenous vincristine

Haematological: bone marrow suppression. A reduced white cell count is usually apparent by day 6 and may last for up to 3 weeks.

CNS: neuropathy may occur after 2 weeks and last for up to 2 months before resolution is observed. Loss of reflexes is the earliest sign of neuropathy. Paraesthesia, ataxia, peripheral nerve palsies causing wrist drop or foot drop, cranial nerve palsies may also occur. Autonomic dysfunction leading to ileus and urinary retention and labile blood pressure can also occur.

Metabolic: hyponatraemia resulting from syndrome of inappropriate antidiuretic hormone secretion (SIADH).

CVS: myocardial infarction has been reported.

Following intrathecal vincristine

This is a catastrophic error which leads to severe ascending neuropathy and is almost invariably fatal.

CNS: lumbar back pain and lower limb weakness occur within 1–2 hours followed by ascending motor paralysis within 2–3 days manifest as flaccid paralysis of the lower limbs with loss of the peripheral reflexes, paraesthesiae. numbness, and slapping gait. Bulbar and cerebral involvement occur within 3–5 days leading to cranial nerve paralysis, loss of gag reflexes, recurrent laryngeal nerve palsy and vocal impairment, and autonomic dysfunction causing urinary retention, ileus, constipation. Encephalopathy, progressive respiratory failure, coma, and death ensue.

Investigations

Monitor FBC, serum U&Es, and liver function tests as for other chemotherapeutic agents.

Management

Intravenous overdose

- Following an intravenous overdose, admit to a critical care bed, e.g. CCU/HDU.
- Regular monitoring of pulse, blood pressure, oxygen saturation, and cardiac rhythm is essential.
- Fluid restriction should be instituted if SIADH develops.
- Pancytopenia should be managed as for other chemotherapeutic agents (see earlier in section).
- No intervention has been shown to be effective in preventing the haematological or neurological effects. Haemodialysis is ineffective for removal.

Intrathecal administration

- Following intrathecal administration, remove as much CSF as is possible (e.g. 20 mL) via the lumbar puncture site and seek urgent neurosurgical advice.
- CSF irrigation with lactated Ringer's solution may be performed through an epidural catheter inserted in the subarachnoid space above the initial lumbar puncture site.
- Ventriculo-lumbar perfusion is performed by insertion of an intraventricular drain or catheter by a neurosurgeon. Continuous CSF irrigation with lactated Ringer's solution is performed at 150 mL/hour with fluid removal through the lumbar access to a closed drainage system.
- Give folinic acid 100 mg intravenously as a bolus, followed by an infusion of 25 mg/hour for 24 hours, followed by folinic acid boluses 25 mg 6-hourly for 1 week.

- Other neuroprotective agents have been suggested, e.g. glutamic acid (10 g intravenous infusion over 24 hours, then 500 mg orally three times daily for 1 month) or pyridoxine (50 mg 8-hourly as an intravenous infusion over 30 minutes) but their role in management is unclear.

Anthracyclines

The anthracyclines are bacterial derivatives which disrupt DNA replication by inhibiting topoisomerase II. They include daunorubicin, doxorubicin, bleomycin, and mitomycin C.

Some are provided as pegylated or liposomal products with effects on pharmacokinetic parameters and adverse effect profile.

Toxicokinetics

Anthracyclines undergo metabolism to form less active metabolites, primarily in the liver. Terminal elimination $t\frac{1}{2}$ are: daunorubicin 55 hours, doxorubicin 30 hours, bleomycin 9 hours, and mitomycin C 17 minutes. Patients with impaired liver function are at increased risk of toxicity.

Investigations

Check FBC, serum U&Es daily. The FBC may be normal initially but pancytopenia may develop over the next 7–12 days. Even if asymptomatic, repeat FBC and U&Es weekly for 4 weeks after the overdose.

Clinical features

Haematological: bone marrow suppression. A reduced white cell count is usually apparent in the 1st week and may last for up to 3 weeks.

CVS: after acute overdose, non-specific ST-T wave abnormalities, arrhythmias, acute heart failure, pericarditis, and myocarditis.

After cumulative doses, anthracyclines cause an irreversible cardiomyopathy leading to congestive cardiac failure. High-risk groups include children and elderly, patients with pre-existing cardiac problems, mediastinal irradiation, or receiving concomitant treatment with cyclophosphamide or other anthracyclines

Management

- Regular monitoring of pulse, blood pressure, oxygen saturation, and cardiac rhythm is essential.
- A chest X-ray should be performed in patients with symptoms and signs of cardiac failure.
- Acute pulmonary oedema should be managed conventionally.
- Pancytopenia should be managed as for other chemotherapeutic agents (see earlier in section).

Acute cardiotoxic effects following an overdose are reversible but no intervention has been shown to be effective in improving the cardiomyopathy associated with cumulative anthracycline use.

Platinum compounds

The platinum compounds include cisplatin and carboplatin which disrupt DNA replication by binding of platinum to DNA.

Toxicokinetics

Platinum compounds undergo elimination primarily by renal excretion. The $t\frac{1}{2}$ are 40–45 minutes for cisplatin and 1–2 hours for carboplatin, however platinum from these compounds is irreversibly bound to plasma proteins and eliminated over several weeks.

Haematological: bone marrow suppression. A reduced white cell count may be delayed and the nadir may occur after 3–5 weeks.

Renal (doses >50 mg/m^2): renal failure due to distal tubular necrosis.

CNS (doses >200 mg/m^2): seizures, encephalopathy, irreversible peripheral neuropathy, visual disturbances including temporary visual loss, optic neuropathy, papilloedema. After exposure to doses greater than 500 mg/m^2, hearing loss may occur.

Investigations

Monitor FBC, serum U&Es, and liver function tests as for other chemotherapeutic agents.

Management

• Adequate hydration with 0.9% saline to maintain a good urine output is essential.
• Sodium thiosulfate may be effective at preventing nephrotoxicity by binding free platinum.
• Haemodialysis does not enhance clearance of platinum but may be necessary in patients with established renal failure.
• Plasmapheresis enhances platinum clearance and may be beneficial if it can be instituted early after exposure.
• Pancytopenia should be managed as for other chemotherapeutic agents (see earlier in section).

Further reading

Aguiar Bujanda D, Cabrera Suárez MA, Bohn Sarmiento U, et al. (2006). Successful recovery after accidental overdose of cyclophosphamide. Ann Oncol, 17:1334

Grush OC, Morgan SK (1979). Folinic acid rescue for folinic acid toxicity. Clin Toxicol, 14:71–8.

Jackson DV Jr, Wells HB, Atkins JN, et al. (1988). Amelioration of vincristine neurotoxicity by glutamic acid. Am J Med, 84:1016–22.

Jakobson AM, Kreuger A, Mortimer O, et al. (1992). Cerebrospinal fluid exchange after intrathecal methotrexate overdose. A report of two cases. Acta Paediatr, 81:359–61.

Jardine LF, Ingram LC, Bleyer WA (1996). Intrathecal leucovorin after intrathecal methotrexate overdose. J Pediatr Hematol Oncol, 18:302–4.

Jung HK, Lee J, Lee SN (1995). A case of massive cisplatin overdose managed by plasmapheresis. Korean J Intern Med, 10:150–4.

O'Marcaigh AS, Johnson CM, Smithson WA, et al. (1996). Successful treatment of intrathecal methotrexate overdose by using ventriculolumbar perfusion and intrathecal instillation of carboxypeptidase G2. Mayo Clin Proc, 71:161–5.

Patel PN (2006). Methylene blue for management of Ifosfamide-induced encephalopathy. Ann Pharmacother, 40: 299–303.

Pelgrims J, De Vos F, Van den Brande J, et al. (2000). Methylene blue in the treatment and prevention of ifosfamide-induced encephalopathy: report of 12 cases and a review of the literature. Br J Cancer, 82:291–4.

Pfeifle CE, Howell SB, Felthouse RD, et al. (1985). High-dose cisplatin with sodium thiosulfate protection. J Clin Oncol, 3:237–44.

Spiegel RJ, Cooper PR, Blum RH, et al. (1984). Treatment of massive intrathecal methotrexate overdose by ventriculolumbar perfusion. N Engl J Med, 311:386–8.

Steger GG, Mader RM, Gnant MF, et al. (1993). GM-CSF in the treatment of a patient with severe methotrexate intoxication. J Intern Med, 233: 499–502.

Thomas LLM, Mertens MJ, von dem Borne AE, et al. (1988). Clinical management of cytotoxic drug overdose. Med Toxicol, 3:253–63.

Quinine

Background

Quinine is an alkaloid extracted from the bark of the cinchona tree. It has long been used as a treatment for malaria in a bark extract. This had antipyretic properties, but pure quinine does not appear to have these. The optical enantiomer of quinine is quinidine, a class 1a anti-arrhythmic drug, which was formerly used quite extensively but is now uncommonly prescribed.

Quinine is widely prescribed as a management for nocturnal cramps, with over 2 million prescriptions per annum in the UK for this indication, despite relatively weak evidence of clinical benefit from clinical trials. Quinine is therefore very widely available in households in the UK. A large number of patients ingesting the drug are not prescribed this themselves, adding to the tragedy that follows a large ingestion. Quinine is particularly hazardous in young children, where the sugar coating on the tablet may give the impression that this is a confection. As few as 4 or 5 tablets can be fatal in a small infant. In adults, doses above 30 mg/kg of quinine base (see Table 7.5) are potentially toxic and require medical assessment and observation. Quinine is also occasionally prescribed for the treatment of falciparum malaria.

Mechanisms of toxicity

Quinine has pharmacological effects principally on sodium and potassium channels similar to those of quinidine (Class 1a effect). In overdose the effects on phase 0 of the polarization of the cardiac muscle results in delayed conduction, while potassium blocking actions result in prolonged repolarization. The ventricular refractory period is increased, conduction velocities decrease, and there is also an effect on the pacemaker cells of the sinoatrial node. This mixture of effects produces cardiac arrhythmias and impaired contractility. In severe overdose cardiac electro-mechanical dissociation may occur, with hypotension and death. These effects are rarely seen at standard therapeutic doses of quinine, but are features of significant overdose.

Quinine is also toxic to the eye, causing blindness by direct effects on the retina which is often irreversible. Early features (also be seen with high-dose antimalarial therapy) may include disturbance of colour vision or blurring of vision. In severe poisoning the periphery of the retinal field is particularly affected and patients who regain some sight having been blind may be left with tunnel vision. Quite subtle peripheral visual loss is relatively common and patients who have had loss of sight as part of their clinical presentation should be seen routinely by an ophthalmologist to have their peripheral vision

formally checked. This is not a medical emergency but is important before the patient is allowed to return to normal daily activities such as driving or operating machinery.

Quinine also causes release of insulin from the pancreas and is recognized to cause hypoglycaemia in patients being treated for malaria, although this is not a common feature in acute overdose.

Quinine tends to exacerbate features of myasthenia gravis and has an oxytocic action on the uterus which is more pronounced in later pregnancy. This may explain the historical use as an abortifacient, even though it is ineffective at concentrations that do not put the mother's life at risk.

Quinine may precipitate severe life-threatening thrombocytopenic purpura due to an immune response to quinine. Doses required to precipitate this immune reaction are extremely low and in sensitive patients merely drinking a glass of tonic water may be sufficient to precipitate a crisis.

Toxicity is therefore seen predominantly following acute overdose, may rarely be seen in accidental ingestion in elderly patients prescribed the drug therapeutically, and may be a complication of high-dose therapy for malaria. Unusually it may occur as a complication of the immune response to quinine resulting in platelet destruction.

Toxicokinetics

After therapeutic doses quinine is absorbed within a few hours, reaching maximum concentrations between 2.5 and 6 hours after ingestion. It's bioavailability is between 75% and 90% and it is highly protein-bound (about 70%) in the circulation. Elimination is predominantly hepatic by metabolism via microsomal oxidases (P450 enzymes) with about 20% of the drug being eliminated unchanged in urine at therapeutic doses. The $t\frac{1}{2}$ is normally around 18 hours, but may be prolonged in overdose, due to a combination of delayed absorption and saturation of hepatic metabolism.

Routine measurement of quinine plasma concentration is not necessary in the management of overdose. There is a relationship between plasma concentration of quinine and clinical effects; serious poisoning is unlikely at plasma concentrations below 10 mg/L of quinine, cardiac arrhythmias and death being seen at concentrations above 15 mg/L.

Clinical trial evidence in volunteers has shown that oral repeat-dose activated charcoal almost doubles the clearance of quinine. Overdose case studies suggest a similar effect. This effect of charcoal may either be due to the gut wall acting as semipermeable membrane allowing the diffusion into the gut lumen and binding of quinine to charcoal or to interruption of entero-hepatic recirculation. Although quinine is excreted more efficiently in acidic urine, the quantities excreted are insufficient to warrant this therapy. Haemodialysis is relatively ineffective and not advised.

Risk factors for toxicity

Children are at particular risk because of the relatively low therapeutic ratio of quinine. Elimination of quinine is delayed in patients with severe hepatic and renal dysfunction including the elderly and it is likely these increase toxicity by increasing the area under the plasma time–concentration curve. Patients with heart disease or who are receiving cardiac drugs may also be at increased risk of toxicity.

Table 7.5 Quinine salts and their quinine base content

Quinine salt	Tablet size (mg)	Quinine base content (mg)
Bisulfate	300	178
Sulfate	125	103
Sulfate	200	165
Sulfate	300	248
Dihydrochloride	300	246
Hydrochloride	300	246

The metabolism of quinine is inhibited by CYP3A4 inhibitors such as erythromycin, ketoconazole, and ritonavir, increasing the risk of toxicity.

Quinine impairs the excretion of digoxin, and this may result digoxin toxicity. It also inhibits the microsomal oxidase enzyme CYP2D6 and may thus delay metabolism of substrates such as codeine, dextromethorphan, flecainide, paroxetine, mexiletine, and metoprolol.

Clinical features

Clinical features of quinine poisoning develop within 3–6 hours of acute ingestion. Initially patients develop classical symptoms of cinchonism, including the following:

- auditory: tinnitus and deafness
- GI: nausea and vomiting, abdominal pain and diarrhoea
- vasomotor: headache, vasodilatation, and sweating— on occasion vasodilatation may be severe enough to cause hypotension.

As poisoning becomes more severe, visual features develop, with blurring of vision an early feature. This may not progress, but in more severe poisoning visual loss or complete blindness will follow. Patients who have taken quinine while intoxicated with alcohol may awake blind. The effects on the eye usually develop 6–15 hours after acute overdose: the pupils became dilated and fixed and this may occur before there is complete loss of light perception. In milder cases patients may present with visual field defects. Constriction of retinal arteries and macular oedema may be seen on fundoscopy. Optic atrophy is a late complication.

The onset of visual features is a warning of the risk of cardiotoxicity, which tends to accompany ocular changes, since both are plasma concentration dependent. ECG changes are common in severe quinine toxicity and manifest as conduction and repolarization abnormalities affecting the QRS and QT intervals and sometimes resulting in broad-complex tachycardia and AV dissociation. The most common arrhythmias associated with quinine are ventricular tachycardias including torsade de pointes. Arrhythmias associated with quinine poisoning are extremely difficult complications to treat and often result in death.

In more severe poisoning neurological features including drowsiness, ataxia, convulsions, and coma may also occur.

Quinine causes hypokalaemia, possibly because of its effects on the sodium channel. The importance of correcting this abnormality is unclear, as theoretically it could be a protective mechanism against arrhythmia.

Thrombocytopenia or haemolysis may occur with chronic therapy but are rare after acute overdose.

Toxicity assessment

Toxicity assessment is based on the history of the ingested dose (see Table 7.5) and careful clinical assessment. As already described, clinical features and plasma concentrations parallel as the severity of the overdose increases. Particular attention is required regarding vision, cardiovascular status, and ECG. Severe toxicity is extremely unlikely to develop in a conscious patient who has no features of cinchonism within 4–6 hours of an acute ingestion.

Accumulation of quinine may occur in patients receiving high intravenous doses of quinine for malaria. Appropriate monitoring procedures need to be put in place to ensure the patient's safety in this situation.

Hypoglycaemia appears to be a feature in this scenario, but is not reported after acute overdose.

Investigations

Patients should be monitored for 12 hours after quinine ingestion. Cardiac rhythm, pulse, BP, serum electrolytes, blood glucose, FBC, and visual acuity should all be recorded. Regular 12-lead ECG recordings are necessary in order to accurately measure changes in the morphology of the ECG waveform.

Management

A clear airway and adequate ventilation should be maintained in all patients. Multiple-dose activated charcoal (50 g (adults) or 1 g/kg (children) every 4 hours enhances elimination and should be given to all patients who have ingested more than 30 mg per kilogram of quinine base (any amount in children <5 years), provided they can protect their airway.

Torsade de pointes should be treated in the first instance with magnesium, e.g. magnesium sulfate 8 mmol intravenously over 30–120 seconds, which may be repeated as necessary. Hypoxaemia, electrolyte disturbance, and acidosis should also be corrected. If this is ineffective the arrhythmia may respond to increasing the underlying cardiac rate using atrial or ventricular pacing to obtain a heart rate of 90–110 beats per minute. Isoproterenol by infusion may also be used to achieve the same cardiac rate if pacing is not possible.

In patients with prolongation of the QRS interval to more than 120 ms, blood gases should be performed and metabolic acidosis corrected with intravenous sodium bicarbonate, aiming to maintain an alkali pH (~7.5) using bolus doses of 50 mmol of sodium bicarbonate. Use of antiarrhythmic drugs will often worsen the arrhythmias associated with quinine.

There is no specific treatment for visual complications; patients require psychological support and should be told that recovery of some vision it is quite likely but not certain. There is no role for any active intervention.

Supportive care is required for patients with coma. Convulsions are treated with intravenous benzodiazepines, e.g. intravenous diazepam (10–20 mg in adults; 0.1–0.3 mg/kg body weight in children) or lorazepam (4 mg in an adult and 0.1 mg/kg in a child).

Use of antidotes and elimination techniques

The only potentially effective method is repeat-dose activated charcoal, which acts by increasing quinine elimination. It is attractive to believe this will reduce the risk of complete blindness, but very difficult to obtain data to support this. A number of other treatments are reported in the old literature, but careful examination of the case stated suggests none are effective. Haemodialysis and haemoperfusion are ineffective.

Further reading

Bateman DN, Blain PG, Woodhouse KW, et al. (1985). Pharmacokinetics and clinical toxicology of quinine overdose: lack of efficacy of techniques intended to enhance elimination. *QJ Med*, 54:125–31.

Bateman DN, Dyson EH (1986). Quinine toxicity. *Adv Drug React Ac Pois Rev*, 4:215–33.

Dyson EH, Proudfoot AT, Bateman DN (1985–1986). Quinine amblyopia: is current management appropriate? *J Tox Clin Tox*, 23:571–8.

Langford NJ, Good AM, Laing WJ, et al. (2003). Quinine intoxication is reported to the Scottish Poisons Information Bureau 1997–2002: a continuing problem. *Br J Clin Pharmacol*, 56:576-8.

Thyroxine and tri-iodothyronine

Background

Thyroxine (levothyroxine, T4) is a naturally occurring hormone secreted by the thyroid gland which is used to treat thyroid deficiency states. Thyroxine is converted in the liver, kidney, and muscle to tri-iodothyronine (liothyronine, T3), which, on a weight-for-weight basis, is about five times more active than thyroxine. Poisoning may follow accidental or deliberate acute ingestion of one or other of these hormones, or may occur in patients prescribed excessive thyroid replacement therapy.

Toxicokinetics

T4 is well absorbed from the upper small bowel with a bioavailability of about 80%, but this may be affected by food and some drugs, e.g. sucralfate. T3 is almost completely absorbed, with an oral bioavailability of about 95%. Time to peak plasma concentration after therapeutic dosing is 2–4 hours for T4 and 2–6 hours for T3. T4 and, to a lesser extent T3, are both heavily bound to plasma proteins, including thyroid binding globulin. Metabolism of thyroid hormones is predominantly in the liver. Following T4 overdose in children the T4 elimination $t\frac{1}{2}$ is shorter (3 days) and the T3 $t\frac{1}{2}$ is longer (6–7 days) than normal, though in adults the T4 $t\frac{1}{2}$ varies between 5–10 days.

Mechanisms of toxicity

Thyroid hormones are essential for normal metabolism, growth and development and have physiological effects on almost all tissues. Thyroid hormones enter the cell via specific membrane transporter proteins. T4 is converted to T3 within the cell. Thyroid hormones, predominantly T3, are transported to the cell nucleus where they bind to a specific thyroid hormone receptor. The thyroid hormone-receptor complex binds with DNA resulting in modulation of gene expression, activation of transcription, increased RNA expression, and synthesis of key proteins including the Na/K ATPase and cardiac myosin proteins. The net effect is an increase in basal metabolic rate associated with increased fat mobilization, gluconeogenesis, and glycogenolysis. This is associated with increased sensitivity to catecholamines and the characteristic clinical features of hyperthyroidism (thyrotoxicosis) such as tachycardia, increased myocardial oxygen demand, tremor, and anxiety.

Risk factors for toxicity

Toxicity may be more marked in patients with underlying heart disease, and in the elderly. Angina or myocardial infarction may be precipitated by overdose in patients with underlying ischaemic heart disease.

Clinical features

Few features are to be expected after a single acute overdose of T4 or T3. Only four of 72 children developed symptoms after an overdose of thyroxine, presumably reflecting the magnitude of their overdose (≤0.5–≥3.0 mg). A retrospective review of 92 children ingesting up to 18.2 mg of thyroxine reported no serious toxicity, although minor symptoms occurred in eight patients. However, those ingesting substantial amounts of thyroxine or tri-iodothyronine will develop typical features of thyrotoxicosis.

Symptoms may develop within a few hours of tri-iodothyronine ingestion, but are not usually maximal for 3–6 days after thyroxine ingestion. Features tend to resolve in about the same time as they take to develop. Palpitations, sinus tachycardia, tremor, anxiety, irritability, insomnia, hyperactivity, sweating, diarrhoea and fever, are most common. Atrial fibrillation and convulsions have also been reported. Myocardial necrosis may occur rarely.

Massive thyroxine poisoning after a pharmaceutical error (T4 70–1200 mg over 2–12 days) led to the development of the classical symptoms of thyrotoxicosis in six patients within 3 days of the first dose. All six patients became comatose, two developed left ventricular failure, and three developed arrhythmias.

A 44-year-old woman who accidentally ingested a 1000 times overdose (400 mg T3 taken over 48 hours) suffered vomiting, palpitations, tachycardia, agitation, confusion, disorientation, hallucinations, aggressive behaviour, convulsions, and hyperpyrexia. Symptoms began 48 hours after beginning the ingestion. She developed pulmonary oedema, cardiac arrhythmias, and myopathy.

There are no long-term complications of acute overdose.

Chronic high doses of thyroxine or tri-iodothyronine may produce pronounced weight loss, anxiety, and accelerated osteoporosis. Myocarditis, cardiac dysrhythmias, tachycardia, cardiac failure, psychosis, and thyroid storm may occur.

Investigations

Free T4 and T3 concentrations (not thyroid-stimulating hormone) should be measured (though not urgently) in blood taken 6–12 hours after ingestion in patients who have taken more than 0.1 mg/kg; the results are useful for planning follow-up. An ECG should be performed if cardiovascular features are present.

Management

Activated charcoal 50 g may be considered in patients who present within 1 hour of a substantial overdose (e.g. >0.1 mg/kg of thyroxine or >10 micrograms/kg of tri-iodothyronine), but efficacy has not been established.

Patients with normal free thyroxine concentrations do not require follow-up, but those with high concentrations should be reviewed 3–6 days after ingestion to exclude delayed-onset hyperthyroidism.

If the features of thyrotoxicosis develop, the patient should be given propranolol 10–40 mg three times daily orally for 5 days. In more severe cases, and if there is no contraindication, propranolol 1 mg over 1 minute IV should be administered and repeated if there is no clinical response, to a maximum of 10 mg. Children should receive propranolol 250–500 micrograms/kg three times daily orally; in severe cases propranolol 25–50 micrograms/kg three times daily IV should be given up to a maximum of 5 mg.

Pyrexia should be treated with paracetamol and IV fluids may be required to correct dehydration. Benzodiazepines may occasionally be required for severe agitation. Anticonvulsant therapy may be necessary in severe cases. In patients who are acutely unwell, use of intravenous hydrocortisone 100 mg three times daily should be considered as this reduces the conversion of thyroxine to the more active T3. Otherwise care is supportive.

Plasmapheresis is not effective in increasing hormone elimination, though plasma exchange with fresh frozen plasma has been shown to be of some benefit. Haemodialysis is ineffective at enhancing thyroid hormone elimination.

Chronic overdose is managed by reducing the prescribed dose and, if necessary, by giving oral propranolol 40 mg three times daily.

Further reading

Binimelis J, Bassas L, Marruecos L, et al. (1987). Massive thyroxine intoxication: evaluation of plasma extraction. *Intensive Care Med*, 13:33–8.

Hack JB, Leviss JA, Nelson LS, et al. (1999). Severe symptoms following massive intentional L-thyroxine ingestion. *Vet Hum Toxicol*, 41:323–6.

Henderson A, Hickman P, Ward G, et al. (1994). Lack of efficacy of plasmapheresis in a patient overdosed with thyroxine. *Anaesth Intensive Care*, 22:463–4.

Jonare Å, Munkhammar P, Persson H (2001). A case of severe levothyroxine poisoning in a child. *J Toxicol Clin Toxicol*, 39:304–5.

Kirkland RT, Kirkland JL, Greger NG, et al. (1984). Thyroid hormone poisoning: therapy questioned. *Pediatrics*, 74:901.

Kulig K, Golightly LK, Rumack BH (1985). Levothyroxine overdose associated with seizures in a young child. *JAMA*, 254:2109–10.

Lewander WJ, Lacouture PG, Silva JE, et al. (1989). Acute thyroxine ingestion in pediatric patients. *Pediatrics*, 84:262–5.

Lin TH, Kirkland RT, Kirkland JL (1988). Clinical features and management of overdosage with thyroid drugs. *Med Toxicol Adverse Drug Exp*, 3:264–72.

Litovitz TL, White JD (1985). Levothyroxine ingestions in children: an analysis of 78 cases. *Am J Emerg Med*, 3:297–300.

Mandel SH, Magnussen AR, Burton BT, et al. (1989). Massive levothyroxine ingestion. *Clin Pediatr*, 28:374–6.

Matthews SJ (1993). Acute thyroxine overdosage: two cases of parasuicide. *Ulster Med J*, 62:170–3.

Nyström E, Lindstedt G, Lundberg P-A. (1980). Minor signs and symptoms of toxicity in a young woman in spite of massive thyroxine ingestion. *Acta Med Scand*, 207:135–6.

Shammas NW, Richeson JF, Pomerantz R. (1994). Myocardial dysfunction and necrosis after ingestion of thyroid hormone. *Am Heart J*, 127:232–4.

Shilo L, Kovatz S, Hadari R, et al. (2002). Massive thyroid hormone overdose: kinetics, clinical manifestations and management. *Isr Med Assoc J*, 4:298–9.

Sola E, Gomez-Balaguer M, Morillas C et al. (2002). Massive tri-iodothyronine intoxication: efficacy of hemoperfusion? *Thyroid*, 12:637–40.

Von Hofe SE, Young RL (1977). Thyrotoxicosis after a single ingestion of levothyroxine. *JAMA*, 237:1361.

Vitamins

Background

Vitamins are naturally occurring substances, present in small amounts in food, which are essential for normal metabolism (Table 7.6). Diets deficient in these essential vitamins can cause various deficiency diseases.

Dietary supplements containing vitamins are readily available for over-the-counter sale. Following a single acute overdose, serious toxicity is unlikely to occur from the vitamin content alone unless very large doses are ingested.

However, many of these preparations may also contain other ingredients such as iron, which may cause toxicity in overdose.

Acute ingestion

In most cases, symptoms other than gastrointestinal upset are unlikely to occur following acute ingestion of vitamins B_1, B_2, B_5, B_9 (folic acid), B_{12}, C, D, E, H, or K.

Parenteral administration of thiamine has been associated with hypersensitivity reactions ranging in severity from very mild to, very rarely, fatal anaphylactic shock.

Systemic toxicity may arise after substantial acute overdoses of vitamin A, B_3, B_6, or B_T, or excessive parenteral administration of vitamin C.

Vitamin A

Acute hypervitaminosis A has been reported following ingestions of vitamin A exceeding 300,000 IU in children and exceeding 600,000 IU in adults.

Clinical features

Features usually develop within 8–12 hours of ingestion.
GI: nausea, vomiting, abdominal pain, loss of appetite, hepatotoxicity.
Neurological: raised intracranial pressure, headache, photophobia, drowsiness, irritability, papilloedema, seizures.
Skin: pruritus and skin peeling (desquamation), which may be delayed.

Table 7.6 Readily available vitamins

Vitamin	Synonym
Vitamin A	Retinol
Vitamin B_1	Thiamine
Vitamin B_2	Riboflavin
Vitamin B_3	Nicotinic acid (niacin)
Vitamin B_5	Pantothenic acid
Vitamin B_6	Pyridoxine
Vitamin B_9 or B_{11}	Folic acid
Vitamin B_{12}	Cyanocobalamin
Vitamin B_T	L-carnitine
Vitamin C	Ascorbic acid
Vitamin D_2	Ergocalciferol
Vitamin D_3	Colecalciferol
Vitamin E	Alpha tocopherol
Vitamin H	Biotin
Vitamin K	Phytomenadione

Management

- Activated charcoal may be given within 1 hour of a massive ingestion of vitamin A.
- Asymptomatic patients should be observed for at least 12 hours. FBC, U&Es, creatinine, LFTs, blood glucose, arterial blood gases, and an ECG should be performed. The fundi and visual acuity should be assessed.
- Liaise with neurological/neurosurgical team early in patients presenting with features of raised intracranial pressure.

Vitamin B_3

Nicotinic acid causes release of prostaglandin D_2 and can cause vasodilatory effects and skin flushing at doses exceeding 1 g. It is occasionally used for treatment of hyperlipidaemia.

Clinical features

Skin: severe skin flushing which may be accompanied by itching.
GI: nausea, vomiting.

Management

Activated charcoal may be given within 1 hour of a massive ingestion. Otherwise management is symptomatic. Antihistamines may be helpful for itching.

Vitamin B_6

Acute ingestion is unlikely to cause clinical effects, although an acute permanent sensory peripheral neuropathy has been reported in two patients administered 2 g/kg pyridoxine intravenously and seizures may occur following large overdoses.

Clinical features

Neurological: seizures, loss of proprioception and vibration sense, sensory ataxia, reduced or absent peripheral reflexes.

Vitamin B_T (L-carnitine)

Seizures have been reported after acute ingestion. These should be treated conventionally.

Vitamin C

Vitamin C is absorbed in the small intestine via a saturable active transport mechanism. Uptake of vitamin C to tissues and metabolism to oxalic acid are also saturable processes.

Although precipitation of oxalate crystals in renal tubules is theoretically possible following ingestion of very large doses, this rarely occurs in practice as a result of poor absorption of the excess dose and saturated metabolic pathways.

However, following excessive parenteral administration of vitamin C, particularly in patients with renal impairment, formation of oxalate stones has been reported.

Chronic ingestion

Toxicity is much more frequently associated with consumption of excessive doses of vitamins A, B_3, B_6, D, or E over a prolonged period.

Vitamin A

Chronic toxicity may result after ingestion of 25,000–50,000 IU/day or more for several months or years.

Clinical features

GI: anorexia and gastrointestinal upset are the main features. Hepatotoxicity characterized by hyper-bilirubinaemia and elevated alkaline phosphatase and transaminases may occur and lead to jaundice, cirrhosis, portal hypertension, oesophageal varices and ascites.

Skin/hair: dry and fragile skin, pruritus, erythema, desquamation. Hair thinning and alopecia may develop and curly or kinky hair may regrow.

Skeletal: bone, joint and muscle pain. X-rays may show skeletal hyperostoses and calcification of tendon and ligaments, periosteal thickening, and bone demineralization. Premature epiphyseal closure has been reported in children.

Metabolic: hypercalcaemia may result from increased bone resorption.

Neurological: raised intracranial pressure, headache, visual disturbances, fatigue, irritability, depression.

Management

- Intake of vitamin A should be discontinued.
- Blood should be sent for FBC, U&Es, creatinine, LFTs, calcium, and phosphate.
- Management is symptomatic and supportive according to the clinical features present.

Vitamin B₃

Toxicity has been reported after chronic administration of high doses (2–3 g daily).

Clinical features

Skin: skin flushing and itching.

CVS: hypotension.

GI: fatigue, anorexia, nausea, vomiting. Hepatotoxicity with jaundice and elevated liver enzymes which can rarely progress to hepatic failure and encephalopathy.

Metabolic: lactic acidosis may occur.

Neurological: myopathy has been reported.

Management

Intake should be discontinued and blood sent for liver function tests. Management is symptomatic and supportive.

Vitamin B₆

Sensory peripheral neuropathy may occur after long term ingestion of doses of vitamin B6 exceeding 200 mg/day.

Clinical features

Neurological: numbness, paraesthesia. loss of proprioception and vibration sense, sensory ataxia, reduced or absent peripheral reflexes.

Management

Intake should be discontinued.

Nerve conduction studies may confirm the presence of distal sensory peripheral nerve dysfunction. Nerve biopsy may show widespread non-specific axonal degeneration.

There is no specific treatment for pyridoxine-induced peripheral neuropathy.

Vitamin D

Toxicity may occur following chronic ingestion of excessive doses (e.g. 50,000–150000 IU vitamin D daily in an adult).

Clinical features

The cardinal feature of vitamin D toxicity is hypercalcaemia.

GI: nausea, vomiting, abdominal pain, constipation.

Renal: polyuria and polydipsia, nephrocalcinosis, and impaired renal function.

Cardiac: cardiac arrhythmias, ECG abnormalities include increased PR interval, widened QRS complex, and shortened QT interval.

Management

Intake should be discontinued.

Check serum calcium and U&Es. Measurement of 25-hydroxy cholecalciferol may confirm excess intake. In patients with hypercalcaemia, rehydrate and consider the use of bisphosphonates in severe cases.

Vitamin E

Toxicity may occur following chronic ingestion of doses of vitamin E exceeding 1000 IU/day. Vitamin E antagonizes the effect of vitamin K and may cause coagulopathy in patients who take warfarin or are vitamin K deficient.

Clinical features

GI: nausea, vomiting, abdominal pain, constipation, or diarrhoea.

Neurological: fatigue, headache, and weakness.

Management

- Intake should be discontinued.
- Blood should be sent for INR or prothrombin time.
- Coagulopathy may be reversed with vitamin K.
- Management is symptomatic and supportive.

Further reading

Albin RL, Alpers JW, Greenberg HS, *et al*. (1987). Acute sensory neuropathy from pyridoxine overdose. *Neurology*, 37:1729–32.

Auer BL, Auer D, Rodgers AL (1998). Relative hyperoxaluria, crystalluria and haematuria after megadose ingestion of vitamin C. *Eur J Clin Invest*, 28:695–700.

Coghlan D, Cranswick NE (2001). Complementary medicine and vitamin A toxicity in children. *MJA*, 175:223–4.

Hathcock JN, Hattan DG, Jenkins MY, *et al*. (1990). Evaluation of vitamin A toxicity. *Am J Clin Nutr*, 52: 183–202.

James MB, Leonard JC, Fraser JJ Jr, *et al* (1982). Hypervitaminosis A: a case report. *Pediatrics*, 69:112–15.

LaMantia RS, Andrews CE (1981). Acute vitamin A intoxication. *South Med J*, 74:1012–14.

Marie J, See G (1953). Benign acute hydrocephalus in infant after administration of a single massive dose of vitamin A. *Ann Paediatr*, 180:308–14.

Morra M, Philipszoon HD, D'Andrea G, *et al*. (1993). Sensory and motor neuropathy caused by excessive ingestion of vitamin B6: a case report. *Funct Neurol*, 8:429–32.

Oren R, Ilan Y (1992). Reversible hepatic injury induced by long-term vitamin A ingestion. *Am J Med*, 93:7034.

Pauling L (1984). Sensory neuropathy from pyridoxine abuse. *N Engl Med J*, 310: 197

Thomson AD, Cook CCH (1997). Parenteral thiamine and Wernicke's encephalopathy: the balance of risks and perception of concern. *Alcohol Alcohol*, 32:207–9.

Winter SL, Boyer JL (1973). Hepatic toxicity from large doses of vitamin B3. *N Engl J Med*, 289:1180–2.

Wong K et al. (1994). Acute oxalate nephropathy after a massive intravenous dose of vitamin C. *Aust NZ J Med*, 24:410–11.

Drugs of abuse

Introduction to problems in the drug user

Background

Recreational drug use is common and may have significant acute and/or chronic health effects. These may be related both to the direct pharmacological/toxicological effects of the drugs involved and/or associated complications related to drug use such as blood-borne virus or bacterial infection related to intravenous drug use.

Categories of recreational drugs

From a toxicological perspective, recreational and illicit drugs can be divided into three broad categories: stimulants, depressants, and hallucinogens. Examples of common drugs from each of these classes are as follows, and are discussed in individual sections in this chapter:

Stimulants

- Cocaine and synthetic cocaine derivatives, e.g. dimethocaine, fluorotropocaine
- Amfetamines and amfetamine-type stimulants, e.g. 3,4-methylenedioxymethamfetmine (MDMA, 'ecstasy'), methamfetamine, para-methoxyamfetamine (PMA)
- Cathinones, e.g. 4-methylmethcathinone (mephedrone), 3,4-methylenedioxymeth-cathinone (methylone)
- Piperazines, e.g. 1-benzylpiperazine (BZP), trifluoromethylphenylpiperazine (TFMPP)
- Piperidines, e.g. 2-diphenylmethylpiperidine (desoxypipradrol), diphenyl-2-pyrrolidinyl-methanol (diphenylprolinol).

Depressants

- Opioids, e.g. heroin, opium and morphine
- gamma-hydroxybutyrate (GHB) and its analogues gamma-butyrolactone (GBL) and 1,4-butanediol (1,4-BD)
- Benzodiazepines, e.g. diazepam, lorazepam, temazepam.

Hallucinogens

- Cannabis
- Synthetic cannabinoid receptor agonists ('Spice'/'K2')
- Ketamine and the ketamine analogues, e.g. methoxetamine
- Lysergic acid diethylamide (LSD)
- Psilocybin ('magic mushrooms').

Epidemiology of recreational drug use

Recreational drugs are commonly used throughout the world. The patterns of use vary both between and within countries. There are also differences in use in certain subpopulations, for example, greater use in those who frequent the night-time economy and other recreational settings (e.g. nightclubs, pubs, music festivals) and in the men who have sex with men (gay) community. In the last 5–10 years there has been increasing use of a range of novel psychoactive substances (often termed 'legal highs'; and sometimes sold under trade names such as 'bath salts', 'plant food', or 'research chemicals').

Classical, established recreational drugs such as cocaine, amfetamines, and heroin are usually supplied through street-level drug dealers. Street-level drug dealers are also increasingly supplying novel psychoactive substances, but these drugs are also commonly supplied through other routes such as Internet 'legal high' websites and high street 'head shops'.

Street names

Street names or colloquial names are often used by users to refer to drugs; these names can cause confusion as the same name can be used for two different drugs (e.g. 'acid' can be used for LSD or amfetamine). Therefore clinicians managing patients who present after recreational drug use should always try and establish the actual name(s) of the drug(s) that a user has taken rather than just the street name(s).

Adulterants

Many recreational drugs are cut or adulterated to add bulk. The adulterants used are either inert bulking agents such as talc, sugars (e.g. lactose, fructose), flour, or active pharmaceutical ingredients (APIs). The APIs used are often chosen to mimic or enhance the effects of the drug (e.g. local anaesthetics such as lidocaine and benzocaine used as cocaine adulterants, quinine as a heroin adulterant), for their physical resemblance to the drug (e.g. phenacetin in crack cocaine) or to facilitate the administration of the drug (e.g. caffeine in heroin or crack cocaine). Adulterants may have important toxic effects, for example, blood dyscrasias associated with levamisole, a common adulterant of cocaine preparations.

A number of studies have demonstrated significant variation in the content of recreational drugs; in addition to adulterants, there can be variation in both the amount of and the actual recreational drug found, such that a drug sold under one name may in fact contain a completely different drug.

It is therefore important that clinicians managing patients with recreational toxicity are alert to the variable content of these drugs and consider that exposure to other recreational drugs or adulterants may be responsible for some of the toxicity seen. This also has potential legal implications for users as substances described on websites and by dealers as being legal may contain illegal, controlled drugs.

Routes of use

Recreational drugs may be used by a variety of routes including: nasal insufflation ('snorting'), smoking, oral ingestion, intravenous ('mainlining') or subcutaneous ('skin popping') injection, and less commonly other routes such as rectal or sublingual administration. The route of use can be important for a number of reasons:

Pharmacokinetic differences

Intravenous administration, smoking, and to a lesser extent nasal insufflation are associated with more rapid systemic absorption/availability of the drug and therefore a more rapid onset of clinical effects than oral ingestion.

Dependence potential

The more rapid onset of action and more intense 'high' associated with intravenous use and smoking result in these routes being generally associated with greater dependence potential than others, such as the oral route.

Secondary complications

Drug users may have poor general health relating to poor nutrition, sleeping rough, or use of tobacco and alcohol, increasing their risk of secondary complications:

- Blood-borne virus infections such as HIV or hepatitis B or C related to sharing drug paraphernalia such as injection needles, smoking pipes, or insufflation straws.
- Bacterial infection related to use of unsterilized injection needles and other injection paraphernalia. *Staphylococcus* and *Streptococcus* species are commonly involved although *Pseudomonas, Serratia, Candida*, and many others may be involved. Infections may be local at the site of injection or systemic, including septicaemia, bacterial endocarditis (especially affecting the right side of the heart), lung abscesses, osteomyelitis, and septic arthritis. Evidence also indicates that risks of community-acquired pneumonia, aspiration pneumonia, and tuberculosis are increased.
- Mucosal damage related to trauma to the nose and/or the local anaesthetic effects of nasal insufflation of drugs such as cocaine.
- Respiratory problems related to heat damage from smoking crack cocaine or heroin and occasionally cannabis.

Hospital admission provides an opportunity to diagnose medical problems, plan appropriate management, and educate users, including about safer drug use.

Patterns of acute toxicity

Each of the three main categories of recreational drugs is associated with a specific pattern of acute toxicity. Some drugs have effects that bridge these categories; nevertheless these categories can be useful as they help to guide the management of patients with acute recreational drug toxicity. This subsection briefly describes patterns of toxicity; further details, including the clinical management of toxicity associated with these drugs is provided in the relevant sections of this book.

Stimulants

These drugs are sympathomimetics and their desired effects and toxicity are both due to an increase in the release of and/or decrease in the re-uptake of sympathetic amines including norepinephrine, serotonin, and dopamine. The different individual drugs and drug classes have differing relative effects on these neurotransmitter systems. This is responsible for the variation in the spectrum of clinical effects seen with different individual drugs/drug classes. Common clinical features seen in patients with stimulant drug toxicity and the more severe complications that can occur are described in more detail in the relevant sections of this chapter.

Depressants

These drugs cause their effects through a range of different pharmacological mechanisms (e.g. opioids at opioid receptors, benzodiazepines at GABA$_A$ receptors, GHB at GABA$_B$ receptors). Toxicity associated with all of these drugs results in central nervous system depression with drowsiness, which may progress to coma, respiratory depression, loss of airway reflexes, aspiration pneumonia, and respiratory arrest. Risk of these complications is increased with high dose, if more than one depressant drug is taken and/or if these drugs are used together with ethanol or other depressants. The other features seen depend on the drug/drug class with opioids causing pin-point pupils and GHB and its analogues causing agitation, vomiting, and convulsions.

Hallucinogens

These drugs are generally of lower inherent toxicity than the stimulants and depressants and although they can cause unpleasant symptoms they are much less likely to cause systemic and/or life-threatening clinical features. Common effects include auditory and visual hallucinations, an altered sense of reality, dissociative effects, paranoia, and drowsiness; agitation, aggression, and hypertension can occur but are rarely severe. If significant systemic toxicity is present, clinicians should consider use of other recreational drugs or alternative explanations for the clinical features.

Chronic toxicity

The chronic toxicity associated with recreational drug use is generally less well characterized than the patterns of acute toxicity associated with these drugs. However, there are some clear associations. These include an increased incidence of psychiatric morbidity such as depression and psychosis in chronic cocaine users, cardiomyopathy and an increased incidence of atheromatous coronary artery disease in chronic cocaine users, and haemorrhagic cystitis and other lower urinary tract pathology associated with chronic ketamine use.

Dependency and withdrawal

Dependence can occur with many of the recreational drugs; this is more likely in frequent users and in those who use drugs outside recreational settings. Generally, these drugs cause psychological dependence rather than physical (pharmacological) dependence. Physical dependence is most likely amongst the depressant class of drugs, e.g. opioids, GHB and its analogues, and benzodiazepines. These can cause significant dependence and an acute withdrawal syndrome on cessation of use of the drug(s). Information on management of withdrawal is provided in the relevant sections of this chapter. Clinicians managing patients with acute recreational drug toxicity should consider whether the user has 'problematic', dependent, drug use and if this is the case consider referral to an appropriate drug service or clinic for support.

Social effects of drug use

Detailed consideration is beyond the scope of this book but drug use may lead to relationship breakdown, job loss and financial hardship, and interfere with education in younger people. Criminal behaviour may result from the need to fund an expensive drug habit. This may include theft or drug dealing, the latter potentially involving clashes with rival dealers. Violent, destructive, or irresponsible behaviour may also occur while under the influence of drugs, which may be associated with accidents, domestic violence, sexually transmitted infections, and unwanted pregnancy.

Further reading

Cole C, Jones L, McVeigh J, *et al.* (2010). *CUT. A Guide to Adulterants, Bulking Agents and Other Contaminants Found in Illicit Drugs.* Liverpool: North West Public Health Observatory. <http://www.cph.org.uk/publication/cut-a-guide-to-the-adulterants-bulking-agents-and-other-contaminants-found-in-illicit-drugs/>.

Gibbons S (2012). 'Legal highs'—novel and emerging psychoactive drugs: a chemical overview for the toxicologist. *Clin Toxicol*, 50:15–24.

Gordon RJ, Lowery FD (2005). Current concepts: bacterial infections in drug users. *N Engl J Med*, 353:1945–54.

Amfetamines and related compounds

Background

A large number of drugs have stimulant, entactogenic, and/or hallucinogenic effects as a result of effects on sympathetic, dopaminergic, and serotoninergic receptor systems. Chemical drug groups sharing these actions with variable potency include phenethylamines (including amfetamines and cathinones), piperazines, and piperidines. Cocaine, ketamine, ergolines (e.g. LSD), and tryptamines also share some of these effects but are described elsewhere (see specific sections in this chapter).

Amfetamine is a substituted phenylethylamine (β-phenylisopropylamine). The terms 'amfetamines' and 'amfetamine-type stimulants' (ATS) are commonly used to describe a group of stimulant (sympathomimetic) recreational drugs which are analogues of amfetamine with various different substitutions on the phenylethylamine structure.

Cathinones are beta ketonated phenethylamines; cathinone and methcathinone are found in the khat plant (see Cannabis and khat, pp. 184–185), but synthetic cathinones, in particular 4-methylmethcathinone (mephedrone), are commonly used recreationally.

Piperazines and piperidines, while not phenethylamines, are covered in this section because they share pharmacological and clinical effects with the amfetamines and cathinones.

Classification

Examples of common or important amfetamines, cathinones, piperazines and piperidines are shown in Table 8.1.

Recreational use

Amfetamines and cathinones may be taken orally, by nasal insufflation or intravenous injection. The piperazines and piperidines are usually taken orally or by nasal insufflation.

Until recently the amfetamines were the most commonly used drugs in this group, particularly MDMA; although the relative use of stimulants in the amfetamine group varies across the world. More recently piperazines (especially 1-benzylpiperazine) and cathinones (especially mephedrone) have been used increasingly. Prior to their widespread use, these drugs, sometimes termed 'legal highs', had not been controlled in many countries and their easy availability via the Internet as well as via retail outlets (e.g. 'head shops') had also facilitated distribution. Mephedrone and other cathinones were commonly sold under the description of 'plant food', 'bath salts', or as 'research chemicals not for human consumption'.

The content of amfetamines and other recreational drugs bought on the street and through other sources such as the Internet and high street 'head shops' is variable. It is therefore important that clinicians managing patients with toxicity are alert to this and consider that the patient may have used other recreational drugs or that adulterants (cutting agents) such as caffeine, lidocaine, or benzocaine may be present and responsible for some of the toxicity seen. Clinicians and drugs users should be aware that drugs sold under one name (e.g. MDMA or amfetamine) may on analysis contain a different drug (e.g. 1-benzylpiperazine or mephedrone) and

Table 8.1 Examples of drugs within the amfetamine, cathinone, piperazine, and piperidine groups

Chemical name	Abbreviations/ common names
Amfetamines	
Amfetamine	'Speed''
Methamfetamine,	'Meth'
	'Crystal meth'
3,4 methlyenedioxymethamfetmine	MDMA,
	'Ecstasy'
3,4 methylenedioxy N-ethylamfetamine	MDEA
	'Eve'
3,4-methylenedioxyamfetamine	MDA
N-methyl-1-(3,4-methylenedioxyphenyl)-2-aminobutane	MBDB
Para-methoxyamfetamine	PMA
	'Death'
Para-methoxymethamfetamine	PMMA
4-chloro-2,5-dimethoxyamfetamine	DOC
4-bromo-2,5-dimethoxyamfetamine	DOB
4-fluoromethamfetamine	
4-methylthioamfetamine	4-MTA
4-bromo-2,5-dimethoxyphenylethylamine	2-CB
Cathinones	
4-methylmethcathinone	Mephedrone
4-methoxymethcathinone	Methedrone
3,4-methylenedioxymethcathinone,	Methylone
4-fluoromethcathinone	Flephedrone
Piperazines	
1-benzylpiperazine	BZP
Trifluoromethylphenylpiperazine	TFMPP
Paramethoxyphenylpiperazine	MeOPP
Meta-chlorophenylpiperazine	mCPP
Piperidines	
2-diphenylmethylpiperidine	2-DPMP
	Desoxypipradrol
diphenyl-2-pyrrolidinyl-methanol	D2PM
	Diphenylprolinol

that substances described on websites and by dealers as being legal may in reality contain legally controlled drugs.

Mechanism of toxicity

Amfetamines and related drugs are sympathomimetic (stimulant) recreational drugs that increase the release of and decrease the re-uptake of sympathetic amines including norepinephrine, serotonin, and dopamine. The different individual agents have differing relative effects on these neurotransmitter systems, which is responsible for the spectrum of clinical effects seen with different individual drugs.

Toxicokinetics

Nasal insufflation and, in particular intravenous, use of these drugs is associated with more rapid-onset clinical effects than oral ingestion. The elimination half-life of amfetamine is pH dependant and is 7–14 hours below and 18–34 hours above a urinary pH of 6.7. Reported half-lives are also available for other drugs in this class including methamfetamine (10 hours), MDMA (7.6 hours), and benzylpiperazine (5.5 hours). Little data is available for the other drugs described in this section, although prolonged clinical effects lasting over 24 hours have been described after use of some of the novel drugs, in particular 2-DPMP and D2PM.

Clinical features

The common symptoms and signs that are seen in amfetamine, cathinone, piperazine, or piperidine toxicity are:
- central nervous system excitation: anxiety, psychomotor agitation, anxiety, hallucinations and delusions
- sweating
- dilated pupils
- tachycardia, palpitations
- hypertension
- bruxism (grinding of the jaws and teeth)
- hypertonia, hyper-reflexia, tremor.

Hypokalaemia, hyperglycaemia, and a metabolic acidosis may also be seen.

Complications

The severe features and complications seen and the likelihood of these developing vary with different agents. As an example, severe agitation and psychosis is more commonly seen with methamfetamine and the piperidines 2-DPMP and D2PM; hyperpyrexia and serotonin toxicity (sometimes referred to as serotonin syndrome) are more common in individuals with acute PMA/PMMA and to a lesser extent acute MDMA (ecstasy) toxicity. Potential complications include:
- seizures
- severe agitation, acute psychosis, delusions, paranoia.
- arrhythmias: narrow complex tachycardias and more rarely ventricular tachycardia or ventricular fibrillation
- aortic dissection
- stroke—related to intracerebral haemorrhage and/or infarction
- mesenteric ischaemia
- chest pain (angina), acute coronary syndrome and myocardial infarction; this is less common that with other sympathomimetic recreational drugs such as cocaine
- hyperthermia: severe hyperthermia can be associated with significant secondary complications including rhabdomyolysis, disseminated intravascular coagulation, acute kidney injury and acute liver dysfunction
- hyponatraemia due to syndrome of inappropriate antidiuretic hormone (SIADH) or water intoxication due to repeated stereotypical behaviour.

Management

Patients with toxicity related to amfetamine, cathinone, or piperazine use should have a 12-lead ECG and monitoring of heart rate, blood pressure, and body temperature.

Agitation and delirium

Patients should be managed in a quiet environment with minimal stimulation. Significant agitation can make it difficult to fully assess and treat patients and puts both the patient and staff at risk. Sedatives such as benzodiazepines are often required. These can be given orally (e.g. diazepam (0.1–0.3 mg/kg body weight) or, in those with more significant agitation, parenterally (e.g. 5–10mg diazepam IV). Large doses (e.g. 1–2mg/kg diazepam) may be required, but this should be given in small boluses titrated against the patient's agitation. Neuroleptics such as haloperidol should generally only be used as second-line agents, after adequate dosing with benzodiazepines, as they can lower the seizure threshold.

Seizures

In patients with seizures it is important to ensure adequate oxygenation, check the blood glucose, and correct acid–base abnormalities. Seizures should initially be treated with parenteral benzodiazepines (e.g. intravenous diazepam 10 mg in adults; 0.25 mg/kg body weight in children) or lorazepam (4 mg in an adult; 0.1 mg/kg in a child). Seizures that are resistant to treatment with benzodiazepines should be managed with intravenous phenobarbital sodium (10 mg/kg at maximum rate of 100 mg/minute; maximum dose 1 g).

Cardiovascular effects

Common cardiovascular features such as tachycardia and hypertension often settle following benzodiazepine administration. Beta-blockers should be avoided as they can result in unopposed alpha-stimulation and worsening hypertension and coronary artery vasoconstriction. Patients with ongoing severe hypertension (e.g. systolic BP greater than 200 mmHg, diastolic BP greater than 120 mmHg) despite adequate sedation with benzodiazepines may require treatment with vasodilators such as nitrates (e.g. intravenous glyceryl trinitrate, starting at 1–2 mg/hour) or alpha-blockers (e.g. phentolamine or phenoxybenzamine).

Hyperthermia

Hyperthermia should be treated aggressively as persistent hyperpyrexia (temperature greater than 39–40° C) is associated with a poor prognosis and a high incidence of secondary complications such as rhabdomyolysis, disseminated intravascular coagulation, acute kidney injury and liver failure. Simple, conventional cooling methods (e.g. cold intravenous fluids, ice packs) should be used initially together with benzodiazepine sedation. Patients with persistent hyperpyrexia greater than 39–40° C despite this initial therapy should be discussed with a clinical toxicologist or poisons centre and further measures such as invasive cooling, dantrolene, or a serotonin antagonist such as cyproheptadine may be considered depending on the amfetamine responsible for the hyperpyrexia.

Further reading

Dargan PI, Sedefov R, Gallegos A, et al. (2011). The pharmacology and toxicology of the synthetic cathinone mephedrone (4-methylmethcathinone). Drug Test Anal, 3:454–63.

Gibbons S (2012). 'Legal highs'— novel and emerging psychoactive drugs: a chemical overview for the toxicologist. Clin Toxicol, 50:15–24.

Greene SL, Kerr F, Braitberg G (2008). Review article: amphetamines and related drugs of abuse. Emerg Med Australas, 20:391–402.

Schep LJ, Slaughter RJ, Beasley DM (2010). The clinical toxicology of metamfetamine. Clin Toxicol, 48:675–94.

Cannabis and khat

Cannabis

Background and therapeutic use

'Cannabis' refers to the *Cannabis sativa* plant, which contains a number of chemicals (>60) known as the cannabinoids. The major active chemical in cannabis, tetrahydrocannabinol (THC), is found mainly in the leaves and flowering tops. Marijuana is the commonly used name to describe the dried leaves and flowers of the cannabis plant. Cannabis resin is obtained by compressing plant material into hard blocks. The typical THC content of outdoor cultivated marijuana or resin was 2–6%, but this may be increased to up to 10% by intensive indoor cultivation methods. Sinsemilla, the flowering tops of intensively cultivated female plants, contains approximately 13% THC and is the predominant form sold in the UK recently.

Cannabis is typically smoked or ingested, although a small number of users may inject cannabis via the intravenous route. Cannabis is usually rolled with tobacco for smoking or vaporized in a smoking device.

The cannabis plant has been grown legally for many years for the fibre known as 'hemp'. Additionally, there is increasing interest in the use of medicinal cannabis in the management of chronic pain and spasticity (particularly associated with multiple sclerosis), control of chemotherapy-related vomiting, and in patients with cancer and HIV to improve appetite. One product is available in the UK (Sativex®), which contains delta-9-tetrahydrocannabinol and cannabidiol.

There are reports of recreational use of cannabis dating back thousands of years. Cannabis is used worldwide recreationally by a considerable proportion of the population. In the 2009/10 British Crime Survey, 30.6% of individuals reported having ever used cannabis, 6.6% had used it in the last year, and 3.9% had used it in the last month.

In recent years reports of use of synthetic cannabinoid receptor agonists (SCRA) have become common. These products, sometimes referred to as 'spice' or 'K2', contain a variety of cannabinoid receptor agonists including JWH-018, JWH-073, JWH-081, JWH-250, CP 47, and WIN 55,212.

Pharmacokinetics

The absorption of cannabinoids from cannabis is dependent on the route of use. Following inhalation of smoked cannabis, there is rapid onset of the desired physiological effects, with peak effects and plasma concentrations occurring within 10 minutes of inhalation. Approximately 10–35% of the smoked cannabinoids are absorbed through this route. Absorption after oral ingestion is less predictable, and typically peak effects occur within 2–4 hours of ingestion; due to first-past metabolism and the effects of gastric acid, only up to 20% of in the ingested amount reaches the systemic circulation. Initially the cannabinoids are distributed to the more vascularized tissues (e.g. brain) before distributing more slowly to fatty tissues. Cannabinoids are very lipid-soluble and accumulate in fatty tissues in chronic users

THC is metabolized by the hepatic cytochrome P450 isoenzyme system (particularly CYP2C) to 11-hydroxy-THC. This metabolite has biological activity similar to that of THC, and is metabolized to the inactive 11-nor-THC carboxylic acid metabolite. Both THC and its active and inactive metabolites are excreted in urine and faeces; although THC is typically not detectable in the urine more than 5–7 days following use, the metabolites may be detectable in the urine for a more prolonged period of time. In chronic users of cannabis, the metabolites may be detected for weeks following the last exposure.

Mechanism of action

Following the discovery that THC was the major active component of cannabis in 1964, the cannabinoid receptors CB1 and CB2 at which cannabis has its activity were not identified until the 1990s. CB1 receptors are located throughout the brain (particularly in the globus pallidus, basal ganglia, substantia nigra, hippocampus, and the cerebral cortex). It is thought that activation of the CB1 receptors by cannabinoids is responsible for the desired euphoria and other effects associated with cannabis use, as well as the nausea and vomiting. The CB2 receptors, thought to be responsible for some of the medicinal use effects of cannabis, are located peripherally.

Acute cannabis toxicity

It is uncommon to see individuals presenting to healthcare facilities following the use of cannabis. Where individuals do present, it is important to ensure that other drug(s) are not responsible for the presentation. The majority of adverse effects are usually managed in the pre-hospital environment by the friends of the individual who becomes unwell.

Typical clinical effects following oral ingestion or inhalation of THC include excitement followed by calmness and euphoria. Undesired features include nausea and vomiting, tachycardia, anxiety, and paranoia/panic. Vomiting is reported to occur more frequently when THC is co-used with ethanol. Vasodilatation may be associated with conjunctival injection, dizziness, and postural hypotension. Cannabis smoking may exacerbate asthma and the risk of myocardial infarction is increased for 1–2 hours after use. Pneumothorax has also been reported. In children, there have been reports of hypotonia and hyporeflexia associated with accidental ingestion of cannabis.

In addition to the unwanted effects just described, there have been reports of fever, rigors, hypotension, renal and hepatic impairment, and myotoxicity following intravenous injection of THC/cannabis.

Clinical experience of toxicity after use of SCRA is limited, but tachycardia, hypertension, hallucinations, and seizures may occur and renal toxicity has also been reported.

Management of acute cannabis toxicity

The management of acute cannabis toxicity is largely supportive. Affected patients should be reassured that the symptoms will settle over time. Anti-emetics may be required for persistent vomiting. For those with significant agitation/anxiety, benzodiazepines may be useful although these should be avoided in children because the risk of paradoxical reactions. Other symptoms/clinical features should be managed appropriately.

Toxicity associated with chronic cannabis use

Long-term use of cannabis is thought to be associated with a number of potential adverse effects. Smoking of cannabis, with or without additional tobacco, is thought to potentially increase the risk of chronic obstructive airways disease with formation of bullae and of respiratory tract carcinomas, although the association has not yet been demonstrated clearly. There are also unconfirmed reported associations with prostate cancer and astrocytoma. There are reports that long-term use is associated with reduced fertility (in both males and females).

Chronic heavy use of cannabis is associated with the development of an 'amotivational syndrome', as well as reduced cognitive function. There is evidence that some individuals develop a dependence syndrome associated with chronic cannabis use, with a withdrawal syndrome on discontinuation of the cannabis use. There is evidence for a link between cannabis use and development of schizophrenia, although data is observational and it is difficult to prove a cause–effect relationship.

Khat

Background and therapeutic use
The khat plant (*Catha edulis*) is an evergreen plant that grows in the horn of Africa and Arabian peninsula. Leaves are chewed by a large proportion of the adult population living in or originating from Somalia and other East African countries. The leaves contain the amfetamine-related stimulants cathinone and cathine, and it is thought that these are responsible for the effects associated with chewing khat leaves.

The khat leaves are chewed over several hours, with the leaves stored in the cheeks in between chewing episodes, and saliva containing the juices from the leaves is swallowed. There is no known medicinal or pharmaceutical use of khat.

Cathinone breaks down to cathine within 48 hours of the leaves being removed from the plant. It is thought that cathinone has greater biological activity than cathine so importers of the leaves need to maintain the freshness of the leaves by freezing and/or ensure rapid importation, for a greater cathinone content. Both cathinone and cathine are structurally related to the synthetic cathinones (e.g. 4-methylmethcathinone, mephedrone) discussed elsewhere in this textbook.

There are significant international differences in the legal control of khat and its major active ingredients cathinone and cathine. In European countries, such as France, the Netherlands, Norway, and Poland, both khat and its major active ingredients are controlled under the relevant national drugs legislation. This will shortly also be the case in the UK, where previously the ingredients were controlled but not the plant or leaves. In the USA, both cathinone and cathine are controlled, and therefore technically the khat plant is also controlled as this contains cathinone and cathine. Finally, in Australia, at this time it remains possible to obtain licences to import khat.

Pharmacokinetics
Cathinone and cathine are phenylethylamines, in common with a number of other stimulant sympathomimetic drugs (e.g. amfetamine), as well as the catecholamines dopamine, epinephrine, and norepinephrine.

On chewing the khat leaves, the released cathinone and cathine are rapidly absorbed. Some is absorbed via the oral mucosa but the majority of the cathinone is absorbed from the gastrointestinal tract after swallowing saliva containing juices from the khat leaves. Cathinone has a relatively short duration of action, and its peak

effects last up to 30 minutes in duration. It is almost completely broken down (98% of ingested/absorbed amount) into norephedrine in the liver. The pharmacology of cathine is less well understood, but it is thought that its duration of action is approximately 3 hours.

Mechanism of action
Both cathinone and cathine block the re-uptake of epinephrine and norepinephrine, and it is thought that these actions are responsible for the 'wakefulness/alertness' that khat users describe. Animal studies have shown that serotonin receptors have high affinity for cathinone, and it is thought that this activity is responsible for the euphoria associated with chewing khat leaves. Finally, cathine is thought to act on adrenergic receptors, resulting in the release of epinephrine and norepinephrine, increasing the effects of the blockade of uptake by both cathine and cathinone.

Acute khat toxicity
The acute toxicity associated with chewing khat is similar to that seen with other stimulant sympathomimetics. Because release of cathinone and cathine requires prolonged chewing of the leaves, this limits the risk of acute toxicity and it is unusual to see individuals with severe khat-related toxicity.

Clinical features of acute khat toxicity are similar to those seen with toxicity associated with other sympathomimetics and include dizziness, tachycardia, hypertension, palpitations/arrhythmias, nausea, dilated pupils, sweating, headache, agitation and aggression, anxiety, pyrexia, urinary retention, and hallucinations. Severe features of toxicity seen with other sympathomimetics (e.g. seizures and cardiovascular toxicity) are, however, rarely seen in relation to khat.

Following use of khat, uses may enter a depressible phase which may be followed by irritability, anorexia, and insomnia which may last 1–2 days and encourage the user to chew khat again to alleviate these features.

Management of acute khat toxicity
The management of acute khat toxicity is dependent on the predominant symptoms and/or signs at the time of presentation. Initially benzodiazepines should be used for khat-related toxicity, particularly agitation, aggression, and anxiety. The management of individuals with more severe features of khat toxicity (e.g. hypertension, arrhythmias, seizures) is similar to described for the management of other sympathomimetic drugs elsewhere in this textbook.

Further reading
Crowther SM, Reynolds LA, Tansey EM (eds) (2010). *The Medicalization of Cannabis*. London: Wellcome Trust Centre for the History of Medicine at UCL. <http://www.ucl.ac.uk/histmed/publications/wellcome_witnesses_c20th_med/wit_40>.

Feyissa AM, Kelly JP (2008). A review of the neuropharmacological properties of khat. *Prog Neuropsychopharmacol Biol Psychiatry*, 32:1147–66.

Grotenhermen F (2007). The toxicology of cannabis and cannabis prohibition. *Chem Biodivers*, 4:1744–69.

Maykut MO (1985). Health consequences of acute and chronic marihuana use. *Prog Neuropsychopharmacol Biol Psychiatry*, 9:209–38.

Patel NB (2000). Mechanism of action of cathinone: the active ingredient of khat (Catha edulis). *East Afr Med J*, 77:329–32.

Cocaine

Background and therapeutic use

Cocaine is in recreational use predominately for its stimulant effects. It has a number of 'street names', which users may use instead of cocaine. These include: 'coke', 'charlie', 'bazooka', 'snow', and 'nose candy'. It should be noted that the use of street names can often be confusing for both the individual user and also for healthcare professionals.

Cocaine is available in two forms: powder cocaine and crack cocaine. Powder cocaine is typically used by nasal insufflation (snorting), but can be absorbed through any mucosal surface and is also sometimes administered by intravenous injection. Crack cocaine, where the hydrochloride base of cocaine is removed making it more heat stable, is typically used by smoking.

Cocaine purity in the UK appears to have decreased considerably over the last few years and there are significant regional differences, both on a national and international level. These differences increase the risk of acute cocaine toxicity when individuals use cocaine that is of greater purity than they are used to. Commonly detected adulterants in cocaine in the UK currently include: phenacetin, lidocaine, benzocaine, levamisole, paracetamol, talc, and sucrose. These adulterants may be associated with an additional risk of toxicity, either in their own right or in combination with the cocaine. The synthetic antihelminthic drug levamisole is a particularly important adulterant as it may cause agranulocytosis in cocaine users.

Pharmacokinetics

Cocaine is rapidly absorbed after any route of exposure. Overall bioavailability is greater than 90% when smoked or used intravenously but approximately 80% when used by nasal insufflation, perhaps due to its vasoconstrictive properties reducing blood flow and therefore absorption. Peak effects typically occur in less than 5 minutes following smoking or intravenous use and within 30 minutes of nasal insufflation. The half-life of cocaine is 45–90 minutes.

Cocaine is metabolized by a variety of metabolic pathways to three main metabolites: benzoylecgonine (formed by hydrolysis), ecgonine methyl ester (formed by plasma cholinesterases), and norcocaine (formed by N–demethylation). These metabolites have differing physiological activity, with norcocaine having similar neurological toxicity to cocaine, while both ecgonine methyl ester and benzoylecgonine are thought to have little physiological activity. The metabolism of cocaine is altered in the presence of ethanol, with production of cocaethylene, which has similar toxicity to cocaine itself but a much longer half-life and therefore duration of action than cocaine.

Mechanism of action

Cocaine has a number of actions, which relate to both its desired stimulant recreational properties, as well as the pathophysiology of its toxicity. Its various mechanisms of action are briefly summarized as follows:

- *Increased synaptic concentrations of sympathetic amines:* this occurs by both inhibition of their reuptake and increased release from synaptic vesicles, increasing presynaptic cytoplasmic concentrations.
- *Blockade of ion channels:* blockade of cardiac sodium channels leads to QRS prolongation and broad complex tachycardias and blockade of neuronal sodium channels predisposes to seizures; blockade of cardiac potassium channels delays cardiac repolarization leading to QTc prolongation and torsade de pointes ventricular tachycardia.
- *Arterial vasoconstriction:* this predominately affects coronary arteries, but can occur any vascular bed, resulting in myocardial ischaemia and hypertension.
- *Other actions:* platelet activation and aggregation, reduction in vasodilating mediators and increase in vasoconstricting mediators, all of which contribute to coronary and other ischaemia.

Clinical features

General

Cocaine, like other sympathomimetic drugs, has a wide range of unwanted effects, across a range of organ systems. These unwanted effects can occur with both use of 'regular' amounts of cocaine and with 'supra-regular' amounts.

Common general features include dilated pupils, sweating, bruxism (continuous grinding of the teeth), euphoria, and agitation.

Severe features of acute cocaine toxicity include severe agitation/anxiety, cardiovascular toxicity (e.g. hypertension, cardiac arrhythmias, acute coronary syndrome), acute cerebrovascular events (both haemorrhagic related to hypertension and ischaemic secondary to cerebral vessel vasoconstriction), gut ischaemia, seizures, and hyperpyrexia. Cardiovascular toxicity and hyperpyrexia are discussed in more detail later in this section.

Seizures can occur due to direct ion channel actions of cocaine, in relation to this sodium channel antagonist activity; alternatively they may be secondary to either cerebral ischaemia or an acute intracerebral haemorrhage.

Hyperpyrexia related to the use of cocaine is due to both direct cocaine-induced myotoxicity and also serotonin syndrome (discussed elsewhere in this textbook).

Cardiac features

- *Hypertension:* the overall prevalence is not known, but hypertension is thought to be relatively common due to cocaine's sympathomimetic actions. Severe acute hypertension (defined as a systolic BP >220 mmHg, diastolic BP >120 mmHg) significantly increases the risk of intracranial haemorrhage.
- *Cardiac arrhythmias:* these range from relatively benign arrhythmias, such as sinus tachycardia, to more life-threatening arrhythmias such as ventricular tachycardia, torsade de pointes, and ventricular fibrillation. Whilst some patients may present with palpitations, some arrhythmias may be associated with sudden cardiac death.
- *Acute coronary syndrome (ACS):* this is due not only to the vasoconstrictive actions of cocaine, but also the other actions already described. The prevalence is not well defined, but the risk is greatest in the first hour following use and remains elevated for several hours after this.
- *Other effects:* acute aortic and/or coronary dissections have been reported.

Investigations

Patients presenting with features of cocaine toxicity should have an ECG performed, together with urea and electrolytes, creatinine and liver function tests. A full blood count is useful to exclude levamisole-associated agranulocytosis. In those with suspected severe toxicity, coagulation, creatine kinase, and arterial blood gases should be assessed.

Management

The management of acute cocaine toxicity is dependent on the predominant symptoms and/or signs at the time of presentation. The management for specific acute cocaine-related problems is discussed as follows.

Agitation/aggression

This should be managed initially with benzodiazepines; haloperidol and other antipsychotics should usually be avoided as they lower the seizure threshold and some may increase risk of torsade de pointes or hyperthermia.

Seizures

Benzodiazepines are the drug of choice for controlling cocaine-related convulsions. Phenytoin should be avoided in cocaine-related seizures as it is also a sodium channel blocker and could further increase the risk of cardiac arrhythmias.

Hyperpyrexia

Rectal/core temperatures higher than 39° C should be considered a medical emergency. Initial treatment consists of benzodiazepines, simple cooling measures, and cold IV fluids; in patients who fail to respond then the use of specific serotonergic agents, such as cyproheptadine together with aggressive external/internal cooling may be required. There is no role for the use of dantrolene in the management of cocaine-related hyperpyrexia.

Hypertension

Acute significant hypertension requires urgent treatment to reduce the risk of intracerebral haemorrhage and other complications. Initial treatment should be with benzodiazepines and intravenous glyceryl trinitrate (GTN). Second-line options include alpha-blockers or calcium channel blockers. Beta-blockers are regarded as absolutely contraindicated, as they may cause unopposed alpha-adrenoceptor stimulation and worsen the hypertension. An ECG indicating underlying left ventricular hypertrophy (LVH) raises the possibility of recurrent episodes of cocaine-induced hypertension and further outpatient investigation may be required.

Arrhythmias

Standard treatment with oxygenation, correction of any underlying electrolyte imbalance, and/or control of cocaine-related sympathomimetic toxicity with benzodiazepines should be used initially in all patients with cocaine-related arrhythmias. Patients with no cardiac output should be treated along standard ALS protocols. Where it is thought that the underlying pathophysiology is myocardial ischaemia, this should be treated as discussed in the following paragraph. Anti-arrhythmic drugs should be avoided where possible; if this is not possible, then both beta-blockers and class IA/IC anti-arrhythmics are contraindicated due to increased risk of toxicity. All patients require a 12-lead ECG to determine the underlying rhythm and to identify any other underlying abnormalities. Sodium channel blockade-related cardiac arrhythmias (e.g. QRS prolongation and ventricular tachycardia), should be treated initially with hypertonic sodium bicarbonate (1–2 mL/kg of 8.4% solution). Lidocaine may be used in resistant cases; there is the theoretical potential that this may increase the risk of seizures. Potassium channel-related cardiac arrhythmias (e.g. QTc prolongation and torsade de pointes) typically are related to peak cocaine plasma concentrations. Therefore it is unusual for them to occur in the hospital environment and where these are noted, clinicians should be aware of the fact that there may be ongoing cocaine absorption (e.g. body packer/body stuffer). Treatment of these arrhythmias is with intravenous magnesium sulfate. For clinically significant tachyarrhythmias of any origin that are resistant to initial treatment regimens, consideration should be given to overdrive pacing.

Acute coronary syndrome (myocardial ischaemia)

Initial investigation of these patients should be by ECG. Studies suggest that in young individuals, a significant proportion of abnormal ECGs are in fact in retrospect 'normal variants'. The current gold standard investigation of cocaine-related ACS is a 12-hour troponin T or I.

The management of cocaine-related ischaemia differs from classical atherosclerotic ACS due to the different underlying pathophysiological processes. Initial management consists of oxygenation, benzodiazepines to reduce sympathetic nervous system stimulation and associated myocardial oxygen demand, aspirin, and vasodilatation with nitrates. Clopidogrel and low-molecular-weight heparins should be considered only in patients who do not have significant hypertension as they may worsen any intracranial haemorrhage that occurs related to the hypertension. For those with ongoing ischaemia the use of second-line vasodilatating agents, such as calcium channel blockers or alpha-blockers, and/or angiography and primary angioplasty should be considered. As noted previously, beta-blockers are contraindicated. In addition to the unopposed alpha-stimulation, studies have shown that they increase cocaine-related coronary artery vasospasm and therefore further reduce coronary artery blood flow.

Further reading

Hoffman RS (2010). Treatment of patients with cocaine-induced arrhythmias: bringing the bench to the bedside. *Br J Clin Pharmacol*, 69:448–57.

McCord J, Jneid H, Hollander JE, et al. (2008). Management of cocaine-associated chest pain and myocardial infarction: a scientific statement from the American Heart Association Acute Cardiac Care Committee of the Council on Clinical Cardiology. *Circulation*, 117:1897–907.

O'Leary ME, Hancox JC (2010). Role of voltage-gated sodium, potassium and calcium channels in the development of cocaine-associated arrhythmias. *Br J Clin Pharmacol*, 69:427–442.

Wood DM, Dargan PI (2010). Putting cocaine use and cocaine-associated cardiac arrhythmias into epidemiological and clinical perspective. *Br J Clin Pharmacol*, 69:443–7.

Wood DM, Dargan PI, Hoffman RS (2009). Management of cocaine-induced cardiac arrhythmias due to cardiac ion channel dysfunction. *Clin Toxicol*, 47:14–23.

Gamma-hydroxybutyrate and related compounds

Background

Gamma-hydroxybutyric acid (GHB) is an endogenous short-chain fatty acid that was initially developed as an anaesthetic agent in the 1960s. It has subsequently been used as a body building agent due to purported anabolic properties. Increasing recreational use, because of purported euphoriant effects, especially in the context of 'rave' parties as a psychedelic drug of abuse led to it being classified as a class C drug in the United Kingdom in 2003. It also has amnesic properties which led to GHB being implicated in some cases of drug-facilitated sexual assault ('date rape'). Sodium oxybate, the sodium salt of GHB, is available in pharmaceutical form as a treatment for narcolepsy.

GHB is as a powder that readily dissolves to form a clear, colourless, and odourless liquid and is often sold in this form to users. Although often referred to as 'liquid ecstasy', it is not structurally or pharmacologically similar to MDMA (Ecstasy)

Gamma butyrolactone (GBL) and 1,4-butanediol (1,4-BD) are precursor molecules of gamma hydroxybutyrate (GHB), both rapidly metabolized by peripheral lactonases and alcohol and aldehyde dehydrogenase respectively to form GHB. These substances, which are clear liquids and available as industrial chemicals, are also misused as substitutes for GHB.

Regular use of GHB, GBL, or 1,4BD is associated with development of tolerance and dependence.

In the United Kingdom GHB, GBL, and 1,4-BD are all controlled as class C drugs under the Misuse of Drugs Act 1971. Sale or supply for the purposes of ingestion is an offence.

Accidental poisoning in children was reported in 2007 from ingestion of toy beads marketed as 'Bindeez,' which contained 1,4-butanediol instead of 1,4-pentanediol.

Mechanism of action

GHB is a precursor of GABA and in high concentrations acts predominantly as an agonist at $GABA_B$ receptors in the cerebral cortex, cerebellum, and thalamus, and possibly also at a GHB-specific receptor in the brain. GHB administration results in inhibition of dopamine and noradrenaline release, increased serotonin turnover, and increased endogenous opioid concentrations.

Toxicokinetics

Following ingestion, GHB is rapidly absorbed and crosses the blood–brain barrier quickly. Peak concentrations occur within 1 hour and onset of clinical effects is within 15–30 minutes. It has a short elimination half-life of 20–50 minutes.

Clinical effects are dose-dependent and are potentiated by ethanol, benzodiazepines, antipsychotics, and other central nervous system depressants. Loss of consciousness occurs at serum concentrations above 50 mg/L and coma above 250 mg/L. Recreational doses are usually above 2.5 g.

GBL is more lipid soluble than GHB and more rapidly absorbed from the GI tract. It is converted to GHB by lactonases with a rapid half-life of about 1 minute and has a longer duration of action.

Because the effects of 1,4 butanediol occur after conversion to GHB by alcohol dehydrogenase, the onset of action may be delayed, particularly if co-ingested with alcohol.

GBL and 1,4BD are approximately equipotent and a typical recreational dose of high purity GBL or 1,4BD is approximately 1 mL.

Following ingestion of GBL or 1,4BD, GHB can be detected in blood samples for 4–5 hours and in urine for 8–10 hours. .

Clinical features

Acute effects

Effects occur within 15–60 minutes after ingestion and 2–15 minutes after intravenous injection. They usually resolve spontaneously within 24 hours. Maximum reported duration 96 hours. Clinical effects are potentiated by co-ingestion of other substances, especially ethanol and other CNS depressants.

GI: nausea, vomiting, hypersalivation, diarrhoea.

CNS: initial euphoria followed by miosis, drowsiness, headache, ataxia, dizziness, confusion, amnesia, urinary incontinence, tremor, myoclonus, hypotonia and agitation, which may be extreme. In severe cases, coma, convulsions, Cheyne–Stokes respiration and respiratory depression may occur, leading to respiratory arrest, which may develop rapidly. Recovery from unconsciousness may also occur abruptly.

CVS: bradycardia, ECG abnormalities including U waves, hypotension (or rarely hypertension) after intravenous use

Metabolic: metabolic acidosis, hypernatraemia, hypokalaemia, and hyperglycaemia.

Other: hypothermia may occur, especially when unconsciousness occurs in a cold environment. Aspiration pneumonia is common in patients who have been unconscious. Rhabdomyolysis may occasionally occur. This may result in renal failure.

Chronic use

Chronic GHB use may lead to a dependence syndrome leading the user to need large doses of GHB at very frequent intervals, e.g. up to hourly.

Acute withdrawal syndrome

The clinical features are similar to the alcohol withdrawal syndrome but features are more prolonged and autonomic features less prominent.

Early (<24 hours): insomnia, tremor, confusion, nausea and vomiting.

Late (>24 hours): tachycardia, hypertension, agitation, seizures and/or myoclonic jerks and hallucinations (both auditory and visual).

Investigations

The following should be measured in patients presenting with clinical features suggesting toxicity:

- oxygen saturation
- U&Es, creatinine, and glucose
- arterial blood gases (when oxygen saturation and/or conscious level is decreased)
- ECG (in patients with severe or cardiovascular features)
- creatine kinase (if rhabdomyolysis is suspected).

Urine toxicology screens do not routinely include GHB and are therefore not helpful for diagnosis.

GHB may be detected in urine for up to 12 hours after use if identification is required for forensic reasons, e.g. cases of drug-facilitated sexual assault.

Management

Acute toxicity

- Ensure clear airway and adequate ventilation in patients with a reduced conscious level. Seek early intensive care advice.
- Intubation, mechanical ventilation, and supportive care are indicated in patients with coma or respiratory arrest.
- Activated charcoal is best avoided in view of the risk of aspiration.
- Agitation may need sedation with benzodiazepines or use of antipsychotic drugs or propofol in extreme cases.
- Metabolic and acid–base disturbances that persist after adequate fluid administration and management of respiratory impairment should be corrected.
- Close monitoring of pulse, BP, respiratory rate, and conscious level (every 15 minutes) and continuous monitoring of the cardiac rhythm should be performed for at least 2 hours after ingestion. Patients who are asymptomatic after 2 hours are unlikely to develop symptoms. Symptomatic patients should be monitored for longer.
- Intravenous atropine may be used to treat bradycardia. Temporary pacing may be considered in the rare patients who fail to respond.
- Frequent or prolonged convulsions may be treated with intravenous diazepam; Phenobarbital sodium is a suitable alternative, although both may further impair conscious level.
- Naloxone has been shown to reverse some effects of GHB in animal models and may be used. However, it is unlikely to be useful alone in severely symptomatic patients and intensive care support should not be delayed.
- In patients with substantially elevated creatine kinase or rhabdomyolysis, early volume replacement and urine alkalinization may be helpful in preventing renal failure.

Enhanced elimination methods such as haemodialysis have no role in the management of GHB poisoning.

Withdrawal syndrome

Benzodiazepines are the first-line therapy for acute GHB withdrawal. The same protocol may be used as for acute alcohol withdrawal initially, but response should be monitored carefully. In severe cases, very high doses of benzodiazepines may be required (e.g. 10–20 mg diazepam at 2–4-hourly intervals).

Patients with extreme agitation who are not responding to high doses of benzodiazepines should be managed in a critical care setting. Barbiturates (e.g. pentobarbital [not licensed for use in the UK]) or propofol have been used in such cases.

Baclofen, a $GABA_B$ receptor agonist which potentiates the effects of GHB, has been suggested as a possible therapeutic option but there is little experience of its use in this situation.

Further reading

Advisory Council on the Misuse of Drugs (2007). *GBL & 1,4-BD: Assessment of Risk to the Individual and Communities in the UK.* <https://www.gov.uk/government/uploads/system/uploads/attachment_data/file/119047/report-on-gbl1.pdf>.

Dyer JE, Roth B, Hyma BA (2001). Gamma-hydroxybutyrate withdrawal syndrome. *Ann Emerg Med*, 37:147–53.

Gunja N, Doyle E, Carpenter K, et al. (2008). Gamma-hydroxybutyrate poisoning from toy beads. *Med J Aust*, 188:54–5.

Snead OC, Gibson KM (2005). Drug therapy: (gamma)-hydroxybutyric acid. *N Engl J Med*, 352:2721–32.

Tarabar AF, Nelson LS (2004). The gamma-hydroxybutyrate withdrawal syndrome. *Toxicol Rev*, 23:45–9

Thai D, Dyer JE, Jacob P, et al. (2007). Clinical pharmacology of 1,4-butanediol and gamma-hydroxybutyrate after oral 1,4-butanediol administration to healthy volunteers. *Clin Pharmacol Ther*, 81:178–84.

Wojtowicz JM, Yarema MC, Wax PM (2008). Withdrawal from gamma-hydroxybutyrate, 1,4-butanediol and gamma-butyrolactone: a case report and systematic review. *CJEM*, 10:69–74.

Wong CGT, Chan KFY, Gibson KM, et al. (2004). Gamma-hydroxybutyric acid: neurobiology and toxicology of a recreational drug. *Toxicol Rev*, 23:3–20.

Zvosec DL, Smith SW, McCutcheon JR, et al. (2001). Adverse events, including death, associated with the use of 1,4-butanediol. *N Engl J Med*, 344:87–94.

Ketamine and related compounds

Background

Ketamine, 2-(2-chlorophenyl)-2-(methylamino)-cyclo-hexanone, first manufactured in the USA in 1962, was developed as a dissociative anaesthetic and remains used for this licensed indication in both human and veterinary medicine. Its anaesthetic effects are described as causing unconsciousness, amnesia, and analgesia whilst sparing airway reflexes and maintaining haemodynamic stability. There is also increasing use of ketamine as an analgesic, especially in palliative care. There is also use in the management of acute severe asthma exacerbations, particularly in the critical care setting.

Ketamine is predominantly used recreationally for its hallucinogenic effects. These effects were described as an 'emergence delirium' in the first clinical trials of ketamine as a dissociative anaesthetic in the 1960s. Reports of the recreational non-medical use of ketamine date from the late 1960s. In the UK, ketamine is been controlled under the Misuse of Drugs Act, 1971 as a class B agent. It has a number of 'street names', including 'Special K', 'K', 'Kit-Kat', and 'Cat Valium'. It should be noted that the use of street names can often be confusing for users and healthcare professionals.

A review of adulterants and bulking agents in illicit drugs found the majority of ketamine to be diverted from legitimate sources and typically unadulterated and relatively pure (>95%). One small study of nine ketamine samples from London nightclubs, as part of an amnesty bin project, detected caffeine as an adulterant in five.

More recently the ketamine analogue methoxetamine (2-(3-methoxyphenyl)-2-(ethylamine) cyclo-hexanone, sometimes referred to by the street names 'MXE', 'MKET', 'MEXY', or 'MOXY', has been marketed as a 'bladder safe alternative' to ketamine (see 'Chronic toxicity' later in this section). Cases of acute toxicity reported from around the UK and Europe suggest it has some acute toxicity effects similar to those of ketamine (particularly dissociative toxicity), but there appear to be additional features such as cerebellar toxicity and sympathomimetic effects (e.g. significant hypertension). It is has been controlled in the UK under the Misuse of Drugs Act, 1971 as a Class B drug since 2013.

Pharmacokinetics

Ketamine is both water- and lipid-soluble and therefore can be used by nasal insufflation, oral ingestion, intravenous/intramuscular injection, or rectal insertion. Recreational doses are between 50 and 300 mg for a single dose; high first-pass metabolism reduces the oral and rectal bioavailability, leading to higher required doses. Peak effects usually occur within seconds/minutes of intravenous or intramuscular injection and within 5–20 minutes of nasal insufflation or oral ingestion. The duration of the desired effect is typically longer following oral ingestion (60–120 minutes) compared to injection (30–45 minutes) or nasal insufflation (45–60 minutes).

Ketamine is metabolized to norketamine by cytochrome P450 mediated N-demethylation, predominately by CYP3A4. This metabolite is then dehydrogenated to dehydronorketamine. The majority of ketamine is excreted in the urine, either as conjugates of ketamine and its metabolites (80%) or as dehydroketamine (16.2%), with little ketamine or norketamine excreted in the urine. The norketamine metabolite of ketamine has

approximately one-third the pharmacological potency of the parent ketamine molecule.

Mechanism(s) of action

Ketamine is reported to have actions at multiple different receptors. Its primary action, however, is that it acts as a glutaminergic N-methyl-D-aspartate receptor (NMDA-R) antagonist in the central and spinal cord. It prevents neuronal calcium influx through non-competitive binding at the phencyclidine-binding site of the NMDA-R. This leads to dissociative anaesthesia through disruption of cortical–cortical and cortical–subcortical signalling and analgesia at both a central and spinal level. Norketamine also has NMDA-R antagonist actions, which potentiates the effects of ketamine.

Agonist actions at opioid receptors make a minor contribution to its analgesic properties. The bronchodilatation seen with ketamine is thought to be due a combination of antagonism of CNS muscarinic acetylcholine receptors, inhibition of acetylcholinesterase and antagonism of endothelin-1-induced bronchial smooth muscle constriction.

Acute toxicity

Clinical features

Neurobehavioural effects

The main clinical features of acute ketamine toxicity relate directly to the desired effects that are associated with its use. The hallucinogenic effects and/or contents of the hallucinations may be unwanted, which users often refer to as 'falling into a K-Hole'. As a result of the hallucinogenic effects, individuals may develop severe agitation, aggression, paranoia, and/or dissociative symptoms.

Risk of physical harm

Ketamine use is associated with a reduction in the awareness of an individual's environment, which can be compounded by the hallucinogenic and analgesic effects of ketamine. As a result, individuals may believe that they are invincible and therefore can put themselves at risk of significant physical harm. Examples include jumping off buildings believing they can fly or walking in front of traffic believing that they won't get hurt. Death can occur as a result of the physical harm sustained.

Cardiovascular toxicity

Therapeutic use of ketamine as an anaesthetic is reported to be associated with tachycardia and hypertension prior to the development of desired anaesthesia. Recreational users of ketamine report tachycardia associated with ketamine use. However, there have been no published reports of significant cardiac arrhythmias as a consequence of either therapeutic or recreational ketamine use. The hypertension seen in individuals with acute ketamine toxicity is often mild and probably directly related to the ketamine-induced agitation/anxiety; it is not as severe as seen with sympathomimetic drugs such as cocaine and amfetamine. There have been isolated reports of pulmonary oedema associated with recreational ketamine use, although it is unclear from the published cases as to whether other factors, including co-used substances, could have been responsible.

Risk of death

Ketamine has a wide therapeutic range, and animal models report that the LD_{50} of ketamine is at least 100 times the therapeutic dose. Post-mortem detection of keta-mine is typically in the presence of one or more other substance which is likely to have had more of a causative effect. Therefore death following the use of ketamine is more likely to be associated with ketamine-related physi-cal harm, rather than direct toxic effects.

Investigations
There are no specific laboratory tests used to assess or guide the management of acute ketamine toxicity. When there is tachycardia and/or hypertension, an ECG is needed to exclude any clinically significant cardiac arrhyth-mia. In those with possible chronic ketamine use, dipstick urinalysis should be performed to exclude haematuria, given the risk of urological toxicity related to chronic keta-mine use (see 'Urological toxicity' later in this section).

Management
The majority of individuals with acute unwanted effects related to the use of ketamine do not present to the emer-gency department for management. Typically they are man-aged by friends and/or pre-hospital medical facilities (e.g. nightclub medical facilities, ambulance services). The man-agement of acute ketamine toxicity is largely supportive, where possible reducing excessive visual and auditory stimu-lation until the acute toxicity has resolved. For those individ-uals with severe symptoms, particularly significant agitation or aggression, use of benzodiazepines may be required.

Chronic toxicity
There are increasing reports of chronic toxicity associ-ated with long-term use of ketamine.

Tolerance and dependence
The majority of ketamine users do so recreationally (e.g. episodic binge style usage). However, there are a minority of users who use ketamine on a more regular dependent-style basis. These individuals often report tol-erance to ketamine, requiring increasing doses to achieve the same desired high. It is thought that this may result from auto-induction of ketamine metabolism, through up-regulation of the relevant cytochrome P450 isoen-zymes. Despite these changes, ketamine is not reported to be associated with a physical withdrawal syndrome on cessation of chronic usage, but individuals may develop psychological dependency, with resultant symptoms on cessation of long-term regular ketamine use.

Neurological and neuropsychiatric toxicity
Animal models (rats and monkeys) have demonstrated that long-term exposure to ketamine is associated with neuronal cell death. Long-term ketamine users report that they have impairment of memory and cognitive function and decreased overall psychological well-being. Additional neuropsychiatric features reported include dissociative symptoms, delusions, and depressive symptoms. It is thought that the risk is directly related to self-reported ketamine usage and may be a result of long-term antagonism of the NMDA-R and/or pre-frontal cortical dopaminergic depletion.

Gastrointestinal toxicity
Regular long-term users of ketamine often complain of vague abdominal pains, often referred to as 'K-cramps'. In a study from Hong Kong, individuals were shown to have *Helicobacter pylori* negative gastritis associated with their symptoms, which appeared to resolve on abstinence of use. Additional gastrointestinal abnormalities reported with long-term use include deranged liver function tests,

choledochal cysts, and benign cystic dilatations of the common bile duct. Similar to the abdominal pain, there is a suggestion from the published literature that these other clinical features improve or resolve with abstinence from ketamine use.

Urological toxicity
There are increasing reports of lower urinary tract symp-toms associated with long-term regular ketamine use. Although these are predominately from China and Hong Kong, where ketamine is the primary stimulant drug used, there are also reports from the UK. Symptoms that users complain of include increased frequency of small volume micturition, dysuria, supra-pubic pain and painful micturi-tion. Clinical findings include reduced bladder volume, bladder wall thickening, detrusor instability, and vesicoure-teric reflux and associated hydronephrosis. Bladder biop-sies demonstrate cystitis with urothelial ulceration and eosinophilic ulceration. The histological findings are similar to carcinoma *in situ*, although it is differentiated as tissue from ketamine users is negative for cytokeratin 20 (CK20). It is thought that these clinical features are directly related to ketamine rather than one or more adulterant or bulk-ing agent in 'street ketamine'. Similar features have been reported in individuals using pharmaceutical grade keta-mine for analgesia in a palliative care setting. Comparative bladder findings have also been reported in mice exposed to ketamine alone for up to 6 months.

Abstinence from ketamine use can be associated with some resolution of symptoms, but there have been no reports of symptoms improving in those who continue to use ketamine. There have been case reports of intra-vesical treatments with compounds such as hyaluronic acid which have been reported to improve symptoms, although there is no standard management recommen-dation at this stage. In those with severe symptoms and/or significant haematuria, there should be consideration as to whether surgical intervention (e.g. cystectomy) is required to alleviate symptoms.

Management
As noted earlier, cessation of long-term ketamine use is not likely to be associated with a physical withdrawal syndrome but users may require support for the man-agement of psychological dependency. In terms of the physical conditions associated with the long-term use of ketamine, it appears that the mainstay of management is abstinence from further ketamine use and then manage-ment of ongoing symptoms after the cessation of use.

Further reading
Cole C, Jones L, McVeigh J, et al. (2010). *CUT: A Guide to Adulterants, Bulking Agents and Other Contaminants Found in Illicit Drugs*. Liverpool: North West Public Health Observatory. <http://www.cph.org.uk/publication/cut-a-guide-to-the-adulterants-bulking-agents-and-other-contaminants-found-in-illicit-drugs/>.

Chu PS, Ma WK, Wong SC, et al. (2008). The destruction of the lower urinary tract by ketamine abuse: a new syndrome? *BJU Int*, 102:1616–22.

Kalsi SS, Wood DM, Dargan PI (2011). The epidemiology and patterns of acute and chronic toxicity associated with recrea-tional ketamine use. *Emerg Health Threats J*, 4:7107.

Poon TL, Wong KF, Chan MY, et al. (2010). Upper gastrointestinal problems in inhalational ketamine abusers. *J Dig Dis*, 11:106–10.

Wood DM, Davies S, Puchnarewicz M, et al. (2012). Acute toxic-ity associated with the recreational use of the ketamine deriva-tive methoxetamine. *Eur J Clin Pharmacol*, 68:853–6.

Psychedelic agents

Background

Substances capable of 'inducing distortion of perception, mood and thought in an otherwise normal sensorium' have been used by man for over 2000 years. There are around 100 potentially hallucinogenic plants, and indigenous peoples have traditionally used some, for example *soma* in ancient India, *teonanacatl* by the Aztecs, *peyote* by the native American church, and *ayahuasca* up to present times in Brazil. Psilocybe ('magic') mushroom use remains common where the species is endemic. More recently, synthetic chemicals capable of altering thought, perception, or mood have been developed and used recreationally by a wider modern population. Discussed in this section are ergolines (e.g. lysergic acid diethylamide or LSD), tryptamines (e.g. dimethyltryptamine (DMT)), phenethylamines (e.g. mescaline), salvinorin A, kratom, and nutmeg. NMDA antagonists (e.g. ketamine), phenylpiperazines, cannabinoid receptor agonists are described elsewhere in this chapter.

Alcohol or drug withdrawal syndromes may be associated with behavioural disturbances and hallucinations and should be considered when the diagnosis is uncertain.

Terminology

The term 'hallucinogen' is widely used but can be misleading because the doses most commonly in recreational use often do not cause hallucinations. Other terms used include psychedelics ('mind manifesting'), psychotomimetics ('psychosis mimicking'), and entheogens ('god within'). The entactogens ('to touch within') such as MDMA (ecstasy) have different psychological and pharmacological properties and should be considered a distinct chemical class.

Mechanism of action

Hallucinations are widely accepted to be due to central nervous system (CNS) serotonin 2A receptor agonism. Animal and human *in vitro* models have demonstrated a close correlation between the serotonin receptor 2A subtype ($5HT_{2A}$) receptor affinity and hallucinogenic activity, which can also be prevented by specific $5HT_{2A}$ antagonists. In addition there are probably roles for CNS glutamate and dopamine. A number of the tryptamines and phenethylamines have sympathomimetic actions mediated by catecholamine release or reuptake inhibition in addition to serotonin receptor agonism and these properties affect the clinical features observed after use.

Acute toxicity

Toxicity of hallucinogenic compounds is highly variable. Chemicals that are predominantly serotonin receptor agonists such as LSD, psilocin, or DMT are of relatively low acute toxicity. Chemicals causing marked serotonin reuptake inhibition or release, monoamine oxidase inhibition or those with sympathomimetic or vasospastic properties may be very toxic, for example, bromo-dragonFLY or dimethoxybromoamfetamine (DOB, see later in section). Acute psychiatric disturbances may be associated with hazardous behaviour with attendant risk of injury or death.

Clinical features

Common features of exposure to psychedelic agents include:

Somatic symptoms: dizziness, weakness, tremors, reduced consciousness, seizures, paraesthesia, mydriasis, blurred vision, hypertension, tachycardia, vasospasm, arrhythmia, chest pain, hyperpyrexia, nausea, diarrhoea, abdominal discomfort, acute hepatic failure, acute kidney injury, rhabdomyolysis and metabolic acidosis.

Perceptual symptoms: altered shapes and colours, difficulty focusing on objects, sharpened or altered sense of hearing and rarely synaesthesias.

Psychic symptoms: alterations in mood, distorted time sense, difficulty in expressing thoughts, depersonalization, true hallucination, agitation, acute psychotic reactions.

Toxicity assessment

Blood pressure, heart rate, temperature, and level of consciousness should be assessed and monitored.

Investigations

U&Es, creatinine, and creatine kinase should be measured. A 12-lead ECG should be taken.

Management

The management of isolated perceptual and psychic symptoms is primarily supportive with reassurance and many will not require hospital assessment.

Activated charcoal may prevent absorption if ingestion has been recent.

Benzodiazepines should be used for pronounced agitation or psychotic features. The use of antipsychotics is controversial because, although effective in controlling agitation and psychosis, there is a risk of lowering seizure threshold and increasing the risk of hallucinogen persisting perception disorder (see later in section).

Sympathomimetic toxicity should be managed conventionally with benzodiazepines, cooling, antihypertensives, anti-arrhythmics, and intravenous fluids.

Vasospasm, associated with some hallucinogenic compounds, may be diffuse and profound and should be managed aggressively, for example, with intra-arterial alpha-adrenergic antagonists and intravenous vasodilators such as nitrates or sodium nitroprusside.

Chronic toxicity

Hallucinogen persisting perception disorder or clinically significant flashbacks may rarely occur and last months to years. The precipitation of psychosis in predisposed individuals is controversial.

Specific agents

Lysergic acid diethylamide (LSD)

LSD or 'Acid,' a semisynthetic ergoline drug, is a highly potent hallucinogen that has been in recreational use since the 1940s. Use was common between 1960 and 1980 but the drug is now less frequently encountered. LSD is commonly provided in small tablets ('microdots') or on small pieces of blotting paper, often with specific decorations or branding, that are placed on the tongue. Typical doses range from 25 to 200 micrograms.

LSD is metabolized in the liver with a half-life of about 2.5 hours. When taken orally, effects appear within about 30 minutes and usually last for 8–12 hours. Typical initial features include dilated pupils, tachycardia, and sometimes hypertension or fever. Visual disturbances are common and cross-sensory perception (synaesthesia) is characteristic, with, for example, noises evoking changes in visual perception. The period under the influence of LSD is commonly referred to as a 'trip'. Hallucinogenic effects may be associated with life-threatening behavioural disturbances. The psychedelic experience associated with LSD can be unpleasant ('bad trip') and this may prompt hospital attendance. Hallucinations and psychosis can occasionally be prolonged over several days and 'flashbacks' may also be reported.

LSD is of low toxicity in overdose, but substantial doses sometimes cause psychosis, tachycardia, hyperthermia, mydriasis, metabolic acidosis, CNS depression, and respiratory depression. Platelet dysfunction with bleeding has also been reported.

Tryptamines
The pharmacology of tryptamines is complex, with these compounds acting as agonists at a range of serotoninergic and other receptor systems. Their action is primarily hallucogenic rather than entactogenic or stimulant.

Natural tryptamines are derived from the amino acid tryptophan and include DMT, psilocin and psilocybin.

Dimethyltryptamine
DMT is not active after oral use due to extensive first-pass metabolism, unless combined with monoamine oxidase inhibitors, such as those also present with DMT in South American Ayahuasca brews. First-pass metabolism can be avoided by insufflation, smoking, or injection. Typical DMT doses range from 15–60 mg. Stimulant effects are seen with low doses with intense visual hallucinations typical after larger doses. The duration of clinical effects depends on dose, but is generally less than 1 hour.

Psilocin
Psilocin and psilocybin are present in hallucinogenic *Psilocybe* ('magic') mushrooms. Psilocybin is converted to psilocin *in vivo*. Typical psilocin doses are 6–20 mg after ingestion of *Psilocybe* mushrooms. Clinical effects occur 20–30 minutes after ingestion and last 4–8 hours. Sympathetic stimulation associated with visual hallucinatory effects predominate.

Synthetic tryptamines
The synthetic 4-substituted tryptamines, e.g. 4-hydroxy-N,N-diethyltryptamine (4-HO-DET), 4-hydroxy-N,N-diisopropyltryptamine (4-HO-DiPT), 4-hydroxy-N-isopropyl, N-methyltryptamine (4-HO-MiPT), and their acetic acid derivatives (e.g. 4-acetoxy-N,N-diethyltryptamine, 4-acetoxy-N, N-diisopropyltryptamine) are reported to have similar actions to psilocin, although available information is limited.

Synthetic substitution of the tryptamine ring in the 5 position using a methoxyl- or hydroxyl- group appears to increase potency. Examples include 5-methoxy-N, N-diisopropyltryptamine (5-MeO-DIPT, 'foxymethoxy'), 5-methoxy-N,N-methylisopropyltryptamine (5-MeO-MIPT), and 5-methoxy-N,N-dimethyltryptamine (5-MeO-DMT). Tachycardia, hypertension, agitation, hallucinations, paranoia, and serotonin syndrome are all reported after use.

Most tryptamines are not associated with life-threatening toxicity, but alpha-methyltryptamine (AMT), which also has stimulant properties and a more prolonged effect (8–14 hours), may be an exception and has been linked with fatalities, although analytical confirmation is not available.

Phenethylamines
The phenethylamines are a diverse group of chemicals; some predominantly stimulant such as amfetamine, some entactogenic such as MDMA, and others with primarily psychedelic effects.

Mescaline
The archetypal natural psychedelic phenethylamine is mescaline (3,4,5 trimethoxyphenethylamine) which is derived from the peyote cactus and is a full agonist at 5-HT_{2A} receptors. It has relatively low hallucinogenic potency, is quite long-acting at approximately 12 hours and has served as the lead compound for the development of new synthetic designer phenethylamines such as DOB. SPECT scan of subjects following mescaline use reveals a pronounced increase in right hyperfrontal cortical blood flow that correlates to reported psychological effects.

Synthetic phenethylamines
Chemical substitutions made to the basic phenethylamine structure by medicinal chemists have led to substances with increased potency, subtly different psychedelic effects, differences in adverse effect and sometimes a 'legal' drug classification position. Methoxy groups added to the aromatic rings of amfetamine or methamfetamine seem to confer particularly marked hallucinogenic activity and give rise to the designer '2C series' or 'D series' drugs respectively. These are stimulant and hallucinogenic. The D series, (e.g. DOB) are more potent and longer lasting in general, are reported to cause profound diffuse vasospasm and are associated with increased morbidity and mortality.

BromodragonFLY (1-(8-bromobenzo(1,2-b;4,5-b') difuran-4-yl)-2-aminopropane) is derived from the D series drug DOB and is noteworthy for being extremely potent (with a dose of 0.5 mg), very long acting (up to 3 days) and apparently associated with significantly greater morbidity and mortality due to profound vasospasm.

Others
Salvinorin A is the psychoactive compound contained in *Salvia divinorum*, a plant in the mint family. It is a κ-opioid receptor agonist without serotonin receptor activity which causes hallucination and synaesthesias with nausea and diuresis as adverse effects.

Mitragynine is the active constituent of kratom which acts at δ and μ opioid receptors and also activates serotoninergic and noradrenergic pathways. It causes hallucination at high doses but also, at lower doses, analgesia, sedation and sometimes stimulation. Addiction is described, with chronic insomnia, anorexia, and weight loss.

Nutmeg contains myristicin, elemicin, and safrole which are psychoactive organic compounds able to activate serotoninergic pathways and inhibit monoamine oxidase enzymes. Euphoria and hallucinations, hypotension, tachycardia, nausea dizziness, and flushing are reported. Nutmeg is not a controlled substance.

Further reading
Bowen JS, Davis GB, Kearney TE, Bardin J (1983). diffuse vascular spasm associated with 4-bromo-2,5-dimethoxyamphetamine ingestion. *JAMA*, 249:1477–9.

Glennon RA, Titeler M, Mckenney JD (1984). Evidence for 5HT2 involvement in the mechanism of action of hallucinogenic agents. *Life Sci*, 35:2505–11.

Halpern JH, Pope HG (2003). Hallucinogen persisting perception disorder: what do we know after 50 years? *Drug Alcohol Depend*, 69:109–19.

Hill SL, Thomas SHL (2011). Clinical toxicology of newer recreational drugs. *Clinical Toxicol*, 49:705–19.

Hollister LE (1984). Effects of hallucinogens in humans. In Jacobs BL (ed), *Hallucinogens: Neurochemical, Behavioural and Clinical Perspectives*, pp. 19–33. New York: Raven Press.

Ismaiel AM, De Los AJ, Teitler M, et al. (1993). Antagonism of 1-(2,5-dimethoxy-4-methylphenyl)-2-aminopropane with a newly identified 5-HT2- versus 5-HT1c-selective antagonist. *J Med Chem*, 36:2519–25.

Nichols DE (2004). Hallucinogens. *Pharmacol Therapeut*, 101:131–81.

Sadzot B, Baraban JM, Glennon RA, et al. (1989). Hallucinogenic drug interactions at human brain 5-HT2 receptors: implications for treating LSD-induced hallucinogenesis. *Psychopharmacol*, 98:495–9.

Opioids

Background

The use of opioid derivatives as drugs of abuse dates back into ancient history. Today large quantities of opium poppies are still grown in Afghanistan and surrounding countries and imported into Europe through Iran and Turkey.

Opioid addicts suffer many dangers resulting from their habit. As an illegal drug obtaining supplies is both expensive and involves criminal elements. The main drug of abuse used is heroin. Street drugs of all sorts are rarely pure and this particularly applies to heroin which is diluted or 'cut' with various impurities at all steps in the supply chain.

To gain the maximum 'hit', addicts will normally use a route that delivers rapid high concentrations to the brain. Many commence by inhaling heated drug ('chasing the dragon'), but economically this is inefficient as drug is lost during the process. Addicts therefore move on to intravenous use with its attendant hazards of overdose due to variability in purity, presence of toxic chemical adulterants, and the presence of pathogenic bacteria.

Opioids used by addicts

The semi-synthetic opioid heroin (diacetyl morphine or diamorphine) is the most common: its main advantage over morphine to the addict is its solubility in acidic aqueous solution. This is often unsterilized lemon juice or citric acid. Street heroin is a potential source of both impurity and infection.

Most countries now adopt drug harm reduction policies by providing addicts with synthetic substitutes for heroin (e.g. methadone or buprenorphine), using alternative drugs (e.g. lofexidine) to reduce craving or prescribing long-acting opioid antagonists (e.g. naltrexone) to encourage abstinence.

Methadone is given orally in solution, usually once a day, often in programmes that require the patient to be directly observed swallowing their medication by the dispensing pharmacist.

Buprenorphine may be given sublingually as it is absorbed rapidly by this route (Subutex®). For opioid addicts a combination of buprenorphine with naloxone is often used (Suboxone®). The ratio is 4 parts buprenorphine: 1 part naloxone, with 2 mg or 8 mg buprenorphine. The naloxone, which is not absorbed via the buccal route, is present to prevent any 'high' from illicit IV use. Buprenorphine is a partial agonist and therefore will counteract the effect of any heroin taken by the patient or the doctor. When introducing it, patients using large quantities of opioid may develop withdrawal symptoms. Buprenorphine is poorly absorbed orally, but is immediately effective intravenously and use via this route may result in an acute withdrawal syndrome.

Methadone and buprenorphine may both be sold on to other addicts. Extreme caution is therefore required when patients present claiming that their methadone has been stolen or lost when receiving prescriptions for longer than 1 day.

Although heroin is the commonest drug use by addicts, in practice any opiate will reduce drug craving. Illicit drug seeking includes ingestion of prescription medications obtained from others and diversion of prescription opioids (see Opioid analgesics, pp. 128–129) is a major public health issue in some countries. Ingestion of modified-release morphine preparations may be particularly hazardous, as

lack of a rapid effect may lead an addict to take more and inadvertently overdose. It is important that clinicians are aware of this potential hazard.

Mechanisms of toxicity

The toxic effects of opioids, including reduced level of consciousness and respiratory depression, are mediated via specific opioid receptors. Heroin and methadone are full agonists and buprenorphine is a partial agonist. Further detail is provided in The opioid syndrome, pp. 85–86. Complications of severe poisoning associated with coma include hypoxic brain injury, aspiration pneumonia, and muscle injury with rhabdomyolysis.

Methadone causes ventricular arrhythmia (torsade de pointes) due to its potassium channel blocking properties. This effect is more likely at doses above 150 mg. The risk of arrhythmia is increased by hypoxaemia or acidosis secondary to reduced respiration.

Toxicokinetics

Heroin

The route of exposure determines time to onset of effects. Inhalation and intravenous injection results in a maximum effect within a few minutes. Intramuscular or subcutaneous injection normally results in peak effects within 1–2 hours. Effects after oral ingestion are delayed, and use of modified-release products results in even slower onset of toxicity. This may occasionally produce severe poisoning including death due to failure to recognize the agent being taken, either by the patient or the doctor. Heroin is rapidly converted to 6-monoacetylmorphine and then morphine, which has a half-life of about 3 hours. The active metabolite of morphine, morphine 6 glucuronide, may accumulate in renal impairment.

Methadone

Absorption is slow with clinical effects peaking at around 6 hours, and a duration of action of 13–20 hours. If used intravenously its onset is far faster and effects on respiration profound. Half-life is long (13–47 hours).

Buprenorphine

Ingestion of buprenorphine is ineffective due to substantial first-pass metabolism, but the drug is absorbed within about 90 minutes after sublingual use. Transdermal patches with delayed release characteristics are also available. The half-life of buprenorphine varies from 6 to more than 40 hours; its strong receptor binding makes it relatively resistant to naloxone.

Risk factors for toxicity

Risk factors for toxicity of opioids are described in The opioid syndrome, pp. 85–86. A major hazard for addicts is use with non-opioid sedatives, particularly benzodiazepines, due to combined effects on central respiratory centres.

Addicts who had been abstinent may put themselves at high risk by injecting doses they had previously been able to take without respiratory arrest. This is a common scenario in patients released from prison.

Patients swallowing drug to avoid arrest or police cells require careful monitoring if large amounts are ingested as absorption from packets is unpredictable (see Body packers and stuffers, pp. 202–203).

Clinical features

Clinical features of opioid intoxication are described in The opioid syndrome, pp. 85–86. Severity depends primarily on agent, route of administration, and dose. If a partial agonist such as buprenorphine is combined with a full agonist, effects of the latter are diminished. Patients may rapidly collapse following intravenous drug use, and this is a common emergency presentation.

Other effects from intravenous drug use
Heroin tastes bitter and quinine has been used as an adulterant. This caused an epidemic of blindness in addicts secondary to quinine toxicity. Other contaminants may be present. Pathogenic bacteria in street drugs may cause infections. *Clostridium* infection may occur in soft tissues, particularly after extravascular injection. More conventional organisms may cause local abscesses or systemic infection, particularly affecting the venous circulation and this may be complicated by right-sided acute bacterial endocarditis and infected pulmonary emboli. Intravenous drug use is also associated with the potential embolization of inadequately dissolved drug or other impurities.

Intravenous drug use causes damage to veins and loss of vascular access. Addicts often resort to larger, less visible veins, particularly femoral sites, forming visible tracts. These are sites of potential infection and use may also cause venous thrombosis. Management of thrombosis in these patients is difficult; warfarin control may be impossible and daily low-molecular-weight heparin may be the only safe anticoagulant option. Another major risk of femoral injection is inadvertent injection of the femoral artery, which can result in vascular spasm, critical limb ischaemia, and amputation.

Chronic smoking of heroin causes a leucoencephalopathy detectable by MRI brain scan.

Toxicity assessment

Assessment of toxicity in opioid poisoning is primarily based on clinical examination and clinical features, including assessment of airway, respiratory, and cardiovascular status. Blood pressure, pulse, respiratory rate, oxygen saturation, temperature, and arterial blood gases should be monitored frequently. A 12-lead ECG should be performed in those exposed to methadone (see also Opioid analgesics, pp. 85–86).

Investigations

Investigation in opioid overdose is aiming at assessing the specific effects of the overdose, the general health of the patient, and where appropriate determining presence or absence of complications and their extent. Investigations should include a full blood count, electrolytes, urea and creatinine, liver function tests, 12-lead ECG and if there is concern about possible aspiration a chest X-ray. In the case of methadone ingestion, or in a patient who is regularly taking methadone and has consumed additional opioids, a 12-lead ECG should be repeated at intervals with careful assessment of QT interval until it is clear that the effects of the methadone have peaked and the patient is recovering. Ideally obtain a urine test for subsequent screening for presence of drugs of abuse.

Management

Management of opioid toxicity is covered in specific sections in Chapters 3 (pp. 63–94) and 5 (pp. 115–130). When managing opioid addicts, several key principles apply:

- The dose or product claimed as being ingested will often not reflect the actual dose or product used.
- Multiple agents may have been used by different routes.
- In addicts ensure that all drugs in their possession are removed.
- The injection site must always be inspected carefully as street drugs are impure and may contain infective organisms. Extravascular injection may result in very serious secondary complications, including local or spreading cellulitis, venous thrombosis, and arterial damage. In patients who 'skin pop' (subcutaneous injection) anaerobic infections, including tetanus, may occur.
- Patients are at high risk of blood-borne infections including hepatitis and HIV and appropriate precautions should be taken.
- Full reversal of toxicity by antidotes may result in patients developing withdrawal features and discharging themselves from hospital inappropriately early. They may subsequently become critically ill or die once the effects of the antidote have worn off. Care should be taken to avoid this scenario by providing enough antidote to overcome respiratory depression, rather than aiming to fully reverse opioid effects.

Methadone ingestion requires specific additional care. A 12-lead on admission is mandatory, and further 12-lead recordings are required if conscious level changes. Measure QT interval and connect to an ECG monitor to establish rhythm. Torsade de pointes should be treated with magnesium sulfate 8 mmol (2 g, or 4 mL of 2 mmol/mL solution) intravenously over 30–120 seconds, repeated twice at intervals of 5–15 minutes if necessary. Hypoxia, electrolyte abnormalities, and acid–base disturbance should be corrected. Alternatively, or if these measures fail, torsade de pointes may respond to increasing the underlying heart rate by atrial or ventricular pacing or by isoprenaline (isoproterenol) infusion to achieve a heart rate of 90–110 bpm. Torsade de pointes is not usually prevented by antiarrhythmic drugs: those which prolong the QT interval (e.g. amiodarone, quinidine) usually make it worse.

Managing other general medical conditions, particularly those causing pain, is problematic as tolerance to opiates means that normal doses of analgesia are inadequate. Differentiating drug seeking behaviour from true pathology can be difficult, particularly in patients who present with 'renal colic' or abdominal pain. Use of NSAIDs may be helpful in such patients

Further reading

Buxton JA, Sebastian R, Clearsky L, et al. (2011). Chasing the dragon – characterizing cases of leukoencephalopathy associated with heroin inhalation in British Columbia. *Harm Reduct J*, 8:3.

Gupta A, Lawrence AT, Krishnan K, et al. (2007). Current concepts in the mechanisms and management of drug-induced QT prolongation and torsade de pointes. *Am Heart J*, 153:891–9.

Krantz MJ, Lewkowiez L, Hays H, et al. (2002). Torsade de pointes associated with very high dose methadone. *Ann Intern Med*, 137:501–4.

Mégarbane B, Hreiche R, Pirnay S, et al. (2006). Does high-dose buprenorphine cause respiratory depression? Possible mechanisms and therapeutic consequences. *Toxicol Rev*, 25:79–85.

Turock MK, Watts DJ, Mude H, et al. (2009). Fentanyl-laced heroin: a report from an unexpected place *Am J Emerg Med*, 27:237–9.

Solvents

Background

Solvents are liquids in which other compounds can be dissolved without chemical changes affecting the compound or solvent. A range of solvents are used for recreational purposes, although not all are manufactured for that purpose. They are found in a number of household and/or industrial products. Volatile hydrocarbons more commonly used as fuels are also subject to abuse and are also considered in this section.

There is a downward trend in the mortality associated with the abuse of solvents in the UK, which is particularly evident in younger individuals. This trend is probably related to changes in the supply (restriction of sale to minors) and in the quantity supplied (reduction in size of individual products).

Classification

The types of solvents (also known as volatile solvents and/or inhalants) can be broadly classified on the basis of their underlying chemical structure:

- aliphatic hydrocarbons: e.g. kerosene, propane, butane
- aromatic hydrocarbons: e.g. toluene, xylene
- ketones: e.g. acetone
- haloalkanes: e.g. trichloroethylene
- nitrites: e.g. alkyl nitrites, nitrous oxide.

The clinical effects and management of inhalational nitrite toxicity are discussed elsewhere in this chapter (see Volatile nitrites, pp. 198–199).

Method(s) of solvent use

Solvents are abused by inhalation. The method for this varies depending on the solvent and the specific product that is being abused.

Typically, some products are placed into a plastic bag (without ventilation holes) and the solvent vapour inhaled from the plastic bag through the mouth ('bagging'). Some individuals will place their whole head inside the bag, to allow repeat inhalations even when they are intoxicated. Solvent may also be used to soak a cloth, which is then held over the nose and mouth as the user inhales deeply ('huffing').

Other products can be inhaled directly from can or canister ('sniffing' or 'snorting'); where there is the possibility of aerosolization of other particulate matter, individuals may inhale the product through cloth to remove these particulates.

Mechanism(s) of action

There is no single mechanism of action that is consistent across all the different chemical groups as just described. In addition, some solvents have not been investigated thoroughly and therefore their mechanism(s) of action are poorly understood. Solvents act on the CNS, where they have effects across a range of different cellular and receptor signalling processes, leading to both the effects desired by users and the toxic effects that may be experienced.

Cardiac arrhythmias associated with sudden death have been reported in some solvent users and may be more common in association with butane or propane. Sensitization of the myocardium to catecholamines is one possible mechanism, although hypoxia may also be responsible.

Toxicokinetics and toxic dose

Solvents are very rapidly absorbed across the respiratory tract epithelium. Typically they are very lipid-soluble and therefore rapidly and easily enter the CNS. The toxic dose for the majority of solvents is not well documented and other factors, such as the circumstances surrounding the use of the solvent(s), also have a significant contributory effect to their overall toxicity. However, it is likely that the toxicity of solvents is a dose-related phenomenon.

Solvents are excreted via the lungs, with some hepatic metabolism. The duration of action and associated toxicity is often short-lived and wears off when the user discontinues inhalation.

Acute toxicity

Clinical features

Solvent use causes euphoria associated with CNS impairment similar to that observed of ethanol intoxication and this is presumably the effect sought by users.

The method of use of solvents described earlier in this section puts an individual at significant risk of asphyxiation. This risk is particularly high when inhalation of the solvent(s) involves placing the whole of the head inside a plastic bag to inhale the solvent. Additionally, prolonged inhalation of a solvent can lead to significant hypoxia.

Because solvents are very rapidly absorbed from the respiratory tract epithelium, some users describe the onset of desired effects as similar to that experienced with intravenous drug use. Typically, therefore, the unwanted toxic effects associated with solvents occur in the pre-hospital environment. Since a significant minority of solvent users do so alone, this further increases the risk, as effective management cannot be offered in a timely manner to prevent further deterioration.

In addition to intoxication, asphyxia, and hypoxia, other unwanted effects associated with solvents include:

- anxiety/agitation, psychosis
- nausea and vomiting
- headache
- laryngospasm
- slurred speech
- ataxia
- drowsiness progressing to reduced level of consciousness and coma
- seizures
- cardiac arrhythmias.

It is thought that the increased incidence of cardiac arrhythmias associated with solvent use explains the risk of sudden unexplained cardiac death in these individuals. Vomiting in individuals with significant drowsiness or coma increases the risk of aspiration and associated complications.

Investigations

There are no specific laboratory tests used to assess the risk of toxicity.

- Oxygen saturation should be measured, with arterial blood gases taken when hypoxia is suggested or there is a reduced level of consciousness.
- An ECG should be taken and ECG monitoring instituted.
- Urea, electrolytes (especially potassium), creatinine, and glucose should be measured.

Management

As the majority of severe life-threatening unwanted effects occur before the affected person reaches hospital, education of users about the dangers of abuse is important. It is especially important to stress that solvent use should not be undertaken when alone as it is important to try and ensure that rapid and effective treatment can be delivered when unwanted effects occur.

The management of unwanted effects is largely supportive and symptomatic with attention paid to airway management and ensuring adequate oxygenation. Seizures may be treated with benzodiazepines in the first instance.

Cardiac arrhythmias associated with solvent use tend to be ventricular in nature and therefore can be rapidly fatal in the pre-hospital environment. When cardiac arrhythmias occur in a hospital environment, electrical DC cardioversion is the treatment of choice. Although there is some limited evidence to suggest that solvents increase myocardial sensitivity to catecholamines, individuals in cardiac arrest should be managed using standard ALS protocols.

Chronic toxicity

Long-term use of solvents, especially toluene, may be associated with chronic toxic features which include the following:

- Chronic neurotoxicity, which may result from damage to myelin. Features include impaired cognition, memory loss and psychomotor impairment. Ataxia, nystagmus, muscle weakness, peripheral neuropathy, tremor, personality changes, confusion and psychosis, may occur.
- Distal renal tubular acidosis associated with hypokalaemia, hypochloraemia, and metabolic acidosis.
- Optic atrophy and hearing impairment have been reported.

Management

The most important management step is to avoid further solvent use. Hypokalaemia and metabolic acidosis should be addressed. Otherwise there is no specific treatment. There may be some improvement in clinical features after abstinence, but permanent effects are likely.

Further reading

Dingwall KM, Maruff P, Fredrichson A, et al. (2011). Cognitive recovery during and after treatment for volatile solvent abuse. *Drug Alcohol Depend*, 118:180–5.

Flanagan RJ, Ives RJ (1994). Volatile substance abuse. *Bull Narc*, 46:49–78.

Long H (2006). Inhalants. In: Flomenbaum NE, Goldfrank LR, Hoffman RS (eds), *Goldfrank's Toxicologic Emergencies*, 8th edition, pp. 1192–201. New York: McGraw-Hill.

Volatile nitrites

Background

Volatile nitrites are organic compounds with the general chemical structure R-ONO, where R is a hydrocarbon (alkyl chain). Examples include amyl nitrite $(CH_3)_2CHCH_2CH_2ONO$ and isobutyl nitrite $(CH_3)_2CHCH_2ONO$. Use of the latter has declined in the UK since sale was prohibited in 2006; many recreational products now contain isopropyl nitrite.

Organic nitrites are potent vasodilators, a property put to medicinal use with amyl nitrite as a treatment for angina in the late 19th and early 20th centuries.

Recreational use of volatile nitrites became popular in the 1970s, sold in bottles or vials as 'poppers' (a name derived from the noise made when the glass vials were crushed to inhale the contents). Bottles of 10–30 mL alkyl nitrites are marketed as room odorizers under a variety of trade names (e.g. Bolt®, Climax®, Liquid Gold®, Rush®) and although they carry the instruction that the contents are 'not to be inhaled' this is invariably the intention of the purchaser.

Mechanisms of toxicity

Many of the 'desirable' effects of volatile nitrite inhalation can be explained clinically by vasodilation, postural hypotension, and reflex tachycardia. Substantial inhalation, or ingestion, additionally may result in methaemoglobin formation as a result of nitrite-induced oxidation of ferrous (Fe^{2+}) to ferric (Fe^{3+}) haem, which cannot participate in oxygen transport.

Methaemoglobin concentrations are normally maintained at around 1% of total haemoglobin by the action of a nicotinamide adenine dinucleotide (NADH)-dependent methaemoglobin reductase, for which the physiological electron carrier is cytochrome b_5. Excess methaemoglobin causes tissue hypoxia, not only because methaemoglobin is incapable of binding oxygen, but also because the oxidation of one or more iron atoms in the haem tetramer distorts the tetramer structure, so that the remaining non-oxidized haem subunits bind oxygen avidly but release it less efficiently.

Toxicokinetics

Absorption is rapid after inhalation, ingestion, and dermal or mucosal exposure, with toxic features appearing with a few seconds of inhalation and within 1–2 hours of ingestion.

Clinical features

Inhalation of volatile nitrites is said to augment sexual pleasure by enhancing and prolonging orgasm and, in men who have sex with men, by relaxing the anal sphincter. Other desirable effects reported include light-headedness, altered perception of reality, momentary loss of identity, and feelings of warmth, happiness, and calm. The potential for temporary detachment from reality has led to increased popularity of isobutyl nitrite and other volatile nitrites by adolescents as a general substance of abuse rather than a 'sex-aid'.

Patients presenting to hospital following volatile nitrite abuse usually do so as a result of symptoms related to hypotension and/or methaemoglobinaemia.

Methaemoglobinaemia is characterized by grey-blue central 'cyanosis', which is often asymptomatic at methaemoglobin concentrations less than 20–25% of total haemoglobin. This discoloration is caused predominantly by the slate-grey colour imparted by the methaemoglobin pigment rather than the presence of deoxygenated haemoglobin. At increasing methaemoglobin concentrations, features reflect impaired oxygen transport to, and liberation at, body tissues. Headache, weakness, and fatigue predominate at methaemoglobin concentrations below 30%, while nausea, dizziness, anxiety, chest pain, and dyspnoea may be observed at concentrations of 30–50%. Impaired consciousness and seizures are likely at methaemoglobin concentrations exceeding 60% and concentrations above 80% may be fatal. Such severe features are unlikely complications of volatile nitrite abuse unless ingested rather than inhaled.

Immune reactions including wheezing, itching, or contact dermatitis may occur after exposure in susceptible individuals. Haemolysis may occur in those with glucose-6-phosphate dehydrogenase (G6PD) deficiency.

Persistent visual loss with phosphenes (flashes of light) and associated with foveal photoreceptor damage has recently been described in organic nitrite users.

Diagnosis

The diagnosis is usually clear if an accurate history is forthcoming but if it is not, two clinical observations may help. First, patients with mild methaemoglobinaemia are often less unwell than one would expect from the severity of the 'cyanosis' present and, secondly, the cyanosis is unresponsive to oxygen therapy.

Standard pulse oximetry is unreliable in the presence of methaemoglobinaemia because the accuracy of the reading depends on the different light absorbant properties of oxygenated and deoxygenated haemoglobin rather than that of methaemoglobin. Until methaemoglobin concentrations are sufficiently high to cause impaired ventilation, arterial blood gas analysis will show normal partial pressures of oxygen and carbon dioxide. If there is significant tissue hypoxia, a metabolic acidosis may be present. Analysers incorporating a co-oximeter will measure methaemoglobin concentrations directly to confirm the diagnosis. Arterial blood gases should be checked in all cyanosed or breathless patients and in those with reduced oxygen saturations on pulse oximetry.

Pulse, blood pressure, and cardiac rhythm should be monitored and a 12-lead ECG carried out.

Management

Further exposure should be prevented and, in the occasional case of widespread skin exposure, appropriate skin decontamination carried out. Symptoms secondary to vasodilation are managed supportively.

Even though methaemoglobin cannot bind oxygen, it is appropriate to administer high-flow oxygen to symptomatic patients with methaemoglobinaemia to maximize oxygen saturation of residual normal ferrous haemoglobin.

If convulsions are frequent intravenous diazepam (0.1–0.3 mg/kg body weight) or lorazepam (4 mg in an adult and 0.05 mg/kg in a child) may be required. Metabolic acidosis should be managed conventionally.

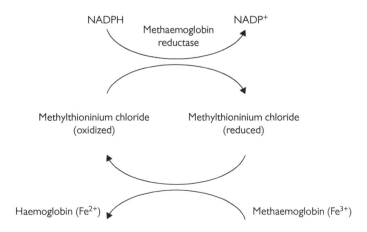

NADP$^+$, oxidized form of nicotinamide-adenine dinulceotide phosphate;
NADPH, reduced form of nicotinamide-adenine dinulceotide phosphate.

Fig 8.1 The reduction of methaemoglobin by methylthioninium chloride.

Antidotes

Methylthioninium chloride (methylene blue), acts as an electron donor to reduce methaemoglobin (Figure 8.1). In otherwise healthy individuals, methaemoglobin concentrations less than 30% usually do not require specific therapy, since such patients have only minor or no symptoms and methaemoglobin will be reduced over several hours by the intrinsic activity of methaemoglobin reductase. However, an anaemic patient may experience symptoms of hypoxia at methaemoglobin concentrations below 30% since even in the absence of methaemoglobinaemia their overall oxygen transporting capacity is reduced. Such patients, or otherwise healthy individuals with methaemoglobin concentrations greater than 30%, warrant treatment with methylthioninium chloride (methylene blue) 1–2 mg/kg (the dose depending on the severity of features) intravenously over 5–10 minutes as a 1% solution (methylthioninium chloride can also be diluted with sodium chloride 0.9% for infusion).

If the methaemoglobin concentration is greater than 50%, methylthioninium chloride 2 mg/kg should be administered. Symptomatic improvement usually occurs within 30 minutes. If there is evidence of continuing chemical absorption or prolonged methaemoglobin formation, a second dose of methylthioninium chloride 1–2 mg/kg may be required.

High doses (typically in excess of 20 mg/kg) of methylthioninium chloride can initiate severe intravascular haemolysis and doses as low as 4 mg/kg may exacerbate the haemolytic effect of oxidizing chemicals. Severe renal impairment is a relative contraindication to methylthioninium chloride administration since elimination is predominantly renal.

Methylthioninium chloride will also be less effective where nicotinamide adenine dinucleotide phosphate (NADPH) availability is reduced, as occurs in the presence of G6PD deficiency and haemolysis and when the chemical initiating methaemoglobin formation itself utilizes NADPH in cyclical methaemoglobin production, as occurs with, for example, dapsone and aniline.

Further reading

Bradberry SM, Whittington RM, Parry DA, et al. (1994). Fatal methemoglobinemia due to inhalation of isobutyl nitrite. *J Toxicol Clin Toxicol* 32:179–84.

Hunter L, Gordge L, Dargan PI, et al. (2011). Methaemoglobinaemia associated with the use of cocaine and volatile nitrites as recreational drugs: a review. *B J Clin Pharmacol* 72:18–26.

Vignal-Clermont C (2010). Poppers-associated retinal toxicity. *N Engl J Med*, 363:1583–5.

Drugs of abuse in sport

Background
The abuse of drugs in a sporting context has become a matter of increasing concern over recent years. Drugs may be taken in an attempt to improve performance or alter body image but some may have serious adverse effects. Use in some gymnasia and body building establishments may be prevalent and start at an early age.

Performance in a particular sport may depend upon either strength or endurance. In some cases, e.g. those involving anabolic agents, drugs may be taken outside the competition season to increase muscle mass, which is then maintained by training. The drug itself may therefore not be present at the time of competition. For other drugs, e.g. beta-blockers, there is a need for them to be present at the time of competition to exert an effect. An effective testing regimen must therefore include both in and out of competition testing.

Regulation
International regulation for many sports is undertaken by the World Anti-Doping Agency (WADA). Their approach includes not only banning particular named substances, but the code of practice also addresses generic techniques which might unfairly enhance performance. Their documents are widely available and include advice for athletes.

Examples of substances and techniques which are prohibited by WADA are shown in Box 8.1. Some substances are prohibited at all times and others specifically in-competition. Some substances are prohibited in particular sports where their use might put others at risk (e.g. alcohol) or decrease tremor (e.g. beta blockers).

Therapeutic use exemption
An athlete may have a medical condition which requires therapy with a substance which would otherwise be banned. This may be allowed as a 'therapeutic use exemption'. However, the circumstances in which this is allowed are regulated carefully and agreed principles of use include the need for treatment and that no additional performance enhancement should occur as a result of the treatment. An example of a substance which would otherwise be prohibited is inhaled salbutamol for asthma.

Box 8.1 Examples of substances and methods prohibited by WADA

Non-approved substances
- Anabolic agents:
  - anabolic androgenic steroids
  - other anabolic agents
- Peptide hormones, growth factors, and related substances
- Beta-2 agonists
- Hormone and metabolic regulators
- Diuretics and masking agents.

Prohibited methods
- Manipulation of blood and blood-components
- Chemical and physical manipulation (e.g. of samples)
- Gene doping.

However, even when used for this purpose, the route of administration, therapeutic doses, and acceptable urinary concentrations may be controlled.

Anabolic agents
Anabolic androgenic steroids may be naturally occurring endogenous substances (e.g. testosterone, dihydrotestosterone) or exogenous agents (e.g. nandrolone, stanozolol). They bind to androgen receptors and increase nitrogen in muscle cells. Administration of testosterone to volunteers produces an increase in strength, but not necessarily the aerobic work-rate. It has also been suggested that anabolic steroids may affect mood, increasing aggression. This may allow athletes to train harder or longer, or give them an in-competition advantage.

Anabolic steroids may be administered orally and/or by injection. Use of combinations is sometimes referred to as 'stacking'.

Acute single administration of anabolic steroids is unlikely to produce toxicity, even if high doses are used, but adverse effects are associated with chronic use. Their virilizing effects, including acne, male pattern hair loss, lowering of the voice, facial hirsuitism, clitoral hypertrophy, and breast atrophy, may explain why use is much less common in women.

Anabolic steroids may alter lipid profile, decreasing high density lipoproteins and increasing low-density lipoproteins, and may also increase blood pressure. Post-mortem findings have suggested premature atherosclerosis, ventricular dilatation, and hypertrophy. A study of body builders found that those using androgenic anabolic steroids had a larger right ventricular diameter and left ventricular mass and depressed diastolic function.

Hepatic side effects include cholestasis and the production of liver tumours. Whilst the majority of tumours are benign, and may regress once use is terminated, there is a risk of potentially fatal haemorrhage into tumours and of malignant transformation.

Prolonged use decreases serum concentrations of luteinizing hormone (LH), and follicle-stimulating hormone (FSH). This causes testicular atrophy and impaired sperm production in men which may take several months to resolve after use ceases. Human chorionic gonadotropin (HCG) may be co-administered to counteract these effects. In women this may inhibit follicle formation and ovulation and can be associated with menstrual irregularities.

Administration to growing children may cause premature fusion of epiphyses and reduced height.

Enhanced oxygen delivery
Techniques employed for increasing oxygen delivery to tissues include red cell transfusions, erythropoietin administration, hypobaric oxygen, high-altitude living, and 'living high–training low'.

Blood doping
This involves administration of red blood cells (sometimes taken from the athlete) to increase the haematocrit and therefore the oxygen-delivering capacity of the blood.

Erythropoietin
Erythropoietin (epoetin, EPO), a 30.4 kDa glycoprotein hormone largely synthesized in the kidneys, is the main regulatory hormone controlling erythrocyte production.

The advent of human recombinant erythropoietin has posed particular regulatory and analytical challenges. It is interesting to note that since the development of more sophisticated detection techniques the haematocrits of some elite endurance athletes has fallen substantially.

Administration of exogenous EPO requires parenteral injection and results in increased red cell mass and haematocrit, and an increase maximal aerobic power (VO_2 max) which, per g/dL of haemoglobin, is the same as that found after transfusion.

Acute overdose of erythropoietin is unlikely to have serious consequences, although chronic administration is associated with increased blood pressure, headaches and elevated thrombotic risk, as in non-EPO users with a high haematocrit. Whilst it is often difficult to ascribe a particular event to a particular drug of abuse, sagittal sinus thrombosis has been reported in a 26-year-old professional cyclist using vitamin A and E supplements, growth hormone, and EPO. Deep venous thrombosis, pulmonary emboli, myocardial infarction, retinal thrombosis, cerebral infarction and cerebral haemorrhage and transient ischaemic attacks have also been reported.

Gene doping
Genetic manipulation now provides the opportunity to transfer genetically modified cells, or nucleic acid analogues. These techniques may result, for example, in the increased production of erythropoietin, resulting in higher haemoglobin concentrations and greater oxygen delivery.

Peptide hormones
As with EPO, other peptide hormones with potential for abuse are present endogenously in varying amounts, so determining abuse can be challenging.

Human chorionic gonadotropin (HCG)
HCG given by subcutaneous injection causes a rise in testosterone and epitestosterone levels, maintaining the ratio between the two steroids. This reduces risk of detection as the ratio may be used to detect exogenous testosterone administration.

Adverse effects of HCG include headache and mood changes. In females, ovarian hyperstimulation syndrome may occur, with nausea, diarrhoea, abdominal bloating, breast tenderness, and ovarian enlargement with cyst formation. This may be accompanied by abnormal liver function tests. Large ovarian cysts are prone to rupture. An association with thromboembolism is also probable.

Luteinizing hormone (LH)
Although in women LH causes changes in oestrogen and progesterone, in men it may increase testosterone production. Adverse effects include headaches, ovarian hyperstimulation syndrome, and thromboembolism.

Human growth hormone (HGH)
Administration of recombinant HGH increases insulin-like growth hormone 1, affects carbohydrate and fat metabolism, and has androgenic properties. Endogenous HGH undergoes pulsatile excretion, and levels change after exercise and stress. This variability and the similarity of exogenous and endogenous HGH present regulatory challenges. Adverse effects include fluid retention, stiffness of extremities, arthralgia, myalgia, and paraesthesia.

Beta-2 agonists
All beta-2 agonists (e.g. salbutamol, clenbuterol) are prohibited at all times under the WADA regulations, with the exception of inhaled salbutamol, salmeterol, and formoterol if these are taken only in particular circumstances,

and also within the manufacturers recommended therapeutic regimen. As well as their effects on respiratory function, when ingested they may increase muscle mass and are sometimes abused by body builders for their anabolic and lipolytic effects. They are associated with serious cardiac effects and myocardial infarction has been reported in a 17-year-old body builder.

Beta-blockers
Beta-blockers reduce tremor and heart rate, which may be beneficial in sports requiring accuracy. They are therefore prohibited during competition for a number of sports including archery, shooting, darts, billiards, and some skiing events. These agents are considered in more detail in Beta adrenoceptor antagonists, pp. 132–133.

Diuretics
Diuretics (e.g. acetazolamide, bumetanide, furosemide) may be used to reduce body weight, conferring an unfair advantage by allowing an athlete to compete in a lower weight category. They may also be used to produce a more dilute urine, thus lowering the concentration of other substances taken illicitly so as to avoid detection. They may therefore be considered as examples of 'masking agents' (see following subsection).

Confounders and masking agents
Taking a substance to mask detection, or to make interpretation of analytical results difficult is forbidden. Diuretics (e.g. furosemide) increase urine volume and reduce the concentration of banned substances in the urine, making detection more difficult. Probenecid reduces the urinary concentration of acidic compounds, 5-alpha-reductase inhibitors reduce the formation and urinary concentration of some anabolic steroid metabolites. Plasma expanders, (e.g. dextran) maintain plasma volume and reduce haematocrit following use of EPO or blood doping.

For some substances, abnormal use may be inferred by comparing the ratio of one substance to another, rather than assessing the concentration alone. For example, administration of testosterone will not only increase testosterone concentrations, but will increase the ratio of testosterone to epitestosterone. Epitestosterone may be administered close to the time of testing to decrease the testosterone to epitestosterone ratio and thus avoid detection.

Further reading
Blazevich AJ, Giorgi A (2001). Effect of testosterone and weight training on muscle architecture. *Med Sports Exerc*, 33:1688–93.

Buckley WE, Yesalis CE, Friedel KE, et al. (1988). Estimated prevalence of anabolic steroids use among male high school seniors. *JAMA*, 260(23):3441–5.

Ekblom B, Berglund B (1991). Effect of erythropoietin administration on mammal aerobic power. *Scand J Med Sci Sports*, 1(2):88–93.

Kadi F, Eriksson A, Holmer S, et al. (1999). Effects of anabolic steroids on the muscle cells of strength trained athletes. *Med Sci Sports Exerc*, 31:1688–93.

Kierzkowska B, Stanczyk J, Kasprzak JD (2005). Myocardial infarction in a 17-year-old body builder using clenbuterol. *Circ J*, 69:1144–6.

Lage JMM, Masdeu J, Rocha E (2002). Cyclist's doping associated with cerebral sinus thrombosis. *Neurology*, 58:665.

Stiger VG, Yesalis CE (1999). Anabolic-androgenic steroid use among high school football players. *J Community Health*, 24:131–45.

World Anti-Doping Agency (2012). *World Anti-Doping Code. The 2013 Prohibited List. International Standard.* <http://www.wada-ama.org/Documents/World_Anti-Doping_Program/WADP-Prohibited-list/2013/WADA-Prohibited-List-2013-EN.pdf> (accessed 29 October 2012).

Body packers and stuffers

Background and definitions

The internal concealment of illicit substances may lead to significant toxicity and/or physical injury.

'Body packers' (also referred to as 'mules' or 'couriers') are individuals who conceal large amounts of well-packaged illicit substances internally, typically heroin or cocaine, usually as part of organized international drug trafficking. 'Body stuffers' spontaneously conceal illicit substances internally, to avoid detection by the police. These are usually less well packaged and in smaller amounts. 'Parachuting' is a technique of recreational drug use in which a single dose of an illicit drug is ingested by wrapping the drug in a covering that is expected to dissolve or unravel in the gastrointestinal tract and release the drug for later absorption and effect.

Body packers

Body packing has become more common due to stricter international border controls and improved drug detection techniques. Most body packers are men, but children and pregnant women have also been used. Common wrapping materials include latex, condoms, foil, plastic, tape, and wax.

Risk assessment

The clinical history may not be accurate due to intoxication or concerns over prosecution, although most body packers are aware of the number and contents of swallowed packages. Determination of the substance involved and ingestion timing is important to assess the risk from package rupture. Cocaine, for example, does not have an effective antidote and packet rupture is life threatening, while heroin presents less of a hazard because there is an antidote, naloxone. Other substances reportedly involved include MDMA, methamphetamine, and cannabis.

Users typically swallow up to 200 individual packages, each one containing 0.5–10 g of drug and rupture of any is potentially life threatening. The wrapping material and technique are relevant to risk assessment and may be sophisticated, with machine produced packages, reducing risk of rupture. For example, in two large case series, involving 1831 cocaine body packers, only 64 (3.5%) were symptomatic. The co-ingestion of substances to increase gastrointestinal transit time should be considered during risk assessment. The presence of clinical features of toxicity or gastrointestinal complication increases risk.

Clinical features

Body packers may present to healthcare services due to packet rupture and subsequent toxicity, gastrointestinal obstruction or perforation, or they may be asymptomatic. Toxicity will be based on the substance ingested. Clinical assessment should include blood pressure, pulse rate, temperature, assessment of conscious level, pupil diameter, respiratory rate, oxygen saturations, abdominal examination, and per rectum examination. Intimate cavity searches should be performed by an appropriately experienced (e.g. forensic) physician.

Investigations

All suspected body packers should undergo radiological assessment, although there is no 'gold standard' method of detecting internally concealed packages. Plain radiographs have reported sensitivity of 47–95%. Supine positioning and the use of contrast may improve accuracy. Packages are typically seen as multiple opacifications within the gastrointestinal lumen. Alternatively the 'halo' or 'double condom' (due to a ring of air trapped between layers of wrapping) or 'rosette' (due to air within the balloon or condom knot) signs may be helpful. False positives occur due to constipation or intra-abdominal calcification. False negative results are also reported; in one series 16 of 48 cocaine body packers who subsequently passed packages had negative plain radiographic assessment. Abdominal computed tomography (CT) may be more sensitive, localize packages more effectively, and even distinguish package contents based on differences in Hounsfield units between cocaine and heroin. In one study ultrasound identified 40 of 42 body packers previously confirmed to have internally concealed packages by plain film. A broadly accepted approach is to perform plain radiograph assessment initially and move to CT if plain films are negative. Low radiation dose CT may have a first-line role but data are limited.

Blood or urine analysis for the detection of illicit substances can be helpful, although may be difficult to interpret. Positive results may be due to microperforation, surface contamination of the package, or previous use of the substance by the individual, but an initial negative analysis that subsequently becomes positive implies packet rupture. It is often difficult to attain these analyses within clinically meaningful time frames. The sensitivity of urine toxicology analysis in confirmed body packers has been reported as 37–52%. A toxicology screen was positive in 71% of cases with packet rupture.

Management

Asymptomatic patients

A conservative approach is favoured over surgical intervention in those without clinical evidence of package rupture or gastrointestinal complications and has a complication rate of approximately 2–5%. The patient should be monitored carefully while commencing whole-bowel irrigation (WBI) with an osmotically balanced oral or nasogastric polyethylene glycol solution (e.g. Klean-Prep® 1.5–2 L per hour). There are numerous case series reporting few complications with this approach but no published data comparing WBI to other conservative approaches, such as oral laxatives. WBI should be continued until all packages are passed. Electrolytes should be checked regularly and corrected as needed.

Indications to switch to a surgical approach are symptoms of toxicity, urine toxicology analysis that was previously negative becoming positive, gastrointestinal complications, or failure to pass packages. The appropriate duration of conservative management before surgical intervention is considered when no packages are produced is unclear, but current practice ranges from 27 hours to 7 days. Endoscopic retrieval of packages is generally not recommended because of the risk of inducing package rupture. Although no clear data showing benefit exists, multiple-dose activated charcoal is recommended by some authors and both heroin and cocaine are well adsorbed. However, in heroin packers, naloxone is likely to be a more suitable therapy while in cocaine packers urgent surgery should be undertaken if package rupture is suspected. Furthermore, charcoal may cause complications in those with subsequent bowel perforation and peritoneal contamination.

Symptomatic patients
Patients with drug toxicity or gastrointestinal complications such as perforation or obstruction require surgical intervention to remove the packages and repair any other complication. If the packages contain heroin or another opioid then a naloxone infusion should be commenced prior to surgery. The optimum surgical procedure depends largely on the location of packages within the GI tract and there is no clear procedural consensus. Colonic packages may be removed by colostomy, but this has a relatively high incidence of complications, e.g. wound infection and dehiscence, presumably due to high colonic bacterial load. Laparotomy and milking packages to the anal canal is therefore recommended by some. Proximal packages can be removed by enterotomy or retrograde milking to the stomach and gastrotomy. The risk of physical trauma due to the milking of packages along the lumen must be compared to the risk of multiple enterostomies. Operative complication rates reported are 6–40%.

Confirmation of package clearance
Following conservative management or surgical intervention elimination of all packages should be confirmed as there are reports of retained packages following both approaches. Observation for 24 hours after two packet-free stools have been passed as well as plain radiographs or abdominal CT are recommended prior to discharge.

Body stuffers

Body stuffing is generally undertaken to conceal evidence from the authorities thereby avoiding detection or arrest and there are key differences compared with body packing. First the quantity of drug is usually significantly less, meaning the clinical risk associated with toxicity is, in general, reduced. However there are case reports of fatalities of body stuffers and each case should be individually assessed for risk and appropriate management. Secondly the quality of wrapping, if present at all, is often inferior and consequently symptoms of toxicity are more common and occur earlier post ingestion. Most body stuffers ingest the illicit substances in thin plastic sandwich bags, in aluminium foil, or unwrapped.

Risk assessment
The history of drug type and quantity ingested, timing, wrapping, and clinical features is critical to understanding the clinical risk to each patient. Unfortunately there is poor correlation between ingestion history and the risk of severe clinical toxicity.

Clinical features
Most body stuffers present early due to symptoms or without symptoms but in the custody of the police. Most cocaine and heroin body stuffers are asymptomatic at presentation whereas most methamphetamine stuffers are symptomatic. Gastrointestinal complications are rare and far less likely than with body packers. In general asymptomatic patients at 4–6 hours post ingestion have favourable outcomes but with exceptions. Most patients who develop severe clinical toxicity have clinical features present at their initial presentation to medical services. Clinical features are determined by the substance ingested.

In a case series of 46 cocaine body stuffers, 34 were asymptomatic, eight had mild toxicity, two had moderate toxicity, and two deaths occurred. In another series of 98 cocaine stuffers there were no deaths but four had seizures. Most had mild or moderate features of toxicity. In 65 heroin body stuffers there were no deaths and 59 were asymptomatic. All those with significant toxicity during their admission had clinical features of toxicity on arrival. Methamphetamine stuffers may have a higher risk of complications; in one report, of 55 cases only 6% were asymptomatic while 29% had severe outcomes such as requirement for intubation. Of these 88% had tachycardia greater than 120/minute or a temperature higher than 38° C on presentation.

Investigations
Abdominal radiographs do not identify packets in most cases and are of little value. CT has been successful in a few cases, but false negatives occur and there are not enough data to recommend use. Toxicology screens, as for body packers, are often difficult to interpret and used with caution in the management of body stuffers.

Management
Most body stuffers are managed with activated charcoal and/or WBI. Although there are no randomized trials to guide management, for cocaine and heroin at least, there seem to be few unfavourable outcomes. The duration of observation is controversial and unclear. In those with symptoms, treatment should continue until clinical toxicity has resolved. In asymptomatic patients, observation for 24 hours is probably reasonable but each patient requires individual risk assessment. In most cases packaging material is not found in faeces and should not be used to determine treatment duration. Naloxone should be used if there are clinical features of opioid toxicity. In most cases surgical intervention will not be required due to small drug quantities and likely package leak. However, body stuffers who have ingested large quantities or well wrapped packets should be managed as for body packers.

Further reading

Booker RJ, Smith JE, Rodger MP (2009). Packers, pushers and stuffers-managing patients with concealed drugs in UK emergency departments: a clinical and medicolegal review. *Emerg Med*, 26:316–20.

de Bakker JK, Nanayakkara PWB, Geeraedts LMG, et al. (2012). Body packers: a plea for conservative treatment. *Langenbecks Arch Surg*, 397:125–30.

Jordan MT, Bryant SM, Aks SE, et al. (2009). A five year review of the medical outcomes of heroin body stuffers. *J Emerg Med*, 36:250–6.

June R, Aks S, Keys N, et al. (2000). Medical outcome of cocaine bodystuffers. *J Emerg Med*, 18:221–4.

Mandava N, Chang RS, Wang J, et al. (2011). Establishment of a definitive protocol for the diagnosis and management of body packers (drug mules). *Emerg Med J*, 28:98–101.

Norfolk GA (2007). The fatal case of a cocaine body stuffer and a literature review – towards evidence based management. *J Forensic Leg Med*, 14:49–52.

Sporer KA, Firestone J (1997). Clinical course of crack cocaine body stuffers. *Ann Emerg Med*, 29:596–601.

Traub SJ, Hoffman RS, Nelson LS (2003). Body packing – the internal concealment of illicit drugs. *N Engl J Med*, 349:2519–26.

West PL, McKeown NJ, Hendrickson RG (2010). Methamphetamine body stuffers: an observational case series. *Ann Emerg Med*, 55:190–7.

Yang RM, Li L, Feng J, et al. (2009). Heroin body packing: clearly discerning drug packets using CT. *South Med J*, 102:470–5.

Common chemical poisonings

Acetone and isopropanol

Acetone

Background

Acetone (dimethyl ketone, 2-propanone, dimethylformaldehyde) (Figure 9.1) is a clear, highly flammable liquid with a characteristic pungent odour and sweet taste. It can be produced endogenously in man from acetyl coA. Acetone is used widely as a solvent in industrial and household products, including paints, nail polish, and nail polish removers; occupational exposure and poisoning is, therefore, well recognized. Poisoning has also occurred following repeated application of a muscle liniment containing 70% (volume/volume) acetone. Since isopropanol (see 'Isopropanol') is metabolized to acetone, the features of systemic poisoning with both chemicals is similar.

Toxicokinetics

Acetone is absorbed rapidly through the lungs and gut. Systemic absorption may also occur via extensive dermal exposure. The principal metabolic pathway is hepatic conversion to pyruvate. Pyruvate enters the gluconeogenic pathway with conversion through oxaloacetate and phosphoenolpyruvate to glyceraldehyde-3-phosphate and glucose-6-phosphate to glucose. Acetone metabolism is saturable and at high concentrations it is also eliminated unchanged in expired air and urine.

Mechanism of toxicity

Systemic toxicity is explained by the ability of acetone to disrupt normal intermediary metabolism leading to hyperglycaemia, plus anaesthetic and CNS depressant actions.

Clinical features

Acetone has an irritating effect on the mucous membranes of the eyes, nose, and throat causing burning and erythema. It has a drying effect on the skin and causes dermatitis. Systemic features may follow prolonged extensive skin contact. Prolonged eye contact with acetone liquid has caused permanent corneal damage.

Nausea, vomiting, hypotension, lightheadedness, headache, excitement, restlessness, chest tightness, ataxia, and incoherent speech are characteristic of intoxication by inhalation or ingestion of larger quantities. Coma, convulsions, and respiratory failure supervene in severe cases and rhabdomyolysis has been described. There is some evidence that vasogenic cerebral oedema contributes to CNS toxicity. Hyperglycaemia may develop, there may be an increased osmolal gap and arterial blood gases may show a high anion gap metabolic acidosis. Hepatic and renal toxicity may occur rarely.

Acetone can be smelt on the breath and readily detected in urine and plasma. The highest reported serum concentration associated with survival is 3900 mg/L. This patient was comatose, required mechanical ventilation and resuscitation with large volumes of intravenous fluid but recovered completely.

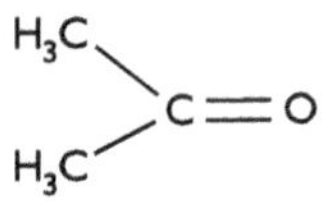

Fig 9.1 . Structure of acetone.

A 30-month-old male ingested approximately 180 mL of nail varnish remover (65% acetone and 10% isopropyl alcohol) and developed coma, convulsions, hypotension, respiratory depression, hyperglycaemia and metabolic acidosis. He made a full recovery with supportive management.

Management

Removal from exposure is the priority following inhalation. Although in vitro studies suggest that acetone is adsorbed to activated charcoal, the value of charcoal in preventing acetone absorption has not been confirmed clinically.

Management of acetone poisoning is otherwise symptomatic and supportive. Hepatic and renal function, arterial blood gases, and blood glucose concentration should be measured.

The osmolal gap (measured minus calculated ($2 \times (Na^+ + K^+)$ + urea + glucose (all in mmol/L)) plasma osmolality should be calculated and is likely to be increased.

In severe cases the serum acetone concentration should be measured.

Hyperglycaemia is unlikely to be sufficiently severe or prolonged to require specific intervention with insulin.

Since the parent compound has a small volume of distribution (0.82 L/kg) and is responsible for toxicity, there is a potential role for haemodialysis in the management of severely poisoned patients in whom the plasma acetone concentrations are high. Acetone clearance during haemodialysis was 165 mL/min in a patient poisoned with isopropanol; 19,899 mg acetone was removed over 3 hours.

Isopropanol

Background

Isopropanol (isopropyl alcohol; 2-propanol) is found in aftershave lotions, disinfectants, and window-cleaning solutions, and is used as a sterilizing agent and 'rubbing' alcohol. It is usually ingested, but inhalation and topical exposure have led to poisoning; there is one report of the accidental use of an isopropanol-containing enema leading to coma and death.

Toxicokinetics

Following ingestion, peak serum isopropanol concentrations are reached after 15–30 minutes. Isopropanol is oxidized to acetone by hepatic alcohol dehydrogenase; hence, fomepizole inhibits isopropanol metabolism. Isopropanol and acetone are both excreted primarily in the urine with minimal amounts being excreted through the lungs; the odour of acetone may be detected on the breath. The elimination half-life of isopropanol is between 5.8 and 7.3 hours but can be prolonged to 16 hours with co-ingestion of ethanol.

Mechanism of toxicity

The effects of isopropanol on the nervous system are similar to those of ethanol, but are probably more severe and more persistent.

Clinical features

Coma and respiratory depression are the major sequelae following substantial exposure. Coma may be prolonged due to the relatively slow metabolism of isopropanol and the subsequent generation of acetone.

Other features following ingestion include haemor-rhagic gastritis (though this has also been reported after topical application), haematemesis, acetone on the breath, hypotension, hypothermia, sinus tachycardia, frequent premature ventricular beats, renal tubular necrosis, acute myopathy, and haemolytic anaemia. Ataxia, headache, dizziness, drowsiness, stupor, hallucinations, areflexia, muscle weakness may occur.

Hypoglycaemia or hyperglycaemia, haemolysis, ketonuria, renal tubular acidosis, hepatic dysfunction, and rhabdomyolysis have been reported.

Development of hypotension is a poor prognostic feature and may herald cardiac arrest.

Skin contact may cause paraesthesia and erythema. Prolonged skin contact may also result in systemic features. Prolonged skin contact has resulted in severe burns and death in a premature infant.

Accidental inhalation may cause mild irritation to the eyes, nose and throat, whereas prolonged inhalation may also result in systemic features.

A 2-year-old child who ingested an unknown amount of isopropanol suffered coma, cardiac and respiratory arrest but recovered with supportive care over a 2-day period. The maximum blood isopropanol concentration was 5200 mg/L.

As little as 24 mL of 70% isopropanol was reported to cause coma in an 18-month-year-old infant. Inadvertent inhalational exposure of 70% solution via a ventilator humidifier over 2 hours resulted in fatality in a 37-week pre-term infant.

Inadvertent infusion of 800 mL of a 35% isopropanol solution caused coma, respiratory depression, and elevated creatine kinase activity in a 19-year-old man.

A 34-week gestation infant with Apgar scores of 2 and 5 was hypotensive, hypotonic, and cyanotic with a weak respiratory effort; she underwent aggressive resuscitation. She developed seizure activity which was treated with phenobarbital. At 1.5 hours of life the isopropanol and acetone concentrations were 1400 mg/L and 160 mg/L respectively. Maternal transfer was confirmed. Her seizures resolved within 24 hours of life, her tone improved, and by the time of discharge she had a normal neurological examination.

Fatalities reported have involved ingestion of more than 550 mL of 70% or higher solutions although survival has been reported following ingestions of over 1000 mL and with blood concentration as high as 5600 mg/L.

Management

There is no evidence that gastric lavage is of value in reducing absorption, nor would this be expected, as absorption is rapid.

The mainstay of treatment is supportive care. In addition, since isopropanol has a small volume of distribution (0.6–0.7 L/kg) and is responsible together with its metabolite, acetone, for toxicity, there is a role for haemodialysis in the management of severely poisoned patients in whom the plasma isopropanol concentrations are very high. Isopropanol clearance during haemodialysis was 137 mL/min; 58,325 mg isopropanol was removed over 3 hours. Acetone is also removed effectively by haemodialysis (see earlier in section).

No advantage is gained by administering fomepizole to block alcohol dehydrogenase, as such treatment will prolong isopropanol elimination and thereby enhance its toxicity.

Further reading

Abramson S, Singh AK (2000). Treatment of the alcohol intoxications: ethylene glycol, methanol and isopropanol. *Curr Opin Nephrol Hypertens*, 9:695–701.

Arts JHE, Mojet J, Van Gemert LJ, et al. (2002). An analysis of human response to the irritancy of acetone vapors. *Crit Rev Toxicol*, 32:43–66.

Burkhart KK, Martinez MA (1992). The adsorption of isopropanol and acetone by activated charcoal. *J Toxicol Clin Toxicol*, 30:371–5.

Dyer S, Mycyk MB, Ahrens WR, et al. (2002). Hemorrhagic gastritis from topical isopropanol exposure. *Ann Pharmacother*, 36: 1733–5.

Gamis AS, Wasserman GS (1988). Acute acetone intoxication in a pediatric patient. *Pediatr Emerg Care*, 4:24–6.

Gaudet MP, Fraser GL (1989). Isopropanol ingestion: case report with pharmacokinetic analysis. *Am J Emerg Med*, 7:297–9.

Gitelson S, Werczberger A, Herman JB (1966). Coma and hyperglycemia following drinking of acetone. *Diabetes*, 15:810–11.

Haviv YS, Safadi R, Osin P (1998). Accidental isopropyl alcohol enema leading to coma and death. *Am J Gastroenterol*, 93: 850–1.

Kallenberg K, Behrens A, Strik H, et al. (2008). MR imaging-based evidence of vasogenic brain edema in a case of acute acetone intoxication. *Am J Neuroradiol*, 29:e16.

Kostusiak V, Bekkal R, Mateu P (2003). Survival after drinking lethal dose of acetone. *Intensive Care Med*, 29:339.

Kumarvel V, Da Fonseca J (2007). Acetone poisoning – a diagnostic dilemma. *Eur J Anaesthesiol*, 24:805–6.

Lacouture PG, Wason S, Abrams A, et al. (1983). Acute isopropyl alcohol intoxication. Diagnosis and management. *Am J Med*, 75: 680–6.

McFadden SW, Haddow JE (1969). Coma produced by topical application of isopropanol. *Pediatrics*, 43:622–3.

Mecikalski MB, Depner TA (1982). Peritoneal dialysis for isopropanol poisoning. *West J Med*, 137:322–5.

Pappas AA, Ackerman BH, Olsen KM, et al. (1991). Isopropanol ingestion: a report of six episodes with isopropanol and acetone serum concentration time data. *J Toxicol Clin Toxicol*, 29:11–21.

Parker KM, Lera Jr TA (1992). Acute isopropanol ingestion: pharmacokinetic parameters in the infant. *Am J Emerg Med*, 10:542–4.

Piatkowski A, Gr€oger A, Bozkurt A, et al. (2007). Acetone associated inhalation injury and rhabdomyolysis. *Burns*, 33:932–4.

Rosansky SJ (1982). Isopropyl alcohol poisoning treated with hemodialysis: kinetics of isopropyl alcohol and acetone removal. *J Toxicol Clin Toxicol*, 19:265–71.

Ross DS (1973). Acute acetone intoxication involving eight male workers. *Ann Occup Hyg*, 16:73–5.

Satoh T, Nakashima H, Matsumura H, et al. (1996). Relationship between acetone exposure concentration and health effects in acetate fiber plant workers. *Int Arch Occup Environ Health*, 68:147–53.

Stremski E, Hennes H (2000). Accidental isopropanol ingestion in children. *Pediatr Emerg Care*, 16:238–40.

Trullas JC, Aguilo S, Castro P, et al. (2004). Life-threatening isopropyl alcohol intoxication: is hemodialysis really necessary? *Vet Hum Toxicol*, 46:282–4.

Van Wijngaarden M, Mock T, Dinwoodie A, et al. (1995). Coma and metabolic acidosis related to the use of muscle liniment. *Crit Care Med*, 23:1143–5.

Vicas IMO, Beck R (1993). Fatal inhalational isopropyl alcohol poisoning in a neonate. *J Toxicol Clin Toxicol*, 31:473–81.

Acids and alkalis

Acids

Background

Acids are substances whose aqueous solutions have a pH less than 7 and have the ability to turn litmus paper red and can react with certain metals and bases to form salts. All acids yield hydrogen ions when dissolved in water and can act as proton donors. They can also accept a pair of electrons to form a covalent bond.

Acids are used in various chemical products to remove and dissolve lime scale. They are also used in metalworking as etching agents and in rust removers. Their strength depends on the chemical structure and the concentration of the solution. Acids provide a certain bactericidal effect, particularly at high concentrations, and are therefore employed in products such as lavatory cleaners. Both organic and inorganic acids are used, the latter are usually stronger.

Hydrochloric acid fumes are heavier than air and can accumulate at ground level and in confined spaces. The UK short-term occupational exposure limit for gas and aerosol mists is 5 ppm (8 mg/m^3) and the long-term exposure limit is 1 ppm (2 mg/m^3).

Mechanisms of toxicity

Acids tend to cause damage to tissues via the free H$^+$ ion. Strong acids, e.g. hydrochloric acid, are corrosive and therefore exposure to any quantity can cause a coagulative necrosis but they have relatively poor tissue penetration compared to alkalis. Weak acids are irritant to mucous membranes and generally of much lower toxicity, e.g. salicylic acid.

The extent of injury following ingestion of acid is dependent on several factors including the strength and viscosity of the compound and the volume involved. Ingestion can lead to tissue injury from both the direct corrosive effects of the acid and an exothermic reaction causing thermal injury.

Clinical features

Ingestion

Acids tend to damage the stomach with ulceration, gangrene, haemorrhage, and perforation. However, in severe cases extensive areas of the gastrointestinal tract may be involved. The presence of oropharyngeal burns does not correlate well with the presence of oesophageal injuries, but generally more extensive oral burns are associated with multiple site involvement. Gastric or oesophageal perforation may occur early in severe cases.

Acids cause immediate pain with burning in the mouth, throat, and stomach. This may be followed by abdominal pain, vomiting, hematemesis, and dyspnoea. Pain and oedema may make swallowing difficult, causing drooling. Airway obstruction from laryngeal and/or epiglottic oedema are features in severe cases. Stridor and respiratory complications (including pneumonitis, pulmonary oedema, ARDS, and pulmonary necrosis) can develop following aspiration of acidic stomach contents.

Systemic features include circulatory collapse, metabolic acidosis, hypoxia, respiratory failure, acute kidney injury, haemolysis, and disseminated intravascular coagulation (DIC).

Stricture formation is a potential late complication, usually occurring between 2 weeks and 2 months post exposure, although it may not be clinically apparent for several years. Severe injury can cause pyloric stenosis and a small, scarred, immobile stomach.

Dermal exposure

Strong acids may cause pain, blistering ulceration, and penetrating necrosis. Coagulation burns may develop, which can be self-limiting and superficial with the destruction of the surface epithelium and submucosa forming a leathery crust that limits the spread of the product. More concentrated and corrosive acids, such as hydrofluoric acid (see Hydrofluoric acid, pp. 247–248), may produce deep burns and there may be systemic absorption requiring more specific management.

Large or prolonged exposure may result in systemic effects.

Inhalation

Following inhalational exposure to the fume or mist produced by some acids, e.g. fuming nitric acid, irritation of eyes and nose with sore throat, cough, chest tightness, headache, fever, wheeze, tachycardia, and confusion may occur. Chemical pneumonitis, tachypnoea, dyspnoea, and stridor due to laryngeal oedema may follow. Pulmonary oedema with increasing breathlessness, wheeze, hypoxia and cyanosis may take up to 36 hours to develop. Chronic inhalation can result in occupational asthma or persistent RADS.

In serious cases, corrosive damage to the mucous membranes of both the upper and lower respiratory tract occurs. Severe inhalation injuries may result in persistent hoarseness, pulmonary fibrosis, and chronic obstructive airway disease.

Ophthalmic exposure

This will depend on the chemical itself and also the time in contact with the eye. The following indicate significant exposure has occurred: pain, blepharospasm, lacrimation, conjunctivitis, palpebral oedema, and photophobia. Acidic solutions may cause corneal burns.

Local injection

The extent of injury following injection of an acid is dependent on several factors including the agent, strength, volume, and the site of injection. Symptoms observed have ranged from local irritation to death.

Local features including pain and swelling at and around the injection site are common. Local reactions with nodule formation and/or soft tissue inflammatory reaction with granuloma formation may occur at the injection site.

Management

Ingestion

- Maintain airway and establish haemodynamic stability.
- In severely affected patients critical care input is essential. Urgent assessment of the airway is required. A supraglottic-epiglottic burn with erythema and oedema is usually a sign that further oedema will occur that may lead to airway obstruction. It is an indication for consideration of early intubation or tracheotomy.
- Do *not* attempt gastric lavage or give neutralizing chemicals as heat produced during neutralization reactions may increase injury.

- The use of intravenous H_2 antagonists or proton pump inhibitors has not been studied in detail but given in the early stages they may help to reduce the extent of injury.
- The use of water or milk (maximum initial volume = 100–200 mL in an adult; 2 mL/kg in a child) as diluents in the management of acid ingestion may be of some symptomatic benefit, but caution is necessary following large ingestions where mucosal damage /perforation may have already developed.
- Monitor BP, pulse, and oxygen saturation. Check FBC, coagulation screen, arterial blood gases, and U&Es. A severe metabolic disturbance is likely to be associated with substantial ingestion. However, while this may be due to the acid ingested, it may also be due to complications such as tissue necrosis.
- Treat haemorrhagic or hypovolemic shock by replacing lost fluids and blood intravenously. Perform erect chest X-ray if perforation is suspected. Parenteral opiate analgesia may be required for pain.
- Early fibreoptic endoscopy by an experienced endoscopist is indicated to grade the severity of the injury in a patient with evidence of oropharyngeal burns, drooling, pain, dysphagia, vomiting, and stridor. Although it was previously recommended that the endoscope should only be passed to the level of the first burn, recent work indicates that complete endoscopy using a flexible endoscope should be carried out to determine the full extent of injury.
- An urgent surgical review is recommended if bowel necrosis or perforation is suspected. Radical early resection of necrotic tissue and intraluminal stenting has been shown to improve survival and reduce the risk of oesophageal stricture formation in patients with alkali burns.
- On discharge, patients with evidence of endoscopic burns should be advised on the possibility of late onset sequelae (stricture) and advised to seek medical attention if symptoms develop. A specialist gastroenterologist should manage those patients who develop strictures.

Dermal exposure
- Avoid contaminating yourself and wear protective clothing if necessary. Carry out decontamination in a well-ventilated area, preferably with its own ventilation system.
- Do not apply neutralizing chemicals as heat produced during neutralization reactions may cause thermal burns and increase injury.
- Contaminated clothing and any particulate matter adherent to skin should be removed and the patient washed with copious amounts of water under low pressure for at least 10–15 minutes, or until pH of skin is normal (pH of the skin is 4.5–6 although it may be closer to 7 in children, or after irrigation). The earlier irrigation begins, the greater the benefit. Pay special attention to skin folds, fingernails, and ears.
- Recheck pH of affected areas after a period of 15–20 minutes and repeat irrigation if abnormal. Burns with strong solutions may require irrigation for several hours or more. Once the pH is normal and stabilised, treat as per a thermal injury.
- Burns totalling more than 15% of body surface area in adults (>10% in children) will require standard fluid resuscitation as for thermal burns.

- A burns specialist should review moderate to severe chemical burns. Excision or skin grafting may be required. Alkalis in particular may penetrate deeply within a few minutes.

Other measures as indicated by the patient's clinical condition.

Inhalation
- The treatment is supportive and depends on the condition of the patient. Remove from exposure and give oxygen.
- Remove contaminated clothing to prevent further exposure. Maintain a clear airway and ensure adequate ventilation. If symptomatic perform a chest X-ray, check ABGs, and perform a peak flow. Asymptomatic patients should be advised to return if symptoms develop over 24–48 hours post exposure.
- All patients with abnormal vital signs, chest pain, respiratory symptoms, or hypoxia should have a 12-lead ECG performed.
- If the patient has clinical features of bronchospasm treat conventionally with nebulized bronchodilators and steroids. Treat pulmonary oedema and/or acute lung injury with CPAP or in severe cases with IPPV and PEEP.
- The role of prophylactic corticosteroids (inhaled or systemic) and antibiotics is controversial, but unlikely to be of benefit. But antibiotics will be required if pneumonia develops.
- Patients with tachypnoea and stridor and those with upper airway damage should be considered for assessment with laryngoscope. Endotracheal intubation, or rarely, tracheostomy may be required for life-threatening laryngeal oedema.

Ophthalmic exposure
- Remove contact lenses if present and immediately irrigate the affected eye thoroughly with water or 0.9% saline for at least 10–15 minutes. Continue until the conjunctival sac pH is normal (7.5–8.0), retest after 20 minutes and use further irrigation if necessary.
- Any particles lodged in the conjunctival recesses should be removed.
- Repeated instillation of local anaesthetics (e.g. tetracaine) may reduce discomfort and help more thorough decontamination.
- Corneal damage may be detected by instillation of fluorescein.
- Mydriatic and cycloplegic agents (e.g. cyclopentolate, tropicamide) may reduce discomfort but should not be used in patients with glaucoma. However, a dynamic risk assessment must be made and it is likely that patients with glaucoma will need to be referred for **urgent** ophthalmological assessment.
- Patients with corneal damage, those who have been exposed to strong acids or alkalis and those whose symptoms do not resolve rapidly should be referred for **urgent** ophthalmological assessment.
- Injection into a small tissue space (e.g. fingers) can (rarely) cause sufficient local reaction to impair blood supply, producing distal ischaemic changes with pain, numbness, stiffness, swelling, and cyanosis. Corrosive effects may lead to severe destruction of surrounding tissues. Intentional injection of 3 mL of HCl into the groin area has resulted in extensive necrosis requiring leg amputation.

- Systemic features may include vomiting, fever, hypotension, tachycardia, electrolyte abnormalities, raised liver enzymes, renal failure, anaemia and haemoglobinuria, ECG abnormalities, and lung damage.

Local injection
- Clean the injection site and treat local swelling and irritation conventionally. Analgesia may be required. Monitor pulse, BP and respiration. Check LFTs, U&Es, ABGs, and FBC. Perform a 12-lead ECG. Perform a chest X-ray if respiratory features develop.
- Early surgical involvement should be considered in all cases. Due to the potential for continued destructive damage, early debridement with exhaustive irrigation may be required.

Alkalis

Background
Alkalis are substances whose aqueous solutions have a pH greater than 7 and have the ability to turn litmus paper blue and can react with an acid to form a salt and water.

They are capable of degrading fats and, to some extent, proteins. This makes them particularly hazardous to the eyes. They therefore have a detergent effect, but are corrosive to skin and mucus membranes. Dishwasher detergents, strong cleansers, oven cleaners, and paint removers are examples of products that often contain alkalis. Examples include sodium hydroxide (NaOH), calcium oxide (CaO), and calcium carbonate ($CaCO_3$).

Sodium hydroxide is strongly corrosive and exposure to any quantity could be dangerous. The UK exposure limit (short term) is 2 mg/m^3.

Mechanisms of toxicity
Strong alkalis are corrosive and therefore exposure to any quantity can be dangerous, e.g. NaOH. Weak alkalis are irritant to mucous membranes and generally of much lower toxicity, e.g. $CaCO_3$. Strong alkalis can directly damage tissue by the saponification of fats and the solubilisation of proteins and collagen. This causes liquefaction burns and necrosis with a softening of the tissues, which can further lead to deep tissue penetration and full-thickness burns.

The extent of injury following ingestion of corrosives is dependent on several factors including the strength and viscosity of the compound and the volume involved. Ingestion can lead to tissue injury from both the direct corrosive effects of the alkali and an exothermic reaction causing thermal injury; this is particularly true following ingestion of strong alkalis where the heat generated on contact with the stomach acid can cause gastric perforation in severe cases.

Clinical features
Ingestion
Alkalis often damage the oesophagus alone, but ingestion of large volumes can also damage the stomach and small intestines. The presence of oropharyngeal burns does not correlate well with the presence of oesophageal damage, but generally more extensive oral burns are associated with multiple site involvement.

For this reason there is often little immediate oral discomfort, but subsequently a burning sensation develops in the mouth and pharynx, together with epigastric pain, vomiting, and diarrhoea. This may be followed by haematemesis and dyspnoea. Pain and oedema may make

swallowing difficult, causing drooling. Haemorrhagic or hypovolaemic shock and airway obstruction from laryngeal and/or epiglottic oedema are features in severe cases.

Oesophageal or gastric perforation may occur in the early stages of severe cases. Stridor and respiratory complications (including mediastinitis, pneumonitis, pulmonary oedema, ARDS, pulmonary necrosis, and aorto-enteric fistula formation as secondary complications of perforation) can develop.

Stricture formation is a potential late complication, usually occurring between 2 weeks and 2 months post exposure, although it may not be clinically apparent for several years. Severe injury can cause pyloric stenosis and a small, scarred, immobile stomach.

Dermal exposure
Strong alkalis may cause pain, ulceration, and necrosis as they can directly damage tissue by the saponification of fats and the solubilization of proteins and collagen. This causes liquefaction burns and necrosis with a softening of the tissues, which can further lead to deep tissue penetration and full-thickness burns. Although pain is usually a key feature, alkali injuries may be initially painless leading to a delay in treatment. Alkali injuries can also progress over several hours and it can be difficult to assess the extent of the resulting burn due to quickly developing skin discolouration. Recurring skin breakdown over extended periods after the initial injury may complicate and delay recovery.

Ocular exposure
Alkaline solutions in particular may penetrate all layers of the eye causing iritis, anterior and posterior synechiae, corneal opacification, cataracts, glaucoma, and retinal atrophy. Alkali burns to the eyes should be considered an ophthalmic emergency.

Management
Ingestion
- Do not attempt gastric lavage or give neutralizing chemicals as heat produced during neutralization reactions may increase injury.
- Early fibreoptic endoscopy by an experienced endoscopist is indicated to grade the severity of the injury in a patient with evidence of oropharyngeal burns, drooling, pain, dysphagia, vomiting, and stridor. Endoscopy should be avoided between 5 and 15 days post exposure, as this is when the oesophagus is at its weakest.
- An urgent surgical review is recommended if bowel necrosis or perforation is suspected. Delay in diagnosis and treatment of transmural oesophagogastric necrosis is the most important factor contributing to mortality. Radical early resection of necrotic tissue and intraluminal stenting has been shown to improve survival and reduce the risk of oesophageal stricture formation in patients with alkali burns.
- On discharge, patients with evidence of endoscopic burns should be advised on the possibility of late onset sequelae (stricture) and advised to seek medical attention if symptoms develop. A specialist gastroenterologist should manage those patients who develop strictures. Corticosteroids have been advocated to reduce the incidence of stricture formation but their value is uncertain. They may decrease the need for surgical repair of strictures arising from second- or third-degree burns if they are used in conjunction with either anterograde or retrograde oesophageal dilation.

- There is a considerable increased risk of squamous cell carcinoma occurring; the mean latent period for development of carcinoma of the oesophagus following alkali ingestion is more than 40 years.

Dermal exposure
- Contaminated clothing and any particulate matter adherent to skin should be removed and the patient washed with copious amounts of water under low pressure for at least 10–15 minutes, or until the skin pH is normal (pH of the skin is 4.5–6 although it may be closer to 7 in children, or after irrigation). Continue irrigation if necessary. Once the pH is normal and stabilized, treat as per a thermal injury. The earlier irrigation begins, the greater the benefit. Special attention should be paid to skin folds, fingernails, and ears.
- As alkalis may penetrate deeply within a few minutes, pain relief is essential.

Ocular exposure
- Remove contact lenses if present and immediately irrigate the affected eye thoroughly with water or 0.9% saline for at least 10–15 minutes. Continue until the conjunctival sac pH is normal (7.5–8.0). Retest after 20 minutes and use further irrigation if necessary. Any particles lodged in the conjunctival recesses should be removed.
- Repeated instillation of local anaesthetics (e.g. tetracaine) may reduce discomfort and help more thorough decontamination. An anaesthetized eye should be covered to protect from traumatic injury.
- Corneal damage may be detected by instillation of fluorescein. Patients with corneal damage should be referred for *urgent* ophthalmological assessment.
- Mydriatic and cycloplegic agents (e.g. tropicamide, cyclopentolate) may reduce discomfort but should not be used in patients with closed angle glaucoma.

Further reading
Andreoni B, Farina ML, Biffi R, et al. (1997). Esophageal perforation and caustic injury: emergency treatment of caustic ingestion. *Dis Esophagus*, 10:95–100.

Brodovsky SC, McCarty CA, Snibson G, et al. (2000). Management of alkali burns. An 11 year retrospective review. *Ophthalmology*, 107:1829–35.

Cattan P, Munoz-Bongrand N, Berney T, et al. (2000). Extensive abdominal surgery after caustic ingestion. *Ann Surg*, 231:519–23.

Cello JP, Fogel RP, Boland CR (1980). Liquid caustic ingestion. Spectrum of injury. *Arch Intern Med*, 140:501–4.

Christesen HBT (1994). Caustic ingestion in adults— epidemiology and prevention. *Clin Toxicol*, 32:557–68.

Crain EF, Gershel JC, Mezey AP (1984). Caustic ingestions. Symptoms as predictors of esophageal injury. *Am J Dis Child*, 138:863–5.

de Jong AL, Macdonald R, Ein S, et al. (2001). Corrosive oesophagitis in children: a 30-year review. *Int J Pediat Otorhinolaryngology*, 57:203–11.

Estrera A, Taylor W, Mills LJ, et al. (1986). Corrosive burns of the esophagus and stomach: a recommendation for an aggressive surgical approach. *Ann Thorac Surg*, 41:276–83.

Ford M (1991). Alkali and acid injuries of the upper gastrointestinal tract. *Contemp Manag Crit Care*, 1:225–49.

Fulton JA, Hoffman RS (2007). Steroids in second degree caustic burns of the esophagus: a systematic pooled analysis of fifty years of human data: 1956–2006. *Clin Toxicol*, 45:402–8.

Gaudreault P, Parent M, McGuigan M (1983). Predictability of esophageal injury from signs and symptoms: a study of caustic ingestion in 378 children. *Pediatrics*, 71:767–70.

Howell JM, Dalsey WC, Hartsell FW, et al. (1992). Steroids for the treatment of corrosive esophageal injury: a statistical analysis of past studies. *Am J Emerg Med*, 10:421–5.

Hsieh CH, Lin GT (2005). Corrosive injury from arterial injection of hydrochloric acid. *Am J Emerg Med*, 23:394–6.

Pelclová D, Navrátil T (2005). Do corticosteroids prevent oesophageal stricture after corrosive ingestion? *Toxicol Rev*, 24:125–9.

Thirlwall AS, Friedman N, Leighton SEJ, et al. (2001). Caustic soda ingestion – a case presentation and review of the literature. *Int J Pediatr Otorhinolaryngol*, 59:129–35.

Thompson JN (1987). Corrosive esophageal injuries. A study of nine cases of concurrent accidental caustic ingestion. *Laryngoscope*, 97:1060–8.

Zargar SA, Kochar R, Mehta S, et al. (1991). The role of fibreoptic endoscopy in the management of corrosive ingestion and modified endoscopic classification of burns. *Gastrointest Endosc*, 37:165–9.

Ammonia

Background

Ammonia (NH_3) is a colourless gas that is lighter than air with a very pungent odour; it occurs naturally and is manufactured. Ammonia gas can be compressed and becomes a liquid under pressure. The odour of ammonia is familiar to most people; it is used in smelling salts, household cleaners, and window cleaning products.

Ammonia easily dissolves in water and most of the ammonia changes to its ionic form: ammonium ions (NH^{4+}) are not gaseous and are odourless. Solutions of ammonia are alkaline and concentrated solutions are corrosive, e.g. ammonium hydroxide, aqueous ammonia, and ammonia solution. Ammonia and ammonium ions can change back and forth in water. In wells, rivers, lakes, and wet soils, the NH^{4+} form is the most common. Ammonia can also be combined with other substances to form ammonium compounds, e.g. ammonium chloride, ammonium sulfate, and ammonium nitrate.

Ammonia is very important to plant, animal, and human life. It is found in water, soil, and air, and is a source of nitrogen for plants and animals. Most of the ammonia in the environment comes from the natural breakdown of manure and dead plants and animals.

Humans are regularly exposed to low levels of ammonia in air, soil, and water. Ammonia exists naturally in the air at levels between 1 and 5 ppb. It is commonly found in rainwater. The ammonia concentrations in rivers and bays are usually less than 6 ppb. Soil typically contains about 1–5 ppm of ammonia. 80% of all manufactured ammonia is used as fertilizer. A third of this is applied directly to soil as pure ammonia. The rest is used to make other fertilizers that contain ammonium compounds, usually ammonium salts. Ammonia is also used to manufacture synthetic fibres, plastics, and explosives. Many cleaning products also contain ammonia in the form of ammonium ions.

Ammonia is essential for mammals and is necessary for making DNA, RNA, and proteins. It also plays a part in maintaining acid–base balance in tissues of mammals.

Toxicokinetics

Ammonia is extremely soluble in water and dissolves in the mucus fluid covering the mucous lining of the respiratory system to produce ammonium hydroxide, a strong base. Following a short-term inhalation exposure, ammonia is almost entirely retained in the upper nasal mucosa. Inhalation of high concentrations of ammonia may exceed the capacity of this mechanism leading to systemic absorption through the lungs.

Although ammonia rapidly enters the eye, systemic absorption is considered not to be quantitatively significant. The toxicity findings after acute skin exposure to ammonia suggest that systemic absorption is not significant by this route either.

Ammonia is absorbed readily through mucous membranes and the intestinal tract but not through the skin. It also rapidly penetrates the eye but as a route of systemic absorption, this is likely to be quantitatively insignificant.

Absorbed ammonia is well distributed throughout body compartments and reacts with hydrogen ions, depending on the pH of the compartment to produce ammonium ions. The ammonium ion is less mobile due to its charged nature. In the liver, ammonium ions are extensively metabolized to urea and glutamine therefore levels of ammonia that reach the circulation are low. Hepatic insufficiency could affect ammonium ion metabolism.

Ammonia reaching the circulation is principally excreted in the urine as urea; excretion of absorbed ammonia in exhaled breath and faeces is not significant. Small amounts of ammonia are excreted via the urine; the average daily excretion for human beings is approximately 2–3 g, about 0.01% of the total body burden. Small amounts of unabsorbed ammonia may also be excreted from the gastrointestinal tract in the faeces.

Mechanisms of toxicity

Ammonia and ammonia solutions are irritant and corrosive. Minor exposures may result in a burning sensation of the eyes and throat and more substantial exposure may cause coughing or breathing difficulties. A one-off exposure (sufficient to cause mild lung or eye irritation) is unlikely to result in long-term health effects. Exposure to high concentrations of ammonia may be potentially fatal.

Anhydrous ammonia gas stored under pressure as a compressed liquid expands rapidly on liberation, resulting in vaporization and a large endothermic reaction. The result may be evaporative freezing of any tissue in contact with the ammonia. The gas can act paradoxically following a release from liquid form because of the rapid cooling and so can form a dense cloud that follows the contours of the ground and does not rapidly dissipate.

Ammonia readily forms ammonium hydroxide on contact with moisture in the air and skin and the resultant hydroxide saponifies lipids of the epidermal fats and cell membranes. The resultant liquefactive necrosis may appear pale and without charring or blistering and may cause an increased depth of injury. The combination of both cryogenic effects with an alkali burn can produce serious injuries.

Clinical features

Inhalation

Inhalation causes irritation of eyes and nose with sore throat, cough, chest tightness, headache, fever, wheeze, tachycardia, and confusion. Chemical pneumonitis, tachypnoea, dyspnoea, and stridor due to laryngeal oedema may follow. Pulmonary oedema with increasing breathlessness, wheeze, hypoxia and cyanosis may take up to 36 hours to develop. Optic neuropathy has been reported following both acute and chronic inhalation. See Table 9.1.

Ingestion

Swallowing of ammonium solutions will typically damage the oesophagus but usually spare the stomach. There is little immediate oral discomfort, but subsequently, a burning sensation develops in the mouth and pharynx, together with epigastric pain, vomiting, and diarrhoea. Oesophageal ulceration with or without perforation may occur with mediastinitis, pneumonitis, cardiac injury, and aorto-enteric fistula formation as secondary complications of perforation. Alkali ingestion may result in stricture formation and there is a risk of malignancy; the mean latent period for development of carcinoma of the oesophagus following alkali ingestion is more than 40 years.

Table 9.1 Summary of toxic effects following acute exposure to ammonia by inhalation

Dose		Features
mg/m³	ppm	
20–35	30–50	Odour threshold
>35	>50	Irritation to eyes, nose and throat
70	100	Rapid eye and upper respiratory tract irritation
174–350	250–500	Tolerated for a few minutes
488	700	Immediately irritating to eyes and throat
>1045	>1500	Pulmonary oedema, coughing, laryngospasm
3480–6965	5000–10000	Rapidly fatal due to airways obstruction

Dermal exposure

Dermal exposure causes direct damage to tissues by the saponification of fats. This causes liquefaction burns and necrosis with a softening of the tissues that can further lead to deep tissue penetration and full thickness burns.

Ocular exposure

Ocular exposure causes pain, blepharospasm, lacrimation, conjunctivitis, palpebral oedema, and photophobia. Alkaline solutions may cause corneal burns and may penetrate all layers of the eye and find their way into the chambers causing iritis, anterior and posterior synechiae, corneal opacification, cataracts, glaucoma, and retinal atrophy.

Delayed effects following an acute exposure

Inhalation exposures to low concentrations for a short period, from which an individual recovers quickly on removal to fresh air, are unlikely to result in delayed or long-term adverse health effects. Substantial inhalation exposures to ammonia may cause long-term health effects, including persistent airway obstruction, cough, exertional dyspnoea, bronchiolitis obliterans, and bronchiectasis, which for some cases may persist for many years. Dysphonia may persist for many months as a result of burns to the aerodigestive tract.

Chronic/repeated exposure

Inhalation—minor respiratory effects have been associated with chronic inhalation exposure to low levels of ammonia.

Ingestion—there are no human data but it is unlikely that chronic exposures to low levels will have a significant adverse health effect.

Management

Remove patient from exposure.

Inhalation

Ensure a clear airway and adequate ventilation. Give oxygen to symptomatic patients. All patients with abnormal vital signs, chest pain, respiratory symptoms, or hypoxia should have a 12-lead ECG performed. If the patient has clinical features of bronchospasm, treat conventionally with nebulized bronchodilators and steroids. Endotracheal

intubation or, rarely, tracheostomy may be required for life-threatening laryngeal oedema. Apply other supportive measures as indicated by the patient's clinical condition.

Dermal exposure

Wash hair and all contaminated skin with copious amounts of water (preferably warm) and soap for at least 10–15 minutes. Decontaminate open wounds first and avoid contamination of unexposed skin. The earlier the irrigation begins, the greater the benefit. Pay special attention to skin folds, axillae, ears, fingernails, genital areas, and feet. Cover affected area with a clean non-adherent dressing. Burns totalling more than 15% of body surface area in adults (>10% in children) will require standard fluid resuscitation as for thermal burns. A burns specialist should review chemical burns. Apply other supportive measures as indicated by the patient's clinical condition.

Ocular exposure

Remove contact lenses if necessary and immediately irrigate the affected eye thoroughly with water or 0.9% saline for at least 10–15 minutes. Patients with corneal damage or those whose symptoms do not resolve rapidly should be referred for urgent ophthalmological assessment.

Ingestion

After ingestion, a clear airway should be established. Opioids are often necessary for analgesia. Dilution and/or neutralization is contraindicated. Urgent endoscopy is required. Urgent laparotomy with resection of necrotic tissue and surgical repair may be lifesaving. Total parenteral nutrition is often required.

Corticosteroids confer no benefit and may mask abdominal signs of perforation; antibiotics should be given for established infection only.

Further reading

Amshel CE, Fealk MH, Phillips BJ, et al. (2000). Anhydrous ammonia burns case report and review of the literature. *Burns*, 26:493–7.

Agency for Toxic Substances and Disease Registry (ATSDR) (2004). *Toxicological profile for ammonia*. Atlanta: ATSDR, US Public Health Service.

Baxter PJ, Aw T-C, Cockcroft A, et al. (2010). *Harrington Hunter's Diseases of Occupations*, 10th edition. London: Hodder.

Beare JD, Wilson RS, Marsh RJ (1988). Ammonia burns of the eye: an old weapon in new hands. *Br Med J*, 296:590.

Brautbar N, Wu MP, Richter ED (2003). Chronic ammonia inhalation and interstitial pulmonary fibrosis: a case report and review of the literature. *Arch Environ Health*, 58:592–6.

Chao TC, Lo DST (1996). Ammonia gassing deaths – a report on two cases. *Singapore Med J*, 37:147–9.

Close LG, Catlin FI, Cohn AM (1980). Acute and chronic effects of ammonia burns on the respiratory tract. *Arch Otolaryngol*, 106:151–8.

Health Protection Agency (2011). *HPA Compendium of Chemical Hazards: Ammonia*. Didcot: CRCE.

Leduc D, Gris P, Lheureux P, et al. (1992). Acute and long term respiratory damage following inhalation of ammonia. *Thorax*, 47:755–7.

Leung CM, Foo CL (1992). Mass ammonia inhalational burns – experience in the management of 12 patients. *Ann Acad Med*, 21:624–9.

Kerstein MD, Schaffzin DM, Hughes WB, et al. (2001). Acute management of exposure to liquid ammonia. *Mil Med*, 166:913–14.

Singh S, Malhotra P, Jain S, et al. (1999). Gastro-esophageal burns following domestic liquid ammonia ingestion: report of two cases. *Assoc Physicians India*, 47:647.

Benzene and toluene

Benzene

Benzene is a colourless, volatile liquid with a pleasant odour. Benzene is used primarily as a solvent in the chemical and pharmaceutical industries, and as a starting material and intermediate in the synthesis of numerous chemicals. As a raw material, it is used in the synthesis of ethylbenzene (used to produce styrene), cumene (used to produce phenol and acetone), cyclohexane, nitrobenzene (used to produce aniline and other chemicals), and chlorobenzenes and other products. Benzene is used as an additive in petrol, but it is also present naturally because it occurs in crude oil and is a by-product of oil-refining processes. It is an ingredient in many paints and varnish removers.

The primary route of human exposure to benzene is inhalation of ambient air. Benzene is present in the atmosphere both from natural sources, which include forest fires and oil seeps, and from industrial sources, which include car exhaust, industrial emissions, and fuel evaporation from petrol filling stations. Occupational exposure may occur during production of benzene or use of substances containing it.

Toxicokinetics

About 10% of inhaled benzene is excreted unchanged in the breath. The remainder is metabolized predominantly by cytochrome P450 2E1 (CYP2E1) to form benzene oxide, which undergoes non-enzymatic rearrangement to form phenol, the major initial product of benzene metabolism. Phenol is oxidized in the presence of CYP2E1 to catechol or hydroquinone, which are oxidized via myeloperoxidase to the reactive metabolites 1,2- and 1,4-benzoquinone, respectively. Several other pathways of benzene oxidase metabolism have been reported.

Mechanisms of toxicity

There is suggestive evidence that one or more benzene metabolites formed in the liver, most probably phenolic metabolites (phenol, hydroquinone, catechol, 1,2,4-benzenetriol, and 1,2- and 1,4-benzoquinone), play a major role in benzene toxicity. There is some evidence that CYP2E1-catalysed benzene metabolism may also occur in bone marrow, a major target tissue of benzene toxicity. Phenolic metabolites can be metabolized by bone marrow peroxidases to highly reactive semiquinone radicals and quinones that stimulate the production of reactive oxygen species. These steps lead to damage to tubulin, histone proteins, topoisomerase II, other DNA associated proteins, and DNA itself.

Clinical features—acute poisoning

Following inhalation, mucous membrane irritation, euphoria, dizziness, weakness, headache, blurred vision, tremor, ataxia, chest tightness, respiratory depression, cardiac arrhythmias, coma, and convulsions can occur. Inhalation of approximately 20,000 ppm has been fatal within 5–10 minutes. A 45-year-old man died after running to shut off a leaking tank containing benzene. The suspected cause of death was a fatal arrhythmia secondary to benzene-induced increased myocardial sensitivity to endogenous catecholamines.

Ingestion may cause nausea, vomiting, and abdominal pain. Systemic toxicity may follow.

Direct skin contact with liquid benzene may produce marked skin irritation. Systemic toxicity may follow.

Three workers died following inhalation and dermal contact with benzene. Their symptoms included second-degree burns to the face, trunk and limbs, alveolar haemorrhage, and pulmonary oedema.

Clinical features—chronic poisoning

The toxic effects of chronic poisoning may not become apparent for months or years after initial contact and may develop after all exposure has ceased.

Anorexia, headache, drowsiness, nervousness, and irritability are well described. Anaemia (including aplastic anaemia), leucopenia, thrombocytopenia, pancytopenia, leukaemia, lymphomas, chromosomal abnormalities, and cerebral atrophy have been reported. Patients have recovered after as long as a year of almost complete absence of formation of new blood cells.

A dry, scaly dermatitis may develop on prolonged or repeated skin exposure to liquid benzene.

Carcinogenicity

Benzene is known to be a human carcinogen. There is an increased incidence of leukaemia (mostly acute myeloid or myelocytic leukaemia but also chronic lymphocytic leukaemia) in individuals exposed to benzene. Some studies found that the risk of leukaemia increased with increasing benzene exposure. Little evidence was found for an association between benzene exposure and multiple myeloma or non-Hodgkin's lymphoma.

Management

Following removal from the contaminated atmosphere, treatment should be directed towards symptomatic and supportive measures. If ingested, gastric decontamination is contraindicated as aspiration is likely to occur.

Toluene

Toluene is used extensively as a solvent in the chemical, rubber, paint, glue, and pharmaceutical industries and as a thinner for inks, perfumes, and dyes.

Toxicokinetics

Following exposure, some 25–40% of toluene is exhaled unchanged via the lungs. The remainder is oxidized by cytochrome P450 enzymes to benzyl alcohol, then to benzaldehyde. Benzaldehyde is in turn metabolized to benzoic acid, primarily by mitochondrial aldehyde dehydrogenase-2. Benzoic acid is metabolized to either benzoyl glucuronide or hippuric acid; the latter is the primary urine metabolite. Ring hydroxylation to cresols is a minor pathway of metabolism. The majority of p-cresol and o-cresol formed is excreted unchanged in urine, though some is excreted as a conjugate. There is controversy as to whether m-cresol is produced as a metabolite of toluene or not, though it has been found in two cases of human poisoning.

Mechanisms of toxicity

Toluene produces CNS depression by a reversible interaction between toluene and the lipid bilayer of nerve membranes and/or reversible interactions with proteins in the membrane. Chronic exposure to high concentrations of toluene causes structural changes in the brain related either to increased breakdown of phospholipids or inhibition of synthesis.

Clinical features—acute poisoning

Acute inhalation results in irritation of the throat and eyes and increased lacrimation. Systemic features, notably euphoria, excitement, dizziness, confusion, headache, nervousness, tinnitus, ataxia, tremor, coma, and amnesia may then occur.

Ingestion gives rise to nausea, abdominal pain, and, rarely, haematemesis from corrosive oesophageal injury. Systemic features may follow.

Skin contact may cause irritation, dryness, erythema, defatting, blistering, and necrotic skin burns if contact is extensive or prolonged. Systemic features may follow.

Eye irritation, coma, slurred speech, headache, sinus tachycardia, and amnesia developed in two men who were exposed to high concentrations of toluene (>7000 mg/m^3 toluene; 1862 ppm for 2–3 hours) while removing glue from tiles in a swimming pool. Their toluene blood concentrations 90 minutes after exposure were 4.1 and 2.2 mg/L respectively.

A 20-year-old man who ingested 30 mL of a mixture of toluene and other hydrocarbons developed drowsiness, dizziness, bradycardia and third-degree AV block.

Ingestion of approximately 60 mL of toluene was reported to be fatal for a 51-year-old man.

Clinical features—chronic exposure

Toluene abuse was first linked with neurological damage in 1961 and characteristically induces cerebellar ataxia, tremor, nystagmus, and titubation. Pyramidal signs and cranial nerve damage, particularly hyposmia and optic atrophy have also been reported and cerebellar and cortical atrophy have been shown by CT. Muscular weakness, presenting as quadriparesis, may be profound and life-threatening and can mimic the Guillain–Barré syndrome; such patients usually have associated severe metabolic disturbances, including hypokalaemia. Cognitive function may also be depressed and dementia has been observed. In less severe cases, school or work performance may be impaired because of apathy and poor concentration. Toluene has also caused a symmetrical peripheral neuropathy.

Haematuria, pyuria, and proteinuria have been described in chronic toluene abusers and may herald renal failure due to glomerulonephritis. In addition, there may be tubular abnormalities, and renal tubular acidosis (usually type 1) is a well-recognized complication possibly as a result of altered permeability of the distal tubule to hydrogen ions with a reduced ability to acidify the urine. The hyperchloraemic metabolic acidosis so induced may be symptomless or present with severe muscular weakness due to hypokalaemia, or with urolithiasis because of hypercalciuria. Fanconi's syndrome has been described, and high anion gap metabolic acidosis has also been reported. Rhabdomyolysis has been observed.

A review of adults who had abused toluene indicated three major patterns of presentation: (1) muscle weakness due to hypokalaemic paralysis, (2) gastrointestinal complaints (abdominal pain, haematemesis), and (3) neuropsychiatric disorders (altered mental status, cerebellar abnormalities, peripheral neuropathy). In addition, hypophosphataemia and hyperchloraemia

were common. Rhabdomyolysis occurred in 40% of cases.

Management

If poisoning results from inhalation, the patient should be removed from the contaminated environment. Gastric decontamination should be considered if very large amounts have been ingested less than 1 hour previously, provided the airway can be protected. Thereafter, treatment consists of symptomatic and supportive measures.

Further reading

Agency for Toxic Substances and Disease Registry (ATSDR) (2007). *Toxicological Profile for Benzene.* Atlanta, GA: Agency for Toxic Substances and Disease Registry.

Ameno K, Fuke C, Ameno S, et al. (1989). A fatal case of oral ingestion of toluene. *Forensic Sci Int,* 41:255–60.

Avis SP, Hutton CJ (1993). Acute benzene poisoning: a report of three fatalities. *J Forensic Sci,* 38:599–602.

Aydin K, Sencer S, Demir T, et al. (2002). Cranial MR findings in chronic toluene abuse by inhalation. *Am J Neuroradiol,* 23:1173–9.

Barbera N, Bulla G, Romano G (1998). A fatal case of benzene poisoning. *J Forensic Sci,* 43:1250–1.

Baskerville JR, Tichenor GA, Rosen PB (2001). Toluene induced hypokalaemia: case report and literature review. *Emerg Med J,* 18:514–16.

Blank IH, McAuliffe DJ (1985). Penetration of benzene through human skin. *J Invest Dermatol,* 85:522–6.

Cámara-Lemarroy CR, Gónzalez-Moreno EI, Rodriguez-Gutierrez R, et al (2012). Clinical presentation and management in acute toluene intoxication: a case series. *Inhal Toxicol,* 24:434–8.

Dickson RP, Luks AM (2009). Toluene toxicity as a cause of elevated anion gap metabolic acidosis. *Respir Care,* 54:1115–17.

Drozd J, Bockowski EJ (1967). Acute benzene poisoning. *J Occup Med,* 9:9–11.

Einav S, Amitai Y, Reichman J, et al. (1997). Bradycardia in toluene poisoning. *J Toxicol Clin Toxicol,* 35:295–8.

IPCS (1993). *Environmental Health Criteria 150. Benzene,* Geneva: World Health Organization.

Kuang S, Liang W (2005). Clinical analysis of 43 cases of chronic benzene poisoning. *Chem Biol Interact,* 153–154:129–35.

Malingre MM, Hendrix EA, Schellens JH, et al. (2002). Acute poisoning after oral intake of a toluene-containing paint thinner. *Eur J Pediatr,* 161:354–5.

Meulenbelt J, de Groot G, Savelkoul TJ (1990). Two cases of acute toluene intoxication. *Br J Ind Med,* 47:417–20.

Midzenski MA, McDiarmid MA, Rothman N, et al. (1992). Acute high dose exposure to benzene in shipyard workers. *Am J Ind Med,* 22:553–65.

National Toxicology Program (2011). *Report on Carcinogens. Benzene.* Durham, NC: US Department of Health and Human Services.

Pace F, Greco S, Pallotta S, et al (2008). An uncommon cause of corrosive esophageal injury. *World J Gastroenterol,* 14:636–7.

Shibata K, Yoshita Y, Matsumoto H (1994). Extensive chemical burns from toluene. *Am J Emerg Med,* 12:353–5.

Snyder R (2002). Benzene and leukemia. *Crit Rev Toxicol,* 32:155–210.

Snyder R, Hedli CC (1996). An overview of benzene metabolism. *Environ Health Perspect,* 104:1165–71.

Tang H, Chu HK, Cheuk A, et al. (2005). Renal tubular acidosis and severe hypophosphataemia due to toluene inhalation. *HK Med J,* 11:50–3.

Tauber JB (1970). Instant benzol death. *J Occup Med,* 12:520–3.

Winek CL, Collom WD (1971). Benzene and toluene fatalities. *J Occup Med,* 13:259–61.

Bromates and chlorates

Bromates

Bromates are highly toxic salts containing the bromate anion BrO_3^-. They are oxidizing agents. The best known examples are sodium and potassium bromate. Sodium bromate was previously used as a neutralizer in home perms but it is being replaced increasingly with less toxic chemicals. Potassium bromate was used as a flour and bread 'improver' (it gave bread maximum volume and an upright shape) but its use for this purpose was banned in the UK in 1989 following concern regarding its carcinogenic potential. Bromates are still in use as laboratory reagents and oxidizing agents. In pure form they exist as white granules, crystals, or a crystalline powder.

Poisoning occurs usually by ingestion. Based on cases in the Japanese literature, the fatal dose is in the range of 12–50 g in adults.

Toxicokinetics

In animal studies some 30% of orally administered bromate was retrieved in urine within 24 hours, partly unchanged and partly as bromide ions (Br^-). Reduction of bromate to bromide is a means of bromate detoxification and is achieved by endogenous sulphydryl containing compounds, such as glutathione and thiosulfate. This process is saturable.

Mechanisms of toxicity

Animal studies suggest that the main mechanism of bromate-induced organ damage is oxidative stress and the generation of reactive oxygen species. Bromate ions are particularly nephrotoxic and ototoxic.

In chronic oral dosing studies in rodents bromates caused cancer of the kidney, thyroid, and peritoneal mesothelium.

Clinical features

Ingestion causes nausea, vomiting, haematemesis, severe abdominal pain, and diarrhoea. Hypotension has been observed, but is not usually severe. Acute kidney injury secondary to tubular necrosis is common and can develop within 12 hours of exposure; in some cases it is irreversible. Haemolytic uraemic syndrome has occurred in association with renal failure.

Convulsions have been reported. A sensorimotor polyneuropathy may develop after severe poisoning, with burning pain and/or paraesthesiae, classically affecting the lower limbs. Nerve conduction studies show demyelination and axonal degeneration. Recovery is usual but may take several months.

Hearing may be impaired within 4–16 hours of ingestion; tinnitus and dizziness are early associated features. Hearing loss is thought to result from oxidative damage within the cochlea. It may be permanent.

Cardiotoxicity and hepatotoxicity have also been reported.

A 78-year-old woman who ingested a cupful of permanent hair-waving solution containing 7% sodium bromate presented with nausea, vomiting, and diarrhoea and went on to develop acute kidney injury requiring haemodialysis but made a full recovery over 4 weeks.

Management

Consider gastric aspiration or lavage within 1 hour of ingestion for any amount provided the airway can be protected.

Hypotension should be corrected by giving an appropriate fluid challenge.

Administration of sodium chloride 0.9% has been shown to reduce the serum half-life of bromide from 12 to 3 days, by competition for renal tubular reabsorption between chloride and bromide ions. For this reason intravenous sodium chloride may be beneficial in cases of bromate poisoning. There are no evidence-based recommendations regarding the rate of infusion, but sodium chloride 0.9% at an infusion rate of 200–500 mL/hour has been suggested for adults.

Since sodium thiosulfate reduces bromate to bromide, administration of 1–5 g (10–50 mL of a 10% solution or 100–500 mL of a 1% solution) has been proposed in severe cases. There is, however, no evidence to confirm the efficacy of this intervention.

Early institution of haemodialysis should be considered in cases of severe toxicity and/or renal failure. Although the role of dialysis in the elimination of bromate has not been the subject of controlled studies, isolated case reports suggest benefit.

Nerve conduction studies are indicated in those who develop symptoms and signs suggestive of a peripheral neuropathy.

Audiometric testing should be performed to assess level of hearing once the patient is clinically stable.

Bromate concentrations cannot be determined easily. Serum bromide determination may be helpful to confirm ingestion where the diagnosis is uncertain but this assay is not widely available.

Chlorates

Sodium and potassium chlorates are highly reactive oxidizing agents, previously used as non-selective herbicides though the licence for this use has been withdrawn in many countries.

Potassium chlorate is used in the production of matchstick heads, fireworks, explosives, mouthwashes, and oxygenating tablets for fish tanks. Sodium chlorate is used as a bleaching agent.

Toxicokinetics

Chlorates are absorbed rapidly from the gastrointestinal tract and renally eliminated predominantly unchanged though with some conversion to chlorite.

Mechanisms of toxicity

Chlorates are potent oxidizing agents and cause devastating oxidative stress to cell membranes, notably red blood cell membranes, resulting in severe intravascular haemolysis. Methaemoglobinaemia occurs due to oxidation of ferrous (Fe^{2+}) haem to ferric (Fe^{3+}) haem. Renal tubular toxicity results both from haemoglobinuria and direct oxidative damage to proximal tubular cells.

Clinical features

The early features include nausea, vomiting, diarrhoea, abdominal pain, and 'cyanosis' secondary to methaemoglobinaemia. The slate grey/blue apparent cyanosis is due, at least initially, to the pigmented colour of methaemoglobin rather than the presence of deoxygenated haemoglobin. Methaemoglobinaemia can be severe, concentrations of 50–80% have been reported. The rate of methaemoglobin formation is relatively slow and clinically significant concentrations can occur insidiously. There may be a delay of up to 12 hours before systemic toxicity manifests with varying degrees of hypoxaemia, general weakness, fatigue, dizziness, confusion, agitation, headache, chest pain, dyspnoea, and ataxia. Rhabdomyolysis, coma, convulsions, and respiratory arrest have been reported.

Significant intravascular haemolysis is a common complication and is usually evident within 6 hours, rendering the urine red or dark in colour. Jaundice may develop. Subsequently disseminated intravascular coagulation secondary to haemolytic anaemia and haemoglobinuria may occur. A decreased platelet count, haematuria, leucocytosis and a metabolic acidosis can be present. Acute kidney injury may ensue due to renal tubular necrosis. Hyperkalaemia resulting from renal failure and exacerbated by haemolysis is expected.

A gardener who sprayed 'a very concentrated' solution of sodium chlorate while a strong wind was blowing reported being aware of it being blown into his face and inhaling it. He also ingested some. Later that day he became nauseated and vomited. The next day he developed abdominal pain, copious vomiting, anuria, and jaundice. Renal failure was confirmed and the blood methaemoglobin concentration was 57%.

Management
Gastric decontamination is best avoided. Activated charcoal does not adsorb chlorates.

The patient should be observed for at least 12 hours. Pulse oximetry is inaccurate in patients with methaemoglobinaemia. Arterial blood gases should be measured to assess both methaemoglobin concentrations, pO_2, and pCO_2 (which may be normal) and acid–base status.

Consider the need for treatment with methylthioninium chloride (methylene blue), particularly if the methaemoglobin concentration is greater than 30%, though antidotal therapy may be indicated at lower concentrations if there are symptoms or signs suggestive of tissue hypoxia (e.g. fits, coma, chest pain, ischaemic ECG) and/or substantial haemolysis. Methylthioninium chloride 1–2 mg/kg body weight as a 1% solution should be given by slow intravenous injection.

Methaemoglobinaemia accompanying severe chlorate poisoning may be unresponsive or only partially responsive to methylene blue. This is because antidotal efficacy is dependent on NADPH availability, which in turn is dependent on the pentose phosphate pathway for which the rate limiting enzyme is glucose-6-phosphate dehydrogenase. Chlorate denaturates glucose-6-phosphate dehydrogenase and haemolysis dilutes the components of the pentose phosphate pathway. NADPH depletion ensues and this not only limits methythioninium chloride efficacy but also increases red cell susceptibility to haemolysis. In these circumstances exchange transfusion may be indicated.

Give high-flow oxygen to maximize oxygen carriage by functioning haemoglobin. Mechanical ventilation may be required in the presence of severe hypoxia.

Measure full blood count, U&Es, total creatine kinase activity, creatinine, liver function and coagulation tests. Intravascular haemolysis can be assessed by measurement of free haemoglobin, haptoglobin, and the reticulocyte count.

Monitor renal and hepatic function and treat failure conventionally. Monitor urine output and obtain urinalysis for haemoglobinuria.

Plasma potassium concentrations should be monitored and reduced if necessary. Haemodialysis will remove chlorate and may also be required for the management of renal failure and hyperkalaemia. Plasmapheresis and plasma exchange/exchange transfusion have also been employed to remove chlorate, circulating free haemoglobin, and red cell stroma and thus help to prevent the development of renal failure.

Further reading

De Vriese A, Vanholder R, Lamiere N (1997). Severe acute renal due to bromate intoxication: report of a case and discussion of management guidelines based on a review of the literature. *Failure Nephrol Dial Transplant,* 12:204–9.

Eysseric H, Vincent F, Peoc'h M, et al. (2000). A fatal case of chlorate poisoning: confirmation by ion chromatography of body fluids. *J Forensic Sci,* 45:474–7.

Gradus D, Rhoads M, Bergstrom LB, et al. (1984). Acute bromate poisoning associated with renal failure and deafness presenting as hemolytic uremic syndrome. *Am J Nephrol,* 4:188–91.

Helliwell M, Nunn J (1979). Mortality in sodium chlorate poisoning. *Br Med J,* 1:1119.

Kurokawa Y, Maekawa A, Takahashi M, et al. (1990). Toxicity and carcinogenicity of potassium bromate–A new renal carcinogen. *Environ Health Perspect,* 87:309–35.

Matsumoto I, Morizono T, Paparella MM (1980). Hearing loss following potassium bromate: two case reports. *Otolaryngol Head Neck Surg,* 88:625–9.

McElwee NE, Kearney TE (1988). Sodium thiosulphate unproven as bromate antidote. *Clin Pharm,* 7:570–1.

Mutlu H, Silit E, Pekkafali Z, et al. (2003). Cranial MR imaging findings of potassium chlorate intoxication. *Am J Neuroradiol,* 24:1396–8.

Petrolini V, Locatelli C, Giampreti A, et al. (2007). Fatal case of sodium chlorate self poisoning. *Clin Toxicol,* 45:361.

Quick CA, Chole RA Mauer SM (1975). Deafness and renal failure due to bromate poisoning. *Arch Otolaryngol,* 101:494–5.

Ranghino A, Costantini L, Deprado A, et al. (2006). A case of acute sodium chlorate self-poisoning successfully treated without conventional therapy. *Nephrol Dial Transplant,* 21:2971–4.

Sashiyama H, Irie Y, Ohtake Y, et al. (2002). Acute renal failure and hearing loss due to sodium bromate poisoning: a case report and review of the literature. *Clin Nephrol,* 58:455–7.

Steffen C, Seitz R (1981). Severe chlorate poisoning: report of a case. *Arch Toxicol,* 48:281–8.

Steffen C, Wetzel E (1993). Chlorate poisoning: mechanism of toxicity. *Toxicology,* 84:217–31.

Trump DL, Hochberg MC (1976). Bromide intoxication. *Johns Hopkins Med J,* 138:119–23.

Uchida HA, Sugiyama H, Kanehisa S, et al. (2006). An elderly patient with severe acute renal failure due to sodium bromate intoxication. *Intern Med,* 45:151–4.

Wang V, Lin KP, Tsai CP, et al. (1995). Bromate intoxication with polyneuropathy. *J Neurol Neurosurg Psychiatr,* 58:516–17.

Carbon disulphide

Background
Carbon disulphide is used as a fumigant for grain and as a solvent, particularly in the rayon industry. It is a clear, colourless, volatile liquid, with an odour like that of decaying cabbage.

Toxicokinetics
The metabolism of carbon disulphide in man has not been established completely. Carbon disulphide is metabolized by cytochrome P450 to an unstable oxygen intermediate, which may either spontaneously degrade to atomic sulphur and carbonyl sulphide or hydrolyse to form atomic sulphur and monothiocarbonate. The atomic sulphur generated in these reactions may either covalently bind to macromolecules or be oxidized to products such as sulfate. The carbonyl sulphide formed may be converted to monothiocarbonate by carbonic anhydrase. Monothiocarbonate may further spontaneously degrade, regenerating carbonyl sulphide or forming carbon dioxide and sulphide bisulphide ion (HS^-). The HS^- formed can subsequently be oxidized to sulfate or other non-volatile metabolites.

Mechanisms of toxicity
Carbon disulphide reacts with free amino groups of proteins and amino acids to form dithiocarbamates, which may in part account for carbon disulphide-induced peripheral neurotoxicity. Dithiocarbamates also inhibit protein synthesis and have been implicated in disturbances of trace metal balance. In contrast, the formation or generation of reactive sulphur may inhibit the microsomal mono-oxygenase system and disturb the metabolism of other endogenous and exogenous compounds.

Clinical features—acute poisoning
Acute poisoning is rare. Absorption occurs through the skin as well as by inhalation.

Acute inhalation may result in irritation of the mucous membranes, blurred vision, nausea and vomiting, headache, delirium, hallucinations, coma, tremor, convulsions, and cardiac and respiratory arrest.

Due to its potent defatting activity, carbon disulphide causes reddening, cracking, and peeling of the skin and a burn may occur if contact continues for several minutes.

Splashes of carbon disulphide in the eye cause immediate and severe irritation.

Mass carbon disulphide poisoning occurred at a viscose rayon factory in Korea in 1988. In 2005, 170 of the exposed workers were compared with carefully matched controls. After adjusting for covariates, carbon disulphide-poisoned subjects had an increased risk of the metabolic syndrome (prevalence ratio 1.57, 95% CI 1.25–1.98).

Clinical features—chronic poisoning
Numerous cohort studies undertaken since the 1930s have demonstrated an increased incidence of cardiovascular disease among workers exposed to carbon disulphide. Despite improvements in ventilation since then, subsequent studies continue to show an increased mortality among this group of workers despite much lower levels of carbon disulphide in the workplace. There is an increased incidence of hypertension, arteriosclerosis, ischaemic heart disease, elevated cholesterol among workers exposed to carbon disulphide. In addition, sleep disturbances, fatigue, anorexia, and weight loss are common complaints. Intellectual impairment, cerebellar signs, diffuse vascular encephalopathy, Parkinsonism, peripheral polyneuropathy, hepatic damage, and permanent impairment of reproductive performance have been described.

Available human studies clearly show that exposure to mean concentrations of carbon disulphide of approximately 31 mg/m³ (10 ppm) and higher cause effects on the cardiovascular and nervous system.

Management
Treatment for acute exposure involves removal from exposure, washing contaminated skin, irrigation of the eyes with water, and supportive measures. Preventive measures to keep carbon disulphide concentrations in the workplace as low as possible are of great importance and should be applied vigorously.

Further reading
Agency for Toxic Substances and Disease Registry (ATSDR) (1996). *Carbon Disulphide*. Atlanta, GA: ATSDR.

Chapman LJ, Sauter SL, Henning RA, et al. (1991). Finger tremor after carbon disulphide-based pesticide exposures. *Arch Neurol*, 48:866–70.

Coppock RW, Buck WB (1981). Toxicology of carbon disulfide: a review. *Vet Hum Toxicol*, 23:5.

Dalvi RR (1988). Mechanism of the neurotoxic and hepatotoxic effects of carbon disulfide. *Drug Metabol Drug Interact*, 6:275–84.

De Laey JJ, De Rouck A, Priem H, et al. (1980). Ophthalmological aspects of chronic CS2 intoxication. *Int Ophthal*, 3:51–6.

Fielder RJ, Shillaker RO (1981). *Toxicity Review. Carbon Disulphide*. London: HMSO.

Frumkin H (1998). Multiple system atrophy following chronic carbon disulfide exposure. *Environ Health Perspect*, 106:611–13.

Gelbke H-P, Goen T, Maurer M, et al. (2009). A review of health effects of carbon disulfide in viscose industry and a proposal for an occupational exposure limit. *CRC Crit Rev Toxicol*, 39(Suppl 2):1–126.

Greim H (ed.) (2005). Carbon disulfide. In The MAK-collection for occupational health and safety. Part I: MAK value documentations, pp. 171–85. Weinheim: Wiley-VCH.

Huang CC, Chu CC, Chen RS, et al. (1996). Chronic carbon disulfide encephalopathy. *Eur Neurol*, 36:364–8.

IPCS (1979). *Environmental Health Criteria 10. Carbon Disulphide*. Geneva: WHO.

Jhun H-J, Lee S-Y, Yim S-H, et al. (2009). Metabolic syndrome in carbon disulfide-poisoned subjects in Korea: does chemical poisoning induce metabolic syndrome? *Int Arch Occup Environ Health*, 82:827–32.

Kim EA, Kang SK (2010). Occupational neurological disorders in Korea. *J Korean Med Sci*, 25(Suppl):S26–35.

Lee E, Kim MH (1998). Cerebral vasoreactivity by transcranial Doppler in carbon disulphide poisoning cases in Korea. *J Korean Med Sci*, 13:645–51.

Peters HA, Levine RL, Matthews CG, et al. (1982). Carbon disulfide-induced neuropsychiatric changes in grain storage workers. *Am J Ind Med*, 3:373–91.

Phillips M (1992). Detection of carbon disulphide in breath and air: a possible new risk factor for coronary artery disease. *Int Arch Occup Environ Health*, 64:119–23.

Spyker DA, Gallanosa AG, Suratt PM (1982). Health effects of acute carbon disulfide exposure. *Clin Toxicol*, 19:87.

Sweetnam PM, Taylor SW, Elwood PC (1987). Exposure to carbon disulphide and ischaemic heart disease in a viscose rayon factory. *Br J Ind Med*, 44:220–7.

World Health Organization (2002). *Concise International Chemical Assessment Document 46. Carbon Disulfide*. Geneva: WHO.

Carbon monoxide

Background
Exposure is most commonly from car exhaust (unleaded petrol cars produce about one-tenth the amount of carbon monoxide (CO) of older cars), and faulty heaters, fires, and industrial accidents.

Toxicokinetics
Carboxyhaemoglobin (COHb) concentration in blood is a function of the CO concentration in inspired air and the time of exposure. Perceptible clinical effects occur within 2 hours of exposure at concentrations as low as 0.01% (100 ppm). Decreased barometric pressure, and any factors that increase the rate of ventilation and perfusion increase uptake of CO (and these are both increased by CO poisoning).

CO is mainly eliminated (unchanged) from the lungs. The half-life of CO in room air is around 4–5 hours. This half-life decreases to approximately 40–80 minutes with administration of '100% oxygen' and to 23 minutes when hyperbaric (2 atmospheres) oxygen is used.

Mechanisms of toxicity
CO binds to haemoglobin at the oxygen binding sites with very high affinity to form COHb. As COHb cannot carry oxygen this leads to reduced oxygen carrying capacity. Due to the cooperative binding of oxygen binding sites, COHb also leads to higher affinity binding for oxygen meaning that oxygen release by the remaining oxygenated Hb is also impaired.

Thus, CO leads to impaired oxygen delivery to tissues and eventually to marked tissue hypoxia when compensatory mechanisms to maintain oxygen delivery fail.

This functional hypoxia produced by CO poisoning is the best understood but not the only explanation for toxic effects. CO also binds to and inhibits mitochondrial cytochrome oxidase thereby directly inhibiting aerobic metabolism (analogous to the effect of cyanide). Further damage may be caused by the marked oxidative stress, free radical production, and inflammation seen when oxygenation improves and CO concentrations fall after severe poisoning, a process roughly analogous to reperfusion injury.

The target organs of CO poisoning are principally the heart and brain. Of particular concern is the potential for delayed neurotoxicity including parkinsonism, memory, and concentration impairment.

The initial clinical effects (at COHb concentrations <40–60%) occur despite compensated hypoxaemia. Oxygen delivery to the brain is maintained by a compensatory increase in cardiac output (as with anaemia).

As COHb concentrations rise, the heart rapidly becomes unable to compensate via higher cardiac output. (Note there is also impaired oxygen delivery and greatly increased oxygen demand for the heart.) Hypotension and reduced cardiac output exacerbate severe tissue hypoxia and death will rapidly occur unless there is intervention. Hypoxic brain damage is readily explainable in this group of patients

Clinical features
The clinical symptoms and signs vary depending on the concentration of COHb. Normal individuals have very low levels but up to 10% COHb may be found in smokers. At levels of 20–40% symptoms typically develop and reflect mild tissue hypoxia and the cardiovascular effects and include headache, breathlessness, tachycardia, confusion, weakness, nausea, and vomiting. At higher concentrations (>50% COHb), tissue hypoxia affecting the CNS (coma, convulsions) and cardiac system (arrhythmias, chest pain from myocardial ischaemia or infarction) develop and death is likely when concentrations exceed 70%. However, the ability of the individual to compensate for the decreased oxygen carrying capacity determines the level at which more severe manifestations become apparent, and those with underlying anaemia, respiratory, cardiac or vascular disease may develop severe toxicity at lower concentrations.

Other coexistent toxic exposures should always be considered; suicide attempts commonly involve drug overdose and smoke inhalation may be associated with cyanide exposure.

Long-term sequelae
The long-term consequences in survivors range from severe brain damage (which is fortunately uncommon) to a much more common syndrome of less severe but persistent problems. These most commonly are largely subjective and affect mood, short-term memory, attention, and concentration. In some cases, these are not noted initially but present later, after initial recovery (typically within a week of the exposure). These are then referred to as delayed neurological sequelae. The best identified risk factors for long-term neurological effects are early and obvious neurological damage or a sustained loss of consciousness during the CO exposure. Neuro-psychological testing may be useful to provide some objective measures of subtle deficits not found with routine bedside mental state examination and also to monitor the progress of these sequelae. The functional prognosis is generally favourable; for example around 80–90% of patients diagnosed with these sequelae are still able to return to full-time work.

Toxicity assessment
COHb concentrations are a rough guide to the severity of exposure. As these are often delayed, it is tempting to perform a backwards extrapolation based on estimated half-life since removal. However, as this is dependent on inhaled oxygen and this is often very poorly quantified, this works well only on those who have had no supplemental oxygen. Further, the correlation with acute and long-term clinical effects is generally poor due to substantial variability in ability to compensate. Thus they can confirm (or possibly exclude) the diagnosis but should not be used as a guide for treatment or long-term prognosis.

A better guide to the severity of exposure is usually found simply from the history of symptoms (loss of consciousness, chest pain) and by examining for evidence of ischaemic damage (neurological signs, ECG changes, troponin). Myocardial injury is very common particularly in those with loss of consciousness, and/or underlying vascular disease. Attributable long-term cardiac consequences are unusual; however, a higher mortality rate has been reported in those with such findings. It is unclear if this partially represents long-term cardiac sequelae or simply underlying cardiovascular risk factors. The S100β levels over the first 6 hours have been suggested to be a potentially useful means of measuring neuronal damage, however to date there are insufficient studies correlating these with sub-sequent clinical outcomes.

A very high lactate that persists after the COHb falls should suggest cyanide toxicity in smoke inhalation.

Management

Provide 100% oxygen by non-re-breather mask (or venti-lator) ASAP. 4–6 hours of 100% normobaric oxygen will remove over 90% of the carbon monoxide.

Assess severity and potential for coexistent poison-ings as previously described—including 12-lead ECG and electrolytes, FBC, and COHb.

If there is impaired consciousness, ensure the airway is maintained with intubation if necessary. Ensure the patient is quiet and resting as unnecessary muscle activity increases oxygen demand.

Obtain serial ECG and cardiac enzymes in patients with a history of sustained loss of consciousness, cardiovascu-lar disease, chest pain, and/or ECG changes.

The main therapeutic goal is to prevent acute and chronic neuropsychiatric consequences. Oxygen is the most important treatment and is always indicated for at least 6 hours. Oxygen toxicity is unlikely with less than 24 hours of treatment. Currently, the evidence for any treatment beyond 100% oxygen is very weak.

Acidosis should not be corrected routinely; in most cases it should rapidly respond to improved oxygenation and ventilation. Acidosis shifts the haemoglobin–oxygen dissociation curve back to the right thereby partially correcting the left-shift and impaired release causes by COHb. Further, aggressive correction may easily lead to rebound alkalaemia as the lactic acidosis usually resolves rapidly.

Hyperbaric oxygen

Administration of hyperbaric oxygen (HBO) at 2.5 atmospheres of pressure decreases the half-life of COHb to approximately 20 minutes. However, given the half-life is only around 40 minutes with 100% oxygen and it usually takes considerably longer than this time to arrange HBO treatment, the biological rationale for HBO being a more effective means of removing CO in practice is limited. It has been suggested it may decrease the risk of neuropsychiatric sequelae due to other mech-anisms not dependent on enhancing CO elimination. However, HBO might also feasibly increase oxidative stress during recovery and also is well known to have other adverse effects including seizures, tympanic mem-brane rupture, sinus and pulmonary complications. It is contraindicated if there has been chest trauma, or if the patient requires close monitoring or is non-cooperative.

The results of hyperbaric oxygen (HBO) vs 100% oxy-gen in six randomized clinical trials to date have overall been unimpressive and conflicting. There have been four negative and two positive studies. The negative studies have had mostly subjective outcome measures of neuro-logical recovery and may feasibly have overlooked clini-cally important benefits. In contrast, there is a high risk of bias introduced during the analysis evident in the positive studies. The largest positive trial was premature stopped 'for benefit' but had numerous assumptions and protocol variations (including a change in the primary outcome) that all favoured showing benefit from HBO.

The role of HBO in the acute management of patients with very severe CO poisoning, such as coma, seizures, severe metabolic acidosis, or cardiac dysfunc-tion is particularly unclear as controlled clinical tri-als have frequently excluded such patients. If rapidly available, HBO may be the most effective mechanism for treating hypoxia in such patients; however, it may also be difficult to use unless a multi-person chamber is available so that medical/nursing care can continue uninterrupted.

In conclusion, HBO has a plausible but not compelling rationale, some risks, and is of unknown effectiveness. It will likely remain so until a large multicentre double blind RCT examining long-term clinical outcomes is per-formed, however, no such trials are currently registered as ongoing. The final recommendations of the American College of Emergency Physicians clinical guidelines com-mittee sum up the current evidence thus:

> HBO is a therapeutic option for CO-poisoned patients; however, its use cannot be mandated. No clinical variables, including COHb levels, identify a subgroup of CO-poisoned patients for whom HBO is most likely to provide benefit or cause harm.

Hyperbaric oxygen in pregnancy

Fetal haemoglobin has a very high affinity for CO, and there is a much longer half-life of CO in the fetal circula-tion even with 100% oxygen. As oxygen tension is already much lower, the fetus is particularly susceptible to CO poisoning. HBO may be more useful in this setting (to shorten the half-life of CO and to deliver oxygen inde-pendent of haemoglobin). HBO appears to be safe in pregnancy although the outcome of significant CO poi-soning in the mother is often fetal death or neurological damage.

Further reading

Annane D, Chadda K, Gajdos P, et al. (2011). Hyperbaric oxygen therapy for acute domestic carbon monoxide poisoning: two randomized controlled trials. Intensive Care Med, 37:486–92.

Buckley NA, Isbister G, Stokes B, et al. (2005). Hyperbaric oxygen for carbon monoxide poisoning -a systematic review. Toxicol Rev, 24(2):75–92.

Buckley NA, Juurlink DN, Isbister G, et al. (2011). Hyperbaric oxygen for carbon monoxide poisoning. Cochrane Database Syst Rev, 4:CD002041.

Henry CR, Satran D, Lindgren B, et al. (2006). Myocardial injury and long-term mortality following moderate to severe carbon monoxide poisoning. JAMA, 295:398–402.

Koren G, Sharav T, Pastuszak A, et al. (1991). A multicenter, prospective study of fetal outcome following accidental car-bon monoxide poisoning in pregnancy. Reproduct Toxicol, 5(5):397–403.

Roughton FJW, Darling RC (1944). The effect of carbon mon-oxide on the oxyhemoglobin dissociation curve. Am J Physiol, 141:17–31.

Smollin C, Olson K (2008). Carbon monoxide poisoning (acute). Clin Evid, 7:2103.

Weaver LK (2009). Carbon monoxide poisoning. N Engl J Med, 360:1217–25.

Wolf SJ, Lavonas EJ, Sloan EP, et al. (2008). Critical issues in the management of adult patients presenting to the emergency department with acute carbon monoxide poisoning. Ann Emerg Med, 51:138–52.

Chlorinated hydrocarbons

Background
Low-molecular-weight chlorinated hydrocarbons such as carbon tetrachloride, methylene chloride, tetrachloroethylene, 1,1,1-trichloroethane, and trichloroethylene are useful solvents.

Carbon tetrachloride
Carbon tetrachloride (tetrachloromethane) was once widely used as a dry-cleaning chemical, degreasing agent, and fire extinguisher but international regulations have now restricted it to laboratory and industrial usage. It is now used as a chemical intermediate, in petroleum refining, in pharmaceutical manufacturing, as an industrial solvent, in the processing of fats, oils, and rubber, and in laboratory applications.

Toxicokinetics
Carbon tetrachloride is absorbed readily from the gastrointestinal and respiratory tract. Dermal absorption is very low. Bioactivation of carbon tetrachloride proceeds by cytochrome P450-dependent reductive dehalogenation. Ethanol-inducible CYP2E1 is the primary enzyme responsible for metabolizing carbon tetrachloride, but others, particularly CYP3A, are also involved at higher concentrations. The trichloromethyl free radical reacts with molecular oxygen, resulting in the formation of trichloromethylperoxyl radicals ($CCl_3OO^\bullet$), which are even more reactive than trichloromethyl radicals. These interact with lipids, causing lipid peroxidation along with the production of 4-hydroxyalkenals. Trichloromethylperoxyl radicals may react further to produce phosgene, which again may interact with tissue macromolecules or with water, finally producing hydrochloric acid and carbon dioxide. Pulmonary excretion of unchanged carbon tetrachloride accounts for up to a third of that inhaled and absorbed.

Mechanisms of toxicity
Carbon tetrachloride depresses the central nervous system. All other toxic effects are related to its biotransformation. The liver and kidney are especially vulnerable because of the abundance of CYP2E1, which is also present in the respiratory and nervous systems, and various isoforms of CYP3A. There is considerable evidence that hepatic injury produced by carbon tetrachloride is mediated by two major processes resulting from bioactivation in the endoplasmic reticulum and mitochondria of centrilobular hepatocytes, which have the highest concentration of CYP2E1; haloalkylation of cellular macromolecules by reactive metabolites, such as trichloromethyl free radicals and trichloromethylperoxyl free radicals, and lipid peroxidation which impairs cellular functions dependent on membrane integrity. Both haloalkylation and lipid peroxidation contribute to loss of cellular functions and subsequent cell death.

Clinical features—acute poisoning
The immediate effects include nausea, vomiting, abdominal pain, and diarrhoea. High concentrations cause dizziness, confusion, coma, respiratory depression, hypotension, and occasionally convulsions. Death may follow from respiratory failure or ventricular fibrillation due to cardiac sensitization to circulating catecholamines. Hepatorenal damage supervenes after a delay of up to 2 weeks. Hepatic enzyme activities increase before jaundice and a tender swollen liver develop. Maximal liver damage probably occurs within 48 hours of an acute exposure and may progress to fulminant hepatic failure.

Acute renal tubular necrosis is common and may develop in the absence of hepatic dysfunction 1–7 days after exposure. Rarely, cerebellar dysfunction, cerebral haemorrhage, optic atrophy, and parkinsonism may occur. Alcohol and previous liver damage render the individual more susceptible.

A plain film of the abdomen may confirm that ingestion has occurred (Figure 9.2).

Clinical features—chronic poisoning
Repeated exposure to low concentrations of carbon tetrachloride may also cause hepatic and renal damage. Hepatic cirrhosis and hepatoma may develop. Prolonged carbon tetrachloride exposure is associated with polyneuritis, various visual disturbances, anaemia including fatal aplastic anaemia, and mild jaundice.

Management
After ingestion, GI decontamination is best avoided because of the risk of aspiration. If the patient presents within 12 hours of exposure acetylcysteine should be given as for paracetamol overdose (see Hepatic failure, pp. 73–74 and Paracetamol, pp. 116–121). Renal and liver failure should be managed conventionally.

Methylene chloride
Until 2010, methylene chloride (dichloromethane) was a common ingredient in paint removers but has now been banned in the EU. It is used as a solvent for plastic films

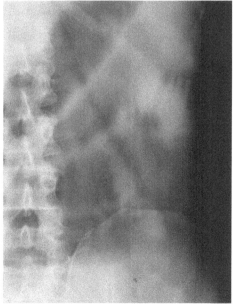

Fig 9.2 Plain abdominal film showing the gut outlined by carbon tetrachloride. Reproduced with permission from Allister Vale.

and cements and also as a degreaser and aerosol pro-pellant. In some European countries, personal defence sprays containing methylene chloride are available.

Toxicokinetics
Methylene chloride is metabolized by two path-ways: by mixed function oxidases to carbon monoxide and by glutathione-S-transferase to carbon dioxide. Carboxyhaemoglobin concentrations of 3–10% are attained commonly following inhalation; exceptionally, concentrations of 40% have been reported.

Mechanisms of toxicity
Methylene chloride itself is responsible for neurotoxic-ity and narcosis, though the features of carbon monoxide poisoning may also contribute to the clinical picture, partic-ularly in the case of ingestion as high concentrations of car-boxyhaemoglobin are likely to be present for several days.

Clinical features
Poisoning usually follows inhalation, though deliberate ingestion is recognized. Exposure to high concentrations of methylene chloride in poorly ventilated areas has resulted in death.

Following inhalation, dizziness, tingling and numbness of the extremities, throbbing headache, cough, breathless-ness, upper respiratory tract irritation, nausea, irritability, sinus tachycardia, hypertension, fatigue, and stupor have been reported. In severe cases, systemic features follow.

Ingestion of methylene chloride causes corrosive injury to the gastrointestinal tract, with rapid onset of systemic features.

Following substantial inhalation or ingestion, systemic features develop: hypotension, respiratory depression, coma, convulsions, pulmonary and cerebral oedema, acute kidney injury, hepatorenal dysfunction, pancreatitis, cardiac arrhythmias and cardiac arrest. Optic atrophy has been reported.

Metabolic acidosis, electrolyte disturbances (hyper-natraemia, hypokalaemia/hyperkalaemia, hypocalcae-mia), transient diabetes mellitus, leucocytosis, raised liver enzyme activities and elevated creatine kinase activity can occur.

Skin contact with liquid methylene chloride can cause second- and third-degree burns. Dermal absorption can occur and prolonged exposure may lead to systemic effects.

Severe and prolonged eye exposure may lead to irri-tant conjunctivitis and lacrimation.

Two patients were admitted to hospital following inhalation of methylene chloride, they had been found unconscious, having suffered a cardiac arrest. One died shortly after admission; the second was intubated and ventilated but did not regain consciousness and died on day 4. His carboxyhaemoglobin concentration peaked at 8% at 8 hours after admission.

Two men were found dead following inhalation for sev-eral hours of high concentrations of methylene chloride in an occupational setting. Both men had carboxyhaemo-globin concentrations of 30%. Post-mortem examination showed diffuse lung congestion and oedema, and erosive multifocal gastritis.

Management
Prompt removal from exposure usually results in com-plete recovery. Thereafter, treatment is symptomatic and supportive and should include the use of supplemental oxygen and ventilation, if required.

Haemorrhagic or hypovolaemic shock should be treated by replacing lost fluids and blood intravenously. Fibreoptic endoscopy by an experienced endoscopist is indicated to grade the severity of the gastrointestinal injury. An urgent surgical review is recommended if per-foration is suspected following corrosive injury.

Tetrachloroethylene
Tetrachloroethylene (perchloroethylene) is a colour-less, non-flammable liquid with a chloroform-like odour. It is used widely as an industrial solvent, particularly for dry-cleaning and degreasing. Poisoning may occur by inhalation or ingestion.

Toxicokinetics
The metabolism of tetrachloroethylene occurs by cytochrome P450-dependent oxidation and CYP2E1, CYP2B1/2, and CYP3A4 are primarily responsible. Tetrachloroethylene oxide is generated, which is con-verted predominantly to trichloroacetyl chloride and chloral. Both chloral and trichloroacetyl chloride are con-verted to trichloroacetic acid, which is the predominant metabolite recovered in urine. Tri- and dichloroacetate are also formed from these metabolites.

Irrespective of the route of exposure, only 1–3% of the absorbed tetrachloroethylene is metabolized to trichlo-roacetic acid; the remainder is exhaled unchanged. That retained is excreted only slowly (half-life ~144 hours). The metabolism of tetrachloroethylene is saturable in humans. A significant portion of tetrachloroethylene is completely metabolized to CO_2 in a dose-dependent manner.

The GSH conjugation pathway is associated with gen-eration of reactive metabolites from tetrachloroethylene selectively in the kidneys.

Mechanisms of toxicity
The mechanisms of tetrachloroethylene liver toxicity involve: (1) modification of signalling pathways, (2) cell death and reparative hyperplasia, and (3) somatic mutation and is believed to be associated with two P450-derived metabolites, tri- and dichloroacetate. Tetrachloroethylene-induced renal toxicity involves mito-chondrial dysfunction, protein alkylation, DNA alkylation, and oxidative stress as initial responses.

Clinical features
Following inhalation or ingestion, there is depression of the central nervous system; nausea and vomiting may occur and persist for several hours. Irritation of the eyes, nose, and throat may occur. Hepatic and renal dysfunc-tion may also develop and ventricular arrhythmias and non-cardiogenic pulmonary oedema have been reported.

Management
After removal from exposure, treatment is supportive and symptomatic.

1,1,1-Trichloroethane (methyl chloroform)
1,1,1-Trichloroethane is a colourless, non-flammable liq-uid of high volatility widely used as a solvent in industry, in the office (e.g. typewriter correction fluid), and at home (e.g. aerosol waterproofing products).

Toxicokinetics
1,1,1-Trichloroethane is rapidly and efficiently absorbed by the lung, skin, and gastrointestinal tract. As the duration of inhalation exposure increases, the per-centage of absorption decreases because steady-state

concentrations are approached in the blood and tissues, and 1,1,1-trichloroethane is metabolized at a low rate. Metabolism appears to play a relatively minor role in the overall disposition of 1,1,1-trichloroethane. The initial oxidation of 1,1,1-trichloroethane to trichloroethanol is thought to be catalysed by the microsomal cytochrome P450 mixed-function oxidase system. The pathway for conversion of trichloroethanol to trichloroacetic acid probably involves the intermediate formation of chloral hydrate and may involve alcohol and aldehyde dehydrogenases or cytochrome P450 mixed-function oxidases. Only a small fraction of the absorbed dose (<10%) is metabolized; a large fraction of the absorbed dose is excreted unchanged in exhaled air, regardless of the exposure route. In humans exposed to 35 or 350 ppm for 6 hours, greater than 91% of absorbed 1,1,1-trichloroethane was excreted unchanged by the lungs, 5–6% was metabolized and excreted as trichloroethanol and trichloroacetic acid, and less than 1% remained in the body after 9 days.

Mechanisms of toxicity
Acute exposures to high 1,1,1-trichloroethane concentrations can cause sudden death in humans due to ventricular fibrillation, myocardial depression, or respiratory arrest. Animal studies show that arrhythmias (that can lead to ventricular fibrillation) can be produced by exogenously administered epinephrine during or immediately after inhalation exposure to 1,1,1-trichloroethane. The studies indicate that the arrhythmias are not caused directly by 1,1,1-trichloroethane, but result from its sensitization of the heart to epinephrine. Concomitant ingestion of ethanol is known to enhance toxicity further.

The mechanism by which high concentrations of 1,1,1-trichloroethane produce mild to moderate hepatotoxicity is not understood.

Clinical features
Following inhalation of a sufficiently large dose, central nervous system depression occurs in proportion to the amount inhaled; hepatic and renal dysfunction may also result. Deaths have followed exposure to very high concentrations in unventilated tanks. In such cases, death may either be due to central nervous system depression, culminating in respiratory arrest, or to fatal arrhythmias (see earlier in section) in the presence of hypoxia.

Inhalation of a weatherproofing aerosol containing 96.6% 1,1,1-trichloroethane has been reported to give rise to transient shortness of breath, constricting chest pain, cough, and myalgia.

Management
The casualty should be removed from the contaminated environment. Thereafter treatment is symptomatic and supportive.

Trichloroethylene

Trichloroethylene is a colourless, volatile liquid used widely as an industrial solvent, particularly in metal degreasing and extraction processes.

Toxicokinetics
Trichloroethylene is absorbed readily from the gut and through the skin and lungs. Following inhalation, it is excreted unchanged in the breath and metabolized via chloral hydrate to trichloroethanol and trichloroacetic acid, which are excreted in the urine.

Mechanisms of toxicity
Trichloroethylene metabolism occurs through two main pathways. Oxidation via the microsomal mixed-function oxidase system (CYP2E1 is particularly important) results in the formation of chloral, probably via an intermediate (possibly trichloroethylene oxide), which readily equilibrates with chloral hydrate via a chlorine migration. Chloral hydrate is metabolized to trichloroethanol and trichloroacetic acid, the major metabolite found in the urine. Trichloroethylene can also be conjugated with glutathione by glutathione S-transferases to S-1,2-dichlorovinyl-L-glutathione.

Clinical features
Following inhalation, ingestion, or dermal absorption, central nervous system depression occurs with nausea and vomiting, hepatic and renal dysfunction, and death. 'Degreaser's flush' (in which the skin of the face and arms becomes markedly reddened) may occur if ethanol is consumed shortly before or after exposure to trichloroethylene. Cranial nerve damage, cerebellar dysfunction, and convulsions have been described.

Carcinogenicity
Trichloroethylene is reasonably anticipated to be a human carcinogen based on limited evidence of carcinogenicity from studies in humans and sufficient evidence of carcinogenicity from studies in experimental animals.

Management
Removal from exposure will reduce central nervous system depression, and thereafter, whether trichloroethylene has been inhaled, ingested, or absorbed through the skin, treatment is supportive and symptomatic.

Further reading

Agency for Toxic Substances and Disease Registry (ATSDR) (1997). *Tetrachloroethylene*. Atlanta, GA: ATSDR.

Agency for Toxic Substances and Disease Registry (ATSDR) (2005). *Carbon Tetrachloride*. Atlanta, GA: ATSDR.

Agency for Toxic Substances and Disease Registry (ATSDR) (2006). *1,1,1-Trichloroethane*. Atlanta, GA: ATSDR.

Bagnasco FM, Stringer B, Muslim AM (1978). Carbon tetrachloride poisoning. Radiographic findings. *NY State J Med*, 78:646.

Buie SE, Pratt DS, May JJ (1986). Diffuse pulmonary injury following paint remover exposure. *Am J Med*, 81:702–4.

Chang YL, Yang CC, Deng JF, *et al*. (1999). Diverse manifestations of oral methylene chloride poisoning: report of 6 cases. *J Toxicol Clin Toxicol*, 37:497–504.

Cohen C Frank AL (1994). Liver disease following occupational exposure to 1,1,1-trichloroethane: a case report. *Am J Ind Med*, 26:237–41.

David NJ, Wolman R, Milne F, *et al*. (1989). Acute renal failure due to trichloroethylene poisoning. *Br J Ind Med*, 46:347–9.

Fagin J, Bradley J, Williams D (1980). Carbon monoxide poisoning secondary to inhaling methylene chloride. *Br Med J*, 281:1461.

Fechner G, Ortmann C, Du Chesne A, *et al*. (2001). Fatal Intoxication due to excessive dichloromethane inhalation. *Forensic Sci Int*, 122:69–72.

Feldman RG, White RF, Currie JN, *et al*. (1985). Long term follow up after single toxic exposure to trichloroethylene. *Am J Ind Med*, 8: 119–26.

Fogel RP, Davidman M, Poleski MH, *et al*. (1983). Carbon tetrachloride poisoning treated with hemodialysis and total parenteral nutrition. *CMAJ*, 128:560–1.

Forbes JR (1944). Carbon tetrachloride nephrosis. *Lancet*, 244:590–2.

Ford ES, Rhodes S, McDiarmid M, *et al*. (1995). Deaths from exposure to trichloroethylene. *JOEM*, 37:749–54.

Garnier R, Bedouin J, Pepin G, et al. (1996). Coin–operated dry cleaning machines may be responsible for acute tetrachloroethylene poisoning: report of 26 cases including one death. J Toxicol Clin Toxicol, 34:191–7.

Gist GL Burg JR (1995). Trichloroethylene – a review of the literature from a health effects perspective. Toxicol Industrial Health, 11:253–307.

Halevy J, Pitlik S, Rosenfeld J (1980). 1,1,1,-Trichloroethane intoxication: a case report with transient liver and renal damage. Clin Toxicol, 16:467.

House RA, Liss GM Wills MC (1994). Peripheral sensory neuropathy associated with 1,1,1-trichloroethane. Arch Environ Health, 49:196–9.

House RA, Liss GM, Wills M, et al. (1996). Paresthesias and sensory neuropathy due to 1,1,1-trichloroethane. JOEM, 38:123–4.

Hughes NJ, Tracey JA (1993). A case of methylene chloride (Nitromors) poisoning, effects on carboxyhaemoglobin levels. Hum Exp Toxicol, 12:159–60.

IPCS (1992). Environmental Health Criteria 136. 1,1,1-Trichloroethane, Geneva: World Health Organization.

IPCS (1999). Environmental Health Criteria 208. Carbon Tetrachloride. Geneva: World Health Organization.

Johns DO, Daniell WE, Shen DD, et al. (2006). Ethanol-induced increase in the metabolic clearance of 1,1,1-trichloroethane in human volunteers. Toxicol Sci, 92:61–70.

Johnson BP, Meredith TJ, Vale JA (1983). Cerebellar dysfunction after acute carbon tetrachloride poisoning. Lancet, 322:968.

Kelafant GA, Berg RA, Schleenbaker R (1994). Toxic encephalopathy due to 1,1,1-trichloroethane exposure. Am J Ind Med, 25: 439–46.

Kobayashi A, Ando A, Tagami N, et al. (2008). Severe optic neuropathy caused by dichloromethane inhalation. J Ocul Pharmacol Ther, 24:607–12.

Köppel C, Lanz H-J, Ibe K (1988). Acute trichloroethylene poisoning with additional ingestion of ethanol – concentrations of trichloroethylene and its metabolites during hyperventilation therapy. Intensive Care Med, 14:74–6.

Kostrzewski P, Jakubowski M Kolacinski Z (1993). Kinetics of trichloroethylene elimination from venous blood after acute inhalation poisoning. J Toxicol Clin Toxicol, 31:353–63.

Laine A, Seppalainen AM, Savolainen K, et al. (1996). Acute effects of 1,1,1-trichloroethane inhalation on the human central nervous system. Int Arch Occup Environ Health, 69:53–61.

Lash LH, Parker JC (2001). Hepatic and renal toxicities associated with perchloroethylene. Pharmacol Rev, 53:177–208.

Leikin JB, Kaufman D, Lipscomb JW, et al. (1990). Methylene chloride: report of five exposures and two deaths. Am J Emerg Med, 8:534–7.

Liss GM (1988). Peripheral neuropathy in two workers exposed to 1,1,1-trichloroethane. JAMA, 260:2217.

Liss GM House RA (1995). Toxic encephalopathy due to 1,1,1-trichloroethane. Am J Ind Med, 27:445–6.

Macdougall IC, Isles C, Oliver JS, et al. (1987). Fatal outcome following inhalation of Tipp-Ex. Scott Med J, 32:55.

Manno M, Rugge M, Cocheo V (1992). Double fatal inhalation of dichloromethane. Hum Exp Toxicol, 11:540–5.

Mathieson PW, Williams G, MacSweeney JE (1985). Survival after massive ingestion of carbon tetrachloride treated by intravenous infusion of acetylcysteine. Hum Toxicol, 4:627–31.

McDonald W, Olmedo M (1996). Accidental deaths following inhalation of methylene chloride. Appl Occup Environ Hyg, 11:17–9.

Mcleod AA, Marjot R, Monaghan MJ, et al. (1987). Chronic cardiac toxicity after inhalation of 1,1,1- trichloroethane. BMJ, 294:727–9.

Memon NA, Davidson AR (1981). Multisystem disorder after exposure to paint stripper (Nitromors). Br Med J, 282:1033.

Miller L, Pateras V, Friederici H, et al. (1985). Acute tubular necrosis after inhalation exposure to methylene chloride. Report of a case. Arch Intern Med, 145:145–6.

Monster AC, Boersma G, Steenweg H (1979). Kinetics of 1,1,1-trichloroethane in volunteers; influence of exposure concentration and work load. Int Arch Occup Environ Health, 42:293–301.

Muttray A, Moll B, Faas M, et al. (2004). Acute effects of 1,1,1-trichloroethane on human olfactory functioning. Am J Rhinol, 18:113–17.

Nager EC, O'Connor RE (1998). Carbon monoxide poisoning from spray paint inhalation. Acad Emerg Med, 5:84–6.

National Toxicology Program (2011). Report on Carcinogens. Durham, NC: US Department of Health and Human Services.

New PS, Lubush GD, Scherr L, et al. (1962). Acute renal failure associated with carbon tetrachloride intoxication. JAMA, 181: 903–6.

Nolan RJ, Freshour NL, Rick DL (1984). Kinetics and metabolism of inhaled methyl chloroform (1,1,1-trichloroethane) in male volunteers. Fundam Appl Toxicol, 4:654–62.

Perace RV (1981). Near-fatal intoxication by 1,1,1,-trichloroethane. Ann Emerg Med, 10:533.

Perbellini L, Olivato D, Zedde A, et al. (1991). Acute trichloroethylene poisoning by ingestion: clinical and pharmacokinetic aspects. Intensive Care Med, 17:234–5.

Perez AJ, Courel M, Sobrado J, et al. (1987). Acute renal failure after topical application of carbon tetrachloride. Lancet, 329: 515–16.

Raphael M, Nadiras P, Flacke-Vordos N (2002). Acute methylene chloride intoxication – a case report on domestic poisoning. Eur J Emerg Med, 9:57–9.

Roberts CJ, Marshall FP (1976). Recovery after 'lethal' quantity of paint remover. Br Med J, 1:20–1.

Ruprah M, Mant TG, Flanagan RJ (1985). Acute carbon tetrachloride poisoning in 19 patients: implications for diagnosis and treatment. Lancet, 325:1027–9.

Scott CS Jinot J (2011). A systematic review and meta-analysis of occupational exposure to trichloroethylene and cancers of the kidney and liver and nonhodgkin lymphoma. Occup Environment Med, 68:A110–11.

Shusterman D, Quinlan P, Lowengart R, et al. (1990). Methylene chloride intoxication in a furniture refinisher. J Occup Med, 32:451–4.

Stewart R, Boettner EA, Southworth RR, et al. (1963). Acute carbon tetrachloride intoxication. JAMA, 183:994–7.

Traiger GJ, Plaa GL (1972). Relationship of alcohol metabolism to the potentiation of CCl4 hepatotoxicity induced by aliphatic alcohols. J Pharmacol Exp Ther, 183:481–8.

Wells GG, Waldron HA (1984). Methylene chloride burns. Br J Ind Med, 41:420.

Winek CL, Wahba WW, Huston R, et al. (1997). Fatal inhalation of 1,1,1-trichloroethane. Forensic Sci Int, 87:161–5.

Winneke G (1981). The neurotoxicity of dichloromethane. Neurobehav Toxicol Teratol, 3:391–5.

Wong CK, Ooi VEC, Wong CK (2003). Protective effects of N-acetyl cysteine against carbon tetrachloride and trichloroethylene-induced poisoning in rats. Environ Toxicol Pharmacol, 14:109–16.

Zarrabeitia MT, Ortega C, Altuzarra E, et al. (2001). Accidental dichloromethane fatality: a case report. J Forensic Sci, 46:726–7.

Chlorine

Background

Chlorine (Cl_2) (CAS 7782-50-5) is a yellow-green, non-combustible gas with a pungent, irritating odour. It is a strong oxidizing agent and can react explosively or form explosive compounds with many common substances. It is moderately soluble in water. Chlorine is heavier than air and may collect in low-lying areas. Odour is not a good indicator of exposure as most people can detect concentrations of 0.2 ppm (some are able to detect 0.02 ppm), which is well below the occupational standards (see later in section).

Mixing household cleaning agents (bleach with acids or ammonia) produces chlorine gas and other active chlorine compounds such as chloramine (NH_2Cl). For example, mixing household bleach (sodium hypochlorite) with acid toilet bowl cleaners produces chlorine gas. Ammonia (NH_3) mixed with bleach results in the release of chloramine.

Chlorine is used extensively in the chemical industry as a starter and intermediate compound. It is highly reactive. It is used in the bleaching of pulp, for disinfecting water, and in waste treatment. It is produced as a by-product of diaphragm cell and mercury electrolytic cell processes. It is used in the manufacture of polyvinyl chloride (PVC) and organochlorine pesticides.

Exposure to workers or the public is usually by the accidental release of chlorine from closed pressurized systems, e.g. road tankers, rail tankers, or industrial complexes. In the UK it is the most common hazardous chemical stored in industrial installations and in the USA it is transported by railroad tankers and although accidents are rare they have a major impact, e.g. Graniteville, South Carolina, 2005, in which nine people died and 5400 people were displaced from their homes leading to a major public health emergency.

Occupational standards

LTEL—long-term exposure limit, 8-hour reference period: not set in UK.

STEL—short-term exposure limit, 15-minute reference period): 0.5 ppm (1.5 mg/m^3) UK.

OSHA PEL = 1 ppm (3 mg/m^3).

NIOSH REL = UK STEL.

Toxicokinetics

Chlorine reacts with water in the respiratory tract to form hydrochloric acid and hypochlorous acid. It can also generate indirectly a reactive oxygen species (ROS), as shown:

1 $Cl_2 + H_2O \leftrightarrow HCl + HOCl$
2 $HOCl \leftrightarrow HCl + ROS$

Mechanisms of toxicity

There are two mechanisms of toxicity of chlorine both involving the formation of free radicals. Chlorine itself is a free radical and very reactive oxidizing agent and can generate a reactive oxygen species as described earlier. The effect of releasing chlorine itself, hypochlorous acid, hydrochloric acid and ROS initiates an inflammatory response in the respiratory tract. Despite its widespread commercial importance since before World War I and its use as a chemical weapon in that conflict little is known

of human exposure data and animal experiments have led to extrapolation to man with additional information form accidental releases.

Chlorine gas is highly corrosive when it contacts moist tissues such as the eyes, skin, and upper respiratory tract. Significant dermal absorption or ingestion is unlikely.

Clinical features

Acute exposure

Where inhalation is the main route and because of chlorine's moderate water solubility, it will act on the upper and lower respiratory tract. It is severely irritating on contact to moist tissues and can be caustic to the eyes, skin, nose, throat, and mucous membranes; exposure can result in severe or permanent eye injury.

Inhalation

Inhalation causes irritation of the nose with sore throat, cough, chest tightness, headache, fever, wheeze, tachycardia, and confusion. Chemical pneumonitis, tachypnoea, dyspnea, and stridor due to laryngeal oedema may follow. Pulmonary oedema with increasing breathlessness, wheeze, hypoxia and cyanosis may take 8–36 hours to develop. Irritation to the mucous membranes in the nose and throat may occur after exposure to low concentrations (see Tables 9.2 and 9.3).

A feeling of suffocation, breathlessness, rhinorrhoea, coughing with white or bloodstained sputum, chest pain and tightness, abdominal pain, nausea, headache, dizziness, and tachycardia may follow more substantial exposures and worsen over several hours. Hoarseness and stridor may develop due to laryngeal oedema. Severe bronchoconstriction and non-cardiogenic pulmonary oedema occur in severe cases.

Symptoms usually occur immediately but less commonly, may be delayed for several hours.

Symptoms generally resolve within 6 hours after mild exposures, but may continue for more than 24 hours after severe exposures. Deterioration may continue for several hours. Exposure to high concentrations of chlorine may be fatal.

It must be noted that the information in Table 9.3 is estimated and in reality if the individual were mobile they would not remain within the chlorine cloud due to its irritating effect and therefore would flee. If, however, the casualty is immobilized or trapped then it is possible to have a prolonged exposure. Moderate or severe

Table 9.3 Summary of toxic effects following acute exposure to chlorine by inhalation

Dose ppm	Signs and symptoms
0.02–0.2	Odour threshold
1–3	Mild irritation to eyes, nose, and throat
3–6	Itching, stinging, and burning of the eyes, lacrimation, blepharospasm, burning of the nose and throat, sneezing, coughing, and bloody nose or sputum
5–10	Moderate upper respiratory irritation
10–20	Intense upper respiratory irritation
30	Chest pain, vomiting, dyspnoea, and cough

Table 9.2 Summary of toxic effects following acute exposure to chlorine by inhalation with respect to time

Dose ppm	Signs and symptoms
1	Change in lung function after 4 hours
14	Severe pulmonary damage after 30 minutes
30–50	Probably fatal after 60 minutes
>430	Probably fatal after 30 minutes
1000	Probably fatal after few breaths

exposure (associated with acute marked airflow obstruction and air-trapping) often results in residual pulmonary dysfunction, most notably hyper-reactive airways disease and low residual volumes. There may be a mixed obstructive and restrictive pattern on spirometry. These long-term sequelae of acute exposure may persist for several years.

Inhalation exposures to low concentrations for a short period, from which an individual recovers quickly on removal to fresh air, are unlikely to result in delayed or long-term adverse health effects. Substantial inhalation exposures to chlorine may cause long-term health effects, including persistent reactive airways dysfunction (RADS), which for some may lead to bronchial hyper-responsiveness and persist for at least 18–24 months.

Dermal exposure
Dermal exposure to concentrated chlorine released under pressure may cause dermal burns and the pressurized liquid can cause frostbite.

Ocular exposure
Ocular exposure causes immediate stinging and burning with lacrimation and blepharospasm. High concentrations will cause ocular burns.

Chronic exposure
Chronic exposure to chlorine gas may cause dyspnoea, palpitations, chest pain, reactive upper airways dysfunction syndrome, dental enamel erosion, and an increased prevalence of viral syndromes. Chronic exposure to 15 ppm produced coughing, haemoptysis, chest pain, and

sore throat. Chronic exposure to chlorine gas can be a cause of occupational asthma.

Management
Remove patient from exposure. Treatment is supportive as there is no antidote or other specific treatment following chlorine exposure. There is no biomarker of exposure to aid the treating physician.

Inhalation
Ensure a clear airway and adequate ventilation. Give oxygen to symptomatic patients. All patients with abnormal vital signs, chest pain, respiratory symptoms, or hypoxia should have a 12-lead ECG performed. If the patient has clinical features of bronchospasm treat conventionally with nebulized bronchodilators and steroids. Endotracheal intubation or, rarely, tracheostomy may be required for life-threatening laryngeal oedema. Apply other supportive measures as indicated by the patient's clinical condition. If the exposure has been substantial then observation of the patient for at least 4 hours would be recommended.

Further reading

Baxter PJ, Aw T-C, Cockcroft A, et al. (eds) (2010). *Hunter's Diseases of Occupations*, 10th edition. London: Hodder.

Bhérer L, Cushman R, Courteau JP, et al. (1994). Survey of construction workers repeatedly exposed to chlorine over a three to six month period in a pulpmill: II. Follow up of affected workers by questionnaire, spirometry, and assessment of bronchial responsiveness 18 to 24 months after exposure ended. *Occup Environ Med*, 51:225–8.

Centers for Disease Control and Prevention. *NIOSH Pocket Guide to Chemical Hazards*. <http://www.cdc.gov/niosh/npg/npgd0115.html>.

Health Protection Agency. *Chemicals and Poisons A–Z Compendium, Chlorine*. <http://www.hpa.org.uk/Topics/ChemicalsAndPoisons/CompendiumOfChemicalHazards/Chlorine/>.

Mitchell JT, Edmonds AS, Cutter SL, et al. (2005). *Evacuation Behavior in Response to the Graniteville, South Carolina, Chlorine Spill*. Quick response research report 178. <http://www.colorado.edu/hazards/research/qr/qr178/qr178.pdf>.

UK Health and Safety Executive (2011). *EH40/2005 Workplace Exposure Limits*, 2nd edition. <http://www.hse.gov.uk/pubns/priced/eh40.pdf>.

Shakeri MS, Dick FD, Ayres JG (2008). Which agents cause reactive airways dysfunction syndrome (RADS)? A systematic review. *Occup Med*, 58;205–11.

Complex glycols (glycol ethers)

Background

Glycol ethers are toxic alcohols are widely used class of high-production-volume chemicals with industrial applications as solvents and chemical intermediates. There are more than 30 in industrial use and they are derivatives of ethylene (E series) or propylene (P series). They may be used alone, or as an ingredient in products such as coatings, cleaners, brake fluids, perfumes and cosmetics, and as solvents found in household cleaners. In poisoning they share many features of the better-known methanol and ethylene glycol (*mono* ethylene glycol). Complex glycols include: glycol ethers (e.g. ethylene glycol monomethyl ether), dialkyl ethers (e.g. ethylene glycol dimethyl ether), and glycol esters (e.g. ethylene glycol monomethyl ether acetate) (Table 9.4). The structures are based on their basic groupings: ethylene-, diethylene-, triethylene-, propylene-, and dipropylene-. Similar derivatives exist for diethylene, propylene, and di-propylene glycols.

Mechanisms of toxicity

Glycol ethers are readily absorbed by inhalation, ingestion, and through the skin. They are metabolized in the liver and toxicity and features depend on this metabolism. Exposures in the workplace may occur, but overall there is little evidence of long-term effects with use of appropriate controls. Concerns exist regarding effects of some glycols on reproductive health. Glycol ethers for which there is evidence of effects on animal reproduction include EGME, EGMEA, EGEE, EGEEA, EGDME, EGDEE, DEGME, DEGDME, and TEGDME.

Toxicokinetics

Glycols are rapidly absorbed and distributed, with peak concentrations usually occurring within 1–2 hours. Metabolism is necessary for the major toxic effects to occur (see earlier in section) and differs in individual glycol ethers. For example, 2-butoxyethanol is conjugated to sulfate and glucuronides, metabolized by alcohol dehydrogenase to an aldehyde and then to butoxyacetic acid, then to carbon dioxide and glycine and glutamate derivatives. In addition it is possible that a small amount is metabolized to ethylene glycol (see Ethylene and diethylene glycols, pp. 240–241) and to oxalate before being excreted (shown in rats, possible in man).

Patients will develop a high osmolal gap as they absorb the glycols over the first few hours. Thereafter, as the glycols are metabolized to acids, the osmolal gap will fall while the patient's anion gap will climb and acidosis worsens. A severely poisoned patient can present early with a normal anion gap and a normal pH or hydrogen ion concentration; however, their osmolal gap may be high. Glycol ethers and their acid metabolites produce a linear increase in plasma osmolality, and osmolal gap with increasing plasma concentration. This change in osmolality may, however, be too small to be clinically useful in cases of acute human glycol ether poisoning.

Clinical features

These depend on the glycol ether; see 'Mechanisms of toxicity'.

Ingestion of large amounts of glycol ethers may cause:
- coma, respiratory depression, convulsions, and severe hypotension

Table 9.4 Ethylene, diethylene and triethylene glycol ethers, illustrating more complex derivatives of ethylene, diethylene and triethylene glycols

Common name	Abbreviation	Chemical name
Ethylene glycol monomethyl ether	EGME	2-Methoxyethanol
Ethylene glycol monomethyl ether acetate	EGMEA	2-Methoxyethyl acetate
Ethylene glycol monoethyl ether	EGEE	2-Ethoxyethanol
Ethylene glycol monoethyl ether acetate	EGEEA	2-Ethoxyethyl acetate
Ethylene glycol monopropyl ether	EGPE	2-Propoxyethanol
Ethylene glycol monobutyl ether	EGBE	2-Butoxyethanol
Ethylene glycol dimethyl ether	EGDME	1,2-Dimethoxyethane
Ethylene glycol diethyl ether	EGDEE	1,2-Diethoxyethane
Diethylene glycol monomethyl ether	DEGME,	2-(2-Methoxyethoxy) ethanol
Diethylene glycol dimethyl ether	DEGDME	2-Methoxyethyl ether
Triethylene glycol dimethyl ether	TEGDME	1,2-Bis(2-methoxyethoxy) ethane

- non-cardiogenic pulmonary oedema
- metabolic acidosis, renal failure
- DIC, hepatotoxicity, reduced haemocrit and haemoglobin, and haematuria, hypocalcaemia, hypokalaemia
- thrombocytopaenia and non-haemolytic hypochromic anaemia.

Glycol ethers irritate the eyes, skin, and the respiratory tract as well as causing nausea, vomiting, and diarrhoea.

Inhalation may cause lacrimation, rhinorrhoea, cough, dyspnoea, and nausea. A high concentration may cause CNS depression.

Skin contact may cause local irritation.

Toxicity assessment

There are two phases to toxicity caused by glycols. In the first, absorption of the chemical is occurring.

Features of toxicity to assess at this stage therefore include:

- evidence of exposure: local irritation, mouth/GI symptoms
- systemic features related to the primary chemical, normally intoxication. NB absence of this feature does not exclude significant toxic hazard.

Glycol ethers and their acid metabolites produce a linear increase in plasma osmolality with increasing plasma concentration. This change in osmolality may be too small to be clinically useful at concentrations expected in many cases of acute human glycol ether poisoning.

In the second phase metabolites form, some of which are potentially toxic, and cause metabolic acidosis and other systemic effects depending on the individual glycol (see 'Toxicokinetics').

Investigations

Assays are not readily available for glycol ethers. Other biochemical measurements such as anion gap or osmolal gap are a more suitable guide to diagnosis. Measure U&Es (including chloride and bicarbonate), FBC, LFTs, glucose, osmolality, and arterial blood gases. Calculate the osmolal gap and anion gap (see Acid–base and electrolyte disturbances in the poisoned patient, pp. 75–76). Changes in these measurements depend on the time interval since ingestion, as acidosis and its consequences require metabolic conversion of the toxic alcohol. Samples taken within 1–2 hours of ingestion may not fully reflect osmolal change, and maximum change in acid–base develops over a period of up to 12 hours as metabolites are formed. Absence of an elevated osmolal gap does not exclude serious poisoning since the osmolal gap begins to fall once glycol ethers are metabolized; it may not be elevated in the later stages of poisoning. A high anion gap metabolic acidosis suggests late presentation substantial metabolism of glycol. A high anion gap metabolic acidosis is not specific to glycol ether ingestion (see Acid–base and electrolyte disturbances in the poisoned patient, pp. 75–76). Absence of a high anion gap metabolic acidosis in early presentation does not exclude toxic risk.

Patients who have biochemistry, osmolality, and arterial blood gases, and normal calculated osmolal and anion gaps, 6 hours after ingestion are unlikely to have significant glycol ether exposure.

Management

Children or adults who have accidentally ingested small amounts should not require treatment.

Ensure a clear airway and adequate ventilation, particularly if there is depression of conscious level.

Consider gastric aspiration if the patient presents within 1 hour of ingestion and the airway can be protected. Charcoal does not adsorb glycol ethers.

Observe for at least 6 hours after ingestion if asymptomatic and 12 hours if symptomatic. Conduct blood tests as delineated in 'Investigations'. Monitor pulse, blood pressure, respiratory rate, cardiac rhythm and urine output. Perform a 12-lead ECG.

Treat hypotension with fluid volume replacement initially, and subsequent management depends on clinical effects of the glycol metabolites.

If metabolic acidosis persists despite correction of hypoxia and adequate fluid resuscitation consider correction with intravenous sodium bicarbonate (see Acid–base and electrolyte disturbances in the poisoned patient, pp. 75–76). Large amounts of bicarbonate, with repeated pH checking, may be required.

Single brief convulsions do not require treatment. Give oxygen, check blood glucose, U&Es, and arterial blood gases, and correct acid–base and metabolic disturbances. If convulsions are frequent or prolonged, control with intravenous diazepam (10–20 mg in adults; 0.1–0.3 mg/kg body weight in children) or lorazepam (4 mg in adults and 0.1 mg/kg in children).

In significant overdose early administration of fomepizole or ethanol will minimize the further metabolism of glycol ethers and the development of clinical and metabolic complications. This means that treatment usually needs to be started before the diagnosis has been confirmed.

Use of antidotes

There are two antidotes available fomepizole and ethanol. Both act by competitively inhibiting alcohol dehydrogenase thereby preventing the further formation of the toxic metabolites (see Ethylene and diethylene glycols, pp. 240–241 and Ethanol and methanol, pp. 236–238). The evidence for use of ethanol and fomepizole is primarily based on treatment of ethylene glycol and methanol poisoning rather than glycol ether poisoning.

Use of elimination techniques

In severe poisoning consider haemodialysis (see Principles of enhanced elimination in the poisoned patient, pp. 40–41) This is effective in removing metabolites and parent glycol ether and can shorten the duration of poisoning in addition to correcting metabolic abnormalities. It may therefore be preferred to prolonged antidotal treatment. Indications include severe metabolic acidosis, renal failure, and severe electrolyte imbalance.

Dialysis should be continued until acidosis and signs of systemic toxicity have resolved. Further elevation of glycol ether concentrations may occur after discontinuing dialysis due to redistribution; recheck U&Es and osmolality 2–4 hours after dialysis has stopped.

Further reading

Boogaard PJ, Swaen GMH (2008). Letter to the editor on a recent publication titled 'Occupation and male infertility: glycol ethers'. Occup Environ Med, published 11 July.

Browning RG, Curry SC (1992). Effect of glycol ethers on plasma osmolality. Hum Exp Toxicol, 11:488–90.

Landry GM, Martin S, McMartin KE (2011). Diglycolic acid is the nephrotoxic metabolite in diethylene glycol poisoning inducing necrosis in human proximal tubule cells in vitro. Toxicol Sci, 124:35–44.

Rambourg-Schepens MO, Buffet M, Bertault R, et al. (1988). Severe ethylene glycol butyl ether poisoning; kinetics and metabolic pattern. Hum Toxicol, 7:187–9.

Cyanide

Background

Cyanide poisoning may result from exposure to industrial chemicals (cyanide salts) and solvents (nitriles), smoke from house fires (hydrogen cyanide gas release from combustion of fabrics), drugs (sodium nitroprusside), and plants containing naturally occurring cyanogenic glycosides (apricot, almond, cassava).

Mechanism of toxicity

Cyanide toxicity results from disruption of mitochondrial oxidative processes and cellular energy production. Due to its high affinity for Fe^{3+} ions, cyanide binds avidly to mitochondrial cytochrome a–a_3 complex to form a stable but reversible complex. The inactivation of cytochrome oxidase leads to uncoupling of mitochondrial oxidative phosphorylation and blocks ATP production. This causes reduced oxygen utilization and tissue hypoxia.

Cellular respiration switches from aerobic to anaerobic metabolism with the production of lactic acid.

Mechanisms of endogenous cyanide detoxification

There are several endogenous mechanisms to detoxify cyanide:

- Rhodanese catalyses the dissociation of the cytochrome oxidase–cyanide complex by sulphur transfer (from endogenous thiosulfate) to cyanide to form thiocyanate which then undergoes renal excretion. The release of cytochrome oxidase leads to resumption of normal aerobic oxidative processes. This accounts for 80% of cyanide detoxification.
- Binding of cyanide to hydroxocobalamin.
- Binding of cyanide to methaemoglobin.
- Binding of cyanide to cysteine and incorporation into choline and methionine.

Clinical feature—acute exposure

Cyanide is highly toxic regardless of route of exposure but onset of toxicity may vary depending on the dose, source, or route of exposure.

Following hydrogen cyanide gas inhalation, toxicity is likely to occur within seconds and death may occur within minutes. Ingestion of soluble cyanide salts can cause toxicity within minutes but may be delayed for up to 1 hour. Continued absorption can produce prolonged toxicity for several hours. Toxicity may be delayed by up to 12 hours after exposure to nitriles and ingestion of plants containing amygdalin. Following dermal exposure, toxicity may occur if a large surface area is affected and may be delayed for several hours.

In patients with smoke inhalation, the presence of soot in the mouth and nose should raise the possibility of cyanide poisoning.

A 'bitter almond' smell on the patient's breath is characteristic (due to excretion of hydrocyanic acid) but 20–40% of people are genetically unable to detect this.

A cherry-red skin colour (reflecting absent tissue oxygen extraction) may be observed. Cyanosis is a late sign and may not be present even in pre-terminal patients.

- *Mild poisoning* occurs at cyanide concentration <1 mg/L (38 micromol/L): nausea, dizziness, headache, anxiety, hyperventilation, confusion, drowsiness, tachycardia, tachypnoea, and palpitations.
- *Moderate poisoning* occurs at cyanide concentration 1–3 mg/L (38–114 micromol/L): vomiting, reduced conscious level, convulsions, hypotension.
- *Severe poisoning* occurs at cyanide concentration >3 mg/L (114 micromol/L): coma, fixed dilated pupils, cardiovascular collapse, cardiac arrhythmias, pulmonary oedema, respiratory failure.

In pre-terminal patients, profound sinus bradycardia or AV dissociation may be present.

A high anion gap metabolic acidosis associated with elevated lactate is usually present in moderate and severe cyanide poisoning. There is a good correlation between the degree of lactic acidosis and the severity of cyanide poisoning. On the other hand, oxygen saturation by pulse oximetry may be high and falsely reassuring since oxygen is still present as oxyhaemoglobin. The reduced oxygen utilization is reflected by a reduced arterio-venous oxygen gradient.

Clinical feature—chronic exposure

Chronic low-dose cyanide exposure commonly presents with features of parkinsonism such as akinesia, dysarthria, and rigidity with evidence of demyelinating lesions affecting the globus pallidus, posterior putamen, and basal ganglia on MRI scan. Spastic paraparesis, ataxia, and deafness may also occur.

Neuropsychiatric sequelae such as headaches, vertigo, convulsions, sleep disturbance, and psychosis may develop.

Optic neuropathy may present as progressive visual loss, loss of red-green colour distinction, visual field changes with central scotoma, optic atrophy, and afferent pupillary defect. This has been reported in smokers (tobacco amblyopia) and in populations where cassava root is a staple food (tropical amblyopia).

Management

Ingestion

Gastric lavage or administration of activated charcoal may be considered in patients presenting within 1 hour of ingestion of cyanide salts, nitriles or cyanogenic glycosides.

Inhalation

The patient should be removed from exposure, and first-aid measures should be instituted. Rescuers should avoid putting themselves at risk and should wear full PPE, including self-contained breathing apparatus.

Dermal exposure

After skin exposure, all contaminated clothing should be removed and double-bagged. Skin should be washed thoroughly with water.

All exposures

Asymptomatic patients and patients with mild symptoms should be observed for at least 6 hours (longer after ingestion of insoluble cyanide salts, nitriles or cyanogenic glycosides)

Patients with symptoms suggestive of moderate-to-severe poisoning should be admitted to and monitored in a critical care environment.

Monitor pulse, blood pressure, respiratory rate, oxygen saturation and cardiac rhythm.

Measure U&Es, arterial blood gases, lactate and whole blood cyanide concentrations in symptomatic patients.

Whole-blood cyanide concentrations may not be readily available. In the presence of relevant clinical features, the finding of a markedly elevated lactate (>7 mmol/L), high anion gap metabolic acidosis, and a reduced arterio-venous oxygen gradient support the diagnosis of cyanide poisoning.

Supportive treatment

Correct metabolic acidosis with intravenous sodium bicarbonate

Correct hypotension with intravenous fluids and use of vasopressors or inotropes as indicated by invasive monitoring.

Antidotal treatment

In mild poisoning oxygen and sodium thiosulfate should be administered. Oxygen and dicobalt edetate should be administered in cases of moderate-to-severe poisoning. If dicobalt edetate is not available give *both* sodium nitrite and sodium thiosulfate intravenously. In smoke inhalation hydroxocobalamin (Cyanokit®) may be used in patients with suspected severe cyanide poisoning, e.g. coma, cardiac arrest, or cardiovascular instability.

Oxygen

The immediate administration of oxygen is of paramount importance, as there is evidence that it prevents inhibition of cytochrome oxidase a$_3$ and accelerates its reactivation. High flow oxygen should be given via a face mask with a rebreather bag or via an endotracheal tube.

Sodium nitrite

Methaemoglobin binds cyanide and, although the affinity of cyanide for methaemoglobin is less than that of cytochrome oxidase a$_3$, the presence of a large circulating methaemoglobin pool diminishes cyanide toxicity by binding cyanide ion before tissue penetration occurs.

Methaemoglobin may be induced effectively by the administration of intravenous sodium nitrite 300 mg (10 mL of 3% sodium nitrite solution) over 5–20 minutes. Children: 4–10 mg/kg (0.12–0.33 mL/kg) up to a maximum of 300 mg or 10 mL. Sodium nitrite should *not* be given again as it may cause severe methaemoglobinaemia.

As the antidotal effect of sodium nitrite is relatively rapid, but methaemoglobin is formed more slowly, the benefit of sodium nitrite may be due in part to its vasodilator action and consequent improvement in tissue perfusion. Inhalation of amyl nitrite was recommended in the past, but it produces only low circulating concentrations of methaemoglobin and is subject to abuse.

Intravenous sodium nitrite is usually given with intravenous sodium thiosulfate. Experimental studies have shown that the antidotal effect of sodium nitrite may be enhanced by co-administration of sodium thiosulfate.

Sodium thiosulfate

Sodium thiosulfate enhances the body's own detoxification mechanisms and is administered intravenously in an adult dose of 12.5 g (25 mL of 50% solution) over 10 minutes. Children: 400 mg/kg (0.8 mL/kg of 50% solution)

However, experimental evidence in a swine model suggests that sodium thiosulfate is ineffective in severe poisoning.

Dicobalt edetate

Experimental work demonstrated not only that dicobalt edetate was capable of resuscitating apnoeic dogs, but also that dicobalt edetate was superior to sodium nitrite and sodium thiosulfate as a cyanide antidote. In addition, dicobalt edetate may cross the blood–brain barrier which is a potential advantage over methaemoglobin-inducing agents such as sodium nitrite and DMAP.

The commercially available preparation contains 13.5–16.5 g/L dicobalt edetate and 1.96–2.40 g/L free cobalt as well as 200 g/L glucose. Thus, each 20 mL ampoule contains dicobalt edetate 270–330 mg (usually assumed to be 300 mg), free cobalt 39–48 mg, and 4g glucose.

Cobalt itself rapidly chelates free and tissue/enzyme bound cyanide to form the cobaltocyanide ion and then the less toxic cobalticyanide ion and monocobalt edetate, which are then excreted renally. Free cobalt appears to complex cyanide up to six times more effectively than dicobalt edetate. The reduction of the plasma free cyanide concentration enhances dissociation of the cyanide–cytochrome oxidase complex, allowing normal cellular respiration to resume.

As free cobalt is toxic, the use of dicobalt edetate in the absence of cyanide poisoning may lead to cobalt toxicity. Adverse reactions including facial and laryngeal oedema, vomiting, urticaria, anaphylactic shock, hypotension, cardiac arrhythmias, and convulsions have been reported from the use of dicobalt edetate in these circumstances. Dicobalt edetate should therefore be given only when the diagnosis is clinically probable. Dicobalt edetate may be administered intravenously in a dose of 300 mg (20 mL of 1.5% dicobalt edetate solution) over 1 minute, with a further 300 mg being given if there is only a partial response or the patient relapses after an initial response.

Hydroxocobalamin

One mole of hydroxocobalamin inactivates 1 mole of cyanide, but, on a weight-for-weight basis, 50 times more hydroxocobalamin is needed than cyanide because hydroxocobalamin is a far larger molecule.

A recent review concluded that there is limited evidence that hydroxocobalamin alone is effective in severe poisoning by cyanide salts. The evidence for the efficacy of hydroxocobalamin in smoke inhalation is complicated by lack of evidence for the importance of cyanide exposure in fires and the effects of other chemicals as well as confounding effects of other therapeutic measures, including hyperbaric oxygen. Evidence that hydroxocobalamin is effective in poisoning due to hydrogen cyanide alone is lacking; extrapolation of efficacy from poisoning by ingested cyanide salts may not be valid. The rate of absorption may be greater with inhaled hydrogen cyanide and the recommended slow intravenous administration of hydroxocobalamin may severely limit its clinical effectiveness in these circumstances.

Hydroxocobalamin 5 g may be given intravenously over 30 minutes; a second dose (5 g) may be required in severe cases. Children: 70 mg/kg over 15 minutes.

Both animal and human data suggest that hydroxocobalamin is lacking in clinically significant adverse effects. However, in one human volunteer study, delayed but prolonged rashes were observed in one-sixth of subjects, appearing 7–25 days after administration of 5 g or more of hydroxocobalamin. Rare adverse effects have included dyspnoea, facial oedema, and urticaria.

Further reading

Baud FJ, Borron SW, Megarbane B, *et al.* (2002). Value of lactic acidosis in the assessment of the severity of acute cyanide poisoning. *Crit Care Med*, 30:2044–50.

Bebarta VS, Pitotti RL, Dixon P, *et al.* (2012). Hydroxocobalamin versus sodium thiosulfate for the treatment of acute cyanide toxicity in a swine (Sus scrofa) model. *Ann Emerg Med*, 59:532–9.

Borron SW, Baud FJ, Mégarbane B, *et al.* (2007). Hydroxocobalamin for severe acute cyanide poisoning by ingestion or inhalation. *Am J Emerg Med*, 25:551–8.

Dart RC (2006). Hydroxocobalamin for acute cyanide poisoning: new data from preclinical and clinical studies; new results from the prehospital emergency setting. *Clin Toxicol*, 44:1–3.

Evans CL (1964). Cobalt compounds as antidotes for hydrocyanic acid. *Br J Pharmacol*, 23:455–75.

Freeman AG (1988). Optic neuropathy and chronic cyanide intoxication: a review. *J R Soc Med*, 81:103–6.

Geller RJ, Ekins BR, Iknoian RC (1991). Cyanide toxicity from acetonitrile-containing false nail remover. *Am J Emerg Med*, 9:268–70.

McKiernan MJ (1980). Emergency treatment of cyanide poisoning. *Lancet*, 2:86.

Meredith TJ, Jacobsen D, Haines JA, *et al.* (eds) (1993). *Antidotes for Poisoning by Cyanide.* Cambridge: Cambridge University Press.

Michaelis HC, Clemens C, Kijewski H, *et al.* (1991). Acetonitrile serum concentrations and cyanide blood levels in a case of suicidal oral acetonitrile ingestion. *Clin Toxicol*, 29:447–58.

Musshoff F, Kirschbaum KM, Madea B (2011). An uncommon case of a suicide with inhalation of hydrogen cyanide. *Forensic Sci Int*, 204:e4–7.

Naughton M (1974). Acute cyanide poisoning. *Anaesth Intensive Care*, 2:351–6.

Paulet G (1957). Valeur des sels organiques du cobalt dans le traitement de l'intoxication cyanhydrique. *C R Soc Biol (Paris)*,151:1932–5.

Paulet G (1958). Intoxication cyanohydrique et chélates de cobalt. *J Physiol (Paris)*, 50:438–42.

Paulet G (1960). *L'Intoxication Cyanhydrique Et Son Traitement.* Paris: Masson SA.

Paulet G (1961). Nouvelles perspectives dans le traitement de l'intoxication cyanhydrique. *Arch Mal Prof*, 22:102–27.

Rosenow F, Herholz K, Lanfermann H, *et al.* (1995). Neurological sequelae of cyanide intoxication – the patterns of clinical, magnetic resonance imaging, and positron emission tomography findings. *Ann Neurol*, 38:825–8.

Singh BM, Coles N, Lewis P, *et al.* (1989). The metabolic effects of fatal cyanide poisoning. *Postgrad Med J*, 65:923–5.

Thompson JP, Marrs TC (2012). Hydroxocobalamin in cyanide poisoning. *Clin Toxicol*, 50:875–85.

Tyrer FH (1981). Treatment of cyanide poisoning. *J Soc Occup Med*, 31:65–6.

Dioxins and polychlorinated biphenyls

Dioxins

Background

Dioxins and dioxin-like chemicals form a large group of chemicals which are structurally related, have a common mechanism of action, and are environmentally and biologically persistent. The group includes polychlorinated dibenzo-p-dioxins (PCDDs), dibenzofurans (PCDFs), and polychlorinated biphenols (PCBs). Although there are 75 congeners of PCDDs and 135 congeners of PCDFs, the term 'dioxin' is generally used to refer to 2,3,7,8-tetrachlorodibenzo-p-dioxin (2,3,7,8-TCDD), the most potent dioxin (Figure 9.3). Dioxins did not exist prior to industrialization except in very small amounts due to natural combustion and geological processes. Dioxins may be produced in municipal solid waste incinerators, medical waste incinerators, pulp and paper mills, and wood burning (both residential and industrial). 2,3,7,8-TCDD was a contaminant of Agent Orange, a herbicide used in the Vietnam war. Dioxins have also been found in the Love Canal area of Niagara Falls and in Seveso, Italy, the latter following an industrial explosion in 1976. Occupational dioxin exposure has also occurred in Amsterdam. Dioxins came to public attention again with the poisoning of President Viktor Yushchenko of Ukraine in 2004.

Toxicokinetics

Very little human data are available. Dioxins can probably be absorbed by oral, inhalational, and dermal routes. In a human volunteer, 87% of an oral dose was absorbed. The half-life of 2,3,7,8-TCDD in human adults is approximately 7 years, though this half-life is shorter in adults exposed to high concentrations of 2,3,7,8-TCDD.

Mechanisms of toxicity

Activation of AhR (the aryl hydrocarbon receptor) by 2,3,7,8-TCDD is hypothesized as the mechanism by which it exerts its carcinogenic and endocrine effects. Activation of the Ah receptor causes a wide spectrum of biological responses considered important to the carcinogenic process, including changes in gene expression, altered metabolism, altered cell growth and differentiation, and disruption of steroid-hormone and growth-factor signal-transduction pathways. 2,3,7,8-TCDD also exerts antioestrogenic responses, for example, by inhibiting 17β-oestradiol-induced cell proliferation, progesterone receptor gene expression, and progesterone receptor binding.

Clinical features

Acute exposure

Transient acute health effects including headache, pruritus, chloracne, fatigue, irritability, inability to have erections or ejaculations, personality changes, abdominal pain, diarrhoea, insomnia, hepatic dysfunction (hepatomegaly and increased ALT, AST and GGT activities) and respiratory irritation have been reported, particularly following occupational exposure. One individual who was exposed to 2,3,7,8-TCDD developed chloracne with pruritus, her face and then her body became densely covered with cysts and she exhibited palmo-plantar keratoderma, epigastric pain, nausea and vomiting, anorexia, and amenorrhoea. Her 2,3,7,8-TCDD concentration was 144,000 pg/g blood fat, the highest concentration reported to date (equivalent to a body burden of 1.6 mg 2,3,7,8-TCDD).

Chronic exposure

Epidemiological studies have found that the risks of all cancers combined, lung cancer, and non-Hodgkin's lymphoma are increased significantly and there is an increase in overall mortality from cancer after chronic exposure to 2,3,7,8-TCDD. Endocrine disruption, including diabetes and thyroid disorders, has also been described. An increased mortality from ischaemic heart disease has been associated with occupational exposure to high 2,3,7,8-TCDD concentrations.

Management

Management is supportive and symptomatic.

Polychlorinated biphenyls

Background

There are no natural sources of polychlorinated biphenyls (PCBs). They are a synthetic family of molecules that consist of 209 isomers formed by the addition of chlorine atoms to a biphenyl nucleus (Figure 9.4). The resulting PCBs are either oily non-volatile liquids or solids. There is little information about the individual isomers of PCBs since they were generally produced as mixtures. For example, in the USA several mixtures (Aroclor 1016, 1242, 1254, 1260, 1268) were commercially produced until 1977.

As PCBs do not degrade easily, even at high temperatures, they were frequently used as insulators and coolants. Their oily nature was responsible for their use as heat-resistant lubricants. Because of their resistance to degradation, and hence environmental persistence, production of PCBs was halted in the USA and in Western Europe in approximately 1977. They continued to be manufactured, however, in Eastern Europe until the 1990s.

Mechanisms of toxicity

Although high-dose animal studies have demonstrated renal and hepatic toxicity, these studies appear to have little relevance to any reasonable human environmental exposure.

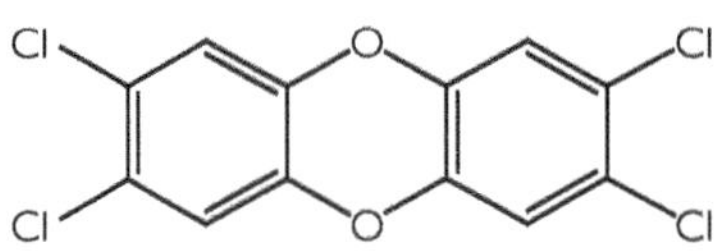

Fig 9.3 2,3,7,8-Tetrachlorodibenzo-p-dioxin (2,3,7,8-TCDD).

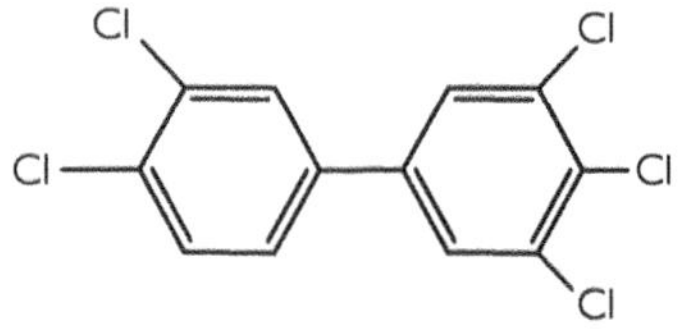

Fig 9.4 3,3',4,4'5-Pentachlorobiphenyl (PCB 126).

Clinical features

The health effects of PCBs in humans, other than rashes, have been poorly characterized. Most of the information on the toxicology of PCBs in humans derives from epidemiological studies on chronically exposed populations. However, the interpretation of many of the studies on PCBs is complicated by the almost inevitable co-contamination with polychlorinated dibenzofurans and polychlorinated dibenzodioxins; the role of these co-contaminants was either not recognized, or not studied, in many instances.

There have been investigations of two major outbreaks of rice oil contaminated with PCBs: the Yusho Cohort which occurred in Japan, and the Yu-Cheng Cohort which occurred in Taiwan in 1979. Approximately 3700 individuals were affected in these two cohorts.

The major concerns regarding the human toxicology of PCBs relate to possible neurobehavioural effects, abnormal thyroid function, immune dysfunction and hepatocellular malignancies. However, there are no convincing studies in humans supporting these associations.

Significant associations between elevated PCB concentrations and diabetes mellitus have been reported but are mostly due to associations in women and in individuals <55 years of age.

Meta-analysis of 12 European mother–child cohorts including more than 7000 pregnancies suggests that low-level PCB exposure impairs fetal growth. On average, birth weight declined by 150 g per 1 microgram/L increase in PCB 153 cord serum concentration, which suggests that low-level exposure to PCBs is inversely associated with fetal growth.

Carcinogenicity

The National Toxicology Program has stated that PCBs are reasonably anticipated to be human carcinogens based on sufficient evidence of carcinogenicity from studies in experimental animals. However, not all PCB mixtures caused tumours in experimental animals. The International Agency for Research on Cancer (IARC) has concluded that PCB 126 was a complete carcinogen in experimental animals and classified it as carcinogenic in humans based on the fact that it acted through the same mechanism as TCDD (dioxin).

Environmental aspects

In the USA, PCBs have been documented to exist in approximately one-third of major hazardous waste sites identified by the Environmental Protection Agency (EPA). They are known to concentrate up the food chain and are found in high concentrations in the fat tissue of fish and aquatic mammals such as seals and whales. However, environmental persistence does not equate to toxicity.

Further reading

ATSDR. Pohl H, Llados F, et al. (eds) (1998). *Toxicological Profile for Chlorinated Dibenzo-p-Dioxins*. Atlanta, GA: Agency for Toxic Substances and Disease Registry, US Public Health Service.

Baan R, Grosse Y, Straif K, et al. (2009). A review of human carcinogens—Part F: chemical agents and related occupations. *Lancet Oncol*, 10:1143–4.

Consonni D, Pesatori AC, Zocchetti C, et al. (2008). Mortality in a population exposed to dioxin after the Seveso, Italy, accident in 1976: 25 years of follow-up. *Am J Epidemiol*, 167:847–58.

Dalderup LM, Zellenrath D (1983). Dioxin exposure: 20 year follow-up. *Lancet*, 2:1134–5.

Faroon O, Jones D, de Rosa C (2000). Effects of polychlorinated biphenyls on the nervous system. *Toxicol Ind Health*, 16:305–33.

Flesch-Janys D, Berger J, Gurn P, et al. (1995). Exposure to polychlorinated dioxins and furans (PCDD/F) and mortality in a cohort of workers from a herbicide-producing plant in Hamburg, Federal Republic of Germany. *Am J Epidemiol*, 142:1165–75.

Geusau A, Abraham K, Geissler K, et al. (2001). Severe 2,3,7,8-tetrachlorodibenzo-p-dioxin (TCDD) intoxication: clinical and laboratory effects. *Environ Health Perspect*, 109:865–9.

Govarts E, Nieuwenhuijsen M, Schoeters G, et al. (2012). Birth weight and prenatal exposure to polychlorinated biphenyls (PCBs) and di-chlorodiphenyldichloroethylene (DDE): a meta-analysis within 12 European birth cohorts. *Environ Health Perspect*, 120:162–70.

Guo YL, Yu M-L, Hsu C-C, et al. (1999). Chloracne, goiter, arthritis, and anemia after polychlorinated biphenyl poisoning: 14-year follow-up of the Taiwan Yucheng cohort. *Environ Health Perspect*, 107:715–19.

IARC (1998). Polychlorinated biphenyls and polybrominated biphenyls – Summary of data reported and evaluation. *IARC Monogr Eval Carcinog Risks Hum*, 18:43–107.

Kimbrough RD, Carter CD, Liddle JA, et al. (1977). Epidemiology and pathology of a tetrachlorodibenzodioxin poisoning episode. *Arch Environ Health*, 32:77–86.

Kimbrough RD, Krouskas CA (2003). Human exposure to polychlorinated biphenyls and health effects: a critical synopsis. *Toxicol Rev*, 22:217–33.

Longnecker MP, Michalek JE (2000). Serum dioxin level in relation to diabetes mellitus among Air Force Veterans with background levels of exposure. *Epidemiology*, 11:44–48.

National Toxicology Program (2011). *Report on carcinogens*. Durham, NC: US Department of Health and Human Services.

Onozuka D, Yoshimura T, Kaneko S, et al. (2009). Mortality after exposure to polychlorinated biphenyls and polychlorinated dibenzofurans: a 40-year follow-up study of Yusho patients. *Am J Epidemiol*, 169:86–95.

Pavuk M, Schecter AJ, Akhtar FZ, et al. (2003). Serum 2,3,7,8-tetrachlorodibenzo-p-dioxin (TCDD) levels and thyroid function in Air Force veterans of the Vietnam War. *Ann Epidemiol*, 13:335–43.

Silverstone AE, Rosenbaum PF, Weinstock RS, et al. (2012). Polychlorinated biphenyl (PCB) exposure and diabetes: results from the Anniston Community Health Survey. *Environ Health Perspect*, 120:727–32.

Smith RM, O'Keefe PW, Aldous KM, et al. (1983). 2,3,7,8-tetrachlorodibenzo-p-dioxin in sediment samples from Love Canal storm sewers and creeks. *Environ Sci Technol*, 17:6–10.

Sorg O, Zennegg M, Schmid P, et al. (2009). 2,3,7,8-tetrachlorodibenzo-p-dioxin (TCDD) poisoning in Victor Yushchenko: identification and measurement of TCDD metabolites. *Lancet*, 374:1179–85.

Steenland K, Piacitelli L, Deddens J, et al. (1999). Cancer, heart disease, and diabetes in workers exposed to 2,3,7,8-tetrachlorodibenzo-p-dioxin. *J Natl Cancer Inst*, 91:779–86.

Sweeney MH, Mocarelli P (2000). Human health effects after exposure to 2,3,7,8-TCDD. *Food Addit Contam*, 17:303–16.

Essential oils

Background

Essential oils are complex mixtures of hydrocarbon compounds extracted from plants. Most are extracted by distillation, though some by solvent extraction. They are volatile, normally lipid-soluble, and colourless. Essential oils are used in fragrances, soaps, aromatherapy, food flavourings, as insect repellents, and in proprietary cough and cold preparations. Some have other claimed medicinal uses, as, for example, menthol on the GI tract as an antispasmodic, or chamomile in managing eczema. Essential oils also have antibacterial properties.

There are several thousand known essential oils, but those normally available commercially contain terpenes, terpenoids, or various aliphatic and aromatic compounds. Some have relatively simple structures, thus oil of wintergreen is methyl salicylate (see Salicylates, pp. 124–127). Essential oils may be available as relatively pure, high concentration, product, usually sold in low volume, or as a small component in carrier oils, which are normally of low toxicity, especially when used in aromatherapy.

Mechanisms of toxicity

Most essential oils are very toxic if ingested in undiluted forms. Main targets for these effects include the liver, kidney and central nervous system (Table 9.5). Thus pennyroyal and clove oil may cause hepatic necrosis while others target the central nervous system causing convulsions or behavioural disturbance. The precise mechanisms of these effects is not all clear, but may involve actions on ion pumps, as seems to be the case for the action of menthol on the gut, or bio-activation to toxic intermediates following metabolism in the liver. Methyl salicylate causes features of salicylate poisoning (see Salicylates, pp. 124–127).

Toxicokinetics

Little information is available on the toxicokinetics of essential oils. As lipid-soluble compounds they are absorbed rapidly, and most undergo metabolism in the liver, as already indicated sometimes this is to toxic metabolites. Methyl salicylate is converted to salicylic acid.

Risk factors for toxicity

Toxic effects are greatest after ingestion of concentrated oils. Children are more at risk because of their size and because of their tendency to explore and consume materials left around the home. Aspiration of oils either in their pure state, or in their carrier oils, may result in pulmonary toxicity and pneumonitis. Dose assessment

is often difficult because of the variability in content of essential oils in different commercial products.

Clinical features

Although different oils are likely to vary in their toxicity, severe toxicity has been reported with several. Essential oils are rapidly absorbed and early symptoms usually occur within 30 minutes but may be delayed up to 4 hours or more. For toxicity related to effects on the liver, a longer time interval will ensue, usually 24–72 hours.

Oils are often sold as mixtures, and it may be difficult to establish the exact cause of symptoms. Thus cardiovascular collapse and multi-organ failure followed an ingestion of approximately 3 L of a mouthwash containing alcohol, eucalyptol, menthol, and thymol in an adult male. Which of these was responsible is a matter of conjecture. Similarly intranasal instillation of a mixed essential oil preparation caused tachypnoea, central cyanosis, wheeze and stridor in a 4-month-old. Tachycardia and excessive oral and nasal secretions also occurred.

Uncertain or mixed ingestion

In a case of uncertain product or mixtures of oils the following features are possible following ingestion: (1) a burning sensation in the mouth and throat, (2) hypersalivation, (3) nausea, vomiting, and diarrhoea. Haematemesis may occur.

Absence of these symptoms makes large ingestions less likely but cannot exclude toxic risk.

Volatile oils may be aspirated into the lungs causing pulmonary complications.

Systemic features

Systemic features may be delayed up to 4 hours after ingestion and include ataxia, dizziness, headache, drowsiness, excitement, delirium, respiratory depression, convulsions, and coma. Hypotension and tachycardia have been reported. In severe poisoning there may be raised liver enzyme activities, increased INR, DIC, renal and liver failure typically with pennyroyal and clove oil. Urine abnormalities such as elevated urine specific gravity, proteinuria, and ketonuria have followed clove oil ingestion. Rhabdomyolysis may occur secondary to convulsions. Hypernatraemia, hypokalaemia, hypoglycaemia, and metabolic acidosis are features in severe poisoning.

Aspiration

Aspiration into the lungs may occur during ingestion or if the patient vomits. Certain physical properties of essential oils, their viscosity and volatility particularly, make them more likely to cause pneumonitis. Symptoms and signs of pulmonary involvement may progress over the first 24 hours and become most severe up to 48 hours post exposure. Features include pyrexia, cough, tachypnoea, and tachycardia. Cyanosis may occur in severe cases. Common chest X-ray findings include infiltrates, non-segmental collapse, and consolidation. Rarely pneumatocoele formation, pneumothorax, pulmonary oedema and ARDS are seen.

Skin contact

Skin contact may cause redness, irritation, and a burning sensation. Contact dermatitis has been reported from exposure to essential oils. Due to their lipophilic nature, absorption across the skin can occur. Systemic toxicity has been reported following significant dermal exposure to eucalyptus oil.

Table 9.5 Some common essential oils—likely toxic chemical content and toxicity

Essential oil	Toxic chemical	Toxic effect
Cinnamon	Cinnamaldehyde	Dermatitis
Clove	Eugenol, eugenyl acetate, caryopheyllene	Hepatic necrosis
Eucalyptus	1,8 Cineole	Seizures
Mentha spp.	Menthol, menthone	Ataxia, myalgia
Pennyroyal	Pulegone	Hepatic necrosis
Wormwood	Alpha- or beta-thujone	Seizures, dementia

Eye contact

Eye contact may cause severe irritation and corneal damage.

Specific clinical features of some individual oils

- Camphorated oil ingestion may cause a burning sensation in the mouth and throat, nausea, vomiting, and diarrhoea. Seizures are a particularly common feature of camphor toxicity and may be delayed up to 9 hours after ingestion Ulceration of the tongue and blistering of the lips is reported. One case of granulomatous hepatitis followed chronic camphor ingestion. Camphorated oil has been withdrawn from sale in UK and USA.
- Cinnamon oil has CNS effects and is less toxic than some other oils, nevertheless approximately 60 mL of cinnamon oil in a 7-year-old caused diplopia, dizziness, drowsiness, vomiting, abdominal cramps, and hypotension. Symptoms persisted for 5 hours with a complete recovery.
- Clove oil caused fulminant hepatic failure and acute kidney injury in a 15-month-old boy who ingested 10 mL of clove oil.
- Pennyroyal caused death from liver failure and cerebral oedema in an infant who ingested pennyroyal oil from home-brewed teas, and other cases of hepatotoxicity are reported with this oil.
- Peppermint oil intravenously (5 mL) led to cyanosis, unconsciousness, and pulmonary oedema. Urticaria, photosensitivity, and contact dermatitis have been reported following topical use of essential oils.

Toxicity assessment

This is based on history, examination, and clinical features. There are no specific laboratory tests. A chest X-ray should be performed if features of aspiration are present.

Investigations

In symptomatic patients U&Es, LFTs, INR and blood glucose should be monitored. Blood gasses should be taken if there are features of respiratory or metabolic effects.

Management of ingestion

Gut decontamination is contraindicated due to the risk of aspiration.

Observe adults and children who have ingested any amount of concentrated essential oil for at least 6 hours post ingestion. Monitor BP, pulse, conscious level, respiratory rate, and oxygen saturations.

In symptomatic patients monitor U&Es, LFTs, INR, and blood glucose and measure blood gasses (arterial or venous).

Maintain a clear airway and ensure adequate ventilation.

Correct hypoglycaemia as quickly as possible. If the patient is awake give oral glucose followed by a carbohydrate meal. In adults: if the patient is drowsy or unconscious give up to 250 mL 10% or 125 mL 20% glucose IV rapidly (titrated to patient responsiveness). Continue an appropriate infusion to maintain consciousness and/or normal blood glucose. If hypoglycaemia persists, 50 mL 50% glucose IV may be given but is irritant to veins and can cause skin necrosis in cases of extravasation.

Hypoglycaemia in children (estimated blood sugar concentration <2.6 mmol/L) should be treated with a 2 mL/kg bolus of 10% glucose followed by an intravenous infusion containing glucose (for example, 0.45% NaCl/10% glucose) at an appropriate rate to maintain adequate blood sugar. Blood sugar concentration should be rechecked at 5-minute intervals until stable at greater than 3 mmol/L. Persistent hypoglycaemia should be treated with repeated boluses of 10% glucose initially, though continuous infusions of higher concentrations of glucose may be required in severe cases. Infusions containing greater than 12.5% glucose normally require central venous access.

Single brief convulsions do not require treatment. Give oxygen, check blood glucose, U&Es and ABG. Correct acid–base and metabolic disturbances as required. If convulsions are frequent or prolonged, control with intravenous diazepam (10–20 mg in adults; 0.1–0.3 mg/kg body weight in children) or lorazepam (4 mg in adults and 0.1 mg/kg in children). If unresponsive to these measures, see Convulsions, pp. 91–92.

If metabolic acidosis persists despite correction of hypoxia and adequate fluid resuscitation consider correction with intravenous sodium bicarbonate. In adults an initial dose of 50 mmol sodium bicarbonate may be given and repeated as necessary, guided by arterial blood gas monitoring (aim for a pH of 7.44) (see Acid–base and electrolyte disturbances in the poisoned patient, pp. 75–76). Hepatotoxicity has been reported following ingestion of some essential oils (particularly clove oil and pennyroyal oil). Acetylcysteine has been used to treat occasional patients but there are no formal studies supporting its benefit.

There are no data to suggest elimination is enhanced by extracorporeal techniques.

Management of aspiration

Maintain a clear airway and ensure adequate ventilation. Give oxygen if indicated. Perform a chest X-ray if symptomatic. Treat pulmonary oedema with CPAP or in severe cases with IPPV and PEEP. The role of prophylactic corticosteroids (inhaled or systemic) and antibiotics is controversial. Antibiotics will be required if pneumonia develops.

Other measures as indicated by the patient's clinical condition. Patients should be advised on discharge to seek medical attention if symptoms subsequently develop.

Management of skin contact

Skin contact

If contact is extensive or prolonged, essential oil may be absorbed through the skin and cause systemic toxicity (see Decontamination, pp. 36–39).

Eye contact

Remove contact lenses if present and immediately irrigate the affected eye thoroughly with water or 0.9% saline for at least 10–15 minutes (see Decontamination, pp. 36–39).

Further reading

Behrends M, Beiderlinden M, Peters J (2005). Acute lung injury after peppermint oil injection. *Anesth Analg*, 101:1160–2.

Eisen JS, Koren G, Juurlink DN, *et al*. (2004). N-acetylcysteine for the treatment of clove oil-induced fulminant hepatic failure. *Clin Toxicol*, 42:89–92.

Holstege CP, Baylor MR, Rusyniak DE (2002). Absinthe: return of the Green Fairy. *Semin Neurol*, 22:89–93.

Khan AJ, Akhtar RP, Faruqui ZS (2006). Turpentine oil inhalation leading to lung necrosis and empyema in a toddler. *Pediatr Emerg Care*, 22:355–7.

Woolf A (1999). Essential oil poisoning. *Clin Toxicol*, 37:721–7.

Ethanol and methanol

Ethanol

Background

Ethanol (alcohol, ethyl alcohol) is widely available as a beverage, is an important constituent of cosmetics, aftershave, hair tonic, antiseptics, mouthwashes, dishwashing detergents, and glass cleaners, and is commonly used as an industrial solvent. Children may be forced to drink alcohol under duress, and this may be associated with sexual abuse.

Toxicokinetics

Ethanol is absorbed rapidly through the gastric and small intestinal mucosae. Peak blood ethanol concentrations usually occur within 30–90 minutes of ingestion. Gastric alcohol dehydrogenase isoenzyme has a role in metabolizing ethanol before absorption, thereby preventing ethanol entering the systemic circulation, particularly following ingestion of moderate amounts of alcohol. Younger women and ethanol abusers of both sexes, have lower gastric alcohol dehydrogenase activity than younger and non-abusing men; therefore, more ethanol is absorbed in these individuals and higher blood alcohol concentrations ensue.

Absorbed ethanol is initially and principally converted to acetaldehyde by a nicotinamide adenine dinucleotide (NAD)-dependent hepatic alcohol dehydrogenase. A small proportion is oxidized by the microsomal ethanol-oxidizing system (MEOS), and the catalase pathway. MEOS activity may be increased by chronic alcohol abuse and by enzyme-inducing drugs; this may explain the greater ethanol tolerance seen in heavy drinkers.

Acetaldehyde, which is toxic, is removed by oxidation via the (oxidized) NAD-dependent enzyme, aldehyde dehydrogenase, to yield acetate and, subsequently, carbon dioxide and water.

About 95% of ingested ethanol is oxidized to acetaldehyde and acetate; the remainder is excreted unchanged in the urine (at a concentration about 1.3 times more than that in the blood), and, to a lesser extent, in the breath (the blood:breath ratio is about 2300:1) and through the skin.

At high blood concentrations (>1000 mg/L) ethanol is eliminated by zero-order kinetics (i.e. the rate of elimination is constant regardless of concentration), so that ethanol concentrations can be expected to decrease at a constant rate of 60–400 mg/L/hour (usually 150 mg/L/hour). Regular social drinkers tend to have higher ethanol elimination rates than non-drinkers, but ethanol abusers with severe liver damage usually eliminate ethanol more slowly.

Mechanisms of toxicity

Ethanol is a CNS depressant that interferes with cortical processes in small doses and may depress medullary function in large doses. The effects of ethanol on the CNS are generally proportional to the blood ethanol concentration, though the precise mechanisms of toxicity responsible for these effects are not yet fully understood. Individuals who are habituated to ethanol may have few symptoms despite massive blood ethanol concentrations. In contrast, teenagers unaccustomed to ethanol may become comatose at more modest blood ethanol concentrations (1000–2000 mg/L).

Ethanol is also a peripheral vasodilator. In the severely intoxicated, it may cause hypothermia and hypotension.

Ethanol metabolism may result in accumulation of free reduced nicotinamide adenine dinucleotide (NADH), with a resultant increase in the NADH:NAD ratio and inhibition of hepatic gluconeogenesis. It can also cause an increase in the lactate: pyruvate ratio, with development of hyperlactataemia. Inhibition of hepatic gluconeogenesis may result in hypoglycaemia, particularly in children or when poisoning follows fasting, exercise or chronic malnutrition.

Clinical features

The features of alcohol poisoning are summarized in Table 9.6 and correlated with blood alcohol concentrations. However, while blood ethanol concentrations are generally useful in helping assess the seriousness of intoxication, they are not always reliable due to individual tolerance. Experienced drinkers may be coherent at blood alcohol concentrations that in others result in the need for ventilatory support. Hence, blood alcohol concentrations should be interpreted in combination with clinical features to provide a more accurate guide to the severity of intoxication.

As ethanol is a CNS depressant and a peripheral vasodilator, coma, hypothermia, and hypotension are observed in those severely poisoned. Acid–base disturbances are also common: respiratory acidosis is observed more

Table 9.6 Features of acute ethanol poisoning related to blood ethanol concentrations

Blood alcohol concentration	Features
<500 mg/L	Talkativeness, subjective feeling of well-being
500–1500 mg/L	Emotional ability and slurred speech
	Mild impairment of visual acuity, muscular coordination and reaction time
1500–3000 mg/L	Blurred vision
	Loss of sensory perception
	Incoordination
	Ataxia
	Slowed reaction time
3000–5000 mg/L	Marked incoordination
	Blurred or double vision
	Sometimes coma and hypothermia
	Occasionally hypoglycaemia and convulsions
≥5000 mg/L	Coma
	Respiratory depression
	Depressed reflexes
	Hypotension and hypothermia
	Death may occur from respiratory or circulatory failure, or as a result of aspiration of stomach contents in the absence of a gag reflex

frequently than metabolic acidosis, and metabolic alkalosis may be observed in those vomiting and hypovolaemic.

Lactic acidosis (usually only mild) is an uncommon but potentially serious complication of acute ethanol intoxication, and occurs particularly in patients with severe liver disease, pancreatitis, or sepsis. Hypovolaemia, which may accompany severe intoxication, predisposes to lactic acidosis.

The magnitude of the metabolic acidosis does not always correlate well with the blood ethanol concentration or the lactate concentration.

Hypoglycaemia typically occurs within 6–36 hours of ingestion of a moderate-to-large amount of ethanol by a previously malnourished individual or one who has fasted for the previous 24 hours. In young children who have not eaten for 8–12 hours, ingestion of even modest amounts of ethanol (e.g. the dregs left after a party) can lead to permanent neurological damage as a result of the development of hypoglycaemia and neuroglycopenia. Convulsions are the most common presenting sign in children with alcohol-induced hypoglycaemia.

Patients with alcohol-induced hypoglycaemia are often comatose, hypothermic, and convulsing, with conjugate deviation of the eyes, trismus and extensor plantar reflexes; the usual features of hypoglycaemia (e.g. flushing, sweating, tachycardia) are often absent.

Acute ethanol poisoning is an uncommon cause of adult death; when fatalities occur, aspiration of gastric contents is an important factor. More often, ethanol potentiates the effects of other drugs taken in overdose. The fatal dose in adults is approximately 5–8 g/kg body weight. The highest survived blood ethanol concentration reported is 15,100 mg/L, while a concentration as low as 2500 mg/L has proven fatal.

Ethanol intoxication is an important cause of accidental death in children under 5 years of age and in children a fatal dose is approximately 3 g/kg body weight.

Management
GI decontamination is unlikely to be of benefit since ethanol is rapidly absorbed and activated charcoal does not significantly reduce the rate of absorption. Supportive measures are all that are required for most patients with acute ethanol intoxication, even if the blood ethanol concentration is very high. Particular care should be taken to protect the airway. In more severe cases, acid–base status should be determined every 2 hours; this may be performed conveniently on a venous sample, unless the patient is hypotensive.

Management of lactic acidosis requires correction of hypoglycaemia, hypovolaemia, and circulatory insufficiency, if present. An infusion of sodium bicarbonate will be necessary in those patients in whom a lactic acidosis persists.

Blood glucose should be determined hourly and the rate of intravenous glucose adjusted accordingly. If blood glucose concentrations decrease despite an infusion of glucose 10%, 50 mL of a 20% solution should be given into a large vein. Ethanol-induced hypoglycaemia is usually unresponsive to glucagon.

Haemodialysis may be considered if the blood ethanol concentration exceeds 7500 mg/L and if a severe metabolic acidosis is present, which has not been corrected by the measures outlined here.

Fructose is of negligible clinical benefit in accelerating ethanol oxidation and may cause acidosis; it should not be used.

Methanol

Background
Methanol is found in antifreeze solutions and windscreen washing fluid and is used widely as a solvent and to denature ethanol.

Toxicokinetics
Methanol is metabolized by alcohol dehydrogenase to formaldehyde. The oxidation of formaldehyde to formate is facilitated by formaldehyde dehydrogenase. Formate is converted by 10-formyl tetrahydrolate synthetase to carbon dioxide and water.

Mechanisms of toxicity
Methanol itself has a relatively low toxicity, but formate accumulates and there is a direct correlation between its concentration and toxicity. The acidosis observed appears to be caused directly or indirectly by formate production. Formate has also been shown to inhibit cytochrome oxidase and is the principal cause of ocular toxicity, though acidosis can increase toxicity further by enabling greater diffusion of formate into cells.

Clinical features
Methanol causes mild and transient inebriation, nausea, vomiting, abdominal pain and mild CNS depression. This is followed by a latent period of 12–24 hours after which uncompensated metabolic acidosis develops (the mortality increases with the severity and duration of acidosis), coma supervenes and visual function becomes impaired; this ranges from blurred vision and altered visual fields to complete blindness. Hyperglycaemia and raised serum amylase activity may ensue. Patients who survive may suffer permanent neurological sequelae, including blindness, rigidity, hypokinesis, and other parkinsonian-like signs. Respiratory arrest, coma, and severe metabolic acidosis are strong predictors of poor outcome.

Management
If there is a suspicion that methanol has been ingested and if presentation is early after exposure, the first priority is to inhibit methanol metabolism using either intravenous fomepizole or ethanol. In addition, if there is a high anion gap metabolic acidosis, or the osmolal gap greater than 10 mosmol/kg without there being another likely cause (e.g. ethanol poisoning), take a sample to measure the methanol concentration (at least 2 hours after ingestion) and *commence an antidote* whilst waiting for the results.

Fomepizole
Fomepizole requires less monitoring, but is more expensive than ethanol. After a loading dose of fomepizole 15 mg/kg over 30 minutes, four 12-hourly doses of 10 mg/kg should be given, followed by 15 mg/kg 12-hourly until the methanol concentration is not detectable. As fomepizole is dialysable, if haemodialysis or haemodiafiltration is employed, fomepizole should be given 6 hours after the first dose and every 4 hours thereafter; alternatively, an infusion of fomepizole 1.0–1.5 mg/kg/hour can be given during dialysis.

If fomepizole is unavailable consider ethanol.

Ethanol
A loading dose of intravenous ethanol 50 g for an adult (50 mL of absolute ethanol in 1 L 5% glucose, that is a 5% ethanol solution) should be given, followed by an intravenous infusion of ethanol, 10–12 g/hour (most easily given as 1 L 5% ethanol solution over 4–5 hours), to

achieve a blood ethanol concentration of approximately 1000 mg/L. Ideally, blood alcohol concentrations should be measured frequently. If haemodialysis or haemodiafiltration is used, greater amounts of ethanol (17–22 g/hour) must be given, because ethanol is readily dialysable. Administration of ethanol should be continued until methanol is undetectable in the blood.

Supportive measures should be employed and metabolic acidosis should be treated conventionally using sodium bicarbonate; several hundred millimoles of bicarbonate will be required in those presenting late after ingestion.

Haemodialysis and haemodiafiltration will enhance methanol and formate elimination and will correct severe metabolic abnormalities and should be employed particularly if presentation is late and marked metabolic acidosis is present.

In addition, folinic acid 30 mg intravenously 6-hourly for 48 hours should be given to enhance formate metabolism.

Further reading

Atassi WA, Noghnogh AA, Hariman R, et al. (1999). Hemodialysis as a treatment of severe ethanol poisoning. Int J Artif Organs, 22:18–20.

Barceloux DG, Bond GR, Krenzelok EP, et al. (2002). American Academy of Clinical Toxicology practice guidelines on the treatment of methanol poisoning. J Toxicol Clin Toxicol, 40: 415–46.

Brent J (2009). Fomepizole for ethylene glycol and methanol poisoning. N Engl J Med, 360:2216–23.

Brent J (2010). Fomepizole for the treatment of pediatric ethylene and diethylene glycol, butoxyethanol, and methanol poisonings. Clin Toxicol, 48:401–6.

Brent J, McMartin K, Phillips S, et al. (2001), Methylpyrazoles for Toxic Alcohols Study Group. Fomepizole for the treatment of methanol poisoning. N Engl J Med, 344:424–9.

Haber PS (2000). Metabolism of alcohol by the human stomach. Alcohol Clin Exp Res, 24:407–8.

Hantson P, Haufroid V, Mahieu P (2000). Determination of formic acid tissue and fluid concentrations in three fatalities due to methanol poisoning. Am J Forensic Med Pathol, 21:335–8.

Hantson P, Mahieu P (2000). Pancreatic injury following acute methanol poisoning. J Toxicol Clin Toxicol, 38:297–303.

Hovda KE, Hunderi OH, Tafjord A-B, et al. (2005). Methanol outbreak in Norway 2002–2004: epidemiology, clinical features and prognostic signs. J Intern Med, 258:181–90.

Hovda KE, Urdal P, Jacobsen D (2005). Increased serum formate in the diagnosis of methanol poisoning. J Anal Toxicol, 29: 586–8.

Jacobsen D, McMartin KE (1986). Methanol and ethylene glycol poisonings: mechanism of toxicity, clinical course, diagnosis and treatment. Med Toxicol, 1:309–44.

Jobard E, Harry P, Turcant A, et al. (1996). 4-methylpyrazole and hemodialysis in ethylene glycol poisoning. J Toxicol Clin Toxicol, 34:373–7.

Johnson HRM (1985). At what blood levels does alcohol kill? Med Sci Law, 25:127–30.

Johnson RA, Noll EC, Rodney WM (1982). Survival after a serum ethanol concentration of 1.5%. Lancet, 320:1394.

Lamminpää A, Vilska J (1990). Acute alcohol intoxications in children treated in hospital. Acta Paediatr Scand, 79:847–54.

Lamminpaa A, Vilska J (1991). Acid-base balance in alcohol users seen in an emergency room. Vet Hum Toxicol, 33:482–5.

Lamminpää A, Vilska J, Korri U-M, et al. (1993). Alcohol intoxication in hospitalized young teenagers. Acta Paediatr, 82:783–8.

Levy R, Elo T, Hanenson IB (1977). Intravenous fructose treatment of acute alcohol intoxication. Effects on alcohol metabolism. Arch Intern Med, 137:1175–7.

Lieber CS (2000). Ethnic and gender differences in ethanol metabolism. Alcohol Clin Exp Res, 24:417–18.

Liesivuori J, Savolainen H (1991). Methanol and formic acid toxicity: biochemical mechanisms. Pharmacol Toxicol, 69:157–63.

McMartin KE, Ambre JJ, Tephly TR (1980). Methanol poisoning in human subjects. Role for formic acid accumulation in the metabolic acidosis. Am J Med, 68:414–18.

McMartin KE, Martin-Amat G, Makar AB, et al. (1977). Methanol poisoning. V. Role of formate metabolism in the monkey. J Pharmacol Exp Ther, 201:564–72.

McRae AL, Brady KT, Sonne SC (2001). Alcohol and substance abuse. Med Clin North Am, 85:779–801.

Norberg A, Jones WA, Hahn RG, et al. (2003). Role of variability in explaining ethanol pharmacokinetics: research and forensic applications. Clin Pharmacokinet, 42:1–31.

Parlesak A, Billinger MHU, Bode C, et al. (2002). Gastric alcohol dehydrogenase activity in man: influence of gender, age, alcohol consumption and smoking in a Caucasian population. Alcohol Alcohol, 37:388–93.

Peters TJ, Preedy VR (1998). Metabolic consequences of alcohol ingestion. Novartis Found Symp, 216:19–34.

Reddy NJ, Sudini M, Lewis LD (2010). Delayed neurological sequelae from ethylene glycol, diethylene glycol and methanol poisonings. Clin Toxicol, 48:967–73.

Skrzydlewska E (2003). Toxicological and metabolic consequences of methanol poisoning. Toxicol Mech Methods, 13:277–93.

Tennant WG, Robertson CE (1987). Alcohol induced hypoglycaemia. Br J Accid Emerg Med, 2:16–17.

Tephly TR (1991). The toxicity of methanol. Life Sci, 48:1031–41.

Zehtabchi S, Sinert R, Baron BJ, et al. (2005). Does ethanol explain the acidosis commonly seen in ethanol-intoxicated patients? Clin Toxicol, 43:161–6.

Ethylene dibromide

Background
Ethylene dibromide (1,2-dibromoethane) is used in agriculture to fumigate soil to control nematodes, wireworms, and other pests. It is also used to treat grain and tree crops so may be encountered in greenhouses, warehouses, mills, and homes.

Toxicokinetics
Ethylene dibromide is rapidly absorbed following ingestion, inhalation, and dermally. It is metabolized mainly in the liver by two routes. Quantitatively the more important is oxidation by P450 enzymes such as CYP2E1, CYP2A6, and CYP2B6, to produce 2-bromoacetaldehyde which, in turn, is metabolized to other products including thiodiacetic acid, thiodiacetic sulphoxide, and S-(2-hydroxyethyl) mercapturic acid. The smaller proportion of ethylene dibromide is conjugated enzymatically with glutathione and the DNA repair protein, O6-alkylguanine alkyltransferase. There are no human excretion data, but excretion is rapid in rats.

Mechanisms of toxicity
Ethylene dibromide is a potent irritant of skin, eyes, and the mucus membranes of the respiratory and gastrointestinal tracts. The acute systemic and long-term effects of ethylene dibromide are due to oxidative metabolites, which bind preferentially to proteins and in doing so cause cell damage. Calcium homeostasis in mitochondria is disrupted resulting in a net efflux of calcium and glutathione from cells. Although in acute poisoning high blood bromide concentrations are found their clinical importance remains unclear.

Clinical features
Ethylene dibromide is highly toxic and ingestion of as little as 1.5 mL (3 g) carried a mortality of 20% in one series of 64 cases; only four individuals did not develop symptoms.

Nausea, vomiting, diarrhoea, and abdominal pain usually develop within a few hours. Blistering and erosions of the lips, mouth, pharynx, and gastric mucosa have been observed. Gastrointestinal bleeding is a feature in some cases. Consciousness may also be impaired at an early stage and, though usually mild, coma is possible. Restlessness is a frequent accompaniment.

Some patients then develop circulatory failure with tachycardia, hypotension and pulmonary congestion and frequently die within 12–24 hours. Indeed, in the largest series, no patient with an unrecordable blood pressure on presentation survived.

Hepatotoxicity and nephrotoxicity are the major features in those that escape cardiovascular collapse but biochemical confirmation may not be obtained until the second or third day post ingestion. Though each may develop independent of the other, they more commonly present together. In a recent series of 31 cases, four patients died. They all had abnormal renal function tests and three had amino and aspartate transaminase activities in excess of 1000 IU/L. The liver may become clinically enlarged and tender and associated with jaundice, elevated transaminase activities, and prolongation of the prothrombin time or INR. Hypoglycaemia was described in over a third of 64 cases and is presumably secondary to hepatocellular necrosis and impaired glycogenolysis.

Hepatic encephalopathy has been reported but the frequency with which it occurred in other series is unclear. Post-mortem examination has shown varying degrees of centrilobular necrosis of the liver.

Renal damage with albuminuria, haematuria, oliguria, a raised plasma creatinine concentration, hyperkalaemia, and metabolic acidosis may require temporary replacement therapy.

Dermal exposure gives rise to burning pain and reddening of the skin followed by swelling and blistering; systemic toxicity may develop. Ocular exposure to ethylene dibromide vapour can cause severe irritation.

Carcinogenicity
The IARC classified ethylene dibromide as 'probably carcinogenic to humans (Group 2A)' because there was sufficient evidence in experimental animals though the evidence in humans was inadequate. The National Toxicology Program has stated that ethylene dibromide is 'reasonably anticipated to be a human carcinogen' as it caused tumours in rats and mice at several different tissue sites and by several different routes of exposure.

Management
Casualties should be removed from a contaminated atmosphere, if appropriate, without placing the rescuer at risk. The patient's soiled clothing, including footwear, should be removed as soon as possible but before performing this task, those involved should be aware that ethylene dibromide can penetrate clothing. Management is then symptomatic and supportive.

Exposed skin should be washed with copious amounts of water and blistered areas treated as thermal burns.

Affected eyes should be irrigated with copious amounts of saline or water for 15 minutes. Instillation of a local anaesthetic may enable adequate decontamination. An ophthalmic opinion should be obtained.

Further reading
Garg PK, Jha D, Agarwal A, et al. (2002). Ethylene dibromide poisoning. *J Assoc Physicians India*, 50:1063–5.

Humphreys SDM, Rees HG, Routledge PA (1999). 1,2-Dibromoethane – a toxicological review. *Adverse Drug React Toxicol Rev*, 18:125–48.

Letz GA, Pond SM, Osterloh JD, et al. (1984). Two fatalities after acute occupational exposure to ethylene dibromide. *JAMA*, 252:2428–31.

Hissink AM, Wormhoudt LW, Sherratt PJ, et al. (2000). A physiologically-based pharmacokinetic (PB-PK) model for ethylene dibromide: relevance of extrahepatic metabolism. *Food Chem Toxicol*, 38:707–16.

Mehrotra P, Naik SR, Choudhuri G (2001). Two cases of ethylene dibromide poisoning. *Vet Hum Toxicol*, 43:91–2.

Nigam M, Godaria I, Varma A, et al. (2010). Ethylene dibromide (EDB) – an underestimated lethal pesticide and its emerging clinico-biochemical trends. *Med Leg Update*, 10:38–41.

National Toxicology Program (2005). 1,2-Dibromoethane (ethylene dibromide). In: *Report on Carcinogens: Carcinogen Profiles*, 11th edition, pp. 1–2. Research Triangle Park, NC: National Toxicology Program.

Singh N, Jatav OP, Gupta RK, et al. (2007). Outcome of sixty four cases of ethylene dibromide ingestion treated in tertiary care hospital. *J Assoc Physicians India*, 55:842–45.

Singh S, Gupta A, Sharma S, et al. (2000). Non-fatal ethylene dibromide ingestion. *Hum Exp Toxicol*, 19:152–3.

Ethylene and diethylene glycols

Ethylene glycol

Ethylene glycol is most commonly used as antifreeze. It may be drunk accidentally by children or intentionally by adults, sometimes as a substitute for ethanol. A lethal dose is of the order of 100 mL by ingestion.

Toxicokinetics

Ethylene glycol is absorbed rapidly from the gut and peak concentrations occur 1–4 hours after ingestion. Ethylene glycol is oxidized by alcohol dehydrogenase to glycolaldehyde. Aldehyde dehydrogenase rapidly converts glycolaldehyde to glycolate. The conversion of glycolate to glyoxylate is slow. A small proportion of glyoxylate is metabolized to oxalate. Calcium ions chelate oxalate to form insoluble calcium oxalate monohydrate crystals; these may be seen in the urine.

Mechanisms of toxicity

Ethylene glycol's toxicity depends predominantly on its metabolites, though the initial inebriation is due to ethylene glycol itself. CNS symptoms occur 6–12 hours after ingestion and coincide with the peak production of glycolaldehyde; aldehydes inhibit many aspects of cellular metabolism. Glycolate is largely responsible for the marked acidosis seen in severe cases; lactate concentrations are generally not very high. Lactate is produced as a result of the large amount of the reduced form of nicotinamide adenine dinucleotide (NADH) formed by the oxidation of ethylene glycol and by inhibition of the tricarboxylic acid cycle by the condensation products of glyoxylate. There is increasing evidence that calcium oxalate monohydrate crystals are the cause of cerebral oedema and renal failure.

Features

The features are summarized in Table 9.7. Although the three stages shown are useful theoretical descriptions of ethylene glycol poisoning, the onset and progression of the clinical course is frequently not as consistent or predictable. After a brief period of inebriation due to the intoxicating effect of ethylene glycol itself, metabolic acidosis develops, followed by tachypnoea, coma, seizures, hypertension, the appearance of pulmonary infiltrates, and oliguric renal failure. If untreated, death from multi-organ failure usually occurs 24–36 hours after ingestion.

Calcium oxalate monohydrate crystalluria is diagnostic and hypocalcaemia is frequent. Leucocytosis is a common but non-specific finding. Severe acidosis, hyperkalaemia, seizures, and coma carry a poor prognosis. Serum glycolate concentrations of 770 mg/L and higher are associated with a poor outcome.

Management

Supportive measures to combat cardiorespiratory depression should be employed and metabolic acidosis, hypocalcaemia, and renal failure should be treated conventionally.

If the patient presents early after ingestion, the first priority is to inhibit ethylene glycol metabolism using either intravenous fomepizole or ethanol. Fomepizole requires less monitoring, but is more expensive than ethanol.

Fomepizole

After a loading dose of fomepizole 15 mg/kg over 30 minutes, four 12-hourly doses of 10 mg/kg should be

Table 9.7 Features of ethylene glycol poisoning

Stage (time course)	Features
Stage 1 (30 minutes–12 hours)	Gastrointestinal and nervous system involvement
	Apparent intoxication with alcohol (but no ethanol on breath)
	Nausea, vomiting, haematemesis
	Coma and convulsions (often focal)
	Nystagmus, ataxia, papilloedema, depressed reflexes, myoclonic jerks, tetanic contractions
	II, V, VII, VIII, IX, X, XII nerve palsies
Stage 2 (12–24 hours)	Cardiorespiratory and metabolic disturbances
	Tachypnoea
	Tachycardia
	Metabolic acidosis
	Myocarditis
	Mild hypertension
	Pulmonary oedema
	Congestive cardiac failure
Stage 3 (24–72 hours)	Renal involvement
	Flank pain
	Renal angle tenderness
	Hypocalcaemia
	Acute tubular necrosis
	Calcium oxalate monohydrate crystalluria

given, followed by 15 mg/kg 12-hourly until the glycol concentration is not detectable. As fomepizole is dialysable, if haemodialysis or haemodiafiltration is employed to remove ethylene glycol, fomepizole should be given 6 hours after the first dose and every 4 hours thereafter; alternatively, an infusion of fomepizole 1.0–1.5 mg/kg/hour can be given during dialysis. This should be continued until glycol is undetectable.

Ethanol

If fomepizole is unavailable, a loading dose of intravenous ethanol 50 g for an adult (50 mL of absolute ethanol in 1 L 5% glucose, that is a 5% ethanol solution) should be given, followed by an intravenous infusion of ethanol, 10–12 g/hour (most easily given as 1 L 5% ethanol solution over 4–5 hours), to achieve a blood ethanol concentration of approximately 1000 mg/L. Administration of ethanol should be continued until glycol is undetectable in the blood. If haemodialysis is used, greater amounts of ethanol (17–22 g/hour) must be given, because ethanol is readily dialysable. Ideally, plasma glycol and ethanol concentrations should be measured frequently until recovery.

Haemodialysis

Haemodialysis and probably haemodiafiltration remove ethylene glycol, glycolaldehyde, and glycolate but not oxalate, and will also correct acid–base disturbances. Haemodialysis and haemodiafiltration should be employed particularly if presentation is late and marked metabolic acidosis is present.

Haemodialysis or haemodiafiltration should be continued until the glycol and glycolate are no longer detectable in the blood.

Diethylene glycol

Diethylene glycol is used as a coolant, as a building block in organic synthesis and as a solvent. It can be also found in some hydraulic fluids and brake fluids. Occupational exposure is by the dermal route but the most common route of exposure is ingestion, often unintentionally as a result of contamination of medicines. Diethylene glycol has been responsible for a number of mass poisonings in Australia, Bangladesh, Haiti, India, Nigeria, South Africa, and the USA.

Toxicokinetics

Diethylene glycol is metabolized in the rat and dog by alcohol dehydrogenase to 2-hydroxyethoxyacetaldehyde and by aldehyde dehydrogenase to 2-hydroxyethoxyacetate (2-HEAA) and a small amount of diglycolic acid. It is considered that 2-HEAA and diglycolic acid are the major metabolites in man.

Mechanisms of toxicity

The metabolic acidosis observed is primarily due to 2-HEAA. Diglycolic acid has been shown to be the metabolite responsible for the development of proximal tubular necrosis.

Features

Nausea and vomiting, headache, abdominal pain, coma, seizures, metabolic acidosis, and acute kidney injury have been reported most commonly. Pancreatitis and hepatitis have been observed, together with cranial neuropathies and demyelinating peripheral neuropathy.

Management

Supportive measures should be employed and metabolic acidosis should be treated conventionally. If presentation is early after exposure, the first priority is to inhibit

diethylene glycol metabolism using either intravenous fomepizole or ethanol. The approach is similar to that used for ethylene glycol. Administration of antidote should be continued until glycol is undetectable in the blood. Ideally, plasma glycol concentrations should be measured frequently until recovery.

It is not known whether 2-HEAA or diglycolic acid is removed by haemodialysis or haemodiafiltration.

Further reading
Besenhofer LM, Adegboyega PA, Bartels M, et al. (2010). Inhibition of metabolism of diethylene glycol prevents target organ toxicity in rats. Toxicol Sci, 117:25–35.

Besenhofer L, McLaren M, Latimer B, et al. (2011). Role of tissue metabolite accumulation in the renal toxicity of diethylene glycol. Toxicol Sci, 123:374–83.

Cheng J-T, Beysolow TD, Kaul B, et al. (1987). Clearance of ethylene glycol by kidneys and hemodialysis. J Toxicol Clin Toxicol, 25:95–108.

Hovda KE, Guo C, Austin R, et al. (2010). Renal toxicity of ethylene glycol results from internalization of calcium oxalate crystals by proximal tubule cells. Toxicol Lett, 192:365–72.

Jacobsen D, Hewlett TP, Webb R, et al. (1988). Ethylene glycol intoxication: evaluation of kinetics and crystalluria. Am J Med, 84:145–52.

Jacobsen D, McMartin KE (1986). Methanol and ethylene glycol poisonings: mechanism of toxicity, clinical course, diagnosis and treatment. Med Toxicol, 1:309–44.

Jacobsen D, Øvrebø S, Østborg J, et al. (1984). Glycolate causes the acidosis in ethylene glycol poisoning and is effectively removed by hemodialysis. Acta Med Scand, 216:409–16.

Landry GM, Martin S, McMartin KE (2011). Diglycolic acid is the nephrotoxic metabolite in diethylene glycol poisoning inducing necrosis in human proximal tubule cells in vitro. Toxicol Sci, 124:35–44.

Moreau CL, Kerns II W, Tomaszewski CA, et al. (1998). Glycolate kinetics and hemodialysis clearance in ethylene glycol poisoning. J Toxicol Clin Toxicol, 36: 659–66.

Porter WH, Rutter PW, Bush BA, et al. (2001). Ethylene glycol toxicity: the role of serum glycolic acid in hemodialysis. J Toxicol Clin Toxicol, 39:607–15.

Reddy NJ, Sudini M Lewis LD (2010). Delayed neurological sequelae from ethylene glycol, diethylene glycol and methanol poisonings. Clin Toxicol, 48:967–73.

Fluoroacetate (sodium fluoroacetate)

Background

Sodium fluoroacetate was selected by screening more than a thousand compounds for rodenticidal action during World War II and introduced into use in the USA in 1946. It was, and still is, referred to as 1080, the laboratory reference number it was given during its assessment. Fluoroacetic acid was isolated in 1944 from *Dichapetalum cymosum*, a South African plant known to be poisonous to farm animals.

Toxicokinetics

Fluoroacetate is absorbed rapidly from the gastrointestinal tract and is widely distributed to tissues. Fluoroacetate is then hydrolysed rapidly, fluoroacetyl CoA is formed, a toxicologically significant quantity of fluorocitrate is synthesized and key intracellular processes are disrupted. Some fluoroacetate is excreted unchanged in the urine.

Mechanisms of toxicity

The toxicity of fluoroacetate stems from its similarity to acetate, which has a pivotal role in cellular metabolism. Fluoroacetate combines with co-enzyme A to form fluoroacetyl CoA, which can substitute for acetyl CoA in the tricarboxylic acid cycle where it reacts with citrate synthase to produce fluorocitrate (Figure 9.5). A metabolite of one of the four possible stereoisomers of 2-fluorocitrate inhibits aconitase, thereby halting further progression of the cycle. As a consequence, energy production is reduced and intermediates of the tricarboxylic acid cycle subsequent to the citrate cycle are depleted.

Among these is oxoglutarate, a precursor of glutamate which is not only an excitatory neurotransmitter in the central nervous system but is also required for efficient removal of ammonia via the urea cycle. Increased ammonia concentrations have been observed in experimental fluoroacetate poisoning and may contribute to the incidence of seizures. Glutamate is also required for glutamine synthesis and glutamine depletion has been observed in the brains of fluoroacetate-poisoned rodents. Reduced cellular oxidative metabolism contributes to a lactic acidosis. Inability to oxidize fatty acids via the tricarboxylic acid cycle leads to ketone body accumulation and worsening acidosis while lowered ATP concentrations inhibit high energy-consuming reactions such as gluconeogenesis.

Fluoroacetate poisoning is associated with citrate accumulation in several tissues, including the brain. This is partly due to aconitase inhibition, for which citrate is the normal substrate. However, fluoroacetate also inactivates the mitochondrial membrane citrate carrier and increases cellular citrate concentrations thereby disrupting several enzyme systems including phosphofructokinase, the key regulatory enzyme of glycolysis. This in turn blocks glucose utilization leading to hyperglycaemia in experimental fluoroacetate poisoning. Hypoglycaemia may also ensue as a consequence of glycogen depletion. Poor glycaemic control does not appear, however, to be a significant problem in fluoroacetate poisoning in man.

Citrate and fluoroacetate are known calcium chelators. Hypocalcaemia is therefore to be expected in fluoroacetate poisoning and both animal and clinical data support hypocalcaemia as a mechanism of fluoroacetate toxicity. It is possible that fluorocitrate-induced seizures are due, at least in part, to calcium being complexed in the spinal cord.

Clinical features

Sodium fluoroacetate poisoning is most common after ingestion. However, systemic toxicity may also occur after inhalation and eye exposure. It is poorly absorbed through intact skin, but may be absorbed through breaks in the skin. Skin and eye exposure may also produce local effects.

Nausea, vomiting and abdominal pain are common within 1 hour of ingestion. Sweating, apprehension, confusion, and agitation soon follow. Both tachycardia and bradycardia have been described. More serious arrhythmias, including supraventricular tachycardia, atrial fibrillation, ventricular tachycardia, ventricular fibrillation, and asystole, have been reported. Non-specific ST and T-wave changes are common, the QT may be prolonged and hypotension may develop.

Seizures are the main neurological feature and may recur, occasionally over a period of days. Consciousness becomes progressively impaired within a few hours of poisoning leading to coma that may persist for several days. Cerebellar dysfunction has been observed.

Serum calcium concentrations have been measured in relatively few cases of human poisoning. In one study, the initial mean total serum calcium concentrations did not differ significantly between seven fatalities and 31 survivors of poisoning. However, later in the course of their hospital stay, 57% of those who died were hypocalcaemic compared with only 36% of survivors (p < 0.01).

Less common features of fluoroacetate poisoning include nystagmus, chewing movements of the jaws, carpopedal spasms, reversible oliguric or non-oliguric renal failure in the absence of hypotension, metabolic acidosis, and increased transaminase activity.

Long-term sequelae have been reported. Cerebellar ataxia lasting for at least 18 months was reported in one patient; memory disturbances and depressive behaviour which resolved were also seen in this patient. Tetraplegia, cogwheel rigidity, grand mal epilepsy, cortical blindness, and divergent strabismus were seen in another patient 9 years after exposure; these features were attributed to cerebral hypoxia at the time of ingestion.

Hypotension, acidaemia, and raised serum creatinine concentrations have been identified as the most sensitive predictors of a fatal outcome, though ventricular arrhythmias, refractory hypotension and secondary lung infections are the main causes of death.

The lethal dose for humans is estimated to be 2–10 mg/kg.

Management

If the patient presents within 1 hour of ingestion of a potentially toxic amount of fluoroacetate, gastric lavage may be performed, or activated charcoal may be given as it binds fluoroacetate, though there is no evidence that lavage or charcoal alters the clinical course.

- The plasma/blood glucose concentration should be measured urgently and hypoglycaemia corrected if found with 10% dextrose.
- If severe hypotension supervenes, rapid administration of intravenous saline 0.9% and a vasopressor such as

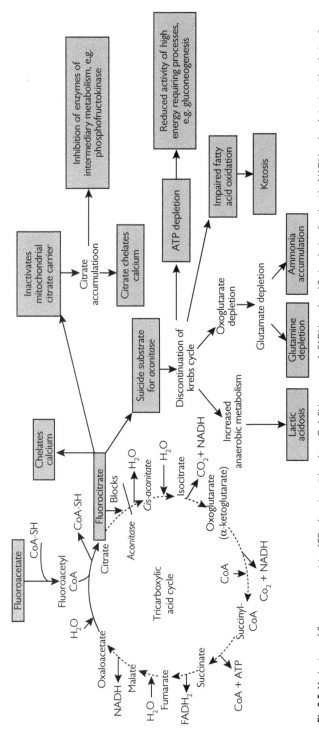

Fig 9.5 Mechanisms of fluoroacetate toxicity. ATP: adenosine triphosphate; CoA-SH: coenzyme A; FADH$_2$: reduced flavin-adenine dinucleotide; NADH: reduced nicotinamide-adenine dinucleotide. Reproduced from Springer, *Toxicological Reviews*, 25, 2006, pp. 213–219, 'Sodium fluoroacetate poisoning', Proudfoot AT et al., with kind permission from Springer Science + Business Media B.V.

norepinephrine 40 micrograms [base]/mL by intravenous infusion at an initial rate of 0.16–0.33 mL/minute, (for children 1 month–18 years give an intravenous infusion at a rate of 20–100 nanograms [base]/kg/minute; max 1 microgram [base]/kg/minute), adjusted according to response, may be necessary.

- Control of convulsions using an intravenous benzodiazepine is clearly vital, as is the establishment and maintenance of a clear airway and adequate ventilation. Give intravenous diazepam 10 mg (child 300–400 micrograms/kg) or lorazepam 4 mg (child 100 micrograms/kg). If repeated convulsions occur, phenytoin 20 mg/kg (max. 2 g) by slow intravenous injection or infusion (with blood pressure and ECG monitoring), at a rate not exceeding 1 mg/kg/minute (max. 50 mg per minute); for a child 1 month–12 years, 20 mg/kg at a rate not exceeding 1 mg/kg/minute (max. 50 mg per minute) as a loading dose.

Metabolic acidosis that is not secondary to hypoxia during seizures requires correction with intravenous sodium bicarbonate. Arrhythmias other than ventricular fibrillation should only be treated if causing peripheral circulatory failure. Renal failure should be managed conventionally.

Though the importance of calcium concentrations in fluoroacetate poisoning is uncertain, the serum calcium should be measured in any patient with severe poisoning and hypocalcaemia should be corrected if it is found.

A number of substances, including ethanol (which inhibits fluorocitrate production), acetate (which is thought to supplement the tricarboxylic acid cycle and to enter cells readily and compete with fluoroacetate for binding to acetyl CoA) and sodium succinate (which is thought to supplement the tricarboxylic acid cycle), alone and in combination, have been assessed experimentally but none has yet been employed in man.

Further reading

Baker T (1952). Acute poisoning with sodium fluoroacetate (compound 1080). JAMA, 149:1520–2.

Brockmann JL, McDowell AV, Leeds WG (1955). Fatal poisoning with sodium fluoroacetate. Report of a case. JAMA, 159:1529–32.

Chi C-H, Chen K-W, Chan S-H, et al. (1996). Clinical presentation and prognostic factors in sodium monofluoroacetate intoxication. J Toxicol Clin Toxicol, 34:707–12.

Chi C-H, Lin T-K, Chen K-W (1999). Hemodynamic abnormalities in sodium monofluoroacetate intoxication. Hum Exp Toxicol, 18:351–3.

Chung H-M (1984). Acute renal failure caused by acute monofluoroacetate poisoning. Vet Hum Toxicol, 26:29–32.

Goncharov NV, Jenkins RO, Radilov AS (2006). Toxicology of fluoroacetate: a review, with possible directions for therapy research. J Appl Toxicol, 26:148–61.

Harrisson JWE, Ambrus JL, Ambrus CM, et al. (1950). Fluoroacetate poisoning. A review and report of a case. Am J Dis Child, 79:310–20.

Höjer J, Hung HT, Du NT, et al. (2003). An outbreak of severe rodenticide poisoning in North Vietnam caused by illegal fluoroacetate. J Toxicol Clin Toxicol, 41:646.

McTaggart DR (1970). Poisoning due to sodium fluoroacetate ("1080"). Med J Aust, 2:641–2.

Peters RA, Spencer H, Bidstrup PL (1981). Subacute fluoroacetate poisoning. J Occup Med, 23:112–13.

Pridmore SA (1978). Fluoroacetate poisoning: nine years later. Med J Aust, 2:269–70.

Proudfoot AT, Bradberry SM, Vale JA (2006). Sodium fluoroacetate poisoning. Toxicol Rev, 25:213–19.

Rammell CG, Fleming P, O'Hara PJ (1977). 1080 poisoning. NZ Med J, 85:295–6.

Reigart JR, Brueggeman JL, Keil JE (1975). Sodium fluoroacetate poisoning. Am J Dis Child, 129:1224–6.

Robinson R, Griffith J, Nahata M, et al (2001). Ingestion of ratbane 1080 sodium monofluoroacetate. J Toxicol Clin Toxicol, 39:477–8.

Robinson RF, Griffith JR, Wolowich WR, et al. (2002). Intoxication with sodium monofluoroacetate (compound 1080). Vet Hum Toxicol, 44:93–5.

Taitelman U, Roy (Shapira) A, Hoffer E (1983). Fluoroacetamide poisoning in man: the role of ionized calcium. Arch Toxicol, Suppl. 6:228–31.

Trabes J, Rason N, Avrahami E (1983). Computed tomography demonstration of brain damage due to acute sodium monofluoroacetate poisoning. J Toxicol Clin Toxicol, 20:85–92.

Formaldehyde and metaldehyde

Background
Both formaldehyde and metaldehyde are organic compounds. Formaldehyde is the simplest aldehyde (CH_2O), whereas metaldehyde is a cyclic tetramer of aldehyde (($CH_3CHO)_4$).

Formaldehyde
Formaldehyde is a naturally occurring compound, which can be synthesized by a number of different routes. Formaldehyde dissolved in water is known as formalin; a saturated aqueous solution, containing approximately 40% by volume formaldehyde, is known as 100% formalin. A typical commercial grade formalin may contain up to 15% methanol to prevent formaldehyde polymerization.

Formaldehyde is used in a number of different industrial uses, including the manufacture of plastics, adhesives, paints, foams and explosives. It is also used as a disinfectant and a biocide. It is used as a tissue fixture for both histological and microbiological specimens, embalming (in addition to its biocide actions) and in DNA/RNA-based studies. Finally, a combination of formaldehyde with concentrated sulphuric acid can be used in 'field tests' to determine whether a suspected recreational drug potentially contains MDMA (3,4-Methylenedioxymetham-phetamine; 'ecstasy') and other related recreational drugs; this field test is known as the Marquis test.

Toxicokinetics
Formaldehyde is oxidized by aldehyde dehydrogenases (predominantly formaldehyde dehydrogenase) to S-formyl glutathione, which is hydrolysed very rapidly by thiolase to formic acid. Formic acid is then oxidized and incorporated into biological molecules via the tetrahydrofolate-dependent, one-carbon, biosynthetic pathway and oxidized further to carbon dioxide and water. Conversion of formate to carbon dioxide is the rate-limiting step in formaldehyde metabolism and the reason for accumulation of formic acid after acute exposure. In addition to eliminating formic acid, the tetrahydrofolic acid-dependent one-carbon pool can also oxidize formaldehyde to formic acid.

Mechanisms of toxicity
Formaldehyde is so soluble in water that it dissolves immediately in any body fluid with which it comes into contact and, in turn, moves into the cells these fluids cover. Whether in surface mucus or in cells, its high tissue reactivity then results in it binding to proteins, nucleic acids, and amino acids and, perhaps most importantly, by covalent reactions with macromolecules. Formaldehyde also reacts readily with free, unprotonated NH_2-groups of amino acids producing methylol derivatives and liberating protons that may be responsible for its irritant effects on mucous membranes. At high concentrations it precipitates proteins.

The metabolic acidosis observed after ingestion of formalin occurs primarily as the result of formation of formic acid, which may also be produced by the metabolism of methanol.

Clinical features—acute poisoning
The features of formaldehyde toxicity depend not only upon the amount and concentration of formaldehyde to which an individual has been exposed, but also on the route of exposure. It should be noted that the upper respiratory tract and the eyes are very sensitive to low concentrations of formaldehyde, and therefore the development of the symptoms described here is a good indicator of exposure, and therefore the need for removal from any potential sources.

Inhalation
Inhalation can be associated with irritant effects to the upper and/or lower airway. Clinical features include bronchospasm and cough, airway oedema, pneumonitis, and adult respiratory distress syndrome (ARDS).

Dermal and ocular exposure
Formaldehyde is associated with localized irritation following either dermal or ocular exposure. In addition, after large dermal exposures, there is the potential for significant systemic absorption and associated systemic toxicity.

Ingestion
Ingestion of 30–60mL of formalin solution is potentially fatal in adults.

Following ingestion individuals may complain of oropharyngeal, chest and abdominal pain, associated with nausea, vomiting, and diarrhoea. There is a risk of GI ulceration and haemorrhage. Typically the greatest injury is seen in the stomach rather than the oropharynx or oesophagus. There have been reports of patients whose stomach has been 'fixed' by the ingestion of formalin.

Systemic toxicity can occur following large ingestions, and features include: drowsiness, reduced level of consciousness, metabolic acidosis which is often severe, respiratory failure, circulatory collapse, seizures, DIC, and hepatic and renal dysfunction.

Clinical features—chronic exposure
There is great concern about the potential for long-term low-dose exposure to formaldehyde, particularly the 'off gassing' from formaldehyde containing insulation and building materials. There have been reports that exposure to concentrations as low as 1 ppm in 'new homes' has been associated with headache, nausea, and other upper respiratory tract irritation symptoms. Additionally, there is some evidence that formaldehyde can be associated with immune-mediated bronchospasm and it can be a dermal sensitizer.

Carcinogenicity
The IARC has concluded that there is sufficient evidence in humans for the carcinogenicity of formaldehyde. Formaldehyde causes cancer of the nasopharynx and leukaemia. Also, a positive association has been observed between exposure to formaldehyde and sinonasal cancer. The detailed evidence to support this classification has now been published both by IARC and by the National Toxicology Program.

Management
The management is largely supportive.

Inhalation
There is no specific management following inhalation exposure; where appropriate a chest X-ray and/or arterial blood gases should be performed to assess the

degree of pulmonary injury. Management should be as directed by the clinical condition of the patient.

Dermal and ocular exposure

Following dermal and/or ocular exposure, the affected area(s) should be thoroughly irrigated, with appropriate dermatological or ophthalmological review as required.

Ingestion

There is no evidence for the use of gastrointestinal tract decontamination in management.

Metabolic acidosis occurs early and is often severe. If it is not responsive to fluid resuscitation and intravenous hypertonic (8.4%) sodium bicarbonate, then haemodialysis or haemodiafiltration should be undertaken.

Appropriate fluid resuscitation and inotropic support should be given, as necessary, particularly in those with circulatory failure.

In patients who have ingested large volumes of formalin, fomepizole should be administered to prevent the metabolism of methanol to additional formaldehyde and formic acid (see Ethanol and methanol, pp. 236–238). In addition, haemodialysis or haemodiafiltration should be undertaken to remove formate. Folinic acid 1 mg/kg intravenously (up to a maximum of 50 mg) 6 hourly for 48 hours should be administered to enhance formate metabolism.

If respiratory failure supervenes, ventilation will be necessary. Seizures should be treated with intravenous benzodiazepines.

Endoscopy should be undertaken early in those with GI bleeding.

Metaldehyde

Metaldehyde is most commonly used as a 'molluscicide', typically in relation to slugs and snails. It is sold under a variety of different trade names, and is sold to be used as pellets (often combined with wheat bait), liquid, or paste. In addition, metaldehyde is also used in solid fuel camping stoves as a 'camping fuel' and in some fireworks. Exposure to more than 400 mg/kg of metaldehyde is potentially life threatening in adults.

Toxicokinetics

Depolymerization to acetaldehyde was long thought to be the route of degradation but the failure to detect acetaldehyde in the plasma of dogs and a man poisoned with metaldehyde suggests that this is not the case.

Mechanisms of toxicity

Contrary to earlier opinion, it is now considered that the features of metaldehyde poisoning are due to the parent compound and not acetaldehyde. Serial plasma concentrations of both metaldehyde and acetaldehyde were measured in nine dogs given metaldehyde 60 mg/kg and six others given the same dose of acetaldehyde. The results and comparison of the morbidity induced in both groups of animals did not support acetaldehyde as the mediator of metaldehyde toxicity. In addition, the features developed by rats poisoned with acetaldehyde did not resemble those caused by metaldehyde and gas chromatography of the serum of others given large amounts of metaldehyde failed to show a peak at the retention time of acetaldehyde. A man poisoned with metaldehyde had measurable serum concentrations of the pesticide over many hours (peak 125 mg/L) but acetaldehyde concentrations did not exceed 1 mg/L in samples taken on presentation and at 11 and 107 hours later.

Clinical features

Ingestion

Nausea, vomiting, abdominal pain, and diarrhoea are common and may occur after a latent period of 1–3 hours. With larger amounts (>100 mg/kg) there may be drowsiness, dizziness, agitation, flushing, increased muscle tone and muscle twitching (including opisthotonos and risus sardonicus) convulsions, impairment of consciousness (which may last several days), metabolic acidosis, respiratory depression, and pyrexia. Increased motor activity may result in rhabdomyolysis.

Hypokalaemia, hyperkalaemia (from rhabdomyolysis), and hypotension have also been reported. Hepatic and renal tubular necrosis may appear after 2–3 days but are unlikely to be severe enough to merit specific treatment.

Inhalation

After inhalation of smoke from a novelty item containing metaldehyde, pneumonitis occurred in a 14-year-old girl with cough, wheeze, pleuritic chest pain, rhinorrhoea, lacrimation, tachypnoea, pyrexia, dizziness, and abdominal pain. A chest X-ray was consistent with ARDS. She recovered fully over a few days.

Management

Is essentially as for formaldehyde.

Ingestion

Animal studies suggest that early use (within 30 minutes) of oral activated charcoal can reduce the absorption of ingested metaldehyde. Based on this, a single dose of 50 g in adults is likely to block absorption of 10 g of metaldehyde. Delayed use beyond 30 minutes is likely to be associated with a reduced therapeutic benefit. Use of activated charcoal may be limited by vomiting, and reduced level of consciousness associated with metaldehyde ingestion. There is a risk of aspiration in these circumstances and appropriate airway protection if required.

Intravenous diazepam should be given to suppress convulsions and a clear airway and adequate ventilation ensured, using endotracheal intubation if necessary. Rhabdomyolysis and its complications are managed conventionally.

Further reading

Bleakley C, Ferrie E, Collum N, et al. (2008). Self-poisoning with metaldehyde. *Emerg Med J*, 25:381–2.

Darkazally N, Judge BS, Rusyniak DE (2003). Early hemodialysis in acute formalin ingestion. *Clin Toxicol*, 41:665.

Eells JT, McMartin KE, Black K, et al. (1981). Formaldehyde poisoning. Rapid metabolism to formic acid. *JAMA*, 46:1237–8.

International Agency for Research on Cancer (2012). Formaldehyde. In: *Chemical Agents and Related Occupations*, Vol. 100 F, pp. 401–35. Lyon: IARC.

Jay MS, Kearns GL, Stone V, et al. (1988). Toxic pneumonitis in an adolescent following exposure to Snow Storm tablets. *J Adolesc Health Care*, 9:431–3.

Keller K H, Shimizu G, Walter FG, et al. (1991). Acetaldehyde analysis in severe metaldehyde poisoning. *Vet Hum Toxicol*, 33:374.

Köppel C, Baudisch H, Schneider V, et al. (1990). Suicidal ingestion of formalin with fatal complications. *Intensive Care Med*, 16:212–14.

Moody JP, Inglis FG (1992). Persistence of metaldehyde during acute molluscicide poisoning. *Hum Exp Toxicol*, 11:361–2.

Shintani S, Goto K, Endo Y, et al. (1999). Adsorption effects of activated charcoal on metaldehyde toxicity in rats. *Vet Hum Toxicol*, 41:15–18.

Hydrofluoric acid

Background

Hydrofluoric acid (HF) (CAS 7664-39-3) is a colourless fuming liquid being a solution of hydrogen fluoride in water. It has an extremely acrid odour with a threshold of between 0.042 and 3 ppm. It can also exist in an anhydrous solid form. Various concentrations are available commercially from 1–100% (anhydrous).

It is used as a catalyst in the petroleum industry, for various fluorination processes, in separating uranium isotopes, in analytical and dye chemistry, in the production of fluorine, and in the production of aluminium fluoride; it is also used to stop the fermentation in brewing. HF is widely used in many industrial settings including the production of integrated circuits, fluorides, plastics, germicides, insecticides, and in etching and cleaning silicone, glass, metal, stone, and porcelain. In addition, it is used in enamelling and galvanizing iron, pickling stainless steel, in the production of petrol, in the production of aluminium, and in adjusting pH in oil well operations and working silk. It is found in automotive cleaning products. HF can be found in many domestic products including air conditioner cleaners, aluminium cleaners, wheel cleaners, and rust removers.

Mechanisms of toxicity

HF is particularly dangerous because of its unique ability among acids to penetrate tissue. HF is a weak acid that exists predominantly in the undissociated state; in this state HF is able to penetrate skin and soft tissue by non-ionic diffusion. Once in the tissues, HF causes liquefactive necrosis of tissues (necrotic material becomes softened and liquefied) and bony erosion. Electrolyte abnormalities result from by fluoride binding with calcium and magnesium.

Clinical features

HF is toxic by dermal, inhalation, ingestion, or ocular exposure. There are specific problems with each of the routes of exposure and systemic effects can occur following any mode of exposure but are more likely following ingestion and/or inhalation.

Dermal exposure

Any exposure can lead to burns, the severity of which depends on the concentration of HF, duration of exposure, and the surface area affected. It is also very important to recognize that pain can be out of proportion to burn appearance. This is due to the F^- binding to tissue Ca^{2+} ions and causes a cascade of K^+ from cells that stimulate nerve endings.

The burns themselves will eventually have the appearance of blue-grey discolouration with significant tissue damage, if not treated promptly. There can also be a delayed reaction following exposure (Table 9.8).

There is a high risk of serious systemic complications if greater than 1% body surface area (e.g. size of hand) is contaminated with a 50% or higher solution of HF; if there are burns to face or neck, with any concentration of HF, because of risk of inhalation (see later in section). Solutions with concentrations as low as 2% may cause burns if they remain in contact with the skin for long enough. Fatalities have been reported from a skin exposure to as little as 2.5% of body surface area (BSA). A patient had a cardiac arrest following a mild partial thickness thigh burn of 3% with a 20% HF solution.

Inhalation

HF causes irritation of the eyes and nose with sore throat, cough, chest tightness, headache, ataxia, and confusion. Dyspnoea and stridor due to laryngeal oedema may follow, depending on the concentration of HF. Haemorrhagic pulmonary oedema with increasing breathlessness, wheeze, hypoxia, and cyanosis may take up to 36 hours to develop. The release of approximately 24 tonnes of HF over a period of 48 hours from a Texas petroleum plant in 1989 led to the hospitalization of 94 residents in the vicinity of the plant due to HF's irritant effects.

Ingestion

There is likely to be burning of the mouth and throat with retrosternal and abdominal pain, which can be severe. The laryngeal involvement may cause oedema, airway obstruction, and difficulty in clearing bronchial secretions, which will lead to hypersalivation. In addition vomiting may occur with increased risk of aspiration. Hematemesis and hypotension are likely following significant ingestion. Oesophageal or gastric perforation may occur in the acute phase. Oesophageal or gastric stricture may develop over weeks or months following ingestion.

Ocular exposure

Any splashes in the eye are serious and can lead to conjunctivitis, chemosis, corneal epithelial coagulation, and necrosis.

Systemic effects

Common systemic features include hypocalcaemia, hypomagnesaemia, hyperkalaemia, and metabolic acidosis. Less common systemic features include myoclonus, tetany, convulsions, CNS depression and cardiac arrhythmias (prolonged QT, VT/VF) which can occur within 90 minutes of exposure.

Management

As HF is so toxic it is vital that first responders and healthcare workers are not put at risk. Removing the patient from further exposure is key but responders should not enter a contaminated area without PPE and self-contained breathing apparatus. If the patient has not been decontaminated, secondary carers must wear appropriate PPE to avoid contaminating themselves. All casualties should have any contaminated clothing removed prior to treatment in a well-ventilated area.

Dermal exposure

• Irrigate the contaminated area with copious volumes of water as soon as possible and for at least 1 minute. Apply

Table 9.8 Summary of dermal effects following exposure to HF

[HF]	Features
<20%	Erythema and pain may be delayed for 24 hours, often not reported until significant tissue injury has occurred
20–50%	Erythema and pain may be delayed for 8 hours, often not reported until tissue injury has occurred
>50%	May produce immediate pain and erythema, rapid destruction of tissues and acute systemic toxicity

calcium gluconate gel repeatedly to the burn as soon as practicable. For burns to the hand the use of a surgical glove containing calcium gluconate gel then pulled over the hand may be effective at reducing pain and retarding skin damage. The pain may need opiate analgesia.
- Hexafluorine™ may be used, though benefit over calcium gluconate has not yet been demonstrated.
- If the burn is small it may respond to local subcutaneous infiltration of a small volume (0.5 mL) of 10% calcium gluconate solution around the wound.
- In severe cases intra-arterial calcium gluconate 10 mL of 10% calcium gluconate diluted in 50 mL dextrose and infused over 3–4 hours into the brachial or radial artery has been used.

NB **Do not give** calcium chloride subcutaneously or intra-arterially as this causes tissue necrosis.

Inhalation
- An urgent assessment of the airway is required to ensure that there is a clear airway and adequate ventilation. Oxygen should be administered. A supraglottic-epiglottic burn with erythema and oedema is usually a sign that further oedema will occur which will lead to airway obstruction and is an indication for early intubation or tracheostomy. Effects may be delayed for some hours.
- If the patient has clinical features of bronchospasm then treat conventionally with nebulized bronchodilators and steroids. Nebulized calcium gluconate 2.5–3.0% has also been recommended, but evidence of its effectiveness is difficult to assess. It is unlikely to cause deterioration and therefore may be worth considering.
- Treat pulmonary oedema and/or acute lung injury with CPAP or in severe cases with IPPV and PEEP.
- There is no consistent evidence available on the prophylactic use of corticosteroids (inhaled or systemic) and antibiotics.
- Monitor the cardiac rhythm in all patients and in any who are symptomatic patients perform an urgent 12-lead ECG and measure the QRS duration and QT interval.
- If possible perform an early erect chest X-ray. This is helpful if the patient deteriorates later.

All patients should have bloods checked to exclude systemic features.

Ingestion
- An urgent assessment of the airway is required to ensure that there is a clear airway and adequate ventilation. A supraglottic-epiglottic burn with erythema and oedema is usually a sign that further oedema will occur which will lead to airway obstruction and is an indication for early intubation or tracheostomy.
- Early complete fibreoptic endoscopy by an experienced endoscopist is indicated to grade the severity of the injury in any patient who is symptomatic or has evidence of oropharyngeal burns (see also Acids and alkalis, pp. 208–211).
- Monitor the cardiac rhythm in all patients and in any who are symptomatic patients perform an urgent 12-lead ECG and measure the QRS duration and QT interval.
- If possible perform an early erect chest X-ray. This is likely to be helpful if the patient deteriorates later.

All patients should have bloods checked to exclude systemic features.

Ocular exposure
- Remove contact lenses if necessary and immediately irrigate the affected eye thoroughly with water or 0.9% saline for at least 30 minutes. Experimental evidence suggests that Hexafluorine® may be of value. There is no evidence of the efficacy of calcium gluconate and there is some evidence that it may be toxic to the conjunctiva. Calcium gluconate is therefore *not* recommended.
- It is important to give adequate pain relief both locally, e.g. repeated instillation of local anaesthetics such as tetracaine, and systemically, e.g. opiates. This will enable thought decontamination and examination. Mydriatic and cycloplegic agents (e.g. cyclopentolate, tropicamide) may also help with pain relief but should *not* be used in patients with glaucoma.
- Corneal examination will be facilitated with the use of fluorescein. Patients with corneal damage, and patients who have been exposed to strong concentrations and those whose symptoms do not resolve rapidly, should be referred for urgent ophthalmological assessment.

Systemic features

Systemic features need urgent treatment. If the patient has proven hypocalcaemia or clinical symptoms/signs suggestive of severe hypocalcaemia (tetany, arrhythmias, QTc prolongation and convulsions), urgent correction of the hypocalcaemia is needed. In adults give either 5–10 mL of 10% calcium chloride or 10–30 mL 10% calcium gluconate IV. In severe cases 40 mL of a 10% calcium gluconate infusion over 1 hour will be required. In children administer either 0.2 mL/kg of 10% calcium chloride or 0.5 mL/kg 10% calcium gluconate solutions IV over 5 minutes.

Correct hypomagnesaemia by giving 8 mmol magnesium sulfate IV over 1–2 minutes in adults.

Treat hyperkalaemia conventionally but stabilize the myocardium urgently by intravenous calcium salts.

If metabolic acidosis persists despite correction of hypoxia and adequate fluid resuscitation, consider correction with intravenous sodium bicarbonate. Rapid correction is particularly important if there is prolongation of the QRS or QT intervals.

Further reading

Baxter PJ, Aw T-C, Cockcroft A et al. (eds) (2010). *Hunter's Diseases of Occupations*, 10th edition. London: Hodder.

Beiran I, Miller B and Bentur Y (1997). The efficacy of calcium gluconate in ocular hydrofluoric acid burns. *Hum Exper Toxicol*, 16:223–8.

Lee DC, Wiley JF 2nd, Snyder JW 2nd (1993). Treatment of inhalational exposure to hydrofluoric acid with nebulised calcium gluconate. *J Occup Med*, 35:470.

McCulley JP (1990). Ocular hydrofluoric acid burns: animal model, mechanism of injury and therapy. *Trans Am Ophthalmol Soc*, 88:649–84.

Spöler F, Frentz M, Först M, et al. (2008). Analysis of hydrofluoric acid penetration and decontamination of the eye by means of time-resolved optical coherence tomography. *Burns*, 34:549–55.

Trevino MA, Herrmann GH, Sprout WL (1983). Treatment of severe hydrofluoric acid exposure. *J Occup Med*, 25:861–3.

Wing JS, Sanderson LM, Brender JD, et al. (1991). Acute health effects in a community after a release of hydrofluoric acid. *Arch Environ Health*, 46:155–60

Wu M-L, Deng J-F, Fan J-S (2010). Survival after hypocalcemia, hypomagnesemia, hypokalemia and cardiac arrest following mild hydrofluoric acid burn. *Clin Toxicol*, 48:953–5.

Hydrogen sulphide

Background

Hydrogen sulphide (H_2S) (CAS 7783-06-4) is a colourless, flammable gas with a characteristic 'rotten egg' smell. It can occur naturally in crude petroleum, natural gas, volcanic gases, and hot springs. It can also result from bacterial breakdown of organic matter. It is also produced by human and animal wastes. It is therefore commonly encountered in places such as sewers, sewage treatment plants (H_2S is often called *sewer gas*), manure stockpiles, mines, and the holds of fishing ships. Bacteria found in the mouth and gastrointestinal tract produce H_2S from bacteria decomposing materials that contain vegetable or animal proteins. H_2S can also result from industrial activities, such as food processing, coke ovens, paper mills, tanneries, and petroleum refineries.

With a vapour density of 1.19, H_2S is approximately 20% heavier than air, so this invisible gas will collect in depressions in the ground and in confined spaces. The use of direct reading gas detection instrumentation should be required before entering confined spaces such as manholes, tanks, pits, and reaction vessels that could contain an accumulation of H_2S gas.

Toxicokinetics

H_2S is rapidly absorbed by the lungs into the bloodstream. It is rapidly and widely distributed throughout the body. There is some limited absorption through the gastrointestinal tract and the skin but this is small compared to the respiratory system. Metabolism of H_2S occurs by oxidation, methylation, or reaction with metalloproteins and the principal product is sulfate which is excreted rapidly from the body in the form of sulfate in urine.

Mechanisms of toxicity

It is an irritant gas with systemic asphyxiant effects, and reversibly inhibits cytochrome oxidase, which impairs cell respiration. It is particularly irritating to the eyes and respiratory tract. Although the odour threshold has been reported to be around 0.011 mg/m^3 (0.008 ppm) in naïve subjects, olfactory paralysis occurs at greater than about 100 ppm (140 mg/m^3). The loss of odour perception is an important factor in toxicity as a few breaths greater than 700 mg/m^3 (500 ppm) can be lethal (Table 9.9).

Table 9.9 Relationship between H_2S exposure concentrations and features

Dose ppm (mg/m^3)	Features
0.008 (0.011)	Odour threshold
2 (2.8)	Bronchial constriction in asthmatic individuals
5–10 (7–14)	Increased blood lactate concentration, decreased skeletal muscle citrate synthase activity, decreased oxygen uptake
4–21 (5–29)	Eye irritation
20 (28)	Fatigue, loss of appetite, headache, irritability, poor memory, dizziness
>100 (>140)	Olfactory paralysis
>402 (>560)	Respiratory distress
>500 (>700)	Death

Clinical features

Following inhalation, respiratory tract irritation, bronchitis, rhinitis, dyspnoea, pharyngitis, and pulmonary oedema have been reported. Systemic effects include vomiting, drowsiness, diarrhoea, tremor, headache, muscular weakness, nystagmus, seizures, dizziness, tachycardia, agitation, and hypotension.

Exposure to concentrations greater than 500 ppm (700 mg/m^3) can be fatal. Respiratory failure is the most common cause of death. Neurological effects at high exposure have included nausea, headache, delirium, disturbed equilibrium, poor memory, neurobehavioral changes, olfactory paralysis, loss of consciousness, tremors, and convulsions. In those surviving exposure to high concentrations some of the neurological effects may be permanent or persistent. Cardiac arrhythmias as well as hypertension have been reported. Healthy individuals can tolerate moderate exposures to H_2S but there is some evidence that asthmatics are more sensitive, with bronchoconstriction and headache seen at 2 ppm (2.8 mg/m^3).

Chronic exposure has resulted in fatigue, poor memory, dizziness and irritability.

Dermal and ophthalmic exposures

Dermal exposure can lead to limited skin effects including discoloration, pain, itching, and erythema.

Ophthalmic exposure may lead irritation, photophobia, inflammation, conjunctivitis, lacrimation, keratitis, conjunctival hyperaemia, and blepharospasm. Recovery is usually complete but there may be permanent damage. A significantly higher prevalence of eye complaints has been reported in workers repeatedly exposed to H_2S hydrogen sulphide concentrations above 3.7 ppm (5 mg/m^3) compared to unexposed workers.

Management

Remove patient from exposure without the rescuers being put at risk. Treatment is supportive as there is no antidote or other specific treatment.

Ensure a clear airway and adequate ventilation. Give oxygen to symptomatic patients. All patients with abnormal vital signs, chest pain, respiratory symptoms or hypoxia should have a 12-lead ECG performed. If the patient has clinical features of bronchospasm treat conventionally with nebulized bronchodilators and steroids. Endotracheal intubation may be required for life-threatening laryngeal oedema. Apply other supportive measures as indicated by the patient's clinical condition.

Further reading

Agency for Toxic Substances and Disease Registry (ATSDR) (2006). *Toxicological Profile for Hydrogen Sulfide*. Atlanta, GA: US Department of Health and Human Services.

Baxter PJ, Aw T-C, Cockcroft A *et al.* (eds) (2010). *Hunter's Diseases of Occupations*, 10th edition. London: Hodder.

Burnett WW, King EG, Grace M, *et al.* (1977). Hydrogen sulphide poisoning: review of 5 years' experience. *CMAJ*, 117:1277–80.

Health Protection Agency (2011). *Compendium of Chemical Hazards: Hydrogen sulphide*. Didcot: CRCE. <http://www.hpa. org.uk/topics/chemicalsandpoisons/compendiumofchemical hazards/hydrogensulphide/>.

International Programme on Chemical Safety (IPCS) (2003). *Hydrogen Sulfide. Concise International Chemical Assessment Document 53*. WHO: <http:// www.hpa.org.uk/topics/chemicals andpoisons/compendiumofchemicalhazards/hydrogen sulphide/>.

Hydrocarbons

Background

The term hydrocarbons is often used synonymously with petroleum distillates. Both terms refer typically to the products of crude oil refining. Crude oil is a naturally occurring mixture of aliphatic (e.g. propane, cyclopropane, and isobutane) and aromatic (benzene-derived) hydrocarbons. Crude oil refining initially involves distillation into fractions with different boiling points. The end products may be chemical mixtures (such as petrol and kerosene) or pure single compounds such as butane and benzene.

Volatile compounds such as propane, butane, and liquefied petroleum gas (a mixture of propane, butane, and isobutane) are the fractions with the lowest boiling points with automotive fuels (petrol), white spirit, and other solvents, kerosene, diesel oil, mineral oils, greases and waxes hydrocarbon fractions with progressively higher boiling points. A schematic representation of the main fractions of crude oil separation is shown in Figure 9.6.

The toxicology of hydrocarbons is complicated by inconsistent use of terminology. For example, while strictly the term petroleum distillates refers to all chemical mixtures derived from crude oil, it is sometimes used synonymously with kerosene. The term paraffin may also be used for kerosene but chemically a paraffin is any aliphatic saturated hydrocarbon so that methane (CH_3), butane (C_2H_6), propane (C_3H_8), etc. are all paraffins. It is also important to distinguish between *naphtha* which refers to the volatile flammable hydrocarbon mixture that distils from crude oil below the volatile gases but above kerosene, and *naphthalene* that is a distinct compound formed of two benzene rings.

See separate sections for Chlorinated hydrocarbons (pp. 221–224); dinitrophenol, pentachlorophenol, phenol (Phenol and related compounds, pp. 257–259); Naphthalene and paradichlorobenzene (p. 254), toluene (Benzene and toluene, pp. 214–215); polychlorinated biphenyls (Dioxins and polychlorinated biphenyls, pp. 232–233); Xylenes (p. 264).

Toxicokinetics

Volatile hydrocarbons are rapidly absorbed via inhalation. Absorption of less volatile fractions by ingestion is related inversely to molecular weight with approximately 60% absorption for hydrocarbons containing around 14 carbon atoms, 5% for C-28 hydrocarbons, and little or no absorption for hydrocarbons with more than 32 carbon atoms. Kerosene typically contains 6–16, diesel 8–21, and paraffin waxes 20–40 carbon atoms per molecule. Skin absorption increases with increasing lipid solubility, surface area, and duration of contact. Well-hydrated skin is more permeable to hydrocarbons as is skin which has sustained a breakdown in integrity. Dermal absorption may contribute significantly to toxicity following exposure to some hydrocarbons including phenol and carbon tetrachloride.

The distribution of absorbed hydrocarbon molecules is dependent on their tissue to blood partition coefficient (the concentration ratio between blood and tissue) with accumulation in tissues that have coefficients greater than one. Toluene, for example, accumulates in body fat because its fat:blood partition coefficient is 60.

Hydrocarbons are usually metabolized in the liver to more polar compounds which are eliminated in urine or bile. Butane, for example, is metabolized to a variety of compounds including butanol, butanediol, and hydroxybutanone. The metabolites of some hydrocarbons are in themselves toxic. For example, methylene chloride is metabolized to carbon monoxide and carbon dioxide and hexane to 2,5-hexanedione which is neurotoxic.

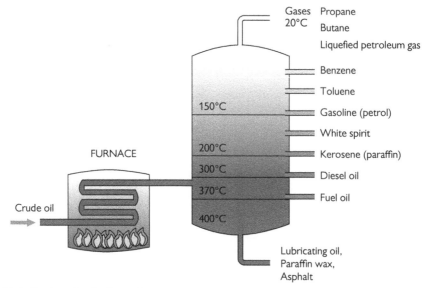

Fig 9.6 Principal fractions of crude oil separation.

Mechanisms of toxicity

The underlying mechanisms of hydrocarbon toxicity relate closely to their physical properties. Lower boiling point mixtures such as liquefied petroleum gas and petrol are of high volatility and low viscosity. They vaporize readily and pose an important inhalational hazard. They are highly lipid-soluble so are easily absorbed across cell membranes including the blood–brain barrier. The central nervous system is thus a major target organ. In addition, their low viscosity increases the likelihood of inadvertent aspiration. In contrast, higher boiling point hydrocarbon mixtures such as diesel and mineral oils are less volatile and more viscous. They do not therefore pose a risk of central nervous system toxicity and are not easily aspirated.

Clinical features

Inhalation

Inhalation of highly volatile hydrocarbons such as lique-fied petroleum gas causes narcosis and asphyxia. Deaths have occurred. Inhalation of petrol fumes may also lead to asphyxiation if exposure is to high concentrations in an enclosed space. Lower exposures cause headache, dizziness, nausea, drowsiness, incoordination, and euphoria. Confusion and disorientation may ensue. In severe cases coma, convulsions, and cardiac arrhythmias occur, the latter due to sensitization of the myocardium to catecholamines. Rare complications include pulmonary oedema and haemolytic anaemia. Sudden cardiac death is recognized. Kerosene is not usually a significant hazard by inhalation but exposure to high concentration in an enclosed space may result in dizziness, drowsiness, headache, and fatigue.

Ingestion

Nausea, vomiting, and diarrhoea may follow ingestion of kerosene. A double gastric fluid level may be visible on X-ray, the lower being the aqueous and the higher the hydrocarbon portion in the stomach. The greatest hazard, however, from kerosene ingestion is the associated risk of pulmonary aspiration causing choking, coughing, wheeze, breathlessness, and possibly cyanosis, hypoxia, fever, and leucocytosis. The chest X-ray may show shadowing in the mid or lower zones. These symptoms and signs may progress over 24–48 hours. Rarely pleural effusions or pneumatocoeles develop. After substantial kerosene ingestion, systemic uptake may result in the features typical of the narcotic effects of more volatile hydrocarbons with central nervous system depression, convulsions, and cardiac arrhythmias.

The most common scenario for petrol toxicity is accidental ingestion in the context of siphoning. Petrol is poorly absorbed from the gastrointestinal tract but there is a risk of aspiration with a similar clinical course to that seen with kerosene.

Topical exposure

Splashes or spills of petrol on the skin usually evaporate without adverse effects. In contrast, prolonged skin contact may cause a severe chemical burn and inappropriate repeated skin contact may cause a chronic dermatitis due to defatting of the skin. Kerosene is a skin irritant and causes dryness and skin cracking due to its defatting action. There may be pain, erythema, and blistering.

Injection

Injection of hydrocarbons subcutaneously or intramuscularly causes local pain and inflammation. Necrosis may ensue precipitated by the defatting action of the compound. Compartment syndrome and rhabdomyolysis may follow. Intravenous injection poses a high risk of pulmonary toxicity which presents as an acute chemical pneumonitis.

Management

Inhalation

Remove subject to fresh air and administer oxygen. Measure arterial blood gases in patients who are unconscious or have reduced oxygen saturations on pulse oximetry. Perform an ECG and cardiac monitor all symptomatic patients for at least 6 hours. Management is otherwise symptomatic and supportive with conventional management of arrhythmias and seizures.

Ingestion

Where there is a potential risk of aspiration observe in hospital for at least 6 hours even if asymptomatic at presentation. A chest X-ray at or beyond 6 hours is recommended in all these patients. It is safe to discharge patients 6 hours after ingestion of kerosene or petrol if they are asymptomatic, have no clinically abnormal signs in the chest, and a chest X-ray is normal. Treat bronchospasm with bronchodilators. There is no good evidence that prophylactic corticosteroids or antibiotics are of benefit. Corticosteroid therapy may even increase the risk of infectious complications by promoting bacterial colonization of the lungs.

Topical exposure

Decontaminate with copious lukewarm water. Do not allow smoking nearby. There may be a risk of fire. Treat symptomatically. Severe chemical burns will require specialist review. Excision and/or skin grafting may be required.

Injection

The site of soft tissue injection with a hydrocarbon requires urgent debridement, if necessary with incision and drainage. Surgical assessment is advised in all cases. Give tetanus prophylaxis. Treat complications including rhabdomyolysis conventionally. Cases of intravenous hydrocarbon injection should be managed as a chemical pneumonitis.

Further reading

Amoruso MA, Gamble JF, McKee RH, et al. (2008). Review of the toxicology of mineral spirits. Int J Toxicol, 27:97–165.

Belonwu RO, Adeleke SI (2008). A seven-year review of accidental kerosene poisoning in children at Aminu Kano Teaching Hospital, Kano. Niger J Med, 17:380–2.

Eskandarlou M, Moaddab AH (2010). Chest wall necrosis and empyema resulting from attempting suicide by injection of petroleum into the pleural cavity. Emerg Med J, 27:616–18.

Gurkan F, Bosnak M (2005). Use of nebulized budesonide in two critical patients with hydrocarbon intoxication. Am J Ther, 12:366–7.

Seymour FK, Henry JA (2001). Assessment and management of acute poisoning by petroleum products. Hum Exp Toxicol, 20:551–62.

Thalhammer GH, Eber E, Zach MS (2005). Pneumonitis and pneumatoceles following accidental hydrocarbon aspiration in children. Wien Klin Wochenschr, 117:150–3.

Vaziri ND, Smith PJ, Wilson A (1980). Toxicity with intravenous injection of naphtha in man. Clin Toxicol, 16:335–43.

WHO EMRO Pediatric Hydrocarbon Study Group, Bond GR, Pièche S, et al. (2008). A clinical decision rule for triage of children under 5 years of age with hydrocarbon (kerosene) aspiration in developing countries. Clin Toxicol, 46:222–9.

Isocyanates

Background

Isocyanates are synthetic organic chemicals that contain the isocyanate radical ($N=C=O$) as the common structural element. There are several thousand different isocyanates, but relatively few are used extensively. The most important isocyanates commercially are shown in Table 9.10. Three diisocyanates account for more than 90% of commercial use: 4,4-methylenediphenyl diisocyanate (MDI), toluene diisocyanate (TDI) which is available in two isomeric forms 2,4-TDI and 2,6-TDI, and hexamethylene diisocyanate (HDI). The most common commercial form of toluene diisocyanate is an 80:20 mixture of 2,4-TDI and 2,6-TDI, while the commercially available form of 4,4-methylenediphenyl diisocyanate contains a small amount of the 2,4 isomer in addition to the 4,4′ isomer.

Pre-polymerized oligomers of the diisocyanates, which still contain free isocyanate groups, are increasingly being used. Aliphatic isocyanates, such as hexamethylene diisocyanate (HDI), are mostly used in paints and coatings (e.g. car paints) due to the excellent resistance to abrasion and superior weathering characteristics, such as gloss and colour retention. Aromatic isocyanates, such as 4,4-methylenediphenyl diisocyanate (MDI) and toluene diisocyanates (TDI) are used as foams, adhesives, sealants, elastomers and binders. Polyurethane foams are a major end use of aromatic isocyanates. Exposure to isocyanates is also possible in tasks which involve heating of polyurethanes or polyurethane-coated products, such as welding, flame cutting, and sawing.

Methyl isocyanate is an intermediate in the synthesis of carbamate pesticides; it has also been used in the production of rubbers, adhesives. In the Bhopal incident of 1984 approximately 27 tonnes of methyl isocyanate was released at the Union Carbide pesticide plant in Bhopal, India. The mortality was between 2500–6000 and over 200,000 people were debilitated by the exposure. Studies have shown chronic illnesses such as pulmonary fibrosis, bronchial asthma, chronic obstructive pulmonary disease, emphysema, recurrent chest infections, keratopathy, and corneal opacities in exposed cohorts.

The exposure hazard, and ultimately therefore the toxicity of a particular isocyanate, is related directly to its molecular weight and volatility. Highly volatile, low-molecular-weight isocyanates, such as toluene diisocyanates and methyl isocyanate, are far more toxic than those isocyanates, such as 4,4-methylenediphenyl diisocyanate (MDI), which have to be heated to form vapours.

Table 9.10 Most important isocyanates commercially

Chemical name	Common abbreviation
Methyl isocyanate	MIC
4,4-Methylenediphenyl diisocyanate	MDI
Hexamethylene diisocyanate	HDI
Isophorone diisocyanate	IPDI
2,4-Toluene diisocyanate	TDI
2,6-Toluene diisocyanate	TDI

Toxicokinetics

Isocyanates are mainly absorbed via the respiratory tract, but absorption through the skin is also possible, notably in contact with liquid isocyanates. Isocyanates are readily metabolized to the corresponding amines, which are rapidly excreted in the urine as such, and as acetylated products.

Biological monitoring methods, based on the analysis of the amines in post-shift urine have been published for MDI and TDI.

Mechanisms of toxicity

It has been shown that the noxious effects of isocyanates are caused by activation of Ca^{2+} influx and membrane currents in sensory neurons. These responses are mediated by transient receptor potential ankyrin 1 (TRPA1), an ion channel serving as a detector for reactive chemicals.

While isocyanate asthma closely mirrors other type I immune hypersensitivity ('allergic') disorders, one important characteristic of hypersensitivity ('allergen'-specific IgE) is absent in a large portion of affected individuals. This variation from common environmental asthma (which typically is induced by high-molecular-weight allergens) is important for two reasons. First, allergen-specific IgE is an important mediator of many of the symptoms of bronchial hyper-reactivity in 'allergic asthma'. Lack of allergen specific IgE in isocyanate-hypersensitive individuals suggests differences in pathogenic mechanisms, with potentially unique targets for prevention and therapy. Secondly, allergen-specific IgE forms the basis of the most commonly used diagnostic tests for hypersensitivity (skin prick and RAST).

Clinical features

Inhalation

Inhaled diisocyanates have been reported to cause four different respiratory reactions:

- Toxic bronchitis and asthma caused by inhalation of an isocyanate in very high concentrations. Exposure to TDI in an atmospheric concentration of 0.5 ppm causes irritation of the mucosal surfaces in the eyes, nose and throat. Persistent asthma and airway hyper-responsiveness following a single inhalation of TDI in toxic concentrations has also been reported.
- Bronchial asthma caused by sensitization to diisocyanates.
- Accelerated decline of forced expiratory volume in 1 second (FEV_1). The rate of decline of FEV_1 in an isocyanate manufacturing plant workforce was similar in non-smokers with high cumulative exposures to TDI to the rate observed in smokers in both the high- and low-exposure groups. The rate in non-smokers with low cumulative exposure was not different from that expected for non-smokers. No additive effect of TDI with smoking was observed.
- Extrinsic allergic alveolitis, which has been reported particularly in workers exposed to MDI but also to HDI.

Inhalation of isocyanates has a primary irritant effect on all parts of the respiratory tract, with burning and irritation of the nose and throat, laryngitis, cough, which may be paroxysmal and may or may not produce sputum, breathlessness, chest pain, and severe bronchospasm. In severe cases, pulmonary oedema may ensue, usually after an interval of 12–48 hours.

Neurological symptoms including dizziness, headache, insomnia, euphoria, anxiety, difficulty in concentration, poor memory, confusion, cerebellar ataxia, and unconsciousness have been reported after acute inhalation of toluene diisocyanate vapour. Poor memory, personality change, irritability, or depression may persist for several years.

Nausea, vomiting, and abdominal pain may also occur after isocyanate vapour inhalation.

Forty workers at a glove manufacturing plant in Sri Lanka were exposed to TDI-contaminated latex and developed headache, nausea, vomiting, abdominal pain, a burning sensation of the eyes, conjunctival irritation, photophobia, corneal ulceration, cough, wheeze, breathlessness, reduced peak flow, and 'inflammation of the skin'. Euphoria, anxiety, cerebellar ataxia, memory loss, muscle pain and elevated creatine kinase activity were also observed.

Thirty-five firemen were involved in a fire in a factory in Somerset, UK, in which polyurethane foam was made. There were exposed to the fumes of toluene di-isocyanate from two large storage tanks which were damaged during the fire, resulting in massive spillage. Thirty-one of the 35 men who were seen after the fire developed tightness in the chest, dyspnoea, or cough; 16 men complained of nausea, vomiting, or abdominal pain. These symptoms were present either at the time of the fire or during the next day. Twenty-three men complained of neurological symptoms after a single severe exposure to toluene diisocyanate. Effects of exposure were immediate in five men and consisted of euphoria, ataxia, and loss of consciousness. These men and nine others complained of headache, difficulty in concentration, poor memory, and confusion during the next 3 weeks. Four years later it was found that nine further men had experienced symptoms that they had not been aware of at 3 weeks. In all, 13 men still complained of poor memory, personality change, irritability, or depression after 4 years. Psychometric testing showed a selective defect for relatively long-term recall in those with persistent symptoms at 4 years.

Dermal exposure
Liquid isocyanates produce a marked transient inflammatory reaction with redness, irritation, and dermatitis.

Ocular exposure
Transient smarting, burning, or prickling sensation and lacrimation may occur after exposure to low isocyanate concentrations, especially following chronic exposure. Severe lacrimation, blepharospasm, conjunctivitis, keratitis, corneal oedema, and photophobia, have been observed after exposure to high vapour concentrations.

Ingestion
No human data have been published but nausea, vomiting and abdominal pain are likely. It is also possible that some of the systemic features observed after inhalation could also be observed after ingestion.

Carcinogenicity
The National Toxicology Program has concluded that toluene diisocyanates are reasonably anticipated to be human carcinogens based on sufficient evidence of carcinogenicity from studies in experimental animals.

Management

Inhalation
Treatment is symptomatic and supportive after removal from exposure.

If the patient has clinical features of bronchospasm treat conventionally with nebulized bronchodilators and steroids. Give oxygen, as required. Monitor arterial blood gases and perform a chest X-ray if symptomatic.

Treat pulmonary oedema and/or acute lung injury with CPAP or in severe cases with IPPV and PEEP.

Observe until at least 8 hours after exposure. Patients who have not developed respiratory features by this time may be discharged with advice to return if features develop because there is a small risk of delayed asthmatic symptoms.

Dermal exposure
The patient's skin should be washed with soap and water under low pressure for at least 10–15 minutes. Particular attention should be paid to mucous membranes, moist areas such as skin folds, fingernails, and ears.

Ocular exposure
If symptomatic, immediately irrigate the affected eye thoroughly with water or 0.9% saline for at least 10–15 minutes. If symptoms persist check for corneal damage by instillation of fluorescein and refer for ophthalmological assessment if necessary.

Ingestion
Gastric decontamination should not be attempted. Treatment is symptomatic and supportive.

Further reading

Andersson N, Ajwani MK, Mahashabde S, et al. (1990). Delayed eye and other consequences from exposure to methyl isocyanate: 93% follow up of exposed and unexposed cohorts in Bhopal. *Br J Ind Med*, 47:553–8.

Axford AT, McKerrow CB, Parry Jones A, et al. (1976). Accidental exposure to isocyanate fumes in a group of firemen. *Br J Indus Med*, 33:65–71.

Bessac BF, Sivula M, von Hehn CA, et al. (2009). Transient receptor potential ankyrin 1 antagonists block the noxious effects of toxic industrial isocyanates and tear gases. *FASEB J*, 23:1102–14.

Dhara VR, Dhara R (2002). The Union Carbide disaster in Bhopal: A review of health effects. *Arch Env Health*, 57:391–404.

Hannu T, Estlander T Jolanki R (2005). Allergic contact dermatitis due to MDI and MDA from accidental occupational exposure. *Contact Dermatitis*, 52:108–9.

Le Quesne PM, Axford AT, McKerrow CB, et al. (1976). Neurological complications after a single severe exposure to toluene di-isocyanate. *Br J Indus Med*, 33:72–8.

Moscato G, Dellabianca A, Vinci G, et al. (1991). Toluene diisocyanate-induced asthma: clinical findings and bronchial responsiveness studies in 113 exposed subjects with work-related respiratory symptoms. *J Occup Med*, 33:720–5.

National Toxicology Program (2011). *Report on Carcinogens. Toluene Diisocyanates*. Durham, NC: US Department of Health and Human Services.

Nielsen J, Sango C, Winroth G, et al. (1995). Systemic reactions associated with polyisocyanate exposure. *Scand J Work Environ Health*, 11:51–4.

Siribaddana SH, Wijesundera A, Fernando R (1998). Toluene diisocyanate exposure in a glove manufacturing plant. *Clin Toxicol*, 36:95–8.

Wisnewski AV Jones M (2010). ProCon debate: is occupational asthma induced by isocyanates an immunoglobulin E-mediated disease? *Clin Exp Allergy*, 40:1155–62.

Naphthalene and paradichlorobenzene

Background

Naphthalene is used widely in industry as a chemical intermediate. It was used as a constituent of mothballs and as a soil fumigant, but these uses were discontinued due to concerns regarding naphthalene toxicity. Paradichlorobenzene is now the active ingredient in mothballs.

Toxicokinetics

Naphthalene is fat-soluble and absorbed effectively following ingestion, inhalation of vapour, and skin contact. Dermal absorption is enhanced with the use of baby oil. Poisoning has occurred from wearing nappies and clothes that have been stored with naphthalene mothballs.

Paradichlorobenzene can also be absorbed systemically by all routes of exposure though dermal absorption is slow. Both chemicals are metabolized to epoxides by the liver and then by phase II metabolism to conjugates which are eliminated via the kidneys.

Mechanisms of toxicity

The epoxide metabolite of naphthalene causes intravascular haemolysis, via oxidative damage to red blood cells. Haemolysis has also been described following paradichlorobenzene ingestion. The mechanism of CNS toxicity has not been elucidated but is likely to involve oxidative stress.

Clinical features—acute poisoning

Ingestion

Naphthalene ingestion causes nausea, vomiting, abdominal pain, diarrhoea, headache, confusion, sweating, fever, tachycardia, tachypnoea, and agitation. Coma and convulsions ensue in severe cases. Haemolysis and haemoglobinuria leading to acute kidney injury may occur after 3–5 days, particularly in patients with glucose-6-phosphate dehydrogenase (G6PD) deficiency who are more susceptible to haemolytic oxidative stress. Fatalities have occurred. The urine may be dark brown or black in colour, due to haemoglobinuria and the presence of naphthalene metabolites. Methaemoglobinaemia occurs rarely.

Acute haemolytic anaemia has also been reported following ingestion of mothballs containing paradichlorobenzene.

Dermal exposure

Both chemicals are irritating to the skin and prolonged contact, particularly with concomitant use of baby oil, has led to systemic features.

Eye exposure

Irritation and possible injury from particles in the eye.

Clinical features—chronic poisoning

Ingestion

Chronic ingestion of paradichlorobenzene containing mothballs has caused cerebellar toxicity and dementia.

Inhalation

Inhalational naphthalene abuse has caused behavioural changes, nausea, vomiting, and hepatic failure. Peripheral neuropathy and chronic renal failure have also been reported.

Accidental inhalation of naphthalene by a 15-year-old pregnant girl caused haemolytic anaemia and methaemoglobinaemia. She gave birth to a child with the same features. The newborn infant recovered after mechanical ventilation and exchange transfusion.

An 18-year-old woman who had inhaled mothball fumes for 10 minutes daily for 6 months and chewed on half a mothball daily for 2 months, presented with an icthyosis-like rash, cerebellar ataxia, and signs of intracranial hypertension. Her sister, who had inhaled but not ingested the same mothballs, had similar though less marked features. Symptoms resolved in both cases in the months following removal from exposure.

Eye exposure

Chronic exposure to vapour has caused corneal damage and opacities.

Management

Ingestion

Since there is in vitro evidence that charcoal adsorbs naphthalene, it is reasonable to administer oral activated charcoal (50 g in an adult), to any patient presenting within 1 hour of mothball ingestion. Observe asymptomatic patients for at least 4 hours. Management is otherwise supportive.

Extracorporeal renal support may be required in patients who develop renal failure. Treat methaemoglobinaemia with intravenous methylthioninium chloride (methylene blue) 1–2 mg/kg. In patients with severe G6PD deficiency methylthioninium chloride may not be effective in treating methaemoglobinaemia and can induce haemolytic anaemia. Exchange transfusion is the treatment of choice in these cases.

Antioxidant therapy with oral ascorbic acid and acetylcysteine have been used on the basis that oxidative stress is the primary mechanism of toxicity but there is insufficient evidence to advocate these treatments.

Further reading

Feuillet L, Mallet S, Spadari M (2006). Twin girls with neurocutaneous symptoms caused by mothball intoxication. N Engl J Med, 355:423–4.

Fradin Z, Stein GY, Varon M, et al. (2005). A Naphthalene induced fatal haemolysis in G6PD deficiency. HAEMA, 8: 286–288.

Kong JT, Schmiesing C (2005). Concealed mothball abuse prior to anesthesia: mothballs, inhalants, and their management. Acta Anaesthesiol Scand, 49:113–16.

Kumar N, Dale LC, Wijdicks EF (2009). Mothball mayhem: relapsing toxic leukoencephalopathy due to p-dichlorobenzene neurotoxicity. Ann Intern Med, 150:362–3.

Kurz JM (1987). Naphthelene poisoning: critical care nursing techniques. Dimens Crit Care Nurs, 6:264–70.

Lim H C, Poulose V, Tan HH (2009). Acute naphthalene poisoning following the non-accidental ingestion of mothballs. Singapore Med J, 50: 298-301.

Molloy EJ, Doctor BA, Reed MD, et al. (2004). Perinatal toxicity of domestic naphthalene exposure. J Perinatol, 24:792–3.

Pysher T, Olson A, Drederick D, et al. (1984). Fatal hepatopathy due to chronic inhalation of naphthalene. Lab Invest, 50:10.

Santucci K, Shah B (2000). Association of naphthalene with acute hemolytic anemia. Acad Emerg Med, 7:42–7.

Todisco V, Lamour J, Finberg L (1991). Hemolysis from exposure to naphthalene mothballs. N Engl J Med, 325: 1660–1.

Weintraub E, Gandhi D, Robinson C (2000). Medical complications due to mothball abuse. South Med J, 93:427–9.

Nitrogen and nitrogen oxides, and smoke inhalation

Nitrogen and nitrogen oxides

Background
Nitrogen is a colourless, odourless gas. The oxides of nitrogen are listed in Box 9.1. Nitric oxide (NO) and nitrogen dioxide (NO_2) occur naturally. In ambient air, NO is oxidized to NO_2. NO_2 exists principally as nitrogen tetroxide (N_2O_4); at higher ambient temperatures, more NO_2 than N_2O_4 is present. Combustion of fossil fuels yields NO and NO_2 (a largely insoluble, brown, mildly irritating gas). Fermentation of silage produces high concentrations of NO_2 within 2 days of filling the silo. It is also a by-product of many industrial processes.

Mechanisms of toxicity
NO_2 is the most toxic nitrogen oxide. It is a strong oxidant and thus reacts with various biomolecules, directly or via the formation of free radicals, inducing pulmonary damage. NO_2 has a low solubility in water. As a result little dissolves in the upper airway mucus, so that the lower respiratory tract is exposed to relatively high concentrations.

Clinical features
Nitrogen is a colourless, odourless gas. It causes hypoxic asphyxia by displacing oxygen.

The features following acute exposure to high concentrations of NO_2 depend on the concentration and duration of exposure to the gas. Since NO_2 is only a mild upper respiratory tract irritant, modest acute exposure (<50 ppm; <100 mg/m^3) for a short time often produces no immediate symptoms, although throat irritation, cough, transient choking, tightness in the chest, and sweating have been observed.

Exposure for longer than 1 hour to greater than 50 ppm (>100 mg/m^3) can induce pulmonary oedema. Even very brief exposure to more than 250 ppm (500 mg/m^3) may cause life-threatening pulmonary damage. Three American astronauts who were exposed to about 250 ppm of NO_2 for 4–5 min owing to the inadvertent firing of the reaction control system in the Apollo-Soyuz spacecraft had radiological evidence of pulmonary oedema the day after splashdown.

Exposure to massive concentrations of NO_2, such as that found in a silo, can produce severe acute lung injury, which may be fatal. The clinical findings are dyspnoea, tachypnoea, hypoxaemia, decreased lung compliance, and diffuse pulmonary infiltrates on chest radiography.

In less severe cases, the onset of symptoms may be delayed for a few hours (typically 3–36 hours) and the patient then develops dyspnoea, chest pain (which may be pleuritic), haemoptysis, tachycardia, headache,

conjunctivitis, generalized weakness, and dizziness (which may be due to hypotension).

Emission of substantial amounts of NO_2 from malfunctioning ice resurfacing machines in closed arenas have led to several outbreaks of acute respiratory illness among players, cheerleaders, and spectators. In one incident, at least 116 individuals were affected. Cough, haemoptysis, chest pain, headache, and dyspnoea were the predominant features experienced during and within 48 hours of attending an ice hockey game. In many subjects the cough persisted for more than 2 weeks, although simple respiratory function tests revealed no persistent deficit in lung function. Bronchiolitis obliterans may develop within 2–6 weeks of NO_2 exposure.

Dermal and ophthalmic exposures
Spillage of liquid nitrogen on the eyes or skin causes extreme cooling, leading to cold burns.

Environmental exposures
Large meta-analyses of studies on the short-term health effects of NO_2 have been carried out. These results indicate a positive association between daily increases of NO_2 and natural, cardiovascular, and respiratory mortality. The findings are consistent with an independent effect of NO_2, which may be a more relevant health-based exposure indicator than particulate matter.

Management
Patients must be admitted for observation. If arterial blood gases and chest radiography remain normal in the first 12 hours, patients can be discharged and followed up as outpatients. If a patient experiences increasing dyspnoea after discharge, they should be readmitted immediately.

In severe cases, supplemental oxygen and bronchodilators should be administered but in many cases mechanical ventilation with PEEP offers the best hope of reducing the mortality. There is no clinical evidence that prophylactic administration of antibiotics or free radical scavengers reduces the clinical effects or improves survival. Administration of corticosteroids does not reduce mortality and may increase morbidity.

Smoke

Background
Smoke consists of a suspension of small particles in hot air and gases which are generated by thermal decomposition and combustion. It has particulate and gaseous phases. The particles consist of carbon and they are coated with combustion products such as organic acids and aldehydes. The gaseous phase of smoke has an extremely variable composition, depending on the materials involved in the fire. Carbon dioxide and carbon monoxide (see Carbon monoxide, pp. 219–220) are always present and usually constitute the bulk of this fraction. Other toxic gases commonly contained in the gaseous phase, though not necessarily in high concentration, include acrolein, ammonia, chlorine, hydrogen bromide, hydrogen chloride, hydrogen cyanide, oxides of nitrogen, phosgene, phosphorus pentoxide, and sulphur dioxide. Several of these are discussed elsewhere in this chapter.

Thermal decomposition of polyurethane foams and synthetic polymers containing acrylonitrile produces

---

Box 9.1 Nitrogen oxides

Nitrous oxide: N_2O
Nitric oxide, nitrogen monoxide: NO
Nitrogen dioxide: NO_2
Nitrogen trioxide: NO_3
Nitrogen tetroxide: N_2O_4 (dimer of NO_2)
Dinitrogen trioxide: N_2O_3
Dinitrogen pentoxide: N_2O_5
NOx: a collective name for NO, NO_2 and N_2O_4

substantial quantities of free hydrogen cyanide gas and other organic cyanides. Characteristics of fires involving plastics are extremely high temperatures (plastic possesses a heat of combustion 2.5 times that of other combustible materials), very high burning rates, and high-density smoke.

Polyvinyl chloride (PVC) produces smoke 4–14 times more dense than that from fires involving constructional timber under similar conditions. On complete combustion each kilogram of PVC can produce about 0.4 kg of hydrogen chloride gas. Other important products of PVC combustion include carbon monoxide, chlorine, and phosgene, together with benzene, naphthalene, toluene, xylenes (see specific sections in this chapter) and vinyl chloride.

Mechanisms of toxicity

The adverse effects of smoke result not only from its chemical composition but also from the fact that the particulate and gaseous fractions are space-occupying and they can rapidly fill an enclosed space at the expense of air. The duration of exposure and the occurrence of that exposure in a confined space are two factors that determine the severity of the pulmonary consequences of smoke inhalation. Thermal injury to the lungs does not play a significant role since, under usual circumstances, heat does not enter the trachea because of the rapid cooling that occurs in the larynx.

Clinical features

The main effects are asphyxia and severe pulmonary irritation and oedema. The release of carbon monoxide, hydrogen cyanide and carbon dioxide in an enclosed space may result in death from asphyxia.

Smaller particles, acids and aldehydes cause lacrimation, burning of the throat, and nausea and vomiting when swallowed. Highly water-soluble gases (e.g. hydrogen chloride, sulphur dioxide) cause immediate irritation to the upper respiratory tract, whereas gases with low solubility (e.g. chlorine, nitrogen dioxide, phosgene) penetrate further into the lung and cause injury to the distal airways and alveoli.

Thus, features range from mild irritation of the eyes and upper airways to severe tracheobronchitis, bronchospasm, pulmonary oedema, and bronchopneumonia, which may result in pulmonary insufficiency and death.

Laryngitis and laryngeal oedema can also occur and may progress to complete laryngeal obstruction over a period of several hours. Acute hypoxaemia may be associated with the occurrence of frequent ventricular premature beats. Tissue hypoxia due to an elevated carboxyhaemoglobin concentration may lead to chest pain and cardiac arrhythmias in subjects with pre-existing ischaemic heart disease.

There is some evidence that smoke inhalation may lead to prolonged airway hyper-responsiveness and asthma.

Management

- After removal of the casualty from further exposure to smoke, resuscitation should be undertaken, if necessary. Supplemental humidified oxygen should be administered, together with a nebulized bronchodilator such as salbutamol, as necessary.
- A carboxyhaemoglobin concentration should be obtained (see Carbon monoxide, pp. 219–220, if raised) and arterial blood gases should be measured; in severe case serial blood gas analyses may need to

be undertaken for at least 48 hours after admission to hospital.

- If there is any likelihood of exposure to burning plastics, the possibility of cyanide poisoning should be considered and, if present, treated with an antidote (see Cyanide, pp. 229–231).
- Early fibre optic laryngoscopy or bronchoscopy may assist the diagnosis and enable the severity of any sub-glottal injury to be determined. There is no incontrovertible evidence that the early administration of high-dose corticosteroids protects against pulmonary injury.

Further reading

Alarie Y (1985). The toxicity of smoke from polymeric materials during thermal decomposition. *Ann Rev Pharmacol Toxicol*, 25:325–47.

Altomare A, Kirkland K, McLellan R, et al. (2012). Exposure to nitrogen dioxide in an indoor ice arena – New Hampshire, 2011. *MMWR Morb Mortal Wkly Rep*, 61:139–42.

Anon (1990). Ice hockey lung: NO2 poisoning. *Lancet*, 335:1191.

Baud FJ, Barriot P, Toffis V, et al. (1991). Elevated blood cyanide concentrations in victims of smoke inhalation. *N Engl J Med*, 325:1761–6.

Berglund M, Bostroem CE, Bylin G, et al. (1993). Health risk evaluation of nitrogen oxides. *Scand J Work Environ Health*, 19(Suppl. 2):1–72.

Chiusolo M, Cadum E, Stafoggia M, et al. (2011). Short term effects of nitrogen dioxide on mortality and susceptibility factors in ten Italian cities: the EpiAir Study. *Environ Health Perspect*, 119:1233–8.

Clark WR (1992). Smoke inhalation: diagnosis and treatment. *World J Surg*, 16:24–9.

De Lange DW Meulenbelt J (2011). Do corticosteroids have a role in preventing or reducing acute toxic lung injury caused by inhalation of chemical agents? *Clin Toxicol*, 49:61–71.

Demling RH (1993). Smoke inhalation injury. *New Horizons*, 1:422–35.

Haponik EF (1993). Clinical smoke inhalation: pulmonary effects. *Occup Med*, 8:430–68.

Hedberg K, Hedberg CW, Iber C, et al. (1989). An outbreak of nitrogen dioxide-induced respiratory illness among ice hockey players. *JAMA*, 262:3014–17.

Karlson-Stiber C, Hojer J, Sjoholm A, et al. (1996). Nitrogen dioxide pneumonitis in ice hockey players. *J Int Med*, 239:451–6.

Kinsella J, Carter R, Reid WH, et al. (1991). Increased airways reactivity after smoke inhalation. *Lancet*, 337:595–7.

Lee-Chiong TL, Jr (1999). Smoke inhalation injury. When to suspect and how to treat. *Postgrad Med*, 105:55–62.

Liu D, Tager IB, Balmes JR, et al. (1992). The effect of smoke inhalation on lung function and airway responsiveness in wildland fire fighters. *Am Rev Respir Dis*, 146:1469–73.

Lowry T, Schuman LM (1956). Silo-filler's disease – a syndrome caused by nitrogen dioxide. *J Am Med Assoc*, 162:153–60.

Moisan TC (1991). Prolonged asthma after smoke inhalation: A report of three cases and a review of previous reports. *J Occup Med*, 33:458–61.

Muller B (1969). Nitrogen dioxide intoxication after mining accident. *Respiration*, 26:249–61.

Orzel RA (1993). Toxicological aspects of firesmoke: polymer pyrolysis and combustion. *Occup Med*, 8:414–29.

Ruddy (1994). Smoke inhalation injury. *Pediatr Clin North Am*, 41:317–36.

Shusterman D, Alexeeff G, Hargis C, et al. (1996). Predictors of carbon monoxide and hydrogen cyanide exposure in smoke inhalation patients. *J Toxicol Clin Toxicol*, 34:61–71.

Shusterman DJ (1993). Clinical smoke inhalation: systemic effects. *Occup Med*, 8:469–503.

Phenol and related compounds

Phenol

Background
The chemical formula of phenol ('carbolic acid') is shown in Figure 9.7. At room temperature it exists as white crystals that turn pink or red on exposure to air. They have a characteristic pungent odour. Phenol is used in the manufacture of resins and in the chemical and pharmaceutical industry for its germicidal properties and as an indicator dye. It is a component of explosives, paints, rubber, textiles, adhesives, soap, and wood preservatives. Exposure may occur not only directly in its production and use but also indirectly, for example, in residential wood burning and from cigarette smoke.

Toxicokinetics
Phenol is highly lipid-soluble and absorbed rapidly by all routes of exposure. Phenol vapour can readily penetrate the skin. It distributes widely. Most absorbed phenol is conjugated in the liver, lung, and gastrointestinal tract mucosa with glucuronic acid and sulfate and eliminated via the kidneys.

Mechanisms of toxicity
Phenol binds covalently to tissue and plasma proteins and denatures them.

Clinical features—acute exposure
Since phenol is so well absorbed systemic toxicity may occur following exposure by any route though the initial presentation and severity of systemic features will vary.

Ingestion
Following ingestion systemic toxicity will typically be preceded by nausea, vomiting, and abdominal pain. Depending on the concentration of the solution corrosive injury may result in bleeding, perforation, and subsequent stricture formation.

Dermal exposure
If phenol is spilt on the skin, pain is followed promptly by numbness as phenol destroys afferent nerve endings. The skin becomes blanched, and a dry opaque eschar forms over the burn. When the eschar sloughs off, a brown stain remains. The severity of skin damage will depend on the concentration of the solution. Even dilute phenol solutions (1–2%) may cause severe burns if contact is prolonged. A worker who accidentally fell into a shallow vat of 40% phenol for a few seconds suffered 50% burns and developed acute tubular necrosis and respiratory distress but survived.

Eye exposure
Eye contact with concentrated phenol solutions causes corrosive damage.

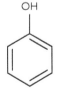

OH

Fig 9.7 Phenol.

Inhalation
The low volatility of phenol limits its hazard by inhalation. However, airborne exposure has caused respiratory tract irritation and in severe cases non-cardiogenic pulmonary oedema.

Systemic toxicity
Initial signs of systemic toxicity include sweating, headache, tinnitus, and dizziness. An initial rise in blood pressure is followed by hypotension precipitated by phenol-induced loss of vasoconstrictor tone. Loss of consciousness, respiratory depression, coma, seizures, and shock may ensue. Fatalities have occurred.

Phenol poisoning is associated with grey or black urine, and though this is due in part to metabolites of phenol, Heinz body haemolytic anaemia, methaemoglobinaemia, and hyperbilirubinaemia contribute.

Clinical features—chronic exposure
Repeated occupational exposure by inhalation has been associated with anorexia, weight loss, weakness, myalgia, impairment of renal and hepatic function, and patches of dark skin pigmentation (ochronosis).

The IARC has determined that there is inadequate evidence for the carcinogenicity of phenol and deemed it 'not classifiable' in this regard.

Management

Ingestion
Fluid resuscitation and prompt assessment of the extent of corrosive damage is crucial following ingestion. Management is otherwise supportive. Follow-up may be required to assess for the development of stricture formation.

Topical exposure
Rapid thorough decontamination is the priority in cases of skin and eye exposure. Expert burns management advice should be sought early.

Inhalation
Management is supportive.

Pentachlorophenol

Background
Pentachlorophenol is a lipid-soluble chlorinated aromatic compound that is stable and persistent in the environment and, partly for that reason, its use has now been discontinued in many countries. The single most important role for pentachlorophenol was as a wood preservative but it was also used as an herbicide, insecticide, and molluscicide and was incorporated into an extensive array of other commodities such as ropes, canvas, brick walls, paints, adhesives, and insulating material.

Toxicokinetics
Pentachlorophenol is metabolized mainly in the liver. The first stage involves dechlorination to produce tetrachlorohydroquinone which is excreted as glucuronide and sulfate conjugates. Further oxidation results in the production of 1,4-benzoquinone and semiquinones. Pentachlorophenol is eliminated only very slowly.

Mechanisms of toxicity
Uncoupling of oxidative phosphorylation is probably the principal mechanism. Pentachlorophenol binds to

mitochondria and their proteins and induces structural changes in mitochondria compatible with such uncoupling. Pentachlorophenol may also attack cell membranes by binding to the hydrophobic interior of the bilayer and altering permeability to hydrogen ions. In *in vitro* studies micromolar concentrations of pentachlorophenol induced the classical p53 apoptotic pathway and up-regulated genes related to the detoxification of reactive oxygen species and glutathione metabolism.

Following long-term exposure pentachlorophenol competes with thyroxine for binding sites on serum proteins and therefore has anti-thyroid actions. In addition, pentachlorophenol suppresses antibody production.

Clinical features

Pentachlorophenol may be absorbed by inhalation, by the dermal and oral routes and topical injury may occur to the eye and skin.

The features of systemic pentachlorophenol poisoning include a feeling of being very hot, lethargy, weakness, apprehension, delirium, intense sweating, tachypnoea without cyanosis, tachycardia, and hyperthermia. A rectal temperature of 42.8° C was recorded in one man shortly before he died. Nausea, vomiting, abdominal pain, and intense thirst have also been reported. Less common complications include limb pains, metabolic acidosis, hyperglycaemia, pancreatitis, hepatomegaly, jaundice, and acute kidney injury. Intravascular haemolysis has also been reported and *in vitro* studies have shown that it can be abolished by albumin which may explain why it is a rare complication.

Terminal 'spasms', muscle twitching, jerking limbs, and convulsions have been described and death may follow within a few hours of the onset of symptoms. Marked rigor mortis is a feature and its onset may be so immediate that resuscitation is impeded. Pulmonary oedema, cerebral oedema and fatty change in the liver and kidneys have been found in fatal cases.

Methaemoglobinaemia (10%) was found in a single infant poisoned with pentachlorophenol, but there was concomitant exposure to trichlorocarbanilide, a known methaemoglobin inducer.

Management

There is no antidote to poisoning with pentachlorophenol and supportive measures, particularly those aimed at reduction of hyperthermia, are of paramount importance. Decontamination appropriate to the route of exposure should be carried out.

Aggressive fluid resuscitation should be initiated, using cooled fluids in those with hyperthermia. Seizures and severe agitation should be controlled with a benzodiazepine, such as intravenous diazepam 10 mg (child 300–400 micrograms/kg) or lorazepam 4 mg (child 100 micrograms/kg). If benzodiazepines do not control agitation or seizures, then paralysis, intubation, and ventilation should be considered. External cooling measures with ice or cooling blankets should be initiated to control hyperthermia; if these measures fail dantrolene 1 mg/kg intravenously should be administered. If fluid therapy fails to maintain the blood pressure an inotropic sympathomimetic should be given, such as dobutamine 2.5–10 micrograms/kg/minute (child 2–20 micrograms/kg/minute) or dopamine 2–5 micrograms/kg/minute (child 3–20 micrograms/kg/minute).

As the metabolism of pentachlorophenol is extensive and the fraction excreted unchanged so small, enhancing its elimination by forced diuresis is unlikely to contribute significantly to recovery. Pentachlorophenol is highly protein-bound (up to 96%) and haemodialysis is therefore unlikely to be of any benefit.

Dinitrophenol

Background

Dinitrophenol (2,4-dinitrophenol) was used in the manufacture of munitions during World War I (it is a precursor for 2,4,6-trinitrotoluene, TNT). Since then, it has also been used as a dye, wood preservative, herbicide, and photographic developer. It was discovered that the human consumption of dinitrophenol led to significant weight loss and it was popularized as a weight loss drug via the Internet.

Toxicokinetics

Nitro reduction is the major metabolic pathway for dinitrophenol elimination and 2-amino-4-nitrophenol is the major mono-reduced metabolite. Approximately eight times more of this metabolite is formed than 4-amino-2-nitrophenol, the other main metabolite, which together account for 50% of dinitrophenol elimination. Both monoamines have elimination half-lives considerably longer than their parent, though 2-amino-4-nitrophenol has an apparent half-life almost twice as long as 4-amino-2-nitrophenol. At least in mice a significant amount of 4-amino-2-nitrophenol, an identified mutagen, appears in plasma.

Mechanisms of toxicity

Dinitrophenol causes uncoupling of oxidative phosphorylation and stimulates glycolysis; the latter increases carbohydrate consumption markedly which allows for rapid weight loss. The discrepancy between the stimulation of glycolysis and the inhibition of oxidative phosphorylation results in a rapid rise in the production of pyruvic acid, leading to an increased production of lactic acid. Potassium accumulates as the concentration of dinitrophenol increases and this process continues even after cellular respiration is inhibited; hyperkalaemia has contributed to toxicity.

Clinical features

The oral route is the most common route of exposure, though the dermal route is the most common route of unintentional exposure and may lead to systemic features. Systemic features may also occur if contaminated air is breathed at dinitrophenol-containing waste sites or from incineration fumes.

The average time to presentation in the reported cases of intentional dinitrophenol poisoning was 7–8 hours, with the onset of symptoms reported as early as 3 hours after exposure; the average time to death was 14 hours. To date, there have been 62 deaths attributed to dinitrophenol poisoning.

Early features following ingestion include nausea, vomiting, abdominal pain, and possibly diarrhoea.

The usual presenting complaint of the patient is that of profuse sweating which may be stained yellow. The initial fever is not associated with a change in heart rate or blood pressure. The classic systemic features observed are a combination of hyperthermia, sinus tachycardia, diaphoresis and tachypnoea. Agitation, restlessness, abnormal behaviour, headache, fatigue, thirst, hyperpyrexia, and dehydration are common. Hypertension, and dysrhythmias may occur. Metabolic (lactic) acidosis may complicate. In severe cases pulmonary oedema, cyanosis, shock, confusion, convulsions, cardiovascular collapse, and pulseless electrical activity are observed. Rhabdomyolysis, hyperkalaemia and acute kidney injury can develop 12–72 hours post exposure. Hepatic injury with jaundice has also been reported.

Preceding death, the patient is often profoundly hyperthermic, suffering from massive cardiovascular collapse and there may be associated methaemoglobinaemia. There have been frequent reports of a rapid (within minutes) onset of generalized rigidity after death, which has been attributed to the release of calcium from the cytosol due to the depletion of ATP.

The lowest published lethal ingested dose is 4.3 mg/kg; the highest reported dose associated with survival was a woman who took 2.4 g with no complications.

Dermal and eye exposures

Dermal exposure can cause yellow staining of the skin and mild corrosive effects.

Ophthalmic exposure may cause yellow discoloration of the sclera with conjunctival injection and irritation.

Management

Patients exposed to dinitrophenol particularly by ingestion should be observed for at least 12 hours, as no patient has been reported to be asymptomatic beyond 10 hours after acute poisoning. During this time, their body temperature, cardiac rhythm, heart rate, and oxygen saturation should be monitored carefully.

Aggressive fluid resuscitation should be initiated, using cooled fluids in those with hyperthermia. Seizures and severe agitation should be controlled with a benzodiazepine, such as intravenous diazepam 10 mg (child 300–400 micrograms/kg) or lorazepam 4 mg (child 100 micrograms/kg). If benzodiazepines do not control agitation or seizures, then paralysis, intubation, and ventilation should be considered. External cooling measures with ice or cooling blankets should be initiated to control hyperthermia; if these measures fail dantrolene 1 mg/kg intravenously should be administered. If fluid therapy fails to maintain the blood pressure an inotropic sympathomimetic should be given, such as dobutamine 2.5–10 micrograms/kg/minute (child 2–20 micrograms/kg/minute) or dopamine 2–5 micrograms/kg/minute (child 3–20 micrograms/kg/minute). Cardiopulmonary resuscitation was performed in some cases for up to an hour, but has never led to a return of spontaneous circulation. Methaemoglobinaemia concentrations should be measured and if the concentration exceeds 30% should be treated with intravenous methylthioninium chloride (methylene blue) 1–2 mg/kg.

Further reading

Armstrong RW, Eichner ER, Klein DE, et al. (1969). Pentachlorophenol poisoning in a nursery for newborn infants. II. Epidemiologic and toxicologic studies. *J Paediatr*, 75:317–25.

Bartlett J, Brunner M, Gough K (2010). Deliberate poisoning with dinitrophenol (DNP): an unlicensed weight loss pill. *Emerg Med J*, 27:159–60.

Bentur Y, Shoshani O, Tabak A, et al. (1998). Prolonged elimination half-life of phenol after dermal exposure. *J Toxicol Clin Toxicol*, 36:707–11.

Cheng WN, Coenraads PJ, Hao ZH, et al. (1993). A health survey of workers in the pentachlorophenol section of a chemical manufacturing plant. *Am J Ind Med*, 24:81

Foxall PJ, Bending MR, Gartland KP (1989). Acute renal failure following accidental cutaneous absorption of phenol: application of NMR urinalysis to monitor the disease process. *Hum Toxicol*, 8:491–6.

Grundlingh J, Dargan P, El-Zanfaly M, et al. (2011). 2,4-dinitrophenol (DNP): a weight loss agent with significant acute toxicity and risk of death. *J Med Toxicol*, 7:205–12.

Gupta S, Ashrith G, Chandra D, et al. (2008). Acute phenol poisoning: a life-threatening hazard of chronic pain relief. *Clin Toxicol*, 46:250–3.

Horch R, Spilker G, Stark GB (1994). Phenol burns and intoxications. *Burns*, 20:45–50.

Hryhorczuk DO, Wallace WH, Persky V, et al. (1998). A morbidity study of former pentachlorophenol-production workers. *Environ Health Perspect*, 106:401–8.

Jiang J, Yuan Z, Huang W, et al. (2011). 2, 4-dinitrophenol poisoning caused by non-oral exposure. *Toxicol Industrial Health*, 27:323–7.

Jorens PG, Schepens PJC (1993). Human pentachlorophenol poisoning. *Hum Exp Toxicol*, 12:479–95.

McFee RB, Caraccio TR, McGuigan MA, et al. (2004). Dying to be thin: a dinitrophenol related fatality. *Vet Hum Toxicol*, 46:251–4.

Müller D, Weller JP, Breitmeier D, et al. (2007). Two lethal poisonings with fat burner containing 2,4-dinitrophenol in Germany. *Clin Toxicol*, 45:358.

Proudfoot AT (2003). Pentachlorophenol poisoning. *Toxicol Rev*, 22:3–11.

Robert TA, Hagardorn AN (1985). Plasma levels and kinetic disposition of 2,4-dinitrophenol and its metabolites 2-amino-4-nitrophenol and 4-amino-2-nitrophenol in the mouse. *J Chromatogr B: Biomed Sci App*, 344:177–86.

Sangster B, Wegman RCC, Hofstee AWM (1982). Non-occupational exposure to pentachlorophenol: clinical findings and plasma-PCP-concentrations in three families. *Hum Toxicol*, 1:123–33.

Smith JE, Loveless LE, Belden EA (1996). Pentachlorophenol poisoning in newborn infants – St Louis, Missouri, April–August 1967 (classical article). *MMWR Morb Mortal Wkly Rep*, 45:545–9.

Uhl S, Schmid P, Schlatter C (1986). Pharmacokinetics of pentachlorophenol in man. *Arch Toxicol*, 58:182–6.

US Environmental Protection Agency, Barron MA (eds) (2002). Toxicological review of phenol (CAS No. 108-95-2). In: *Support of Summary Information on the Integrated Risk Information System (IRIS)*. Washington, DC: Environmental Protection Agency.

Young JF, Haley TJ (1978). A pharmacokinetic study of pentachlorophenol poisoning and the effect of forced diuresis. *J Toxicol Clin Toxicol*, 12:41–8.

Phosgene

Background

Phosgene is a colourless gas with a choking odour of mouldy hay. When compressed or refrigerated it forms a yellowish liquid. As it is heavier than air it can accumulate in low-lying areas.

It is used extensively in industry in the manufacture of isocyanates, dyes, pesticides, and pharmaceuticals.

Toxicokinetics

Phosgene dissolves slowly in water, but when this occurs, it hydrolyses to form carbon dioxide and hydrochloric acid.

Mechanisms of toxicity

Phosgene and its decomposition product, hydrochloric acid, cause direct irritation to mucous membranes.

The extent of respiratory injury from phosgene exposure is mainly determined by exposure dose (the product of the atmospheric concentration in the breathing zone and the exposure duration) rather than concentration alone. A lethal dose of phosgene is estimated to be approximately 300 ppm-minutes or higher.

Clinical features

Due to its gaseous nature, inhalation and ocular exposure are most likely, though dermal penetrating burns have been observed from liquid phosgene. Ingestion is a most unlikely route of exposure since liquid phosgene rapidly vaporizes when released.

Three distinct clinical phases are recognized following inhalation:

1 The initial phase is characterized soon after exposure by airway and mucous membrane irritation, leading to coughing, choking, tearing, and pain and tightness in the chest. The presence or absence of initial symptoms does not reflect the severity of poisoning as pulmonary oedema may still develop up to 24 hours (rarely 72 hours) later in individuals who show minimal or no immediate effects.

These initial symptoms may be followed by non-specific secondary symptoms, such as headache, nausea, and vomiting, which are thought to be due to psychological factors and not a direct effect of phosgene.

2 In the second phase, which can last from 1–24 hours, patients are often asymptomatic.

3 In the third phase, pulmonary oedema and respiratory failure may develop. Rarely, in very severe cases, circulatory collapse may also follow.

Most survivors make a complete recovery, although exertional dyspnoea and reduced physical fitness may occur for several months after exposure, particularly in those with chronic obstructive pulmonary disease.

The majority of patients who die do so within 48 hours of exposure.

Dermal and eye exposures

Direct contact with liquid phosgene under pressure can cause frostbite as well as severe irritation and corrosive damage. Eye exposure can cause eye irritation, photophobia, and excessive lacrimation.

Management

- The casualty should be removed from exposure by rescuers who themselves are protected from exposure. Contaminated clothing should be taken off, and the patient washed with copious amounts of water for at least 10–15 minutes, to prevent further exposure. If there are ocular symptoms, contact lenses should be removed and the affected eye(s) should be irrigated immediately with water or 0.9% saline for at least 10–15 minutes.
- All exposed patients should be assessed at hospital and those with confirmed exposure or symptoms need to be observed for at least 24 hours.
- A clear airway and adequate ventilation must be maintained. The oxygen saturation and pulmonary function should be monitored and a chest X-ray performed 12–24 hours after exposure, or earlier if symptoms develop. Serial X-rays may be of value in diagnosing pulmonary oedema before clinical features are present.
- If the oxygen saturation falls below 94%, the patient should receive the lowest concentration of supplemental oxygen to maintain their SaO_2 in the normal range. Once patients require oxygen, nebulized β_2-agonists (e.g., salbutamol 5 mg by nebulizer every 4 hours) may reduce lung inflammation if administered within 1 hour of exposure, though the benefit of delayed administration has not been investigated.
- There is no evidence that nebulized corticosteroids are of benefit. If presentation is less than 6 hours after exposure an IV bolus of high-dose corticosteroid (e.g. methylprednisolone 1 g) should be given.
- Early elective intubation using the ARDSnet (Acute Respiratory Distress Syndrome Network) protective ventilation strategy should be considered as this improved mortality by 22% compared with traditional mechanical ventilation in a multinational, multicentre trial of some 300 patients with acute lung injury/ ARDS. The ARDSnet study incorporated low tidal volume ventilation with increased PEEP and FiO_2. Experimental studies have shown that this approach lessens the severity of phosgene-induced lung injury and significantly improves survival.
- The role of prophylactic antibiotics is controversial, though antibiotics should be given if pneumonia develops.

Further reading

Collins JJ, Molenaar DM, Bowler LO, et al. (2011). Results from the US industry-wide phosgene surveillance: the Diller Registry. JOEM, 53:239–44.

Diller WF (1985). Late sequelae after phosgene poisoning: a literature review. Toxicol Ind Health, 1:129–36.

Grainge C, Jugg BJ, Smith AJ, et al. (2010). Delayed low-dose supplemental oxygen improves survival following phosgene-induced acute lung injury. Inhal Toxicol, 22:552–60.

Grainge C, Rice P (2010). Management of phosgene-induced acute lung injury. Clin Toxicol, 48:497–508.

Parkhouse DA, Brown RF, Jugg BJ, et al. (2007). Protective ventilation strategies in the management of phosgene-induced acute lung injury. Mil Med, 172:295–300.

Sciuto AM, Hurt HH (2004). Therapeutic treatments of phosgene-induced lung injury. Inhal Toxicol, 16:565–80.

Smith A, Brown R, Jugg B, et al. (2009). The effect of steroid treatment with inhaled budesonide or intravenous methylprednisolone on phosgene-induced acute lung injury in a porcine model. Mil Med, 174:1287–94.

The Acute Respiratory Distress Syndrome Network (2000). Ventilation with lower tidal volumes as compared with traditional tidal volumes for acute lung injury and the acute respiratory distress syndrome. N Engl J Med, 342:1301–8.

Strychnine

Background
Strychnine is an alkaloid isolated from *Strychnos nux-vomica*, *Strychnos ignatti*, and *Strychnos tiente*. Strychnine salts (hydrochloride, nitrate, and sulfate) are odourless white powders which have a bitter taste but can also exist as hard and transparent crystals.

Strychnine was used as a rodenticide in the UK until September 2006 when use for this purpose was banned in the European Union. Strychnine is still permitted for use as a below-ground pesticide to control rodents in the United States where most formulations contain 0.5% strychnine.

Historically strychnine was used as a 'tonic'. It has been found as a contaminant in herbal preparations and drugs of abuse such as cocaine, heroin and amfetamines.

The minimum lethal oral dose in adults is 50–100 mg (1–2 mg/kg body weight). Increased muscle tone and twitching have been reported following oral doses of 5–7 mg while ingestion of 10–20 mg caused convulsions and respiratory arrest in a 13-month-old boy who ultimately survived.

Toxicokinetics
Strychnine is absorbed rapidly from the gastrointestinal tract, nasal mucosa, and following injection, but much more slowly via the dermal route where delays of up to 12 hours have occurred before features develop. Strychnine is poorly protein bound and distributed widely. It is metabolized by oxidation primarily by hepatic enzymes. The metabolites are believed to be of relatively low toxicity. Approximately 5–20% is excreted unchanged in the urine within 24 hours of ingestion. Elimination following ingestion is a first order process with a half-life of 10–16 hours.

Mechanisms of toxicity
Strychnine selectively blocks the uptake of the inhibitory neurotransmitter glycine at receptor sites on postsynaptic motor neurons located in the brain and spinal cord, thereby producing CNS stimulant and convulsant effects.

Clinical features
Features often develop within 15–30 minutes following ingestion, and as quickly as 5 minutes following inhalation or intravenous injection. Systemic features can be delayed up to 12 hours following dermal exposure though may be preceded by tingling or irritation in the exposed area.

Initial symptoms following ingestion include nausea and vomiting and abdominal pain. Following exposure by all routes there may be a sense of increased awareness, apprehension, diaphoresis, chest tightness, lethargy, muscle stiffness (particularly of the neck and facial muscles, with the latter causing trismus and risus sardonicus) and myalgia, tremor, agitation, hyper-reflexia, tachypnoea, tachycardia, and hypertension; bradycardia and hypotension have also been reported.

In severe cases muscle twitching may precede the onset of convulsions, which may be precipitated by visual, touch, or auditory stimuli. Rhabdomyolysis may follow repeated convulsions and be associated with the development of compartment syndrome and renal failure.

Opisthotonus, mydriasis, proptosis, nystagmus, blurred vision, and loss of vision have been described. Bilateral conjugate and dissociated deviation of the eyes has been observed in one case of ingestion. Short-term memory impairment due to hypoxic brain damage has been reported.

Non-specific ST and T-wave changes on ECG and QTc and QRS prolongation secondary to hypocalcaemia have been described. Hypokalaemia and acute pancreatitis has been reported rarely.

Death is usually due to asphyxia from respiratory or cardiac arrest, which may occur during a convulsion.

Management
- Asymptomatic patients should be observed for a minimum of 6 hours after exposure though require no specific treatment.
- Management of symptomatic patients is supportive. Secure a clear airway as soon as possible. This may be difficult if muscle tone is increased or convulsions are occurring and it may be necessary to paralyse and ventilate the patient.
- The benefit of gastric decontamination is uncertain. Consider activated charcoal (50 g for adults; 1 g/kg for children) if the patient presents within 1 hour of ingestion of any amount and the airway can be protected. Paralysis and administration via a nasogastric tube is likely to be required prior to administration. Gastric lavage is contraindicated as a convulsion may supervene during the procedure or be precipitated by the procedure.
- Keep the patient at absolute rest to minimize muscle spasms and avoid stimuli which may precipitate convulsions.
- Treat convulsions, rhabdomyolysis, renal failure, cardiac and metabolic disturbances conventionally.

Extracorporeal techniques will not enhance the elimination of strychnine, as it has a large volume of distribution (13 L/kg).

Strychnine can be assayed in biological fluids and tissues. Seek specialist advice.

Further reading
Blain PG, Nightingale S, Stoddart JC (1982). Strychnine poisoning: abnormal eye movements. *J Toxicol Clin Toxicol*, 19:215–17.

Dargan PI, Webster E, Jones AL (2001). Strychnine poisoning: a case report with toxicokinetic data. *J Toxicol Clin Toxicol*, 39: 508.

Edmunds M, Sheehan TMT, Van't Hoff W (1986). Strychnine poisoning clinical and toxicological observations on a non-fatal case. *J Toxicol Clin Toxicol*, 24:245–55.

Greene R, Meatherall R (2001). Dermal exposure to strychnine. *J Anal Toxicol*, 25:344–7.

Heiser JM, Daya MR, Magnussen AR, et al. (1992). Massive strychnine intoxication: serial blood levels in a fatal case. *J Toxicol Clin Toxicol*, 30:269–83.

Lindsey T, Hara J, Irvine R, et al. (2004). Strychnine overdose following ingestion of gopher bait. *J Anal Toxicol*, 28:135–7.

O'Callaghan WG, Joyce N, Counihan HE, et al. (1982). Unusual strychnine poisoning and its treatment: report of eight cases. *Br Med J*, 285:478.

Palatnick W, Meatherall R, Sitar D, et al. (1997). Toxicokinetics of acute strychnine poisoning. *J Toxicol Clin Toxicol*, 35:617–20.

Sgaragli GP, Mannaioni PF (1973). Pharmacokinetic observations on a case of massive strychnine poisoning. *J Toxicol Clin Toxicol*, 6:533–40.

Sulphur dioxide

Background

Sulphur dioxide (SO_2) (CAS 7664-09-5) is a colourless non-flammable gas that is heavier than air with a very irritating odour. Most people can smell sulphur dioxide at concentrations of 0.3 to 1 ppm. It is a common air pollutant and is produced naturally by active volcanoes and forest fires. The majority of SO_2 in the environment is due to the combustion of fossil fuels at large industrial sites. Other sources include motor vehicle exhaust gases, domestic boilers, and fires.

Its main industrial use is as a chemical intermediate in the production of sulphuric acid. It is also used as a fumigant, a food preservative, and as a bleaching agent. SO_2 has also been used in the purification of petroleum products.

Exposure is most likely to occur by the inhalational route due to fires or faulty industrial processes.

Sulphur dioxide easily dissolves in water to form sulphurous acid:

$$SO_2 + H_2O \leftrightarrow HSO_3^- + H^+$$

It is a weak acid and the major component of acid rain. Sulphur dioxide gas is an irritant and mildly corrosive. Minor exposures may result in a burning sensation of the eyes and throat and more substantial exposure may cause coughing or breathing difficulties. A one-off exposure (sufficient to cause mild lung or eye irritation) is unlikely to result in long-term health effects. Exposure to high concentrations of SO_2 may be potentially fatal due to airway obstruction or from asphyxiation if exposure is in a poorly ventilated, enclosed, or low-lying area. Exposure to pure SO_2 is likely to be rare unless in the industrial setting as it will tend to be mixed with other gases and pollutants (e.g. PM_{10}) in the outdoor environment.

Occupational standards

No exposure limits are set in UK although there is an industry agreement to try and keep the levels below 1ppm.

OSHA PEL (permissible exposure limit) = 5 ppm (averaged over an 8-hour work shift).

NIOSH IDLH (immediately dangerous to life or health) = 100 ppm.

AIHA ERPG-2 (maximum airborne concentration below which it is believed that nearly all persons could be exposed for up to 1 hour without experiencing or developing irreversible or other serious health effects or symptoms that could impair their abilities to take protective action) = 3 ppm.

Toxicokinetics

Sulphur dioxide is soluble in water and dissolves in the mucus fluid covering the mucous lining of the respiratory system to produce sulphurous acid, a weak acid. Following a short-term inhalation exposure, SO_2 is almost entirely retained in the upper nasal mucosa. Inhalation of high concentrations may exceed the capacity of this mechanism leading to systemic absorption through the lungs. There is no specific biomarker of exposure available to the treating physician.

Although SO_2 is an irritant to the eye and mucous membranes, systemic absorption is considered not to be quantitatively significant.

Clinical features

Toxic mainly by inhalation, although dermal or ocular exposure may occur. Ingestion is not thought to be likely or significant.

Acute exposure

Inhalation causes irritation of eyes and nose with sore throat, cough, chest tightness, and a feeling of suffocation. Bronchospasm, pneumonitis, and pulmonary oedema can occur. Moderate-to-high doses by inhalation can cause gastrointestinal symptoms including nausea, vomiting, and abdominal pain, and corrosive damage to the respiratory tract. Asthmatics may experience increased airway resistance with SO_2 concentrations less than 0.1 ppm when exercising. Healthy adults experience increased airway resistance at 5 ppm, sneezing and coughing at 10 ppm, and bronchospasm at 20 ppm. Respiratory protection is needed for exposures greater than 20 ppm. Exposures of 50–100 ppm may be tolerated for more than 30–60 minutes, but higher or longer exposures can cause death from airway obstruction. Children may receive larger doses due to greater lung surface area to body weight ratios and increased minute volumes to weight ratios.

It should be noted that some individuals are very susceptible to the presence of sulphur dioxide and overreact to concentrations, which, in most people, elicit a much milder response. This hyper-reactive response occurs the first time the individual is exposed and is therefore not an acquired immune or hypersensitivity response. Exposure to high concentrations of sulphur dioxide can lead to reactive airway dysfunction syndrome (RADS).

Ingestion of the gas is unlikely but swallowing of sulphurous acid will be the same as ingestion of a weak acid (see Acids and alkalis, pp. 208–211).

Dermal/ocular exposure causes severe irritation to the mucus membranes at concentrations of greater than 10–20 ppm.

Sulphur dioxide gas stored under pressure as a compressed liquid expands rapidly on liberation, resulting in vaporization and a large endothermic reaction. The result may be evaporative freezing of any tissue in contact with the liquid.

Chronic/repeated exposure

Respiratory effects have been associated with chronic inhalation exposure to low concentrations of sulphur dioxide. These include wheeze and asthma.

Genotoxicity

There is no human evidence.

Carcinogenicity

It has not been classified as carcinogenic by the IARC.

Reproductive and developmental toxicity

There are no human data.

Management

Remove patient from exposure. If a patient has been exposed only to sulphur dioxide gas and has no eye or skin irritation decontamination is not required. There is no biomarker of exposure to aid the treating physician.

Inhalation

Treatment is supportive of respiratory function. Ensure a clear airway and adequate ventilation. Give oxygen to symptomatic patients. All patients with abnormal vital signs, chest pain, respiratory symptoms, or hypoxia should have a 12-lead ECG performed. If the patient has clinical features of bronchospasm treat conventionally with nebulized bronchodilators and steroids. Endotracheal intubation, or rarely, tracheostomy may be required for life-threatening laryngeal oedema. Apply other supportive measures as indicated by the patient's clinical condition. If the exposure has been substantial then observation of the patient for at least 4 hours would be recommended.

Dermal exposure

This will be unlikely but treat as a weak acid exposure to the mucous membranes as outlined in Acids and alkalis, pp. 208–211. Decontamination with water, if necessary, and supportive treatment is the mainstay. A burns specialist should review chemical burns if clinically significant but this is unlikely with sulphurous acid. Apply other supportive measures as indicated by the patient's clinical condition.

Ocular exposure

This will be unlikely but treat as a weak acid exposure to the eyes as outlined in Acids and alkalis, pp. 208–211.

Remove contact lenses if necessary and immediately irrigate the affected eye thoroughly with water or 0.9% saline for at least 10–15 minutes.

Patients with corneal damage or those whose symptoms do not resolve rapidly should be referred for urgent ophthalmological assessment as there may be other factors involved.

Delayed effects following an acute exposure

Inhalation exposures to low concentrations for a short period, from which an individual recovers quickly on removal to fresh air, are unlikely to result in delayed or long-term adverse health effects. Substantial inhalation exposures may cause long-term health effects, including RADS. Bronchospasm might be triggered in people who have chronic pulmonary diseases, such as asthma and emphysema.

Further reading

Agency for Toxic Substances and Disease Registry (2013). *Medical Management of Sulfur Dioxide*. Atlanta, GA: ATSDR. <http://www.atsdr.cdc.gov/mmg/mmg.asp?id=249&tid=4>.

Baxter PJ, Aw T-C, Cockcroft A, et al. (eds) (2010). *Hunter's Diseases of Occupations*, 10th edition. London: Hodder.

Health and Safety Executive (2011). *EH40/2005. Workplace Exposure Limits*, 2nd edition. London: HSE. <http://www.hse.gov.uk/pubns/priced/eh40.pdf>

Piirilä, PL, Nordman, H, Korhonen, OS, et al. (1996). A thirteen-year follow-up of respiratory effects of acute exposure to sulfur dioxide. *Scand J Work, Environ Health*, 2:191–6.

Shakeri, MS, Dick, FD, Ayres, JG (2008) Which agents cause reactive airways dysfunction syndrome (RADS)? A systematic review. *Occup Med*, 58:205–11.

US Environmental Protection Agency (2012). *Acid Rain*. <http://www.epa.gov/acidrain/what/>.

Xylenes

Background
Commercial 'xylene' contains a mixture of the three xylene isomers, ortho-xylene (~5–10%), para-xylene (5–10%) and meta-xylene (65–85%), toluene (14%), ethyl benzene (20%) and other, non-aromatic chemicals. Xylene is used widely in paints, lacquers, pesticides, gums, resins, adhesives, and the paper coating industry.

Toxicokinetics
The biotransformation of xylenes in humans proceeds primarily by the oxidation of a side-chain methyl group by mixed function oxidases in the liver to yield toluic acids (methylbenzoic acids). These toluic acids conjugate with glycine to form toluic acids (methylhippuric acids) that are excreted into the urine. Of the xylene absorbed, about 95% is metabolized to methylhippuric acid and 70 to 80% is excreted in the urine within 24 hours. If not metabolized, xylenes are quickly eliminated in exhaled air. Peak blood concentrations occur 1–2 hours after ingestion and the elimination half-life is 20–30 hours. Ingestion of a moderate dose of ethanol (0.8 g/kg) by volunteers prior to inhalation of meta-xylene (6.0 or 11.5 mmol/m³) for 4 hours caused a marked alteration in xylene kinetics. After ethanol intake the blood xylene concentration rose about 1.5–2.0-fold and urine methylhippuric acid excretion declined by about 50%, suggesting that ethanol decreased the metabolic clearance of xylene by about one-half during xylene inhalation.

Mechanisms of toxicity
The lipophilic effects of xylenes, which dissolve lipid membranes, are responsible for the irritant effects on eyes, mucous membranes and skin. In addition, the lipophilicity of xylenes is responsible for their narcotic and anaesthetic properties, which are similar for the three isomers, which are not fully understood but are probably related to intercalation of the chemical into neuronal cell membranes, changing membrane properties that affect transmission of nerve impulses. The mechanism could either be by a disruption of the lipid environment in which membrane proteins function or by direct interaction with the hydrophobic/hydrophilic conformation of proteins in the neuronal membrane. The mechanism for by which xylenes affect the kidneys is also unknown, but may be related to formation of reactive metabolites and subsequent irritation or direct membrane fluidization.

Clinical features
Xylenes are very lipophilic, and are rapidly absorbed by all routes of exposure. Systemic toxicity can occur through all routes of exposure.

Nose and throat irritation have been reported following exposure to mixed xylene concentrations of 200 ppm for 3–5 minutes, to meta-xylene concentrations of 50 ppm for 2 hours, and to para-xylene concentrations of 100 ppm for 1–7.5 hours/day for 5 days.

At air concentrations as low as 50 ppm, CNS effects, including excitement, flushing of the face, headache, and dizziness, occur. Dizziness was reported by the majority of subjects exposed to 690 ppm mixed xylene for 15 minutes, but in only one of six persons exposed at 460 ppm.

With increasing xylene concentrations other effects occur including drowsiness, tremor, confusion, coma, ataxia, respiratory depression, narcosis, and catecholomine-induced ventricular arrhythmias. Hepatorenal damage also has been described.

Impaired short-term memory, impaired reaction time, performance decrements in numerical ability, and alterations in equilibrium and body balance have been reported. Exposure to 100 ppm mixed xylene for 4 hours resulted in prolonged reaction time and exposure to 299 ppm mixed xylene for 70 minutes during exercise resulted in impaired short-term memory and reaction time.

Dermal exposure to xylenes causes skin irritation, dryness and scaling of the skin, and vasodilation. Immersion of the hand in liquid xylene may result in erythema and a burning feeling, with some scaling of the skin.

A 30-year-old man injected 8 mL of xylene intravenously in a suicide attempt. After 10 minutes he developed acute respiratory failure for which he required intubation and mechanical ventilation with PEEP and high FiO₂ but survived.

Management
Once rescued from exposure, treatment is symptomatic and supportive.

Further reading
Abu Al Ragheb S, Salhab AS, et al. (1986). Suicide by xylene ingestion. A case report and review of literature. Am J Forensic Med Pathol, 7:327–9.

Agency for Toxic Substances and Disease Registry (2007). Xylene. Atlanta, GA: ATSDR.

Akisu M, Mir S, Genc B, et al. (1996). Severe acute thinner intoxication. Turk J Pediatr, 38:223–5.

Anon (1989). Xylene. IARC Monogr Eval Carcinog Risks Hum, 47:125–56.

Ansari EA (1997). Ocular injury with xylene – a report of two cases. Hum Exp Toxicol, 16:273–5.

Bakinson MA, Jones RD (1985). Gassings due to methylene chloride, xylene, toluene, and styrene reported to Her Majesty's Factory Inspectorate 1961–80. Br J Ind Med, 42:184–90.

Draper TH Bamiou DE (2009). Auditory neuropathy in a patient exposed to xylene: case report. J Laryngol Otology, 123:462–5.

Fishbein L (1985). An overview of environmental and toxicological aspects of aromatic hydrocarbons. III. Xylene. Sci Total Environ, 43:165–83.

Gonzalez-Reche LM, Schettgen T, Angerer J (2003). New approaches to the metabolism of xylenes: verification of the formation of phenylmercapturic acid metabolites of xylenes. Arch Toxicol, 77:80–5.

Greim H (ed) (2001). Xylene (all isomers). In: Greim H (ed), Occupational Toxicants: Critical Data Evaluation for MAK Values and Classification of Carcinogens, pp. 257–88. Weinheim: Wiley-VCH GmbH.

Gupta BN, Kumar P, Srivastava AK (1990). An investigation of the neurobehavioural effects on workers exposed to organic solvents. J Soc Occup Med, 40:94–6.

IPCS (1997). Environmental Health Criteria 190. Xylenes. Geneva: World Health Organization.

Klaucke DN, Johansen M, Vogt RL (1982). An outbreak of xylene intoxication in a hospital. Am J Ind Med, 3:173–8.

Morley R, Eccleston DW, Douglas CP, et al. (1970). Xylene poisoning: a report on one fatal case and two cases of recovery after prolonged unconsciousness. Br Med J, 3:442–3.

Riihimäki V, Savolainen K, Pfäffli P, et al. (1982). Metabolic interaction between m-xylene and ethanol. Arch Toxicol, 49:253–63.

Sevcik P, Hep A, Peslova M (1992). Intravenous xylene poisoning. Intensive Care Med, 18:377–8.

Poisoning due to metals, and their salts

Antimony

Background

Antimony (Stibium, Sb) is a lustrous grey metalloid that occurs naturally in many minerals, often as the sulphide stibnite (Sb_2S_3). It belongs to the same periodic group as arsenic which it resembles chemically though antimony is much less toxic. Antimony forms organic and inorganic compounds in the trivalent and pentavalent states. Elemental antimony is used in alloys with lead, tin, and copper. Antimony compounds are used in flame retardants, fireworks, matches, pigments, and glass. They have also been used as parasiticidal drugs for the treatment of conditions such as schistosomiasis. Toxicologically significant antimony exposures occur predominantly in an occupational setting including metal smelting, coal-fired power plants, and refuse incineration. Stibine gas (SbH_3) is toxicologically important because exposure can cause intravascular haemolysis. It is formed by the reaction between acids and antimony alloys or the electrolysis of solutions where antimony is present in the cathode.

Toxicokinetics

Antimony compounds may be absorbed by inhalation or ingestion. Trivalent antimony accumulates in red blood cells whereas pentavalent antimony is found predominantly in plasma.

Some pentavalent antimony is reduced to the trivalent form in the liver. Elimination is mainly in the urine, with small amounts appearing in faeces via bile after conjugation with glutathione. Antimony in bile undergoes entero-hepatic circulation.

Mechanisms

Like many other metals the principal mechanisms of antimony toxicity involve interaction with endogenous sulphhydryl groups.

Clinical features—acute poisoning

Inhalation

Dust and fumes of antimony and its compounds are irritant to the respiratory tract and mucous membranes causing conjunctivitis, laryngitis, pharyngitis, tracheitis, rhinitis, and bronchitis. There may be radiological evidence of pneumonitis which resolves upon removal from exposure.

In addition to respiratory tract irritation, seven men exposed to antimony trichloride fumes also experienced abdominal pain, anorexia, and vomiting. Similar symptoms plus diarrhoea, headache, and dizziness have been experienced by smelter workers exposed to antimony fumes.

Ingestion

One hundred and fifty children who drank lemon which had been refrigerated for 20 hours in a large agate pot experienced nausea, vomiting, and diarrhoea due to leaching of antimony from the agate lining.

Four adults presented with severe diarrhoea and vomiting having mistaken 'tartar emetic' (antimony potassium tartrate) for 'cream of tartar'. Three made an uneventful recovery but the fourth died from haemorrhagic gastritis complicated by cardiorespiratory failure.

Topical exposure

Antimony compounds are skin irritants.

Clinical features—chronic poisoning

Inhalation

Chronic occupational exposure to antimony and its compounds may cause 'antimony pneumoconiosis'. Typical radiological findings include diffuse, dense, punctate non-confluent opacities predominately in the middle and lower lung fields, sometimes associated with pleural adhesions. Cough and exertional breathlessness are the symptoms most frequently reported, sometimes in association with wheeze, chest pain, and malaise.

Perforation of the nasal septum has been described in antimony workers who were co-exposed to arsenic.

Topical exposure

Dermatitis following contact with antimony compounds is well described although this is not usually a problem after contact with the metal. Typical lesions arise on the arms, legs, and in the flexures, sparing the face, hands, and feet. Papules and pustules predominate around sweat and sebaceous glands with areas of eczema and lichenification. These 'antimony spots' occur mainly in the summer.

Parenteral administration

Treatment with parenteral antimonial compounds is associated frequently with nausea, vomiting, anorexia, myalgia, and arthralgia. Abdominal pain, a metallic taste, diarrhoea, reversible elevations in hepatic enzyme activities, uveitis, and retinal haemorrhage are recognized. ECG changes including T-wave inversion or amplitude reduction, QT interval prolongation and ST segment abnormalities may occur but usually reverse when treatment is discontinued. Less common adverse effects include hepatic necrosis, renal tubular acidosis, acute tubular necrosis, pancreatitis, optic atrophy, and bone marrow hypoplasia.

Carcinogenicity

The carcinogenic potential of antimony in man is difficult to evaluate since co-exposure to arsenic is common. The International Agency for Research on Cancer (IARC) has classified antimony trioxide in group 2B, that is 'possibly carcinogenic to humans' and antimony trisulphide in group 3 that is 'not classifiable as to its carcinogenicity to humans'.

Management

Management of antimony poisoning is by removal from exposure and supportive measures. Though there are no controlled studies in man, present evidence favours DMSA as the chelating agent of choice.

Further reading

Greim H (2007). Antimony and its inorganic compounds (inhalable fraction). In: Greim H (ed), The MAK-Collection For Occupational Health and Safety. Part I: MAK Value Documentations, Vol. 23, pp. 1–73. Weinheim, Germany: Wiley-VCH.

Hepburn NC, Nolan J, Fenn L, et al. (1994). Cardiac effects of sodium stibogluconate: myocardial, electrophysiological and biochemical studies. QJM, 87:465–72.

Lauwers LF, Roelants A, Rosseel PM, et al. (1990). Oral antimony intoxications in man. Crit Care Med, 8:324–6.

McCallum RI (1989). The industrial toxicology of antimony. The Ernestine Henry lecture 1987. J R Coll Physicians Lond, 23:28–32.

Potkonjak V, Pavlovich M (1983). Antimoniosis: a particular form of pneumoconiosis. I. Etiology, clinical and X-ray findings. Int Arch Occup Environ Health, 51:199–207.

Arsenic and arsine

Background
The toxicity of arsenic depends on the chemical form involved and whether exposure is acute or chronic. Arsine is a colourless, non-irritating extremely flammable gas with a garlic-like odour. Arsine is also explosive. Arsine is produced when arsenic or arsenic-containing compounds react with acid or water.

Elemental arsenic is a grey crystalline metalloid that is often found naturally in conjunction with sulphur and metals. It is used for strengthening alloys of copper and lead, in electroplating, semiconductor manufacturing, and in the production of glass and ceramics.

Arsenic forms organic and inorganic compounds in two valency states—arsenic(III) and arsenic(V). Trivalent arsenic is some 60 times more toxic than pentavalent arsenic. However, most absorbed pentavalent arsenic is converted in vivo to the trivalent form.

Inorganic arsenic compounds
Inorganic arsenic(V) salts that contain $AsO_4{}^{3-}$ are known chemically as arsenates. Arsenates are the main form of arsenic to contaminate groundwater, an important source or arsenic poisoning in Asia. Such contamination can be naturally occurring due to contact with arsenic-rich rocks or from industrial or pesticide pollution. Arsenates were previously used in insecticides and fungicides although are no longer licensed for these purposes in the UK.

Inorganic arsenic(III) salts that contain $AsO_3{}^{3-}$ or $AsO_2{}^-$ are known chemically as arsenites. Arsenic trioxide (As_2O_3) is also an inorganic arsenic(III) compound and is commercially important as a precursor of other industrial compounds. Arsenic trioxide is licensed for the treatment of acute promyelocytic leukaemia in patients who have failed to respond to first-line therapy.

Inorganic arsenic compounds may also be found in Chinese and Indian traditional medicines and rarely in some other herbal supplements.

Inorganic arsenical compounds may generate arsine gas (see later in this section) when in contact with acids, reducing metals, sodium hydroxide, and aluminium.

Organic arsenic compounds
Organic arsenic compounds were used as chemical weapons during World War I as either Adamsite (dibenzo-1-chloro-1,4 arsenine) or Lewisite (chlorovinyl-2-arsenic dichloride). Organic arsenic compounds have been used previously as pesticides.

Methylation of inorganic arsenic is a naturally occurring detoxification process for arsenic and results in the accumulation of organoarsenic compounds (e.g. arsenobetaine) in some fish and vegetables.

Toxicokinetics
The bioavailability of ingested elemental arsenic is likely to be considerably less than the absorption of arsenic from arsenic salts.

Arsenic compounds exist in air as particulate matter. The extent of absorption following inhalation depends on the solubility of the arsenic compounds and the size of the particles. Overall absorption following inhalation is about 30–34%.

Absorption may also occur through the skin if exposure is prolonged/repeated or if the dermal barrier is damaged.

Arsenic is widely distributed. Arsenic compounds can pass the blood–brain and placental barriers.

Metabolism occurs primarily in the liver and involves two processes depending on the compound. First, pentavalent arsenic compounds (arsenates) are reduced, for example, by glutathione, to trivalent arsenic compounds (arsenites). Secondly, trivalent inorganic arsenic is methylated in the liver to monomethylarsonic (MMA) acid which is further methylated to dimethylarsinic acid (DMA).

Short-term studies in man indicate that daily intake in excess of 0.5 mg progressively, but not completely, saturates the capacity to methylate inorganic arsenic.

The main route of elimination is the kidney with DMA excreted unchanged, MMA slightly (~13%) methylated to DMA prior to excretion and inorganic arsenic excreted as approximately 25% unmethylated, 25% MMA and 50% DMA. There is considerable genetic variation in arsenic metabolism.

Biliary elimination of arsenic has been demonstrated in rats and is more important as a means of eliminating arsenic(III) than arsenic(V).

In man the majority of a single dose of ingested arsenic is excreted in urine within 85 hours. The whole-body half-life of arsenic in six human volunteers fitted a three-compartment system, with 65.9% of orally administered arsenic acid having a half-life of 2.1 days, 30.4% a half-life of 9.5 days, and 3.7% a half-life of 38.4 days (mean values).

Mechanisms of toxicity
Trivalent arsenic enters cells by diffusion or specific transmembrane transporters and binds to sulphydryl groups, resulting in the dysfunction of numerous key enzymes including pyruvate dehydrogenase with subsequent disruption of oxidative phosphorylation. Pentavalent arsenic enters cells through phosphate transport proteins and subsequently may be reduced to trivalent arsenic or substitute for inorganic phosphate in metabolic reactions including glycolysis, again leading to uncoupling of oxidative phosphorylation and loss of ATP formation. Chronically, inorganic arsenic and its methylated metabolites disrupt cell proliferation and survival signalling pathways, cause DNA damage and inhibition of DNA repair resulting in an increased risk of cancer. Paradoxically, the anticarcinogenic effects of arsenic trioxide have been attributed to the induction of apoptosis and the inhibition of microtubule formation.

Clinical features—acute poisoning
Ingestion
Features of poisoning are similar following exposure to arsenic or any arsenic salt but are generally less severe when exposure has been to an organic arsenic compound.

Following ingestion features usually start within 2 hours and commonly include abdominal pain, vomiting, and diarrhoea. There may be no other features following a small ingestion of organic arsenic salts. In more severe cases, particularly following ingestion of inorganic arsenic salts, the severity of gastrointestinal fluid loss may precipitate hypovolaemic shock and acute tubular necrosis.

Trivalent arsenic compounds such as arsenic trioxide are particularly irritant to the gastrointestinal mucosa and may cause haemorrhagic gastroenteritis.

The most severely poisoned patients progress within hours to multi-organ involvement. Features include deterioration in hepatic and renal function, coagulopathy, haemolysis, rhabdomyolysis, non-cardiogenic pulmonary oedema (adult respiratory distress syndrome), myelosuppression (classically pancytopenia), and cardiac involvement (myocardial depression, ST segment changes, prolonged QT interval, ventricular tachycardia, torsade de pointes, or ventricular fibrillation). Neurological features include CNS depression, convulsions, encephalopathy, and a peripheral neuropathy. The latter is typically a symmetrical sensorimotor neuropathy, sometimes resembling the Guillain–Barré syndrome and may be seen up to 5 weeks after exposure. Pancreatitis has also been reported.

Inhalation

Arsenic compounds are irritant to the upper airways and can produce laryngitis, bronchitis, and rhinitis. Perforation of the nasal septum has also occurred.

Inhalation of arsenic has also led to nausea, vomiting, and diarrhoea. It was assumed that arsenic particles were transported to the larynx by mucociliary clearance and then reached the gastrointestinal tract as a result of swallowing. Acute encephalopathy (hallucinations, increased excitability, emotional lability, memory loss, difficulties in learning new information) has been reported after occupational exposure, but ingestion of arsenic cannot be excluded as the main route of exposure.

Features of systemic toxicity may also occur (see earlier in section).

Dermal exposure

Arsenic compounds are irritant. Typical responses following skin contact include erythema and swelling, with papules and blisters in more severe cases. Exposure to arsenic dusts in the workplace have also caused contact dermatitis. Features of systemic toxicity would only be expected following prolonged skin exposure or if the skin integrity was already damaged prior to skin contact.

Seven patients unintentionally applied a 30% arsenic solution to their entire body instead of benzyl benzoate to treat scabies. Hours later they developed severe burns, blisters, bullae, and generalized erythema. Systemic features of arsenic poisoning followed. Three patients died and three developed polyneuropathy.

Eye exposure

There are limited data on ocular exposure but features expected include pain, lacrimation, blepharospasm, conjunctivitis, photophobia, visual disturbance, and corneal damage.

Clinical features—chronic exposure

Features of chronic low-level exposure (also called arsenicosis) include anorexia, weight loss, abdominal pain, diarrhoea, and headache. Skin changes are characteristic and include hyperkeratosis of the palms and soles, hyperpigmentation ('raindrop' pattern on the trunk and extremities), exfoliative dermatitis, and alopecia. Mees' lines (transverse white lines on nails) may appear. A peripheral sensorimotor neuropathy may be present. Complete respiratory muscle paralysis and a phrenic neuropathy have been reported. Hepatic features include jaundice, hepatomegaly, and non-cirrhotic portal fibrosis. Cardiovascular effects include black foot disease, a form of peripheral vascular disease characterized by severe systemic arteriosclerosis, and dry gangrene which, in extreme cases, leads to spontaneous amputations of affected extremities. Haematological features include anaemia or pancytopenia. Muscle fasciculation, muscle wasting, and ataxia have also been described.

Chronic arsenic exposure has been associated with an increased incidence of diabetes mellitus, cerebrovascular disease, and chronic lung diseases including chronic obstructive pulmonary disease, and bronchiectasis.

Prolonged or repeated exposure is associated with increased risk of cancer of the skin, lung, liver, bladder, kidney, and prostate.

Analytical confirmation of the diagnosis

Arsenic poisoning is most easily investigated by urine analysis. In most circumstances a single void or 'spot' urine specimen is sufficient; 24-hour collections are preferable only prior to and during chelation therapy.

Seafood, fish, or seaweed are rich in complex organic arsenic species, which are of little toxicological significance, but can result in total urine arsenic concentrations which are elevated, sometimes spectacularly so. In individuals not exposed to inorganic arsenic and who have not consumed sea-food, fish or seaweed within the last 7–10 days, the urine arsenic excretion is usually less than 10 micrograms/g creatinine (<15 nmol/mmol creatinine) or less than 10 micrograms (0.13 micromoles) arsenic/24 hours if a 24-hour urine collection is made. Asking a patient to refrain from these foods will restrict this phenomenon.

It is most important that the laboratory undertaking the analysis is able to perform some degree of arsenic speciation, the minimum being the capability to report a 'total non-dietary arsenic' result, i.e. a value which excludes the complex organic forms of the element. It should be noted, however, that the major metabolites of inorganic arsenic (MMA and DMA) may also be minor components of 'marine' dietary arsenic and, as such, be present in detectable quantities in urine.

Blood arsenic concentrations are less useful as a primary index of exposure as the element and its metabolites are cleared rapidly from the blood. However, blood should be collected when no urine is available and (together with urine) when acute poisoning is suspected. It may also be useful in the follow up of confirmed cases of significant chronic exposure. Normal whole blood arsenic (inorganic plus its metabolites) concentration is less than 10 micrograms/L (<130 nmol/L).

Analysis of arsenic in hair or nails generally is not useful in acute diagnosis.

Management

Where the practical expertise exists, consider gastric aspiration/lavage in adults within 1 hour of a potentially life threatening ingestion of an arsenic compound, providing the airway can be protected. Activated charcoal is unlikely to be of benefit.

Save blood (whole blood not serum) and urine for arsenic concentration determination. Consider the need for chelation therapy with DMPS or DMSA in patients who are symptomatic and/or have elevated urine arsenic concentrations (see 'Chelation therapy').

Check full blood count, U&Es, creatinine, and liver function tests. Monitor urine output and perform urinalysis.

A 12-lead ECG should be performed in all patients and chest X-ray in patients who have respiratory symptoms.

Ingested arsenic and arsenic salts may be visible on abdominal X-ray.

Commence intravenous fluids in patients with diarrhoea and vomiting. Correct electrolyte disturbances and consider need for blood transfusion if haemorrhagic gastroenteritis present.

Vasopressors may be required in the most severely hypotensive patients.

Treat convulsions, arrhythmias, and non-cardiogenic pulmonary oedema conventionally.

Haemodialysis or haemodiafiltration may be required for the clinical management of patients with established renal failure. Although haemodialysis has been used in a number of cases of acute arsenic poisoning, the amount of arsenic removed in the dialysate was small. This is consistent with rapid clearance of arsenic from the blood to tissues.

Patients with bone marrow suppression may require red cell and platelet transfusion. Consider the need for GM-CSF in patients with severe neutropenia.

Perform nerve conduction studies in patients with a peripheral neuropathy. These typically show reduced conduction velocity consistent with axonal degeneration.

Inhalation, dermal, and eye exposure
Removal from the source of exposure is the priority.

Management is otherwise supportive. Treat systemic features as previously described.

Save urine and whole blood for arsenic concentration determination.

Chelation therapy
Consider the need for chelation therapy in patients who are symptomatic and/or have elevated blood/urine arsenic concentrations. Note that it is important to distinguish dietary from non-dietary arsenic.

Dimercaprol has been used in the management of arsenic poisoning in the past but its use has been associated with a number of adverse effects and it has now been superseded by DMPS (unithiol) and DMSA (succimer) which have been shown to increase urine arsenic excretion and decrease blood arsenic concentrations following experimental and clinical exposures. There are insufficient data to determine which chelating agent is the agent of choice, but limited evidence favours DMPS. Most data have related to the treatment of poisoning with inorganic arsenicals.

The intravenous dose of DMPS is 30 mg/kg/day for 5 days, which may be repeated if necessary after 5–7 days. If the intravenous formulation is not available, consider oral DMPS. Since the bioavailability of oral DMPS is only 39%, oral DMPS would need to be administered in a dose of 77 mg/kg/day for 5 days to achieve the same serum concentrations as DMPS 30 mg/kg/day intravenously. A further treatment course may be given after 5–7 days. Seek expert advice.

Treatment in 5-day courses should continue until there is relief of systemic clinical features. If possible, monitor the patient's blood and urine arsenic concentrations during and following chelation therapy to determine whether a further course of chelation is necessary.

Adverse reactions to DMPS include skin reactions (rash, urticaria), mucous membrane reactions (ulcers), and elevation in body temperature. Rapid IV administration has been associated with vasodilatation and transient hypotension.

DMSA has been used for chelation in acute and chronic arsenic poisoning, though is less efficacious than DMPS. The oral dose is 30 mg/kg/day (can be given in either a single or three divided doses) for 5 days, repeated after 5–7 days, if necessary.

Few side effects have been reported following DMSA use but include nausea, transient increase in ALT activity and, rarely, a mucocutaneous eruption.

Arsine
A colourless, non-irritating extremely flammable gas with a garlic-like odour. Arsine is also explosive. Available in cylinders and used in organic synthesis and in semiconductor manufacture. Arsine is produced when arsenic or arsenic-containing compounds react with acid or water. Many exposures occur occupationally as a result of the accidental formation of arsine as a by-product during processes in the chemical and metallurgical industries.

Mechanism of toxicity
The mechanisms of arsine toxicity are not fully understood. Arsine enters red blood cells, binds to oxyhaemoglobin and induces severe acute haemolysis and impairment of oxygen transport. Several mechanisms for haemolysis have been proposed. These include a direct reaction between arsine and oxyhaemoglobin at the haem binding site, with destabilization and degradation of haemoglobin, the release of haemin (ferriprotoporphyrin chloride) and precipitated globin protein (as Heinz bodies) resulting in structural damage to the red cell membrane. It has also been proposed that arsine-induced red cell membrane damage is secondary to the formation of reactive oxygen species which combine with haemoglobin, though there is evidence that this process does not contribute significantly to haemolysis. Arsine also reacts with the sulphydryl groups on red blood cell membranes including those of Na^+K^+-ATPase, causing impaired ion balance, so that red blood cells swell and haemolyse. It is unlikely, however, that Na^+K^+-ATPase is the primary target for arsine. Arsine binds with oxidized haemoglobin causing marked intravascular haemolysis. Haemoglobinuria and acute renal tubular necrosis then develop.

Toxicokinetics
Arsine is rapidly absorbed through the respiratory tract. Oxidation to trivalent arsenic occurs in body fluids with some further oxidation to pentavalent arsenic, though ultimately most arsenic(V) is reduced to arsenic(III). Trivalent arsenic is methylated in the liver to monomethylarsonate and dimethylarsinate. The metabolites are excreted mainly in urine with relative amounts: monomethyl arsonate > dimethyl arsinate > trivalent arsenic > pentavalent arsenic.

Clinical features
The onset of features is often delayed for several hours following inhalation. Features include headache, malaise, thirst, dizziness and breathlessness followed by nausea and vomiting, abdominal pain, paraesthesiae/dysaesthesiae and severe haemolysis. Weakness with muscle cramps and occasionally hypotension may occur.

Painless dark red urine (due to the presence of haemoglobin) generally develops within 4–6 hours of exposure. Bronze/orange discolouration of the skin and orange-red staining of the conjunctiva and sclera may occur as a result of haemolysis and is probably due to the presence of circulating degradation products of haemoglobin in plasma.

After 24–48 hours, fever, anaemia, jaundice, enlargement of the liver, hyperkalaemia, prolongation of the prothrombin time (INR) and pulmonary oedema may ensue.

Peaked T waves on ECG (most probably secondary to hyperkalaemia), leucocytosis, and reticulocytosis often develop. Hyperbilirubinaemia, an increase in serum LDH concentration, and a reduced haptoglobin concentration are present in patients with significant haemolysis.

Acute hepatic and renal failure may occur. Mild methaemoglobinaemia is recognized but is unlikely to be clinically significant.

Peripheral neuropathy with weakness, myalgia, and paraesthesiae may persist; horizontal white lines on the nails (Mees' lines) may appear.

Urine and blood arsenic concentrations will be elevated.

Management

If haemolysis is severe, the use of red cell exchange and plasma exchange may be more beneficial than red cell exchange alone, though plasma exchange alone is also effective in the treatment of intravascular haemolysis. Blood transfusion will be required in cases of severe haemolysis. If renal failure ensues, haemodialysis/haemodiafiltration/haemofiltration should be undertaken. Dimercaprol and DMSA are of no value.

Further reading

Aposhian HV, Aposhian MM (2006), Arsenic toxicology: five questions. *Chem Res Toxicol*, 19:1–15.

Aposhian HV, Zheng B, Aposhian MM, *et al.* (2000). DMPS-arsenic challenge test. II. Modulation of arsenic species, including monomethylarsonous acid (MMAIII), excreted in human urine. *Toxicol Appl Pharmacol*, 165:74–83.

Apostoli P, Alessio L, Romeo L, *et al.* (1997). Metabolism of arsenic after acute occupational arsine intoxication. *J Toxicol Environ Health*, 52:331–42.

Blackwell M, Robbins A (1979). Arsine (arsenic hydride) poisoning in the workplace. NIOSH Current Intelligence Bulletin 32. *Am Ind Hyg Assoc J*, 40:A56–61.

Cheraghali AM, Haghqoo S, Shalviri G, *et al.* (2007). Fatalities following skin exposure to arsenic. *Clin Toxicol*, 45:965–7.

Danielson C, Houseworth J, Skipworth E, *et al.* (2006). Arsine toxicity treated with red blood cell and plasma exchanges. *Transfusion*, 46:1576–9.

DePalma AE (1969). Arsine intoxication in a chemical plant. Report of three cases. *J Occup Med*, 11:582–7.

Dueñas-Laita A, Pérez-Miranda M, González-López MA, *et al.* (2005). Acute arsenic poisoning. *Lancet*, 365:1982.

Fowler BA, Weissberg JB (1974). Arsine poisoning. *N Engl J Med*, 291:1171–74.

Guha Mazumder DN (2008). Chronic arsenic toxicity & human health. *Indian J Med Res*, 128:436–47.

Guha Mazumder DN, Ghoshal UC, Saha J, *et al.* (1998). Randomized placebo-controlled trial of 2,3-dimercaptosuccinic acid in therapy of chronic arsenicosis due to drinking arsenic-contaminated subsoil water. *J Toxicol Clin Toxicol*, 36:683–90.

Hatlelid KM, Brailsford C, Carter DE (1996). Reactions of arsine with hemoglobin. *J Toxicol Environ Health*, 47:145–57.

Hatlelid KM, Carter DE (997). Reactive oxygen species do not cause arsine-induced hemoglobin damage. *J Toxicol Environ Health*, 50:463–74.

International Agency for Research on Cancer (2004). Arsenic in drinking water. In: *IARC monographs of the Evaluation of Carcinogenic Risks to Humans*, Vol. 84, pp. 41–267. Lyon: IARC.

International Programme on Chemical safety (2001). *Environmental Health Criteria 224. Arsenic and Arsenic Compounds*, 2nd edition. Geneva: World Health Organization.

International Programme on Chemical safety, Czerczak S (eds) (2002). *Concise International Chemical Assessment Document No. 47. Arsine: Human Health Aspects*. Geneva: World Health Organization.

Kim LHC, Abel SJC (2009). Survival after a massive overdose of arsenic trioxide. *Crit Care Resusc*, 11:42–5.

Kitchin KT (2001). Recent advances in arsenic carcinogenesis: modes of action, animal model systems, and methylated arsenic metabolites. *Toxicol Appl Pharmacol*, 172:249–61.

Lenz K, Hruby K, Druml W, *et al.* (1981). 2,3-dimercaptosuccinic acid in human arsenic poisoning. *Arch Toxicol*, 47:241–3.

Moore DF, O'Callaghan CA, Berlyne G, *et al.* (1994). Acute arsenic poisoning: absence of polyneuropathy after treatment with 2,3-dimercaptopropanesulphonate (DMPS). *J Neurol Neurosurg Psychiatr*, 57:1133–5.

Pakulska D, Czerczak S (2006). Hazardous effects of arsine: a short review. *Int J Occup Med Environ Health*, 19:36–44.

Phoon WH, Chan MOY, Goh CH, *et al.* (1984). Five cases of arsine poisoning. *Ann Acad Med Singapore*, 13:394–8.

Pullen-James S, Woods SE (2006). Occupational arsine gas exposure. *J Natl Med Assoc*, 98:1998–2001.

Rael LT, Ayala-Fierro F, Carter DE (2000). The effects of sulfur, thiol, and thiol inhibitor compounds on arsine-induced toxicity in the human erythrocyte membrane. *Toxicol Sci*, 55:468–77.

Romeo L, Apostoli P, Kovacic M, *et al.* (1997). Acute arsine intoxication as a consequence of metal burnishing operations. *Am J Ind Med*, 32:211–16.

Song Y, Wang D, Li H, *et al.* (2007). Severe acute arsine poisoning treated by plasma exchange. *Clin Toxicol*, 45:721–7.

Stenehjem A-E, Vahter M, Nermell B, *et al.* (2007). Slow recovery from severe inorganic arsenic poisoning despite treatment with DMSA (2.3-dimercaptosuccinic acid). *Clin Toxicol*, 45:424–8.

Teitelbaum DT, Kier LC (1969). Arsine poisoning. Report of five cases in the petroleum industry and a discussion of the indications for exchange transfusion and hemodialysis. *Arch Environ Health*, 19:133–43.

Vantroyen B, Heilier J-F, Meulemans A, *et al.* (2004). Survival after a lethal dose of arsenic trioxide. *J Toxicol Clin Toxicol*, 42:889–95.

Wax PM, Thornton CA (2000). Recovery from severe arsenic-induced peripheral neuropathy with 2,3-dimercapto-1-propanesulphonic acid. *J Toxicol Clin Toxicol*, 38:777–80.

Wilkinson SP, McHugh P, Horsley S, *et al.* (1975). Arsine toxicity aboard the Asiafreighter. *Br Med J*, 3:559–63.

Winski SL, Barber DS, Rael LT, *et al.* (1997). Sequence of toxic events in arsine-induced hemolysis in vitro: implications for the mechanism of toxicity in human erythrocytes. *Fundam Appl Toxicol*, 38:123–8.

Zilker T, Felgenhauer N, Pfab R, *et al.* (1999). Little effect of haemodialysis and CAVHDF on the elimination of arsenic compared to DMPS treatment. *J Toxicol Clin Toxicol*, 37:400–1.

Cadmium

Background

Cadmium is a heavy metal found naturally in zinc containing ores. Cadmium toxicity was first recognized in the 19th century in zinc smelter workers. Cadmium is found as a number of salts, e.g. cadmium oxide, chloride, and sulfate. Cadmium is used in the production of plastics, pigments, and dyes; the production of nickel-cadmium/lithium-cadmium batteries; cement manufacture; and in soldering and electroplating. Clinically significant exposure generally results from occupational inhalational exposure or hobbies involving cadmium products. This is more likely to occur when workers are employed in enclosed areas with poor ventilation and with poor occupational hygiene.

Environmental cadmium exposure generally results from eating food grown in soil contaminated with cadmium in industrial areas.

Toxicokinetics

Cadmium is poorly absorbed (5–20%) after oral ingestion, with poorer absorption at higher dose. Oral absorption is increased by iron/calcium deficiency and decreased by zinc/magnesium co-ingestion. Cadmium is well absorbed (50–75%) after inhalational exposure. There is limited absorption of cadmium through intact skin. Cadmium is highly protein bound and carried in red blood cells. It distributes to the liver and kidneys where it binds metallothionein. Within the kidneys it is concentrated in proximal tubular cells. Cadmium has a long half-life of up to 10 years.

Mechanisms of toxicity

Cadmium increases the formation of reactive oxygen species, increasing oxidative stress. It binds sulphydryl groups, inhibits mitochondrial metabolism, and interferes with intracellular calcium and zinc transport. Cadmium has a high affinity for metallothionein; metallothionein-bound cadmium is less toxic than free cadmium, particularly within the kidneys.

Clinical features—acute poisoning

Inhalational exposure to cadmium can result in severe, potentially fatal, toxicity. Low-dose (0.01–$0.15mg/m^3$) inhalational exposure can result in irritant upper respiratory tract symptoms (e.g. cough, throat irritation). There may be a delay in symptoms of up to 6–24 hours followed by headache, fever, cough, and dyspnoea. This can progress to a pneumonitis over the next 1–4 days particularly with high-dose exposure. Severe acute lung injury can develop with hypoxia and pulmonary infiltrates leading to respiratory failure and death. Those exposed to greater than 1–$5mg/m^3$ can develop other early complications including hypotension, arrhythmias, metabolic acidosis, and multi-organ failure. Those who survive an episode of acute cadmium pneumonitis can develop pulmonary fibrosis and/or emphysema.

Clinically significant, acute, oral cadmium ingestions are rare. Small ingestions can cause irritant effects including vomiting and diarrhoea. Larger ingestions can cause haemorrhagic gastroenteritis and systemic toxicity with hypotension, facial/pulmonary oedema, metabolic acidosis, and acute kidney injury.

Cadmium is not absorbed significantly through intact skin and so skin exposure does not result in systemic toxicity; it can, however, be associated with skin irritation.

Clinical features—chronic poisoning

This generally occurs as a result of excess occupational cadmium exposure over more than 5–10 years. However, historically there have been a number of outbreaks of environmental cadmium exposure. The most significant resulted from cadmium contamination of water and rice crops from a mine near the Jinzu River, Japan in the 1950s. This resulted in an epidemic of 'itai itai' (painful osteomalacia and chronic renal failure).

Renal cadmium accumulation results in tubular effects, initially causing low-molecular-weight proteinuria ($beta_2$ microglobulin, retinol binding protein). In more advanced cases glomerular dysfunction can occur with frank proteinuria progressing to chronic renal failure. Chronic cadmium exposure is associated with nephrolithiasis.

Cadmium can disrupt calcium homeostasis and vitamin D metabolism resulting in osteomalacia, osteoporosis, and increased fractures.

Neurological toxicity including extrapyramidal features and olfactory disturbance has been reported.

Long-term follow-up of workers with chronic inhalational cadmium exposure has had conflicting results. It is not clear whether chronic cadmium exposure is associated with restrictive lung defects or emphysema. Pulmonary effects may occur with repeated moderate acute cadmium toxicity causing pneumonitis and subsequent fibrosis.

Carcinogenicity

The IARC classifies cadmium as a human carcinogen. It is associated with an increased risk of lung and possibly prostate cancer.

Management

Patients with significant inhalational cadmium toxicity should be monitored closely for delayed-onset pulmonary effects. Patients may require ventilation and conventional acute lung injury management. There is no evidence that corticosteroids or prophylactic antibiotics are of benefit.

Supportive care of patients with significant oral cadmium exposure may require anti-emetics, fluid resuscitation, and standard management of complications such as hypotension and acute kidney injury. Patients with large-dose exposure may potentially benefit from chelation with agents such as 3,4-dimercaptosuccinic acid (succimer; DMSA) or sodium calcium edetate.

Further reading

Barnhart S, Rokenstock L (1984). Cadmium chemical pnuemonitis. Chest, 86:789–91.

Cantilena LR, Klassen CD (1982). Decreased effectiveness of chelation therapy with time after acute cadmium poisoning. Toxicol Appl Pharmacol 1982;63:173–180.

Johri N, Jacquillet G, Unwin R (2010). Heavy metal poisoning: the effects of cadmium on the kidney. Biometals, 23:783–92.

Liu J, Liu Y, Habeebu SS, Klaasen CD (1998). Susceptibility of MT null mice to chronic CdCL2-induced nephrotoxicity indicates that renal injury is not medicated by the CdMT complex. Toxicol Sci, 46:197–203.

Nogawa K, Kido T, Shaikh ZA (1992). Dose-response relationship for renal dysfunction in a population environmentally exposed to cadmium. IARC Sci Publ, 118:311–18.

Chromium

Background

Most naturally occurring chromium exists as chromite in which chromium is in the Cr^{3+} state which is relatively non-toxic. In contrast, many industrial applications (especially metal finishing and pigments) use chromates in which chromium is in the Cr^{6+} oxidation state which is both highly toxic and a confirmed human carcinogen (see later in section). Even industries utilizing predominantly Cr^{3+} (leather tanning, some metal finishing and pigment manufacture) or Cr^0 (ferrochromium alloys and stainless steel) may incur exposure to Cr^{6+} as a precursor, a by-product or an impurity. A schematic representation of the principal pathways of chromium processing is shown in Figure 10.1. Some commonly encountered chromate (Cr^{6+}) compounds include sodium dichromate ($Na_2Cr_2O_7$), sodium chromate (Na_2CrO_4), potassium dichromate ($K_2Cr_2O_7$), and ammonium dichromate ($[NH_4]_2Cr_2O_7$).

Toxicokinetics

Hexavalent chromium compounds are highly reactive, powerful oxidizing agents that are reasonably well absorbed by all routes of exposure. Some reduction of ingested Cr^{6+} occurs in the stomach. Absorbed chromates (CrO_4^-) readily cross cell membranes through anion channels. In contrast, trivalent chromium is much less reactive and less well absorbed though absorption does still occur. Trivalent chromium crosses cell membranes only by phagocytosis or complexed with transferrin. Within cells reduction of Cr^{6+} to Cr^{3+} occurs. Elimination of absorbed chromium is predominantly renal.

Mechanisms of toxicity

Although hexavalent chromium salts are recognized to be far more toxic than trivalent chromium salts, paradoxically trivalent chromium is the final perpetrator of chromium-induced carcinogenicity. This occurs both via Cr^{3+} binding to cellular and nuclear proteins and as a result of oxidative damage to lipids, proteins and DNA caused by reactive oxygen species produced during the intracellular reduction of Cr^{6+} to Cr^{3+}.

Clinical features—acute poisoning

Inhalation

Inhaled soluble hexavalent chromium compounds, such as sodium and potassium chromate and dichromate and chromic acid (hexavalent chromium oxide) mist, are highly irritant to mucous membranes causing inflammation of the nasal mucosa, hoarseness, cough, bronchospasm, and dyspnoea. Headache, chest pain, pulmonary oedema, and cyanosis may ensue.

Ingestion

Ingestion of highly water-soluble hexavalent chromium compounds leads within minutes to nausea, vomiting, abdominal pain, diarrhoea, and a burning sensation in the mouth, throat, and stomach; gastrointestinal haemorrhage is a frequent complication. Methaemoglobinaemia, haemolysis, disseminated intravascular coagulation, and renal and hepatic failure have been reported.

Topical exposure

Chromic acid splashes produce severe burns. Percutaneous absorption may lead to kidney and liver failure; fatalities have occurred.

Clinical features—chronic poisoning

Inhalation

Inhalation of hexavalent chromium compounds has led to atrophy, ulceration, and perforation of the nasal septum. Pharyngeal and laryngeal ulcers may also occur. Asthma may be precipitated by exposure to fumes. Lung fibrosis, bronchitis, emphysema, and proximal tubular damage have resulted from occupational exposure.

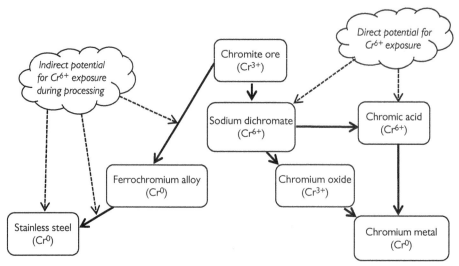

Fig 10.1 Principal pathways of industrial chromium processing and sources of hexavalent chromium exposure.

Topical exposure

'Chrome ulcers' may develop after repeated topical exposure to hexavalent chromium compounds. Hexavalent chromium compounds are also skin sensitizers and contribute to the development of cement dermatitis and contact dermatitis from paint primer, tanned leather, tattoo pigments, and matches.

Carcinogenicity

Hexavalent chromium is classified by the IARC in group I, that is, a confirmed human carcinogen. This involves both genotoxic and non-genotoxic mechanisms associated with the intracellular reduction of Cr^{6+} to Cr^{3+}. Occupational inhalation of Cr^{6+} is associated with an increased incidence of lung cancer and there is ongoing controversy regarding acceptable inhaled Cr^{6+} limits in the workplace. There is also evidence that excess chromium ingestion via contaminated drinking water is associated with increased mortality from lung and stomach cancer though the threshold for this effect remains unknown.

Management

Management of occupational chromium poisoning is primarily by avoiding exposure via instigation of appropriate health and safety measures including, where applicable, monitoring of airborne hexavalent chromium concentrations. Systemic uptake of chromium can be assessed by measuring blood and urine chromium concentrations.

Inhalation

Management of chromic acid mist inhalation is supportive with oxygen, bronchodilators, and mechanical ventilation as required. Chemical pneumonitis associated with pulmonary oedema should be treated with continuous positive airway pressure or in severe cases with intermittent positive pressure or positive end-expiratory pressure ventilation. Antibiotics will be required if pneumonia develops.

Ingestion

Corrosive ingestion requires prompt vigorous resuscitation and early grading by endoscopy or CT scan with contrast. Early surgical excision of necrotic tissue may be lifesaving. Management is otherwise supportive. The amount of chromium removed by haemodialysis or haemodiafiltration is small and these measures only increase chromium clearance significantly in patients with established renal failure. Successful liver transplantation has been performed in a case of fulminant hepatic failure complicating ingestion of potassium dichromate. Plasmapheresis has been advocated in the treatment of severe systemic chromium poisoning following its use in a patient exhibiting signs of liver and renal toxicity after ingesting some 10 g sodium dichromate. An initial serum chromium concentration was 1820 micrograms/L (normal range <0.52 micrograms/L) and fell to 468 micrograms/L after a 2 L plasma exchange. The patient survived without organ damage. Unfortunately the chromium contents of the plasmapheresis filtrate was not measured. On the basis of this limited experience, early plasmapheresis can be considered in serious cases of hexavalent chromium poisoning, though the high cellular uptake of chromium will limit its overall efficacy.

The role of ascorbic acid is controversial. Animal studies have suggested that parenteral ascorbic acid administered up to 2 hours post ingestion may reduce nephrotoxicity but administration beyond 3 hours resulted in increased toxicity. Based on these data high-dose parenteral ascorbic acid may be considered shortly after exposure but there is insufficient evidence in clinical practice to justify its routine use. The suggested dose is 5–10 g IV within 2 hours of ingestion. Later administration may enhance toxicity by accelerating intracellular hexavalent to trivalent chromium reduction. In addition, high doses of ascorbic acid risk oxalate nephropathy.

The use of dimercaprol, acetylcysteine, and DMPS as chelating agents has been suggested in the management of systemic hexavalent chromium poisoning but their efficacy is unproven. Sodium calcium edetate (1.2–3 g) did not enhance urine chromium excretion in one study of 16 non-chromium poisoned patients. A single dose of sodium calcium edetate 1 g was associated with a fourfold increase in dialysate chromium concentration in a case of potassium dichromate poisoning, but the combined dialysis and renal excretion over the first 400 hours of hospitalization was only 0.16% of the ingested dose.

Topical exposure

Decontamination with copious water is the priority. Early aggressive excision of exposed skin is advocated in all but the most minor chromic acid burns, in order to minimize systemic hexavalent chromium uptake. There are clinical data to support the topical application of 10% ascorbic acid to increase the rate of healing of hexavalent chromium-induced dermatitis and ulceration. The proposed mechanism is reduction of the skin surface of Cr^{6+} to Cr^{3+}. There are however insufficient data to advocate the routine use of ascorbic acid systemically or topically in the treatment of chromic acid burns.

Further reading

Barceloux DG (1999). Chromium. *J Toxicol Clin Toxicol*, 37:173–94.

Beaumont JJ, Sedman RM, Reynolds SD, et al. (2008). Cancer mortality in a Chinese population exposed to hexavalent chromium in drinking water. *Epidemiology*, 19:12–23.

Bradberry SM, Vale JA (1999). Therapeutic review: is ascorbic acid of value in chromium poisoning and chromium dermatitis. *J Toxicol Clin Toxicol*, 37:195–200.

Hruby K, Donner A (1987). 2,3-Dimercapto-1-propanesulphonate in heavy metal poisoning. *Med Toxicol*, 2:317–23.

Iserson KV, Banner W, Froede RC, et al. (1983). Failure of dialysis therapy in potassium dichromate poisoning. *J Emerg Med*, 1:143–9.

Kolacinski Z, Kostrzewski P, Kruszewska S, et al. (1999). Acute potassium dichromate poisoning: a toxicokinetic case study. *J Toxicol Clin Toxicol*, 37:785–91.

Kolacinski Z, Kruszewska S, Winnicka R, et al. (2004). Toxicokinetics of chromium elimination in hemodialysis and forced diuresis based on a case of potassium dichromate intoxication. *J Toxicol Clin Toxicol*, 42:514.

Lin C-C, Wu M-L, Yang C-C, et al. (2009). Acute severe chromium poisoning after dermal exposure to hexavalent chromium. *J Chin Med Assoc*, 72:219–21.

Ryu HH, Jeung KW, Lee BK, et al. (2010). Caustic injury: can CT grading system enable prediction of esophageal stricture? *Clin Toxicol*, 48:137–42.

Stift A, Friedl J, Laengle F (1998). Liver transplantation for potassium dichromate poisoning. *N Engl J Med*, 338:766–7.

Wasser WG, Feldman NS, D'Agati VD (1997). Chronic renal failure after ingestion of over-the-counter chromium picolinate. *Ann Intern Med*, 126:410.

Waters RS, Bryden NA, Patterson KY, et al. (2001). EDTA chelation effects on urinary losses of cadmium, calcium, chromium, cobalt, copper, lead, magnesium, and zinc. *Biol Trace Elem Res*, 83:207–21.

Copper salts

Background

Copper is a component of several enzymes, including tyrosinase and cytochrome oxidase, and is essential for the utilization of iron. Copper salts exist with copper in 1+ or 2+ valency states. Copper(I) compounds tend to be insoluble in water and include copper sulphide, copper cyanide, and copper fluoride. Copper(II) salts are generally water-soluble and include copper carbonate, copper sulfate, and copper chloride. Copper salts are used in fungicides, algicide fertilizers, electroplating, dyes, inks, disinfectants, and wood preservatives.

Acute copper poisoning usually results from the ingestion of contaminated foods or from accidental or deliberate ingestion of copper salts.

Toxicokinetics

Following ingestion copper transport across the intestinal mucosa is facilitated by cytosolic metallothionein, with subsequent transfer of albumin-bound copper to the liver via the portal circulation. Within the liver copper is incorporated into caeruloplasmin which serves as a means of copper detoxification with subsequent excretion via a lysosome-to-bile pathway. An impaired or overloaded biliary copper excretion system results in hepatic copper accumulation, as occurs in Wilson's disease and copper poisoning. Free copper can penetrate the erythrocyte membrane as indicated by the markedly higher whole blood than serum copper concentration within the first few hours following ingestion.

Studies among vineyard sprayers provide evidence that inhaled copper sulfate can be absorbed. Copper sulfate can also be absorbed through the skin.

Mechanisms of toxicity

Free reduced copper(I) can bind to sulphydryl groups and inactivates enzymes such as glucose-6-phosphate dehydrogenase and glutathione reductase. In addition, copper may interact with oxygen species (e.g. superoxide anions and hydrogen peroxide) and catalyse the production of reactive toxic hydroxyl radicals. Copper(II) ions can oxidize haem iron to form methaemoglobin.

Clinical features—acute poisoning

Ingestion

Ingestion causes profuse vomiting with abdominal pain, diarrhoea, headache, dizziness, and a metallic taste. Gastrointestinal haemorrhage, intravascular haemolysis, methaemoglobinaemia, rhabdomyolysis, coma, convulsions, and hepatorenal failure may ensue and fatalities have occurred. Body secretions may have a green or blue discoloration.

Dermal exposure

Copper salts are mild irritants to intact skin. Systemic copper uptake may result from repeated application to broken skin. Contact dermatitis has been reported.

Eye exposure

Copper salts are irritant to the eye and may cause corneal necrosis and opacification if crystals remain in the conjunctival sac.

Clinical features—chronic poisoning

Chronic copper poisoning has been reported predominantly as 'vineyard sprayer's lung' in those spraying fungicides containing copper sulfate. Features include progressive dyspnoea, cough, wheeze, myalgia, malaise, anorexia, micronodular and reticular opacities on chest X-ray (which may coalesce), and a restrictive lung function defect. Lung biopsy may show pulmonary granulomata and fibrosis. Other features include hepatic copper-containing granulomas, hypergammaglobinaemia and hepatomegaly. There is no convincing evidence that copper is carcinogenic in humans.

Investigations

Blood copper concentrations correlate well with severity of intoxication following acute ingestion: a concentration of less than 3 mg/L indicating mild-to-moderate poisoning while greater than 8 mg/L implies severe intoxication. Serum caeruloplasmin concentrations will also be increased in acute copper salt poisoning.

Management

Ingestion

Vomiting occurs invariably following the ingestion of many copper salts. Gastric lavage should not be attempted. Supportive measures are paramount. Ensure adequate fluid resuscitation. Early endoscopy or CT scan with contrast is recommended if corrosive damage is suspected. An early surgical opinion should be sought if there are clinical signs of an acute abdomen or deep ulcers and/or areas of necrosis on endoscopy or CT. Methaemoglobinaemia should be treated with intravenous methylthioninium chloride 1–2 mg/kg.

Oral D-penicillamine 1.5–2 g daily enhances urinary copper elimination in patients with Wilson's disease but confirmed benefit in acute copper salt poisoning has not been demonstrated.

Experimental studies suggest dimercaptopropane sulphonate (DMPS) may be the most effective antidote in copper poisoning. In practice the presence of acute kidney injury in severely poisoned patients often limits the value of antidotes which enhance urine copper excretion. It is advisable to seek expert clinical toxicological advice if chelation therapy is being considered.

Extracorporeal elimination techniques do not significantly enhance copper elimination. Exchange transfusion has been undertaken successfully in patients with copper sulfate-induced haemolysis.

Inhalation

Remove from exposure. Treat symptomatically. There is no established role for steroid therapy in these patients.

Dermal and eye exposure

Thorough decontamination should be followed by symptomatic and supportive measures.

Further reading

Barceloux DG (1999). Copper. J Toxicol Clin Toxicol, 37:217–30.

Malik M, Mansur A (2011). Copper sulfate poisoning and exchange transfusion. Saudi J Kidney Dis Transpl, 22:1240–2.

Sharma A (2010). Acute copper sulfate poisoning: a case report. Indian J Forensic Med Toxicol, 4:4–5.

Stark P (1981). Vineyard sprayer's lung – a rare occupational disease. J Can Assoc Radiol, 32:183–4.

Takeda T, Yukioka T, Shimazaki S (2000). Cupric sulfate intoxication with rhabdomyolysis, treated with chelating agents and blood purification. Intern Med, 39:253–55.

Fluoride (sodium fluoride)

Background

Fluoride (F⁻), the anion of fluorine, is encountered primarily in fluoride compounds, of which the most important are sodium fluoride (NaF), calcium fluoride (CaF_2), and hydrofluoric acid (HF). Hydrofluoric acid is considered separately (see Hydrofluoric acid, pp. 247–248).

Sodium fluoride is added to water supplies, mouthwashes, and toothpastes to protect against dental decay. Fluoride toothpaste contains between 1000 and 1450 ppm fluoride ion (as 0.22–0.312 % w/w sodium fluoride); each mg of sodium fluoride containing 0.45 mg fluoride ion. Calcium fluoride is an industrial compound used in the manufacture of hydrofluoric acid, glass, steel, and in iron processing.

Sodium fluoride is potentially toxic by inhalation and ingestion; the effects are dose dependent. In contrast, calcium fluoride is much less toxic as it is practically insoluble in water and is very poorly absorbed in man. The remainder of this section relates to sodium fluoride.

Toxicokinetics

Fluoride ions released from sodium fluoride are well absorbed following ingestion and inhalation, and are rapidly and widely distributed in both intracellular and extracellular water, though at steady state some 99% of the total body burden of fluoride is retained in bones and teeth. Fluoride is eliminated renally.

Mechanisms of toxicity

Fluoride ions modify a number of enzyme activities. Fluoride has also been shown to inhibit DNA and protein synthesis, impair cell proliferation, and be directly cytotoxic at high concentrations. Some manifestations of toxicity (notably cardiac conduction disturbances) are secondary to fluoride-induced hypocalcaemia (see later in section). Substantial ingestions of sodium fluoride can lead to the formation of hydrofluoric acid within the stomach as a result of reaction with gastric hydrochloric acid.

Clinical features—acute poisoning

Ingestion
Ingestion of less than 5 mg/kg body weight fluoride ion is unlikely to result in symptoms though nausea, vomiting, or diarrhoea may occur. Patients who have ingested 5–10 mg/kg fluoride ion are likely to develop gastrointestinal symptoms but they usually resolve within 24 hours.

With larger fluoride ion ingestions corrosive injury to the gastrointestinal tract ensues, the severity depending on dose. Nausea, vomiting, hypersalivation, abdominal pain, and diarrhoea are likely. In the most severe cases haemorrhagic gastroenteritis occurs and perforation of the gastrointestinal tract is possible. Hypovolaemic shock, respiratory failure and coma may follow (see Hydrofluoric acid, pp. 247–248).

Hypocalcaemia occurs as a result of formation of calcium fluoride and this, along with associated hypomagnesaemia and hyperkalaemia, leads to cardiac conduction disturbances (notably QT prolongation) and an increased risk of ventricular arrhythmias, particularly torsades des pointes. Hypocalcaemia may lead to paraesthesiae, carpopedal spasms, hyperactive reflexes, tetany, and convulsions.

Inhalation
Inhalational exposure may occur in welding (sodium fluoride is widely used in fluxes) or in chemical processing. While acute exposure to high concentrations may cause respiratory tract irritation, most clinical experience of inhalation is in the context of chronic exposure.

Clinical features—chronic poisoning

Chronic fluorosis may occur following prolonged exposure to high fluoride concentrations in water or food or following chronic occupational inhalation. Initial increased bone brittleness and reduced tensile strength may proceed to bone pain, stiffness, limited movement, and in severe cases crippling deformities.

Increased density and coarsened trabeculation of bone and calcification in ligaments, tendons and muscle insertions may be detected on X-ray. Other features include renal impairment and a variety of abnormalities of thyroid function.

Management

Ingestion
An urgent assessment of the airway is required to ensure that there is a clear airway and adequate ventilation. Early fibreoptic endoscopy is indicated to grade the severity of the injury in any patient who has abdominal pain or haematemesis. Monitor the cardiac rhythm in all patients and in any who are symptomatic patients perform an urgent 12-lead ECG and measure the QRS duration and QT interval. All patients should have bloods checked to exclude systemic features. Hypocalcaemia, hypomagnesaemia, and hyperkalaemia should be corrected conventionally.

Inhalation
Remove from exposure. Management is supportive.

Further reading

Arnow PM, Bland LA, Garcia-Houchins S, et al. (1994). An outbreak of fatal fluoride intoxication in a long-term hemodialysis unit. *Ann Intern Med*, 121:339–44.

Augenstein WL, Spoerke DG, Kulig KW, et al. (1991). Fluoride ingestion in children: A review of 87 cases. *Pediatrics*, 88:907–12.

Bayless JM, Tinanoff N (1985). Diagnosis and treatment of acute fluoride toxicity. *J Am Dent Assoc*, 110:209–11.

Cummings CC, McIvor ME (1988). Fluoride-induced hyperkalemia: the role of Ca2+-dependent K+ channels. *Am J Emerg Med*, 6:1–3.

Eichler HG, Lenz K, Fuhrmann M, et al. (1982). Accidental ingestion of NaF tablets by children - report of a poison control center and one case. *Int J Clin Pharmacol Ther Toxicol*, 20:334–8.

Heifetz SB, Horowitz HS (1986). Amounts of fluoride in self-administered dental products: safety considerations for children. *Pediatrics*, 77:876–82.

IPCS. Liteplo R, Gomes R, Malcolm H (eds) (2002). *Environmental Health Criteria 227. Fluorides*. Geneva: World Health Organization.

Lantz O, Jouvin MH, De Vernejoul MC, et al. (1987). Fluoride-induced chronic renal failure. *Am J Kidney Dis*, 10:136–9.

McIvor ME. Acute fluoride toxicity. *Drug Saf*, 5:79–85.

Monsour PA, Kruger BJ, Petrie AF, et al. (1984). Acute fluoride poisoning after ingestion of sodium fluoride tablets. *Med J Aust*, 141:503–5.

Susheela AK, Bhatnagar M, Vig K, et al. (2005). Excess fluoride ingestion and thyroid hormone derangements in children living in Delhi, India. *Fluoride*, 38:98–108.

Lead

Background

Lead has many industrial uses including battery manufacture, solders, pigments, and radiation shielding. Its use as an additive in household paint has ceased but lead-containing paint is still found in UK properties built before the 1960s. In addition, some industrial outdoor paints are still allowed to contain lead due to the weather resistance lead affords.

Occupational exposure is usually by inhalation of lead dust or fumes in lead-using industries or during demolition of old properties. Non-occupational lead exposure can arise from inhalation during property renovation but usually involves ingestion. Important sources of ingested lead are 'traditional' remedies (adults) and old paintwork (children). Cooking with lead-glazed earthenware and contaminated soil or water are other potential sources.

Retained lead particles from pellets or bullets may result in lead poisoning, particularly if the lead source lies in synovial fluid or a highly vascular area.

Toxicokinetics

Between 10% and 80% of ingested or inhaled lead is absorbed into the bloodstream, with children more efficiently absorbing lead than adults, and inhalation a more efficient route of uptake than ingestion. Absorption of lead by inhalation requires generation of respirable-size particles (<5 microns) or lead fume; the latter is generated only by processes that heat lead above 500° C. Lead absorption is also enhanced in the presence of iron or calcium deficiency.

Nearly all lead in blood is contained within red blood cells where it binds to the enzyme δ-aminolaevulinic acid dehydratase (ALAD). Lead is distributed widely and in steady state fits a three-compartment model (Table 10.1).

Elimination is predominantly renal (at least 75%) with some loss also in bile, hair, nails, and sweat. Lead readily crosses the placenta and accumulates in the fetus.

Mechanisms of toxicity

The bivalent lead ion Pb^{2+} can complex with important functional chemical groups including -COOH, -NH$_2$ and -SH and so disrupt the function of enzymes and other biologically important molecules. Lead also can substitute for divalent metallic cations, particularly calcium and zinc. The chemical similarity between lead and calcium explains why more than 90% of the total body burden of lead is in the skeleton.

Among the most important enzymes disrupted by lead are those involved in haem synthesis (Figure 10.2). Inhibition of δ-aminolaevulinate (ALA) dehydratase (the rate limiting enzyme of the haem synthetic pathway) leads to accumulation of ALA. ALA resembles gamma-aminobutyric acid (GABA) and stimulation of GABA receptors is thought to be an important mechanism of lead-induced neurotoxicity. Inhibition of ferrochelatase (Figure 10.2) results in increased concentrations of red cell zinc protoporphyrin (ZPP), measurement of which has

been used as an indication of lead toxicity. Lead also inhibits the enzyme erythrocyte pyrimidine-5'-nucleotidase which is responsible for clearing nucleotides from developing red cells. Accumulation of these molecules in the red cells of lead poisoned patients is detectable as basophilic stippling. Such cells have a reduced life span and face early splenic destruction, a further contributing factor to lead-associated anaemia.

The ability of lead to bind thiol (SH) groups contributes to cellular oxidative stress by depletion of reduced glutathione with increased production of free radicals and the resulting risk of lipid and protein peroxidative damage.

Lead also can complex with the negatively charged polar groups of phospholipid membranes, causing disruption of membrane structure and function. Important manifestations include damage to the myelin sheaths of nerves and the specialized membranes of the blood–brain barrier.

The multiple roles of calcium in cell structure and function provide many potential targets for lead toxicity. The nervous system is particularly vulnerable since calcium contributes to neuronal differentiation, myelination, synapse development and function. The fact that vital neuronal development occurs primarily in early life probably explains the acute sensitivity of the developing brain to lead-induced damage. The ability of lead to substitute for calcium also means it can contribute to the initiation of programmed cell death (apoptosis) for which high intracellular calcium concentrations is an important trigger.

Clinical features

Lead poisoning frequently presents with non-specific features including headache, lethargy, poor concentration/memory difficulties, abdominal pain (usually diffuse but may be colicky), and constipation which may be very severe and contribute substantially to abdominal pain. Anaemia develops as a result of impaired haem synthesis and reduced red cell lifespan. Encephalopathy occurs only with very severe poisoning and is more common in children than adults. Renal effects include reversible proximal tubular dysfunction and, in more severe cases, irreversible interstitial fibrosis and progressive renal insufficiency. Chronic lead poisoning is characterized by foot or (rarely) wrist drop, attributable to a peripheral

Table 10.1 Three-compartment lead distribution

Compartment	Body burden %	t½
Blood	1	35 days
Soft tissues	0.5	40 days
Bone	98.5	10–15 years

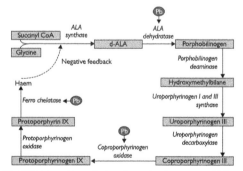

Fig 10.2 Haem biosynthetic pathway showing enzymes inhibited by lead. Reprinted from *Medicine*, 40, 3, Sally M Bradberry, 'Lead and Mercury', pp. 133–134, Copyright 2012, with permission from Elsevier.

primary motor neuropathy, though this manifestation is now uncommon.

It is increasingly recognized that there is no 'safe' blood lead concentration, particularly in young children, with evidence of cognitive impairment even at blood lead concentrations below 10 micrograms/dL (0.48 micromol/L). In children whose maximal blood lead concentrations remained less than 10 micrograms/dL, IQ declined by 7.4 points as lifetime average blood lead concentrations increased from 1 to 10 micrograms/dL.

In adults too there is accumulating evidence that blood lead concentrations previously deemed non-hazardous, do pose risks to health. For example, subclinical reductions in peripheral nerve conduction velocities have been observed in those with blood lead concentrations around 30 micrograms/dL (1.45 micromol/L), renal tubular dysfunction has been detected at blood lead concentrations around 40 micrograms/dL (1.93 micromol/L), and subclinical deficits of neurocognitive function have been observed among lead workers with blood lead concentrations in the range 20–50 micrograms/dL (1–2.4 micromol/L).

Transplacental transfer of lead from mother to fetus leads to reduced fetal viability, reduced birth weight, and premature birth. Male blood lead concentrations around 40 micrograms/dL (1.93 micromol/L) have been associated with reduced semen quality.

Diagnosis and management

Diagnosis may be prompted by the presence of anaemia and basophilic stippling on the blood film and is confirmed by measurement of the whole blood lead concentration (normal <10 micrograms/dL; 0.48 micromol/L). Lead is radio-opaque and ingested or retained lead containing foreign bodies will be visible on X-ray. In chronic lead poisoning the body burden can be estimated using X-ray fluorescence though this is not available widely.

Removal from exposure is the priority. The decision to use chelation therapy is based on the blood lead concentration and the presence of symptoms. If the blood lead concentration is less than 50 micrograms/dL (2.4 micromol/L), the patient is asymptomatic and not pregnant, it is reasonable to monitor the impact of cessation of exposure. The blood lead concentration should be repeated after 2–4 weeks.

All patients with blood lead concentrations of 50 micrograms/dL (2.4 micromol/L) or higher should be considered for chelation therapy. Parenteral sodium calcium edetate 75 mg/kg/day has been the chelating agent of choice for over 50 years but oral DMSA (succimer) 30 mg/kg/day is of similar efficacy. Both chelating agents significantly increase urine lead excretion and reduce blood lead concentrations. DMSA has the potential advantages over sodium calcium edetate that it can be administered orally, has not been associated with nephrotoxicity (though this is rare with sodium calcium edetate at doses not exceeding 80 mg/kg/day) and does not chelate zinc to a clinically significant extent. Sodium calcium edetate typically chelates more lead in the first 48 hours of treatment than does DMSA and although there is no significant difference in lead clearance between the two agents by 4 days' treatment sodium calcium edetate remains the treatment of choice for lead encephalopathy.

DMSA did not improve scores on tests of cognition, behaviour and neuropsychological function in children with blood lead concentrations of less than 45 micrograms/dL. This is explained by the fact that largely irreversible damage has occurred before treatment begins and emphasizes again the crucial role of exposure prevention.

During chelation therapy blood lead concentrations and urine lead excretion should be monitored and a good urine output ensured, if necessary by the administration of supplemental intravenous fluid.

Occupational legislation

The increasing recognition that even low lead exposures are potentially hazardous to health puts substantial pressure on both the lead utilizing industry and governmental bodies responsible for occupational health and safety. The risk management strategy is of necessity a trade-off between the health and environmental benefits of risk reduction and the costs to society of using resources to obtain those benefits.

Legislation to control lead exposure in the workplace varies between countries. In the UK, under the Control of Lead at Work Regulations 2002 and the Approved Code of Practice (ACOP) 2002, employers are required to assess the risks posed to their employees by lead. The risk assessment may include air lead concentration measurements but these are not required for processes known already to be associated with significant lead exposure. Where an employee's occupational lead exposure is deemed significant, they are placed under medical surveillance that involves regular monitoring of blood lead concentrations. In the UK in 2012 a blood lead concentration (in adult males) of 35 micrograms/dL (1.7 micromol/L) is the so-called 'biological initiator value' that triggers regular monitoring. Within the EU the biological initiator value varies between 20–60 micrograms/dL (1–3 micromol/L). In the UK employers are required to investigate circumstances leading to blood lead concentrations of 50 micrograms/dL (2.4 micromol/L) and higher and to suspend an individual from duty if the blood lead concentration reaches 60 micrograms/dL. The biological initiator value for women of reproductive capacity is 20 micrograms/dL (1 micromol/L), with action and suspension values of 25 micrograms/dL (1.2 micromol/L) and 30 micrograms/dL (1.45 micromol/L) respectively.

Further reading

Araki S, Sato H, Yokoyama K, et al. (2000). Subclinical neurophysiological effects of lead: a review on peripheral, central, and autonomic nervous system effects in lead workers. Am J Ind Med, 37:193–204.

Bradberry S, Sheehan T, Vale A (2009). Use of oral dimercaptosuccinic acid (succimer; DMSA) in adult patients with inorganic lead poisoning. QJM, 102:721–32.

Bradberry S, Vale A (2009). Dimercaptosuccinic acid (succimer; DMSA) in inorganic lead poisoning. Clin Toxicol, 47:617–31.

Bradberry SM, Vale JA (2009). A comparison of sodium calcium edetate (edetate calcium disodium) and succimer (DMSA) in the treatment of inorganic lead poisoning. Clin Toxicol, 47:841–58.

Canfield RL, Henderson CR, Jr., Lanphear BP (2003). Intellectual impairment and blood lead levels – the authors reply. N Engl J Med, 349:501–2.

Pergande M, Jung K, Precht S, et al. (1994). Changed excretion of urinary proteins and enzymes by chronic exposure to lead. Nephrol Dial Transplant, 9:613–18.

Rogan WJ, Dietrich KN, Ware JH, et al. (2001). The effect of chelation therapy with succimer on neuropsychological development in children exposed to lead. N Engl J Med, 344:1421–6.

Telisman S, Cvitkovic P, Jurasovic J, et al. (2000). Semen quality and reproductive endocrine function in relation to biomarkers of lead, cadmium, zinc, and copper in men. Environ Health Perspect, 108:45–53.

Manganese

Background

Manganese (CAS 7439-96-5) is a grey-white, silvery, hard, brittle, lustrous transition metal. It is a widely distributed, abundant element, constituting 0.085% of the earth's crust. Manganese is found in minute quantities in water, plants, and animals. Manganese is an essential trace element and is needed for normal prenatal and neonatal development. It also plays a role in bone mineralization, protein and energy metabolism, metabolic regulation, protection against free radicals, and the formation of glycosaminoglycans. It also has a control and regulatory function for some enzyme systems including transferases and hydrolases.

It can be found in more than 100 mineral forms. Mineral forms of manganese that are most common are oxides (pyrolusite, manganite, psilomelane, and hausmannite), silicates (braunite and rhodonite), sulphides (manganese blend and hauserite), and carbonates (manganoan calcite and rhodocrosite). Manganese can exist in inorganic and organic forms; inorganic forms in the oxidation states Mn(II), Mn(III), or Mn (IV) are most often encountered in the environment and in the workplace.

Metallic manganese is primarily used in the manufacture of steel and as an ingredient in the production of ferrous and non-ferrous alloys. More than 90% of the world's manganese consumption is associated with iron and steel production. Manganese reagents are used to reduce oxygen and sulphur and thus remove sulphides and oxides during steel, cast iron, and non-ferrous metal production. As an alloying agent, it imparts increased strength, hardness, and abrasion resistance in finished steel. Manganese can also be combined with aluminium, copper, nickel, silver, and titanium; these alloys are mainly used in chemical/electrical resistance applications. Manganese is used for electrode coating in welding rods and fluxes, for rock crushers, paints, varnishes, inks, dyes, matches, and fireworks, as decolourizers and colouring agents in the glass and ceramics industry and in railway points and crossings. Manganese salts are utilized in fertilizers, as driers for linseed oil, for glass and textile bleaching, and for leather tanning. Manganese chloride is used as a catalyst, in dry-cell batteries, and as an animal feed supplement. An organic manganese compound (manganese ethylene bisdithiocarbamate) is contained in the fungicide Maneb.

Clinical features—acute poisoning

Inhalation

Inhalation of fumes with high concentrations of manganese can rarely cause metal fume fever (see Metal fume fever, p. 283). This mimics a flu-like illness with muscle aches and pain, fever, weakness, cough, vomiting, and sore throat with dryness. Symptoms often occur after several hours following exposure and are self-limiting and disappear after 24–48 hours.

Ingestion

Manganese is less toxic than most metals and so ingestion is unlikely to lead to any acute health effects. There may be some gastrointestinal irritation with large oral doses.

Clinical features—chronic poisoning

Inhalation (and possibly ingestion)

Chronic manganese poisoning occurs after significant inhalational exposure (in the occupational setting welders in particular are at increased risk) and possibly ingestion (from manganese in water and foodstuffs).

Early features include headache, lethargy, irritability, and occasionally psychosis. Seizures, myoclonic involuntary movements, and impaired cognition have also been observed.

Later features include generalized muscle weakness, speech impairment, incoordination, and impotence. Tremor, paraesthesia, and muscle cramps may also be present.

Advanced stages show hypersalivation, inappropriate emotional reactions and parkinsonian symptoms. This has been referred to as 'manganism' and was first reported in 1837 by John Couper in five men who were employed in grinding manganese dioxide in the manufacture of chlorine. There have been many reports in the literature since those first cases.

Although there is evidence that neurological signs and symptoms may be improved after removal from exposure, in most cases they tend to persist or even progress even in the absence of additional exposure.

Investigations

Blood manganese concentrations may be useful to confirm exposure; however, normal reference ranges may not be available and can be difficult to interpret. It is likely that levels above 50 ng/mL whole blood will indicate significant exposure.

Management

This is supportive. Extrapyramidal features may respond to standard parkinsonism treatment regimens, including levodopa, but typically patients with manganism do not respond in the same way.

Sodium calcium edetate has been used to enhance urine manganese excretion but whether this is associated with clinical improvement is controversial.

Further reading

Bingham E, Cohrssen B (eds) (2012). Patty's Toxicology. Hydrocarbons and Organic Nitrogen Compounds. New York: John Wiley & Sons.

Cotzias GC Horiuchi K Fuenzalida, S, et al. (1968). Chronic manganese poisoning Clearance of tissue manganese concentrations with persistence of the neurological picture. Neurology, 18:376.

Franco-Uría A, López-Mateo C, Roca E, et al. (2009). Source identification of heavy metals in pastureland by multivariate analysis in NW Spain. J Hazard Mater, 165:1008–15.

Huang CC, Chu NS, Lu CS, et al. (1998). Long-term progression in chronic manganism: ten years of follow-up. Neurology, 50:698–700.

Ky SQ, Deng HS, Xie PY, et al. (1992). A report of two cases of chronic serious manganese poisoning treated with sodium para-aminosalicylic acid. Br J Ind Med, 49:66–9.

Lee JW (2000). Manganese intoxication. Arch Neurol, 57:597–9.

McMillan G (2005). Is electric arc welding linked to manganism or Parkinson's disease? Toxicol Rev, 24:237–57.

Nordberg GF, Fowler BA, Nordberg M, et al. (eds) (2007). Handbook on the Toxicology of Metals, 3rd edition. Burlington, MA: Elsevier.

Stellman J (1998). Encyclopaedia of Occupational Health and Safety, 4th edition, Vols 1–4. Geneva: International Labour Organization.

Mercury and mercury salts

Background and uses

Mercury is the only metal that is liquid at room temperature. It exists in three states:
- elemental/metallic Hg
- mercurous Hg_2^{2+}
- mercuric Hg^{2+}.

Metallic mercury is a highly mobile, silvery, dense liquid which is volatile even at room temperature. It is used in thermometers, barometers, manometers, sphygmomanometers, dental amalgams, and fluorescent lamps. Mercury forms inorganic mercuric and mercurous salts and organic compounds.

Inorganic mercuric salts have a number of industrial and pharmaceutical uses. For example, mercuric chloride ($HgCl_2$) is used in electroplating and other metal processes as well as in wood, anatomical and biological sample presentation, as a constituent of skin lightening creams, and (historically) as an antiseptic, anticancer drug, and a fungicide. Mercurous chloride (Hg_2Cl_2) is a component of calomel electrodes, calomel paper, and is mixed with gold paint for use on porcelain. It was used formerly as a fungicide, in teething and 'nappy rash' powders, in the treatment of syphilis, as a laxative, diuretic, cathartic, and cosmetic. In Chinese medicine mercurous chloride has been used topically as an antiseptic and orally as a general tonic.

Organic mercury compounds include short-chain alkyl (e.g. methylmercury, ethylmercury), long-chain alkyl (e.g. methoxyethyl), and aryl (e.g. phenylmercury) compounds.

Many organic mercury compounds are man-made but methyl mercury occurs naturally as a result of methylation of inorganic mercury in soil or sea-beds. Historically, organomercury compounds have been used in agriculture as fungicides in, for example, seed dressings. In 1992 all organomercury-containing pesticides were banned under the EC 'Prohibitive Directive'. Ethyl and methyl mercury are the most toxic organomercury compounds since they are well absorbed; dimethyl mercury is particularly toxic.

Toxicokinetics

Elemental mercury

Mercury vapour is highly lipid-soluble and readily traverses cell membranes. Some 80% of inhaled vapour is retained and rapidly oxidized to Hg^{2+} by the enzyme catalase found in most tissues. Prior to oxidation elemental mercury (Hg^0) can cross the blood–brain barrier. Oxidation of Hg^0 within the CNS serves to 'trap' mercury in the brain and explains the susceptibility of the CNS to mercury vapour poisoning.

Liquid mercury is very poorly absorbed (<1%) following ingestion with most passing directly through the gastrointestinal tract.

Mercury compounds

Mercurous salts are less well absorbed following ingestion than are mercuric salts. Organic mercury salts are generally well absorbed and can utilize transmembrane amino acid carriers to facilitate wide distribution. Some organic mercury compounds, e.g. methylmercury, undergo entero-hepatic circulation as complexes with glutathione which are eventually dealkylated by intestinal flora with faecal elimination of the liberated inorganic mercury.

All other systemically absorbed mercury is ultimately metabolized to Hg^{2+} ions and eliminated renally.

Mechanisms of toxicity

The toxicity of all mercury compounds is dependent predominantly on binding to sulphydryl groups, on structural proteins, receptors, enzymes, DNA, and RNA. In the case of elemental mercury and inorganic salts this occurs via the mercuric (Hg^{2+}) ion. While the toxicity of organic mercury compounds is also largely dependent on interactions with sulphydryl groups, the lipid solubility of these compounds facilitates their penetration of lipid bilayers and hence their ability to reach a wider range of cellular targets.

Clinical features

The clinical presentation of mercury poisoning is influenced by the chemical form, the amount involved, the route of exposure, and whether the exposure was a single acute episode or repeated. The CNS is particularly susceptible to mercury poisoning.

Elemental mercury

Inhalation

Acute mercury vapour inhalation causes headache, cough, nausea, a metallic taste, dyspnoea, and chest pain. Chemical pneumonitis may ensue. Repeated exposure to low mercury vapour concentrations presents typically with characteristic neurological features including fine tremor, lethargy, memory loss, insomnia, personality changes, and ataxia. Other features include stomatitis, gingivitis, hypersalivation, and renal tubular damage. Mixed motor and sensory peripheral neuropathy may develop.

Ingestion

Ingestion of metallic mercury is not usually a significant toxicological hazard because less than 1% is absorbed.

Dermal exposure

Discoid eczema, hyperhyridosis, skin erythema, and pruritus can develop following dermal exposure.

Eye exposure

Ocular exposure may lead to conjunctivitis and ocular irritation. The lens may be discoloured grey or brown. Blurred vision, photophobia, reduction of the visual field, altered colour perception and depth of vision are also possible.

Injection

There may be pain, swelling, redness, and abscess formation at the site following subcutaneous injection and granuloma formation may occur. Systemic toxicity may develop with nausea, fever, paraesthesiae and tremor. X-rays may show multiple metallic opacities.

Intravenous administration may result in embolization to the lung and symptoms of pulmonary embolus with pleuritic chest pain, dyspnoea, and hypoxia.

Inorganic mercury salts

Ingestion

Divalent mercuric (Hg^{2+}) salts are substantially more corrosive to the gastrointestinal tract than are monovalent mercurous (Hg^+) salts.

Features following mercuric salt ingestion include burning of the mouth and throat, abdominal pain, nausea, vomiting and/or haematemesis, and diarrhoea which may also be bloody. Oropharyngeal oedema may be sufficiently severe to require tracheostomy. Dehydration, circulatory collapse, and coma may ensue. Acute colitis and intestinal mucosal necrosis are recognized. Fatalities have occurred. Other features described in the acute phase of poisoning include ECG changes (atrial fibrillation, broadening of the QRS complex), transient pancytopenia and increased transaminase, amylase and total creatine kinase activities though these are likely, at least in part, to be secondary to the metabolic disturbances present rather than direct inorganic mercury toxicity.

Patients surviving the acute gastrointestinal phase of mercuric mercury poisoning may go on to develop other features of systemic mercury toxicity, manifest predominantly with renal glomerular and neurological damage (see 'Systemic toxicity').

Mercurous chloride (calomel) used as a teething powder caused 'pink disease' (acrodynia) which is a hypersensitivity reaction characterized by fever, irritability, photophobia, an erythematous desquamating rash, hyperkeratosis of the palms and soles and lymphadenopathy. Systemic features of mercury poisoning may occur following acute or chronic exposures to mercurous salts (see 'Systemic toxicity'). A similar clinical picture has arisen from the use of mercurous chloride in Chinese medicines used as general tonics.

Mercury containing batteries have been banned for a number of years in many countries. Accidental ingestion of batteries containing inorganic mercury salts (e.g. mercuric oxide) may result in local corrosive effects if the battery casing is damaged, though systemic symptoms of mercury poisoning are unlikely.

Dermal exposure

Dermal exposure to inorganic mercuric compounds, notably 'cinnabar' (mercuric sulphide) used as a red dye in tattoos, has caused contact dermatitis and granulomatous reactions. Skin lightening creams and soaps containing calomel (mercurous chloride) or mercuric chloride are still encountered and there are numerous cases of these cosmetics causing systemic mercury toxicity (see 'Systemic toxicity'), particularly after repeated exposures.

Injection

Intravenous injection of mercuric chloride approximately 5 mg/kg daily for 6–12 days caused death from renal necrosis and associated pulmonary oedema.

Mercuric chloride solutions used for intraperitoneal lavage in cancer chemotherapy have also caused death from haemorrhagic colitis and acute tubular necrosis.

Systemic toxicity

Mercuric ions (Hg^{2+}) that reach the circulation from any route of exposure, including the initial exposure being to mercurous salts, accumulate predominantly in proximal tubular cells causing acute tubular necrosis. In addition, in cases of mercuric salt ingestion, reduced renal perfusion associated with hypovolaemic shock also contributes to the onset of renal failure. Substantial or repeated exposure may result in glomerular damage manifest as the nephrotic syndrome with proteinuria and oedema. A type IV hypersensitivity granulomatous interstitial nephritis developed in a patient who recovered from acute tubular necrosis complicating ingestion of a mercuric salt.

Neurological features (presumably due to gradual accumulation of mercury in the CNS) including weakness, irritability, weight loss or failure to thrive (young children), hypersalivation, tremor, and paraesthesiae may also occur.

Reversible hyperintense lesions in the subcortical white matter have been observed on brain MRI in a child with systemic mercury toxicity following topical exposure to a skin whitening cream containing both mercuric and mercurous chloride.

Organic mercury salts

Ingestion

Ingestion of aryl mercury salts such as phenylmercury causes nausea, vomiting, and abdominal pain, with risk of severe irritant effects following substantial ingestions. Systemic mercury poisoning may ensue.

Most cases of human poisoning from alkyl mercury compounds result from ingestion of contaminated foods over a long period. In such patients there is often a latent period of several weeks before the development of systemic, predominantly neurological, features. These include a fine tremor, drowsiness, dizziness, cerebellar ataxia, dysarthria, hyper-reflexia, muscle weakness, memory loss, headache, irritability, confusion, personality changes, insomnia, hearing impairment, blurred vision, diplopia, optic atrophy, constriction of the visual fields, leading to blindness in severe cases, seizures and coma. Fatalities have occurred. There may be pain and paraesthesiae around the mouth and in the limbs, the latter indicative of a peripheral neuropathy.

Gastrointestinal features may accompany or precede neurological features and include nausea, vomiting, diarrhoea, gingivitis, hypersalivation, abdominal pain, and anorexia.

Other reported features include sweating, arthralgia, renal tubular dysfunction, and an erythematous vesicular rash.

Mercury readily crosses the placenta and is extremely toxic to the fetus.

Chronic exposure to methylmercury has been associated with an increased incidence of liver cancer, cirrhosis, renal disease, and cerebral haemorrhage.

Two important epidemics of methylmercury poisoning have occurred in Minamata, Japan and Iraq.

The epidemic of methylmercury poisoning ('Minamata disease') occurred in Minamata, Japan in the 1950s as a result of effluent containing methylmercury being discharged into the Bay by an acetaldehyde manufacturing plant. Consequently, methylmercury bioaccumulated in aquatic species and poisoning followed consumption of contaminated seafood. A second outbreak of Minamata disease occurred in the early 1960s, in the Niigata region, Japan, as a result of methylmercury wastewater being discharged into the Agano River. These two incidents resulted in several thousand cases of methylmercury poisoning.

Fatalities that occurred acutely were due to encephalitis with coma, convulsions, and paralysis. By November 1999, 2263 cases of Minamata disease had been identified in the region of the first outbreak and of these 1368 patients had died. In those exposed chronically to lower concentrations of methylmercury the incidence of liver cancer, cirrhosis, renal disease, or cerebral haemorrhage was significantly higher (p <0.01) than in the general population of Japan.

Infants born to women exposed to methylmercury showed features similar to those of cerebral palsy with growth and mental retardation, hearing impairment, limb deformity, pyramidal symptoms and signs including loss of primitive reflexes, ataxia, hyperkinesia, seizures, dysarthria, strabismus, hypersalivation, and swallowing and learning difficulties.

In Iraq in 1972, 459 of 6000 patients admitted to hospital with methylmercury poisoning following the ingestion of contaminated seed grain used to make bread died; the diagnosis was confirmed analytically.

There was a typically a latent period between cessation of exposure and the development of symptoms. In one study of 125 cases the latent period varied between 16 and 38 days. The earliest and most common symptom reported was paraesthesiae of the extremities or perioral area (~77.5%). Also reported were visual (~53.8%) and hearing (~17.5%) disturbances, ataxia (~62.5%) and dysarthria (~40.0%). The severity of features was dose-dependent. Patients consuming contaminated bread over a short period of time exhibited only paraesthesiae whereas longer periods of consumption resulted in more severe clinical manifestations.

Some children exposed prenatally were born with visual problems (blindness in some cases) and developmental delay.

Inhalation
Acute inhalation may cause features of mucous membrane irritation. Repeated or substantial occupational exposures have resulted in systemic toxicity (see ingestion) though such exposures may have involved multiple routes of exposure and the importance of inhalation alone was not clear.

Dermal exposure
Organomercury compounds are mucous membrane irritants at high concentrations. Death from systemic mercury poisoning has occurred following dermal exposure to dimethyl mercury.

Eye exposure
Organomercury compounds, particularly the aryl compounds such as phenylmercury, are mucous membrane irritants and vesicants at high concentrations. Phenylmercuric acetate used as a preservative in eyedrops has caused a microscopic discolouration and change in transparency of the lens called mercurialentis. Corneal calcification has also been described.

Management
Elemental

Inhalation
Removal from the source of exposure and symptomatic and supportive measures are the mainstay of treatment.

Observe all patients for a minimum of 12 hours. Perform a thorough neurological examination, including visual fields, particularly where chronic poisoning is suspected.

Check U&Es, creatinine, liver function tests, full blood count, and perform a peak flow.

Treat pulmonary oedema and/or acute lung injury with continuous positive airway pressure or in severe cases with intermittent positive pressure ventilation and positive end-expiratory pressure.

Monitor blood and urine mercury concentrations and consider the need for chelation therapy. Take expert advice.

Treat patients with renal failure conventionally.

Ingestion
Usually no specific treatment is required. Confirmation of ingestion can be achieved by X-ray.

Dermal exposure
Wash the affected area with copious amounts of water and treat symptomatically. Remember that patients with substantial skin exposure may have inhaled a significant amount of vapour (see earlier in section).

Eye exposure
Decontamination is the priority with ophthalmological referral for those whose symptoms do not resolve rapidly.

Injection
X-ray the site of injection to confirm the presence of mercury.

Perform chest and abdominal X-rays to identify the site of mercury deposition if injected intravenously, intravesically or intravaginally. Consider surgical removal of mercury deposits if feasible, under X-ray control. Seek specialist advice.

Monitor blood and urine mercury concentrations and consider chelation therapy.

DMPS (unithiol) has been shown to increase urine mercury elimination and reduce blood mercury concentrations. Case reports suggest benefit but there are no controlled studies. DMPS can be administered intravenously or orally. Intravenous DMPS should be given to severely poisoned patients. The dose is 30 mg/kg/day for 5 days, which may be repeated if necessary after 5–7 days. If the intravenous formulation is not available, consider oral DMPS. Since the bioavailability of oral DMPS is only 39%, oral DMPS 77 mg/kg/day would need to be administered to achieve the same plasma drug concentrations as with the intravenous preparation. Seek expert advice.

Inorganic mercury

Ingestion
In severely affected patients critical care input is essential. A supraglottic-epiglottic burn with erythema and oedema is usually a sign that further oedema will occur that may lead to airway obstruction. It is an indication for consideration of early intubation or tracheotomy.

Do *not* attempt gastric lavage.

Save blood and urine for mercury concentration determination.

If confirmation of ingestion is required, inorganic mercuric salts may be visible on abdominal X-ray. They can also be visualized by CT.

Treat haemorrhagic or hypovolaemic shock by replacing lost fluids and blood intravenously.

Perform erect chest X-ray if perforation is suspected.

Parenteral opiate analgesia may be required for pain.

The use of antacids, an (intravenous) H_2 antagonist or proton pump inhibitor may help to reduce the extent of corrosive injury.

An urgent surgical review is recommended if bowel necrosis or perforation is suspected.

Early fibreoptic endoscopy by an experienced endoscopist is indicated to grade the severity of the injury in a patient with drooling, severe pain, dysphagia, vomiting, or stridor and those with evidence of oropharyngeal burns.

Whole-bowel irrigation (WBI) has been used in a patient who developed nausea, vomiting, and abdominal pain after deliberately ingesting mercuric oxide 40 g. This patient had only mild gastrointestinal symptoms and radiopaque material was present in the stomach on initial abdominal X-ray. WBI was continued until X-ray evidence of mercuric oxide was absent.

It is reasonable to consider WBI in similar clinical circumstances.

Chelation therapy with DMPS (see earlier in section) may be indicated in inorganic mercury poisoning. Seek expert advice.

Treat renal complications conventionally. Case reports suggest that the amount of mercury removed during haemodialysis or haemofiltration is insignificant though 1 g was retrieved (12.7% of the ingested dose) of mercuric sulfate via continuous veno-venous haemodiafiltration (CVVHDF) in conjunction with DMPS 750–1500 mg daily in one report. Another report also advocated CVVHDF over HD for elimination of the relatively large complex formed between DMPS and mercury in a patient who survived ingestion of a mercuric salt complicated by renal failure.

There are occasional reports of plasma exchange being used to treat inorganic mercury poisoning but the amount of mercury retrieved by this method does not support its use.

Inhalation

Removal from exposure is the priority.

Save blood and urine for measurement of mercury concentrations. Assess for systemic toxicity, particularly renal and neurological features. Consider the need for chelation therapy in those with systemic toxicity.

Dermal exposure

Carry out decontamination in a well-ventilated area, preferably with its own ventilation system.

Save blood and urine for mercury concentration determination. Assess for systemic mercury toxicity, particularly renal and neurological features.

Consider the need for chelation therapy in those with systemic toxicity. Seek expert advice.

Organic mercury

Ingestion

- The benefit of gastric decontamination is uncertain. Consider activated charcoal (50 g for adults; 1 g/kg for children) if the patient presents within 1 hour of ingestion of any amount.
- Save blood and urine for mercury concentration determination in symptomatic patients. Check U&Es and creatinine.
- Perform a neurological examination including visual fields.
- Observe all patients for a minimum of 12 hours.
- Specialist referral is indicated in patients with systemic features of mercury poisoning and in those found to have increased blood or urine mercury concentrations. Chelation therapy with DMPS may be required in these cases.

Inhalation

Removal from exposure is the priority.

Consider the possibility of systemic uptake following substantial/chronic exposures.

Dermal exposure

Decontamination is the priority.

In chronic exposures or where the dermal barrier has been breached by burns, consider the possibility of systemic uptake.

Eye exposure

Decontamination is the priority.

Patients whose symptoms do not resolve rapidly should be referred for urgent ophthalmological assessment.

Further reading

Aguado S, de Quirós JFB, Marín R, et al. (1989). Acute mercury vapour intoxication: report of six cases. *Nephrol Dial Transplant*, 4:133–6.

ATSDR (1999). *Toxicological Profile for Mercury*. Atlanta, GA: Agency for Toxic Substances and Disease Registry, US Public Health Service.

Bakir F, Damluji SF, Amin-Zaki L, et al. (1973). Methylmercury poisoning in Iraq. *Science*, 181:230–41.

Benz MR, Lee SH, Kellner L, et al. (2011). Hyperintense lesions in brain MRI after exposure to a mercuric chloride-containing skin whitening cream. *Eur J Pediatr*, 170:747–50.

Bluhm RE, Bobbitt RG, Welch LW, et al. (1992). Elemental mercury vapour toxicity, treatment and prognosis after acute, intensive exposure in chloralkali plant workers. Part I: history, neuropsychological findings and chelator effects. *Hum Exp Toxicol*, 11:201–10.

Bradberry SM, Sheehan TMT, Barraclough CR, et al. (2009). DMPS can reverse the features of severe mercury vapor-induced neurological damage. *Clin Toxicol*, 47:894–8.

Chan TYK (2011). Inorganic mercury poisoning associated with skin-lightening cosmetic products. *Clin Toxicol*, 49:886–91.

Ekino S, Susa M, Ninomiya T, et al. (2007). Minamata disease revisited: an update on the acute and chronic manifestations of methyl mercury poisoning. *J Neurol Sci*, 262:131–44.

Koh C, Kwong KL, Wong SN (2009). Mercury poisoning: a rare but treatable cause of failure to thrive and developmental regression in an infant. *Hong Kong Med J*, 15:61–4.

MacLehose R, Pitt G, Will S, et al. (2001). Mercury contamination incident. *J Public Health Med*, 23:18–22.

Nierenberg DW, Nordgren RE, Chang MB, et al. (1998). Delayed cerebellar disease and death after accidental exposure to dimethylmercury. *N Engl J Med* 1998; 338:1672–6.

Pai P, Thomas S, Hoenich N, et al. (2000). Treatment of a case of severe mercuric salt overdose with DMPS (dimercapto-1-propane sulphonate) and continuous haemofiltration. *Nephrol Dial Transplant*, 15:1889–90.

Rowens B, Guerrero-Betancourt D, Gottlieb CA, et al. (1991). Respiratory failure and death following acute inhalation of mercury vapor. A clinical and histologic perspective. *Chest*, 99:185–90.

Sanfeliu C, Sebastia J, Cristofol R, et al. (2003). Neurotoxicity of organomercurial compounds. *Neurotox Res*, 5:283–305.

Song Y, Li A (2007). Massive elemental mercury ingestion. *Clin Toxicol*, 45:193.

Triunfante P, Soares ME, Santos A, et al. (2009). Mercury fatal intoxication: two case reports. *Forensic Sci Int*, 184:e1–e6.

Verma S, Kumar R, Khadwal A, et al. (2010). Accidental inorganic mercury chloride poisoning in a 2-year old child. *Indian J Pediatr*, 77:1153–5.

Weinstein M, Bernstein S (2003). Pink ladies: mercury poisoning in twin girls. *Can Med Assoc J*, 168:201.

Yorifuji T, Tsuda T, Inoue S, et al. (2011). Long-term exposure to methylmercury and psychiatric symptoms in residents of Minamata, Japan. *Environ Int*, 37:907–13.

Metal fume fever

Background and uses

Typically metal fume fever arises as a result of inhalation of metal fumes but occasionally exposure to finely ground dust may produce symptoms. Zinc oxide is involved most commonly. Metal fume fever has also been reported with copper, magnesium, cadmium, chromium, and antimony although more recent evidence suggests these metals do not cause metal fume fever.

Occupational inhalation of metal fumes occurs during zinc welding and smelting and causes a dose-dependent inflammatory response in the lung. It is most likely to occur after exposure to freshly formed fumes in occupations involving high heat and metal vaporization.

A review in 1993 estimated that one in five welders had experienced metal fume fever by the age of 30. Despite improvements in occupational standards in the metal industry, cases still occur. For example, 26 cases were reported to the Louisiana Poison Control Center between 2004 and 2006. The Annual Report of the American Association of Poison Control Centers' National Poison Data System reported that across 60 centres in America there were 399 enquiries regarding adults with suspected metal fume fever in 2010.

Toxicokinetics

There is limited information in humans regarding the toxicokinetics of zinc oxide following inhalation. Increased blood and urine zinc concentrations after inhalation of zinc oxide confirm that zinc is absorbed by this route. Occupational studies provide indirect evidence that zinc distributes to tissues to produce systemic effects. Most zinc is complexed to organic ligands rather than as a solution as metallic ion. Zinc is excreted renally.

Mechanisms of toxicity

The precise pathogenesis of metal fume fever is poorly understood. In an experimental model a dose-dependent increase in the polymorphonuclear leucocyte count was demonstrated in bronchoalveolar lavage fluid obtained 22 hours after exposure in nine welders. A later volunteer study confirmed these findings and demonstrated a concomitant increase in bronchoalveolar lavage fluid pro-inflammatory cytokines triggered by zinc oxide inhalation. This supports an underlying immunological process which is likely since the clinical picture is similar to 'farmer's lung' and other forms of extrinsic allergic alveolitis. More recent studies have further supported a cytokine inflammatory response in the lungs suggesting tumour necrosis factor, IL-8, and IL-6 have roles in mediating metal fume fever.

Clinical features

Symptoms may occur up to 24 hours after fume exposure but more typically occur within the first few hours, and resemble an influenza-like illness with cough, dyspnoea, sore throat, and chest tightness in association with headache, malaise, fever, rigors, sweating, arthralgia, sometimes a metallic taste, nausea, vomiting, and blurred vision. Some ingestion of inhaled particles, following mucociliary clearance from the lungs, could account for the gastrointestinal symptoms.

There may be transient chest X-ray changes (usually ill-defined opacities), increased blood lactate dehydrogenase activity (pulmonary isoenzyme), and an elevated serum zinc concentration during the acute illness. A transient leucocytosis has also been reported.

Symptoms of metal fume fever may improve towards the end of the working week (possibly due to the development of short-term immunity) but reappear after the weekend giving rise to the term 'Monday morning fever'.

Management

Management is largely symptomatic and supportive. The prognosis is usually excellent with complete recovery within 1–4 days if exposure ceases although there are occasional reports of on-going symptoms and signs of airways obstruction in individuals with no previous history of asthma.

Symptomatic patients and those with abnormal respiratory physical signs should have a chest X-ray.

Non-steroidal anti-inflammatory drugs are useful for control of pain and fever.

Supplemental oxygen via face mask may be given if required.

Occupational monitoring

Steps should be taken to ensure that exposure to metal fumes does not occur as more serious chronic features could occur with continued exposure.

Occupational monitoring of workplace air metal oxide concentrations is therefore very important in the prevention of metal fume fever. Several studies have attempted to estimate the zinc concentration associated with the symptoms and signs of metal fume fever but the results are difficult to interpret. Occupational exposure to 8–12 mg zinc/m^3 for up to 3 hours or to a mean zinc concentration of 0.034 mg zinc/m^3 for 6–8 hours produced no adverse effects. In another study no symptoms occurred following 8 hours of occupational exposure to 14 mg zinc/m^3 or 20 minutes of exposure in an experimental setting to 45 mg zinc/m^3 (as zinc oxide). By contrast, a more recent study described at least one 'classic' symptom of metal fume fever (fever, chills, dry or sore throat, chest tightness and headache) some 4–8 hours after a 2-hour inhalation of 4 mg zinc/m^3 (5 mg zinc oxide/m^3) in each of four volunteers. These symptoms were not accompanied by lung function changes.

Further reading

Ahsan SA, Lackovic M, Katner A, et al. (2009). Metal fume fever: a review of the literature and cases reported to the Louisiana Poison Control Center. *J La State Med Soc*, 161:348–51.

Bronstein AC, Spyker DA, Cantilena LR, et al. (2011). 2010 Annual Report of the American Association of Poison Control Centers' National Poison Data System (NPDS): 28th Annual Report. *Clin Toxicol*, 49:910–41.

Chaplupka AN, Chalupka S (2008). Metal fume fever. *AAOHN Journal*, 56:224.

Fine JM, Gordon T, Chen LC, et al. (1997). Metal fume fever: characterisation of clinical and plasma IL-6 responses in controlled human exposure to zinc oxide fume at and below the threshold limit value. *J Occup Environ Med*, 39:722–6.

Gordon T, Fine JM (1993). Metal fume fever. *Occup Med (Phila)*, 8:504–17.

Kaye P, Young H, O'Sullivan I (2002). Metal fume fever: a case report and review of the literature. *Emerg Med J*, 19:268–69.

Wong A, Greene S, Robinson J (2012). Metal fume fever – A case review of calls made to the Victorian Poisons Information Centre. *Aust Fam Physician*, 41:141–3.

Phosphorus

Background

Elemental phosphorus exists in several crystalline forms (allotropes), red phosphorus being non-toxic and black phosphorus the most stable. Toxicologically, yellow phosphorus (sometimes referred to as white) is the most important allotrope and the subject of this section because of its high toxicity. It is a waxy white/yellow solid with a garlic-like odour. It has a low melting point and has to be stored under water to prevent spontaneous combustion on contact with oxygen. Combustion produces a yellow flame and dense white smoke of phosphorus pentoxide.

Phosphorus is used in the manufacture of phosphoric acid (which is used to make fertilizers and cleaning products), rodenticides, fireworks and military ammunitions.

The fatal dose of elemental phosphorus is often quoted as 1 mg/kg but deaths have occurred at lower doses. Multi-organ toxicity may follow oral, inhalational, or dermal exposure.

Toxicokinetics

Phosphorus oxidizes spontaneously in contact with air to form phosphorus pentoxide, which, by an exothermic reaction, forms phosphoric acid on contact with water. Hence, dermal and gastrointestinal exposures to phosphorus rapidly become exposures to phosphoric acid. Absorption is facilitated by thermal and corrosive damage to dermal/mucosal surfaces. Increased phosphate concentrations in some patients are consistent with the subsequent dissociation of phosphoric acid to phosphate and hydrogen ions.

Mechanisms of toxicity

Phosphorus damages the rough endoplasmic reticulum where protein synthesis occurs. It therefore impairs the synthesis of proteins including enzymes. Hepatotoxicity is due partly to accumulation of triglycerides in the liver with steatosis and fibrosis as a result of inhibition of the synthesis of very-low-density lipoproteins which are vital to lipid transport. Hypocalcaemia is secondary to hyperphosphataemia. In acute poisoning, thermal injury caused by phosphorus combustion is also important as is corrosive injury that results from the formation of phosphoric acid on contact with warm air and moisture.

The mechanisms by which long-term exposure to phosphorus resulted in necrosis of bone ('phossy jaw') are uncertain but are likely to have involved damaged gums or teeth allowing inhaled or ingested phosphorus direct access to bone.

Clinical features—acute poisoning

Fortunately, the yellow phosphorus-containing products that are available to the public and are ingested (rodenticide pastes and fireworks) contain relatively low concentrations of the element so that burns are uncommon and symptomatic hypocalcaemia rare. The consequences are more serious when exposure is the result of explosion of munitions when concentrations are higher and phosphorus may be carried deep into tissues by shrapnel.

Ingestion

Although classically three stages of phosphorus poisoning have been described (see below), it may be more useful to classify patients based on whether the principal presenting features are gastrointestinal (GI) or involve the central nervous system (CNS). In a review of 91 reported cases those presenting with CNS features had a mortality some three times higher than those presenting with GI features.

In the conventional staging system, features occur as follows:

- Stage 1: features generally begin within minutes of ingestion, but may be delayed, and include nausea, vomiting, abdominal pain, burns of the pharynx, oesophagus, and stomach, which may lead to gastrointestinal haemorrhage. In patients who have ingested a substantial amount of phosphorus, cardiovascular and CNS toxicity develops early, with shock in part due to fluid loss and GI haemorrhage. Restlessness, irritability, lethargy, and drowsiness may be present. Cardiovascular collapse and arrhythmias are the most common cause of death within the first 5 days following ingestion. There may be a garlic odour to breath and stools and the faeces and vomitus may be luminescent.
- Stage 2: in some patients there may be a relatively symptom-free period of 24–72 hours.
- Stage 3: this is marked by clinical deterioration, notably hepatorenal failure, CNS toxicity (restlessness, delirium, coma, convulsions and cerebral oedema), cardiovascular toxicity (hypotension, shock, and arrhythmias), and metabolic complications (metabolic acidosis, hypoglycaemia, hyperphosphataemia, and hypocalcaemia); the mortality is high.

Acute hepatocellular necrosis, sometimes with hepatomegaly and a cholestatic component, is the most important late-onset feature. Some patients are clinically jaundiced within as little as 48 hours after ingestion. The prothrombin time is frequently prolonged. Renal damage with albuminuria, microscopic haematuria, hypercalciuria, and hyperphosphaturia is also a potential complication and preservation of the ability to concentrate and acidify the urine suggests mainly proximal tubule involvement. Renal impairment is seldom of such severity that replacement measures are required.

Where death occurs later than 24 hours post ingestion it is usually due to cerebral oedema and haemorrhage complicating fulminant hepatic failure. The earlier hepatic transaminase activities increase and the greater the magnitude of the rise, the poorer the prognosis. Similarly, patients who develop hypoglycaemia and acidosis within the first 72 hours are less likely to survive.

In survivors, recovery usually occurs over 1–3 weeks.

Inhalation

Headache, upper respiratory tract irritation, and non-cardiogenic pulmonary oedema (which may be delayed in onset) have been described. Acute hepatic damage and other manifestations of systemic toxicity may ensue (see 'Ingestion').

Dermal exposure

Skin exposure to elemental phosphorus causes chemical and thermal burns that usually involve less than 10% of body surface area but more extensive areas are damaged in some cases. Similarly the depth of tissue damage varies with no more than erythema and blistering in some cases to full-thickness lesions in others. Affected skin may be yellowish in colour and may give off a white vapour with a garlic-like odour. Even particles of phosphorus that are driven into deeper tissues may 'smoke'. Contaminated skin luminesces in the dark. Lesions are slow to heal.

After some hours systemic toxicity may become apparent, the features being those described under ingestion. Sudden death in patients with phosphorus burns has in some cases been attributed to hypocalcaemia and hyperphosphataemia triggering fatal arrhythmias.

Eye exposure
Irritation, blepharospasm, photophobia, lacrimation, and conjunctivitis. Particles may cause corneal perforation.

Clinical features—chronic poisoning
Historically, chronic industrial inhalational exposure to phosphorus fumes resulted in symptoms including bronchitis, anaemia, cachexia, and mandibular necrosis ('phossy jaw'). The latter was characterized by local swelling and inflammation with a foul-smelling purulent discharge from necrotic bone with secondary bacterial infection.

Management

Ingestion
Gut decontamination with gastric lavage is not recommended as corrosive damage is likely; activated charcoal does not adsorb phosphorus.

Patients whose level of consciousness is impaired require measures to ensure a clear airway and adequate ventilation.

Hypotension/shock should be corrected vigorously with intravenous fluid and inotropes. If metabolic acidosis is not responsive to fluid resuscitation, give intravenous hypertonic (8.4%) sodium bicarbonate.

Early fibreoptic endoscopy by an experienced endoscopist is indicated to grade the severity of the injury in any patient who is symptomatic or has evidence of oropharyngeal burns.

The cardiac rhythm, blood glucose and calcium concentrations, the prothrombin time, and alanine and/or aspartate aminotransferase activities should be monitored and appropriate action taken when clinically significant abnormalities are detected.

Acute liver failure and acute kidney injury are managed conventionally.

Intravenous acetylcysteine has been advocated in the treatment of phosphorus-induced liver failure but there is no evidence that this is beneficial.

Inhalation
There is no specific management following inhalation exposure; where appropriate a chest X-ray and/or arterial blood gases should be performed to assess the degree of pulmonary injury. Management should be as directed by the clinical condition of the patient. If non-cardiogenic pulmonary oedema develops, mechanical ventilation may be required.

Dermal exposure
White/yellow phosphorus represents a toxic, fire, and explosive hazard. Any solid particles adhering to the skin should be brushed away and stored under water. As phosphorus fluoresces under ultraviolet light, remove loose or imbedded phosphorus particles that are visualized under UV light with tweezers, while keeping the phosphorus-contaminated areas immersed in water. Wash contaminated skin with copious amounts of water under low pressure for at least 10–15 minutes. Continuous irrigation can prevent further oxidation and allow removal of particles from the skin surface without re-ignition. The earlier irrigation begins, the greater the benefit. Pay particular attention to mucous membranes, moist areas such as skin folds, fingernails, and ears. Water- or saline-soaked dressings applied to the affected area will allow transportation of patients without re-ignition of the remaining particles, prior to meticulous surgical debridement of all embedded phosphorus particles under anaesthetic. A burns specialist should be consulted as excision or skin grafting may be required. Burns totalling more than 15% of body surface area (>10% in children) will require standard fluid resuscitation as for thermal burns.

Soiled clothing should be placed in a water-filled sealed container clearly labelled as a biohazard.

Topical silver nitrate (1–3% solutions) has been used in 13 humans with up to 15% body phosphorus burns, one-third of which were full thickness. It is claimed to be successful, produce smaller scars, and prevent the development of laboratory abnormalities but has not been subjected to controlled study.

Further reading
Bowen TE, Whelan TJ, Nelson TG (1971). Sudden death after phosphorus burns: experimental observations of hypocalcemia, hyperphosphataemia and electrocardiographic abnormalities following production of a standard white phosphorus burn. *Ann Surg*, 174:779–84.

Eldad A, Simon GA (1991). The phosphorus burn – a preliminary comparative experimental study of various forms of treatment. *Burns*, 17:198–200.

Elizabeth J, Kelkar PN, Gandhi W (1995). Yellow phosphorus poisoning – an unusual presentation. *JAPI*, 43:371–2.

Fernandez OUB, Canizares LL (1995). Acute hepatotoxicity from ingestion of yellow phosphorus-containing fireworks. *J Clin Gastroenterol*, 21:139–42.

Kaufman T, Ullman Y, Har-Sdhai Y (1988). Phosphorus burns: a practical approach to local treatment. *J Burn Care Rehabil*, 9:474–5.

McCarron M, Gaddis GP, Trotter AT (1981). Acute yellow phosphorus poisoning from pesticide baits. *Clin Toxicol*, 18:693–711.

Simon FA, Pickering LK (1976). Acute yellow phosphorus poisoning. *JAMA*, 235:1343–4.

Song ZY, Lu YP, Gu XQ (1985). Treatment of yellow phosphorus skin burns with silver nitrate instead of copper sulfate. *Scan J Work Environ Health*, 11(Suppl 4):33.

Sutters M, Gaboury CL, Bennett WM (1996). Severe hyperphosphatemia and hypocalcemia: a dilemma in patient management. *J Am Soc Nephrol*, 7:2055–61.

Talley RC, Linhart JW, Trevino AJ, et al. (1972). Acute elemental phosphorus poisoning in man: cardiovascular toxicity. *Am Heart J*, 84:139–40.

Thallium

Background

Thallium is a soft and pliable metal which in elemental form is of low toxicity. However, it is easily converted into compounds which are highly toxic. These include thallium hydroxide, thallium oxide, thallium sulfate, thallium nitrate, and thallium chloride.

Thallium sulfate was previously used as a rodenticide but is now banned for this use in many countries. Thallium salts have also been employed in the manufacture of optical and electrical equipment, as catalysts in organic synthesis, and in isotopic form for medical imaging of the myocardium. Thallium was used to treat venereal diseases and ringworm in the past and many cases of severe thallium poisoning resulted. Fatalities have been observed following the ingestion of 8 mg/kg or more of thallium sulfate, but more usually occur after 10–15 mg/kg.

The success of thallium sulfate as a poison can be explained by its odourless, colourless and tasteless properties combined with extreme toxicity by all routes of exposure.

Mechanisms of toxicity

Though understood incompletely thallium toxicity is known to involve the following mechanisms:

Substitution for potassium

Thallium ions (Tl^+) are able to substitute for potassium and therefore cell membranes are potentially permeable to thallium via potassium channels including the Na^+/K^+-ATPase transport system. At high concentrations thallium inhibits the action of the Na^+/K^+-ATPase pump and can alter membrane physical properties by increasing their surface potential, decreasing the fluidity of their anionic regions, and promoting the rearrangement of membrane lipids.

Interaction with thiol groups

Many of the effects of thallium on biological systems can be explained by the interaction of Tl^+ with thiol groups, for example, of cysteine and glutathione. In particular, the interaction of thallium with reduced glutathione and enzymes involved in the glutathione redox system causes loss of cellular protection against oxidative stress.

Interaction with phospholipid membranes

Tl^+ interacts with the phosphate (PO_4^-) portion of phospholipid molecules within lipid bilayers causing rearrangement of membrane lipids and disruption of membrane transport. Thallium binding to cell membrane protein thiol groups further disrupts transmembrane transport, the function of membrane-bound enzymes and receptors.

Mitochondrial disruption

The mitochondria bear specialized phospholipid membranes that support cellular respiration. Thallium-induced damage to these membranes increases mitochondrial permeability to a number of ions, including calcium. Increased intramitochondrial Ca^{2+} triggers opening of a so-called 'transition pore' in the inner mitochondrial membrane, uncoupling of oxidative phosphorylation, acute loss of ATP utilization and synthesis, and cell death by necrosis.

Toxicokinetics

Absorption of thallous salts, particularly the more soluble salts such as sulfate, acetate, or carbonate, is rapid and complete following ingestion, inhalation, or dermal absorption. Thallium has a volume of distribution in man of 4.23 L/kg.

After intravenous injection the concentration versus time course of thallium shows three phases. In the first phase, which takes about 4 hours, thallium is distributed throughout a central compartment which consists of the blood and highly perfused organs such as the kidneys, liver and muscle. The second phase, from 4–24 hours, is mainly determined by the distribution over a slow exchange compartment which consists mainly of the CNS. The third phase, which becomes effective after 24 hours, is mainly determined by the rate of elimination.

Thallium elimination occurs via the kidneys and in faeces; elimination by both routes is slow, particularly via the gut if thallium-induced constipation is present. The ratio of faecal to urinary elimination is approximately 2:1. Thallium is also excreted slowly via the hair and to a lesser extent the nails. Thallium elimination is complicated by the fact that an extensive entero-enteral cycle exists between absorption and secretion with thallium ions transferred from blood to gut lumen against an electrochemical gradient throughout the gastrointestinal tract.

In one human case of poisoning the half-life was 1.96 days and in another approximately 4 days. In patients treated with Prussian blue and charcoal haemoperfusion the half-lives were 1.0–1.7 days.

Thallium can cross the placenta and is found in breast milk.

Clinical features

Features can develop within a few hours following exposure by any route.

Initial symptoms (if ingested) include nausea, vomiting, abdominal pain, and, less commonly, gastrointestinal bleeding which may be severe. Constipation follows in the majority of patients.

Following all routes of exposure, parotid (sialadenosis) and pancreatic damage may occur and pleuritic chest pain has also been reported. After a few days (usually between 2 and 5), paraesthesiae develop which start in the feet and progress to the hands and fingers; painful and tender extremities ('burning feet syndrome') and ascending sensory neuropathy then supervene.

In severe cases confusion, delirium, convulsions, renal failure, respiratory failure, heart failure, and coma occur; the mortality is high.

If death does not occur within the first week, tremor, ataxia, and (usually lower limb) muscle weakness develops, due to the onset of motor neuropathy, which is usually distal. Thus, patients may have the features of a sensorimotor neuropathy. Reflexes are characteristically preserved early in the course of the disease and are frequently found to be brisk rather than reduced. When tendon reflexes are diminished, the ankle jerks are lost first.

Ocular features include nystagmus, ptosis, and abnormalities of gaze due to involvement of the IIIth, IVth, and VIth cranial nerves. Retrobulbar neuritis, facial paralysis, decreased visual acuity, optic atrophy, and defective colour vision may develop.

Electrophysiological studies show abnormalities of the electroretinogram and a delayed visual evoked response. Experimental studies have shown that the retina, particularly the photoreceptor layer, is susceptible to the effect of thallium and that the degree of impairment depends on the duration of exposure and the dose.

Characteristically, alopecia develops within 1–3 weeks and it is often this sign which leads to the diagnosis being made. If the patient survives, the hair usually regrows, but is often abnormally fine and unpigmented.

In the first week, there is often a sudden onset of acne which may be severe and complicated by necrotic lesions. Sweat glands and sebaceous glands are destroyed and the skin becomes dry and slightly scaly. Nail growth is impaired with the development of ridges, Mees' lines and erosion of the proximal parts of the nails.

Anaemia, leucocytosis, eosinophilia, thrombocytopenia, lymphopenia, and abnormal liver function tests have also been reported.

Ocular exposure

Exposure to thallium dust or spray may irritate the eye though serious local effects are unlikely.

Management

Prevent further absorption by removing soiled clothing and wash contaminated skin with soap and water if dermal exposure has occurred.

Consider gastric lavage if a substantial amount has been ingested within 1 hour.

Measure thallium concentrations in blood or urine in cases of suspected toxicity. Seek expert advice. Blood concentrations of greater than 10 micrograms/L (>50 nmol/L) or urine concentrations of greater than 20 micrograms/L (>100 nmol/L) signify clinically significant exposure.

As thallium ions are excreted into the gastrointestinal tract via the saliva, the bile, and through the intestinal mucosa, it is possible to sequester thallium ions in the gut and prevent reabsorption by the oral administration of colloidally soluble Prussian blue (potassium ferrihexacyanoferrate(II)) 250–300 mg/kg/day (~10 g twice daily for an adult). Thallium ions are exchanged for potassium ions in the lattice of the Prussian blue molecule and are subsequently excreted in faeces. During treatment with Prussian blue, plasma concentrations of thallium fall and urine excretion declines exponentially. In contrast, faecal excretion of thallium is detectable even when urine excretion of the metal has ceased and, therefore, administration of Prussian blue should be continued until thallium can no longer be detected in the faeces.

Though limited human data suggest that Prussian blue may be of benefit in thallium intoxication, neurological damage may be permanent even if chelation therapy has been employed.

It is possible that the administration of intravenous potassium might further enhance the excretion of thallium into the gut. In contrast, oral potassium supplements should theoretically be avoided because they are likely to interfere with the exchange between potassium and thallium ions in the gut and so increase the signs of poisoning, though this has not always been observed.

If Prussian blue is not immediately available use repeat-dose activated charcoal (50 g every 4 hours to a total dose of 200 g). As thallium causes ileus later in the course of poisoning, an osmotic laxative should be administered in conjunction with charcoal.

Monitor pulse, blood pressure, respiratory rate, oxygen saturation, and cardiac rhythm.

Perform a 12-lead ECG in all patients and chest X-ray in patients who are symptomatic.

Check U&Es, creatinine, liver function tests, and a full blood count.

Treat convulsions, bradycardia, and hypotension conventionally.

Other agents such as dithizone and sodium diethyldithiocarbamate (dithiocarb) while enhancing thallium elimination, also cause thallium redistribution and are inherently toxic, and should not be employed.

Peritoneal dialysis, haemodialysis, and haemoperfusion have not been shown to be of clinical benefit in thallium intoxication, though clearance is increased. Although forced diuresis enhances thallium elimination, the presence of thallium-induced renal impairment may preclude its use.

Recovery may take many months and residual neurological problems may persist for many years. Attention to mouth hygiene is important as stomatitis is often present and physiotherapy is valuable in ensuring successful rehabilitation.

Further reading

Al Hammouri F, Darwazeh G, Said A, et al. (2011). Acute thallium poisoning: series of ten cases. *J Med Toxicol*, 7:306–11.

Al-Mashhadani Z, Al-Fatlawy A, Abu Nawas K, et al. (2008). Thallium poisoning from eating contaminated cake – Iraq, 2008. *MMWR Morb Mortal Wkly Rep*, 57:1015–18.

Atsmon J, Taliansky E, Landau M, et al. (2000). Thallium poisoning in Israel. *Am J Med Sci* 2000, 320:327–30.

Hoffman RS (2000). Thallium poisoning during pregnancy: a case report and comprehensive literature review. *Clin Toxicol*, 38:767–75.

Hologgitas J, Ullucci P, Driscoll J, et al. (1980). Thallium elimination kinetics in acute thallotoxicosis. *J Anal Toxicol*, 4:68–75.

Kuo H-C, Huang C-C, Tsai Y-T, et al. (2005). Acute painful neuropathy in thallium poisoning. *Neurology*, 65:302–4.

Meggs WJ, Hoffman RS, Shih RD, et al. (1994). Thallium poisoning from maliciously contaminated food. *Clin Toxicol*, 32:723–30.

Moeschlin S (1980). Thallium poisoning. *Clin Toxicol*, 17:133–46.

Mulkey JP, Oehme FW (1993). A review of thallium toxicity. *Vet Hum Toxicol*, 35:445–53.

Pelclová D, Urban P, Ridzon P, et al. (2009). Two-year follow-up of two patients after severe thallium intoxication. *Hum Exp Toxicol* 2009, 28:263–72.

Rauws AG (1974). Thallium pharmacokinetics and its modification by Prussian blue. *Naunyn Schmiedebergs Arch Pharmacol*, 284:295–306.

Sharma AN, Nelson LS, Hoffman RS (2004). Cerebrospinal fluid analysis in fatal thallium poisoning: evidence for delayed distribution into the central nervous system. *Am J Forensic Med Pathol*, 25:156–8.

Villanueva E, Hernandez-Cueto C, Lachica E (1990). Poisoning by thallium. A study of five cases. *Drug Saf*, 5:384–9.

Wainwright AP, Kox WJ, House IM, et al. (1988). Clinical features and therapy of acute thallium poisoning. *QJM*, 69:939–44.

Zhao G, Ding M, Zhang B, et al. (2008). Clinical manifestations and management of acute thallium poisoning. *Eur Neurol*, 60:292–7.

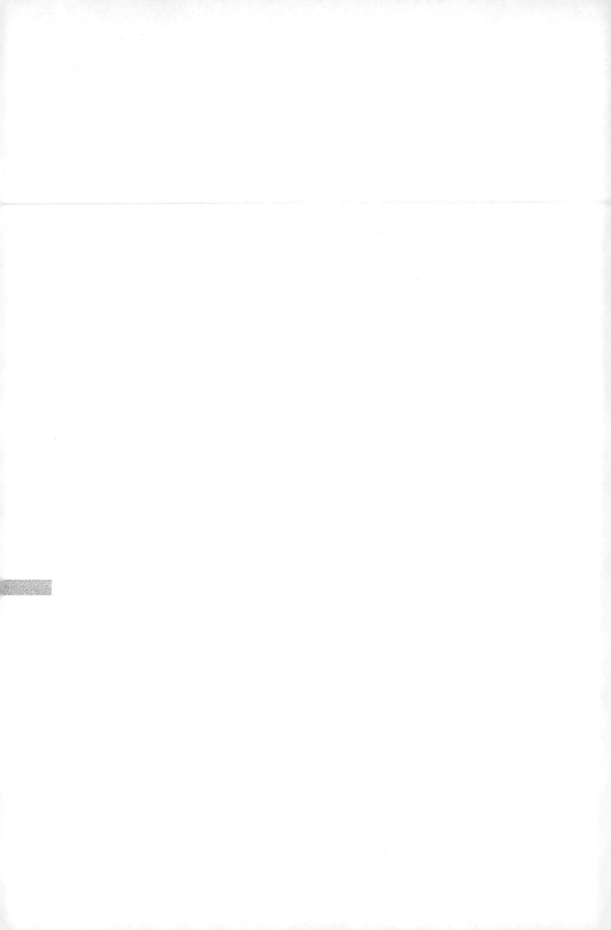

Household products

Detergents

Background

Detergents refer to a class of surfactants (surface active agents) that increase the solubility of contaminants within a solvent. Surfactants contain both polar and non-polar regions that reduce the surface tension of a solvent. In the case of detergents this allows non-polar contaminants, such as grease, to become soluble in water.

Detergents can be classified according to the net charge of the surfactant's functional group:

A. Anionic (e.g. sodium dodecylbenzenesulphonate, which contains $CH_3(CH_2)_{11}C_6H_4SO_2O^-$ ions and is found in washing powders).

B. Cationic (e.g. quaternary amine salts, NH_4^+).

C. Non-ionic polar groups capable of forming hydrogen bonds with water.

Detergent products may consist of one or more of these surfactants. In addition they may also contain disinfectants (see Antiseptics and disinfectants, pp. 292–293); preservatives and other solvents, such as alcohols (see Chapter 9, pp. 205–264).

The majority of cases of poisoning with detergents occur in children under the age of 5 years. In these cases the exposure is usually accidental and occurs in the home. Detergent ingestion in adults tends to be deliberate and subsequent injury is often more severe.

A review of referrals to the UK National Poisons Information Service found that approximately 10% of all telephone enquiries concerned exposure to household products. Detergents accounted for 37% of these enquiries, of which 17% involved liquid detergent capsules, 10% involved dishwasher products, and 10% involved multi-purpose cleaning products.

Liquid detergent capsules (also known as liquitabs or liquid detergent sachets) have been marketed as laundry detergents in Europe since 2001. The capsules or sachets consist of a water-soluble polyvinyl membrane enclosing between 32 and 43 mL of liquid detergent. The detergents are usually a mixture of anionic and non-ionic surfactants along with ethanol (2–5%) and propylene glycol (15–20%) solvents. It should be noted that outside of Europe laundry sachets with greater toxicity are available. A case series from Sri Lanka has described 18 fatalities following ingestion of laundry sachets containing potassium permanganate and oxalic acid.

Dishwasher products, such as sodium silicates, sodium carbonates, and sodium polyphosphates are extremely corrosive and potentially fatal if ingested.

Household liquid detergents containing either anionic or non-ionic surfactants or less than a 10% concentration of cationic surfactant are generally considered to be of low toxicity. Industrial strength detergents of a higher concentration are potentially more caustic however.

Mode of toxicity

The toxicity of older alkali detergents has traditionally been attributed to the alkalinity of the contents. The concentration of surfactant itself may also exacerbate cellular injury. Tissues exposed to alkaline agents undergo liquefactive necrosis characterized by fat saponification, protein dissolution, and cell death as a result of nucleophilic attack by hydroxyl (OH^-) groups. The extent of tissue injury is also dependent on the dose (amount) and

duration of exposure in addition to the type and concentration of detergent.

Clinical features

The clinical features of detergent injury will depend on the route of exposure. A recent study found that the majority of patients are asymptomatic or develop minor features only. Caustics can injure any biological surface that they come into contact with. Exposure may occur through ingestion, eye contact, inhalation, or skin contact. Children may have multiple sites of injury if exposed through bursting liquid detergent capsules.

Gastrointestinal features

These may occur following ingestion. These are usually mild and include vomiting and diarrhoea. In cases where highly caustic detergents, such as dishwasher powders, have been ingested, drooling, dysphagia, and haematemesis may occur. Early and/or severe symptoms coupled with the presence of oropharyngeal lesions suggest the presence of severe oesophageal injury with the risk of perforation or subsequent stricture formation.

Ocular exposure

This most frequently results in conjunctivitis, often accompanied by localized pain. Keratitis has also been recorded and in one case was present 9 days post exposure.

Respiratory features

Respiratory features may arise from aspiration of detergent present in the oropharynx, either at the time of ingestion or secondary to the aspiration of regurgitated gastric contents. Stridor and coughing suggest injury to the upper airway and may herald occlusion secondary to oedema. Bronchospasm or crepitations over the lung fields may suggest aspiration and subsequent risk of a chemical pneumonitis or ARDS, although this appears to be a rare complication.

Skin contact

Skin contact may result in a localized irritation and rash. A true chemical burn may develop following exposure to a caustic detergent. A generalized rash has also been described following the ingestion of liquid detergent capsules by children. It was unclear whether the rash was the result of systemic toxicity or was due to coincidental skin exposure around the time of ingestion.

Systemic features

Cardiovascular collapse and metabolic acidosis may occur secondary to an extensive caustic injury. A reduced level of consciousness, characterized by drowsiness, has been described in children under the age of 2 years following ingestion of liquid detergent capsules. The mechanism of toxicity is unclear but it may reflect the alcohol content of liquid detergent capsules.

General management

Ingestion

Ingestion of detergents usually results in no or minimal symptoms. Minor gastrointestinal systems may be relieved by a small glass of water.

Ingestion of a caustic detergent requires an urgent assessment of the airway and the cardiovascular system. If there is evidence of oedema of the upper airway, early intubation or tracheotomy should be considered. Gastric lavage is contraindicated due to the risk of aspiration and further injury to the upper airway. Chemical neutralization is highly exothermic and should not be attempted due to the risk of thermal injury.

Oesophageal and gastroduodenal endoscopy may be used to evaluate patients following caustic ingestion. Endoscopy may aid the identification of patients requiring surgical intervention and to identify those at risk of developing complications such as stricture or perforation. There is currently little consensus regarding the indications or timing for endoscopy and an early discussion with an upper GI surgeon is recommended in individuals with severe symptoms or following ingestion of a strong alkali. Thoracic CT may assist in determining whether there is local oedema or evidence of mediastinitis.

Surgical advice should also be sought if perforation or necrosis is suspected. Early radical resection of necrotic tissue is associated with improved survival and a lower risk of stricture formation. Corticosteroids have been used to reduce the risk of oesophageal stricture. There is little evidence that they are beneficial and they may even delay or impair wound healing. There is little evidence to recommend prophylactic antibiotic therapy.

Inhalation

Inhalation may occur indirectly through the aspiration of gastric contents. The upper airway should be assessed for potential injury. If there is evidence of oedema of the upper airway, early intubation or tracheotomy should be considered. Injury to the lower airway may result in a pneumonitis or ARDS. A chest X-ray is required if aspiration is suspected. Treatment is supportive. There is no clear evidence to support either the routine use of corticosteroids or prophylactic antibiotic therapy.

Skin

Skin contact with a caustic should be treated by urgent irrigation with water for 10–15 minutes or until the skin pH returns to normal (4.5–7). Any contaminated clothing should be removed. First-aiders should wear appropriate protective equipment to avoid injury. Thereafter the injury should be assessed and treated as a chemical burn.

Eye

Eye contact with a caustic should be treated as an ophthalmic emergency. Alkali solutions can penetrate all layers of the eye and can cause long-term injury such as cataracts, glaucoma, and retinal atrophy.

The eye should undergo urgent irrigation with water or normal saline for 10–15 minutes or until the pH of the conjunctival sac returns to normal (7.5–8.0). A full ophthalmic examination should be conducted, including the use of fluorescein dye to assess for corneal abrasions.

An urgent ophthalmic referral is indicated if any abnormalities are detected, or if the patient remains symptomatic or has been exposed to a strongly alkali solution.

Further reading

Daintith J (ed) (2008). *A Dictionary of Chemistry*. Oxford: Oxford University Press.

Gawarammana IB, Ariyananda PL, Palangasinghe C, et al. (2009). Emerging epidemic of fatal human self-poisoning with a washing powder in Southern Sri Lanka: a prospective observational study. *Clin Toxicol*, 47:407–11.

Kynaston JA, Patrick MK, Shepherd RW, et al. (1989). The hazards of automatic-dishwasher detergent. *Med J Aust*, 151:5–7.

Williams H, Bateman DN, Thomas SH, et al. (2012). Exposure to liquid detergent capsules: a study undertaken by the UK National Poisons Information Service. *Clin Toxicol*, 50:776–80.

Williams H, Moyns E, Bateman DN, et al. (2012). Hazards of household cleaning products: a study undertaken by the UK National Poisons Information Service. *Clin Toxicol*, 50:770–5.

Antiseptics and disinfectants

Background

Antiseptics and disinfectants are chemicals used to kill or inhibit the growth of microorganisms. Antiseptics are intended for use on the skin or mucosal surfaces. Disinfectants are used to decontaminate non-living objects. There is no absolute distinction between the two groups as some chemicals are suitable for both purposes (Table 11.1).

Both antiseptics and disinfectants are available for industrial use or as household products. The distinction is important since industrial grade products tend to have greater concentrations of the active chemical(s) and therefore have a greater potential toxicity.

Domestic poisoning usually occurs in young children under the age of 5 years encountering antiseptic or disinfectants through exploratory behaviour. In these cases the doses ingested tend to be low, partly due to the corrosive nature of the product and also due to the presence of aversant 'bittering' agents in many household products.

The toxicity of individual antiseptics and disinfectants is determined locally by the degree to which it is corrosive to the surface it is applied to. The greater the corrosive actions, then the less likely features of systemic toxicity are to occur. Generally, the disinfectants are more corrosive than the antiseptics. The management of the corrosive effects are considered at the end of this section. The systemic effects are dependent on the chemistry of individual agents and are considered separately in this section, and outlined in Table 11.1. See also Chapter 9, pp. 205–264 for specific chemicals.

Table 11.1 Common antiseptics and disinfectants and their likely toxicity

Chemical	Corrosiveness	Systemic toxicity
Antiseptics		
Ethanol	–	++
Chlorhexidine	+	–/+
Hydrogen peroxide		
Iodine-based	+/++	+/++
Isopropanol	–	++
Propanol	–	++
Disinfectants		
Cresol	++	+++
Dichlorometaxylenol	++	++
Formaldehyde	+++	+++
Hydrogen peroxide	+++	++
Phenol	+++	+++
Quaternary ammonia*	–/+	–/+
Sodium hypochlorite*	–/+	–/+

(–) unlikely; (+) mild; (++) moderate; (+++) severe; (*) concentration dependent (severe if >10%).

Antiseptics

The traditional alcohol solutions (70% ethanol or isopropanol) have been largely replaced by halogenated compounds such as chlorhexidine and iodine. Whilst the localized effects of alcohol antiseptics are minimal they are systemically toxic, central nervous system depression and metabolic disturbances being among the more serious effects (also see Chapter 9, pp. 205–264). It should be noted, however, that tincture of iodine is based in an ethanol solution (50%). The possibility of ethanol toxicity should also be considered.

Chlorhexidine

Chlorhexidine is a bisbiguanide compound that is usually available as a 4% solution. At this concentration it is a mild irritant. Animal studies suggest that chlorhexidine is not systemically toxic occurring following ingestion of up to 150 mg/kg. There is a single case report of hepatitis and oral-oesophageal ulceration following ingestion of approximately 400 mg/kg in man. Gastritis has been reported following chronic ingestion of chlorhexidine.

Iodine

Iodine is used as an antiseptic in solution in its elemental form, or as an iodophor compounded to a high-molecular-weight carrier such as polyvinylpyrrolidone (povidone). The fatal dose of iodine is estimated to be between 2 to 4 g. Clinical features include gastric irritation and erosions, cardiovascular collapse, and, rarely, seizures or renal impairment. Aspiration of iodine-contaminated gastric contents can produce a pneumonitis. The toxicity of iodine is reduced by the presence of food or milk, which increases the conversion of iodine to iodide.

Iodophors limit the release of elemental iodine and are considered to be of lower toxicity. There are cases of cardiovascular collapse following the therapeutic use of povidone in paediatrics and at least one fatality. Burns have also been reported after the use of povidone in surgical patients.

The treatment for iodine or iodophor poisoning is generally supportive management. The thyroid function tests should be requested on admission and the patient reviewed at 4–7 days for features of thyroid dysfunction.

Disinfectants

Phenol

Phenol (carbolic acid), the traditional caustic disinfectant, has been largely substituted by derivative compounds such as cresol and dichlorometaxylenol. Phenol is both locally corrosive and systemically toxic, producing cardiac ventricular arrhythmias, hypotension, metabolic acidosis, methaemaglobin, coma, and respiratory depression. Treatment is supportive.

Cresol

Cresol (cresylic acid or methylphenols) is locally very corrosive and is also topically absorbed through the skin. Systemic features include cardiovascular instability, metabolic acidosis, methaemoglobin (see Chapter 9, pp. 205–264), and initial central nervous system stimulation followed by a decreased level of consciousness and respiratory depression. Treatment is supportive.

Dichlorometaxylenol

Dichlorometaxylenol (chloroxylenol) shares similar features to phenol and cresol toxicity.

Formaldehyde

Formaldehyde is a gas at room temperature. Following inhalation or ingestion of formaldehyde solution, it rapidly reacts with amine groups on proteins and amino acids to liberate hydrogen ions. It is therefore a potent irritant and can cause extensive respiratory tract irritation if inhaled or gastrointestinal injury if ingested. Formaldehyde is also converted to formic acid. Systemic features include a metabolic acidosis with a high anion gap, hypotension, reduced cardiac contractility, and respiratory depression. Treatment is supportive (see Formaldehyde and metaldehyde, pp. 245–246, for more details). Formaldehyde may be prepared in a solution of aqueous methanol. The treatment of concurrent methanol poisoning should also be addressed (see Ethanol and methanol, pp. 236–238).

Hydrogen peroxide

Hydrogen peroxide is an irritant in dilute (3% solution) form and is corrosive at higher concentrations (35% solutions). Hydrogen peroxide reacts with catalase to liberate gaseous oxygen and water. At high concentration the volume of oxygen produced can be significant and may form a gas embolus if it enters the bloodstream. Encephalopathy has also been reported.

Quaternary ammonia

Quaternary ammonia compounds (cationic surfactants) are ammonium chloride derivates. At concentrations less than 10% they are a mild irritant. At higher concentration they are corrosive and may cause extensive damage to the gastrointestinal tract, hypotension, and tachycardia.

Sodium hypochlorite

"Bleach" may be either chlorine-based (containing chlorine or sodium hypochlorite) or oxygen-based (containing hydrogen peroxide, see earlier in this section). Sodium hypochlorite is an irritant at concentrations of less than 10%. Significant toxicity is unlikely unless large concentrations have been ingested (>100 mL). Industrial strength bleaches (>10%) are highly corrosive and can produce significant gastrointestinal injury, with secondary circulatory collapse and metabolic acidosis, if ingested. Bleaches can also react with other cleaning agents to produce chlorine gas (see Chlorine, pp. 225–226).

General management of corrosive injuries

Corrosives can injure any biological surface that they come into contact with. The corrosive effects are a function of both the oxidizing capacity and the pH of the solution. Either strong acids or strong alkalis may cause pain, blistering, penetrating necrosis, and coagulating burns. Cardiovascular collapse and metabolic acidosis may occur secondary to an extensive corrosive injury.

Ingestion

Ingestion of a corrosive should be managed by an urgent assessment of the airway and the cardiovascular system. If there is evidence of oedema of the upper airway, early intubation or tracheotomy should be considered. Gastric lavage is contraindicated due to the risk of aspiration and further injury to the upper airway. Chemical neutralization is highly exothermic and should not be attempted due to the risk of thermal injury. Surgical advice should be sought if perforation or necrosis is suspected. Early radical resection of necrotic tissue is associated with improved survival and a lower risk of stricture formation. There is a risk of perforation associated with early endoscopy. In the event of a serious corrosive injury advice should be obtained from a specialist poisons centre, such as the UK National Poisons Information Service.

Inhalation

Inhalation may occur directly in the presence of a volatile corrosive or indirectly through the aspiration of gastric contents. The upper airway should be assessed for potential injury. If there is evidence of oedema of the upper airway, early intubation or tracheotomy should be considered. Injury to the lower airway may result in a pneumonitis or acute respiratory distress syndrome. Treatment is supportive. There is no clear evidence to support either the routine use of corticosteroids or prophylactic antibiotic therapy.

Skin

Skin contact with a corrosive should be treated by urgent irrigation with water for 10–15 minutes or until the skin pH returns to normal (4.5–7). Any contaminated clothing should be removed. First-aiders should wear appropriate protective equipment to avoid injury. Thereafter the injury should be assessed and treated as a thermal burn.

Eye

Eye contact with a corrosive should be treated with urgent irrigation with water or normal saline for 10–15 minutes or until the pH of the conjunctival sac returns to 7.5–8.0. A full ophthalmic examination should be conducted, including the use of fluorescein dye to assess for corneal abrasions. An urgent ophthalmic referral is indicated if any abnormalities are detected or if the patient remains symptomatic.

Further reading

Catten P, Munoz-Bongrand N, Berney T, et al. (2000). Extensive abdominal surgery after caustic ingestion. *Ann Surg*, 231:519–23.

Massano G, Ciocatto E, Rosabianca C, et al. (1982). Striking aminotransferase rise after chlorhexidine self-poisoning. *Lancet*, 1:289.

Roche SW, Chinn R, Webb S (1991). Chlorhexidine-induced gastritis. *Postgrad Med J*, 67:210–11.

Non-toxic household products

Medical importance

Although a number of products found in the home may be toxic, many are not. However, it is not always immediately apparent to members of the public which products have the possibility to cause harm. For example, many household detergents have a low toxicity, whereas the contents of some liquid detergent sachets may be quite irritant.

Exposure within the home, particularly of small children, may be quite alarming. However, it would be inappropriate for all these potential cases of poisoning to be brought for medical assessment, if all that is needed is reassurance and advice on how to prevent future exposures. Similarly it is important that potentially severe cases are not missed.

Poisons information services may have an important role in advising the public on these 'non-toxic' exposures. Appropriate and timely advice can prevent unnecessary hospital attendances and result in more effective use of resources. Indeed, preventing unnecessary attendances at medical facilities is part of the rationale for the cost-effectiveness of poisons information services, particularly those to which the public have direct access.

Circumstances of exposure

Most commonly it is children less than 5 years old who become exposed to household products. For young children, the exposures are almost invariably accidental: very young children may explore their environment by picking up objects and putting them in their mouths. Assessing the severity of these putative childhood exposures is complicated by the fact that young children are unable to explain what they have done. Some of these accidental exposures may, in fact, be poisoning 'scares' rather than actual exposures. Where ingestion has occurred, the volume ingested by children is often much smaller than is the case seen with deliberate ingestions in older patients.

Consideration should be given to the circumstances of exposure. Accidental exposure in the home may be a sign that children are not living in a safe environment and may be a marker that they are living in a chaotic environment, for example, as a result of parental drug abuse or mental illness. Whilst there is good evidence that child-resistant packaging may be of benefit, evidence for the effectiveness of other interventions to prevent household poisoning is not so clear. An exposure that is trivial in toxicological terms may act as a useful marker that all is not well, and provide an opportunity for a beneficial intervention. Within the United Kingdom, health visitors may be well placed to provide this intervention.

Low-toxicity products

Ingestions of the following products (as formulated in the United Kingdom) rarely result in systemic toxicity and may be regarded as 'low-toxicity' products. The products are often ingested accidentally in small quantities by curious toddlers. Patients (or parents) can usually be reassured if accidentally ingested. The following list details those products which have low toxicity.

General household cleaning products
- Washing up liquids (excluding dishwasher products)
- Fabric conditioners (excluding concentrated products)
- Carpet cleaners
- Washing powders and detergents (excluding concentrated products and liquid detergent sachets).

DIY products
- Emulsion paints
- Wallpaper paste
- Putty.

Cosmetics
- Foundations
- Eye shadows/blushers
- Mascaras
- Lipsticks.

Toiletries
- Soap
- Shampoo
- Handwash/ liquid soap
- Shower gel
- Bubble bath
- Body lotion
- Hand creams
- Moisturizers
- Deodorant
- Shaving foam.

Baby products
- Baby shampoo
- Baby bath
- Baby wipes
- Baby lotion
- Nappy rash creams
- Gripe water/Infacol®.

Pet and plant products
- Cat food
- Dog food
- Fish food
- Flower food
- Baby Bio® plant food
- Plant food.

Arts and crafts products
- Glue stick
- PVA glue
- Crepe paper
- Play-Doh®
- Plasticine®
- Blu-Tack®
- Blackboard chalks
- Felt pens
- Ball point pens
- Pencil lead.

Clinical features

The following are the main clinical features associated with ingestions of these products.

General household products
- Unpleasant taste in mouth
- Gastrointestinal disturbance including nausea, vomiting, or diarrhoea may occur
- Foaming may occur with detergents
- There is a small risk of aspiration if foaming at the mouth occurs.

Cosmetics
- Gastrointestinal symptoms including nausea, vomiting, or diarrhoea
- Theoretical risk of airways obstruction with a solid product.

Toiletries/baby shampoo
- Unpleasant taste in mouth
- Gastrointestinal upset may occur (nausea, vomiting, and diarrhoea)
- There is a small risk of aspiration if foaming at the mouth occurs
- Hand creams and nappy rash creams may cause gastrointestinal upset.

Baby products
Baby wipes have a theoretical potential of causing mechanical obstruction.

Arts and crafts materials
These may be ingested or inhaled as foreign bodies with the potential to cause mechanical obstruction.

Laboratory investigations
Laboratory investigations are not routinely indicated but may need to be considered according to clinical need, e.g. severe vomiting or diarrhoea where biochemical or metabolic disturbance may occur.

Management of ingestions and eye contamination
First-aid treatment
- The patient or parent can usually be reassured.
- Check the packaging of the product in the case of household products to exclude a concentrated product and the presence of a hazard symbol.
- Wash any product off skin paying attention to skin folds and nails.
- If there is product in the eye irrigate with water, if irritation is present continue to irrigate for at least 10–15 minutes.
- If the eye remains irritable after irrigation formal assessment of the eye should be undertaken to assess for corneal injury.
- Ingestions or eye contamination with concentrated products or liquid detergent sachets require urgent medical assessment.

Hospital treatment
Assessment in hospital following accidental ingestion of these products is not usually necessary if the patient is asymptomatic. If there are concerns over the safety or well-being of a child, further assessment and admission is advisable. All non-accidental ingestions require further assessment.

The patient or carers should be advised to seek medical advice should symptoms develop. These include:
- nausea
- vomiting
- diarrhoea
- coughing
- respiratory distress.

Gastric decontamination or induced vomiting with ipecac is *not* recommended. The patient may be encouraged to drink milk or water for the unpleasant taste and to ease gastrointestinal symptoms. In addition, for young children, this may distract them from the incident and provide some reassurance. Simeticone may be used if foaming at the mouth occurs.

Respiratory features requiring urgent assessment
The presence of stridor in a child (particularly in children less than 3 years old) may suggest the presence of an inhaled foreign body. This is often preceded by a history of choking or vomiting.

Supportive treatment
Gastrointestinal symptoms are unlikely to be severe following ingestion of small amounts of these products. Should there be intractable vomiting or diarrhoea intravenous fluid replacement may be necessary along with assessment of urea and electrolytes and replacement as required.

Respiratory symptoms require further clinical assessment a history of foaming at the mouth may suggest a possibility of pulmonary aspiration. A chest X-ray should be performed along with arterial blood gas assessment if clinically indicated.

Drowsiness should not be expected and when present may indicate the ingestion of a more toxic product. In particular, ingestions of liquid detergent sachets have been associated with drowsiness which may be due to the propylene glycol or ethanol content.

Eye injuries
First aid
Eyes should be irrigated with generous volumes of water for at least 10–15 minutes. Topical local anaesthetics can be used to alleviate pain and allow assessment for corneal damage. Examination with a slit lamp and fluorsceine instillation will reveal any corneal injury.

Concentrated products and liquid detergent sachets may cause serious eye damage and symptoms require urgent ophthalmological assessment.

Further reading
Millward LM, Morgan A, Kelly MP (2003). Prevention and reduction of accidental injury in children and older people. Evidence briefing. <http://www.nice.org.uk/niceMedia/documents/prev_accidental_injury.pdf>

NPIS. Low toxicity substance poster: <http://www.nhs-direct.nhs.uk/swallowedorinhaledobjectorsubstance/swallowedsubstance>.

US Dept of Health and Human Services Household products database: <http://householdproducts.nlm.nih.gov/help.htm>.

Pesticides, herbicides, and rodenticides

Organophosphorus insecticides

Background

Organophosphorus insecticides are widely used as agricultural pesticides. They are usually formulated as liquid formulations or granules; the former also contain organic solvents and a surfactant that aid agricultural use.

Toxicity

Organophosphorus insecticides inhibit the synaptic enzyme acetylcholinesterase (AChE). AChE breaks down acetylcholine, curtailing stimulation at cholinergic synapses. By inhibiting AChE, organophosphorus insecticides cause acetylcholine to accumulate, allowing overstimulation of both muscarinic and nicotinic receptors in the autonomic nervous system, central nervous system (CNS), and neuromuscular junction (NMJ).

Organophosphorus insecticides cause relatively long-lived inhibition of AChE compared to carbamates. Spontaneous reactivation does occur slowly, with a half-life of 0.7 hours for dimethyl compounds (see later in section for discussion of alkyl chemistry) and 31 hours for diethyl compounds. However, after a large ingestion of insecticide, reactivated AChE is simply re-inhibited by the organophosphorus insecticide in the blood and extravascular space.

Oximes can reactivate AChE efficiently; again this differs between diethyl and dimethyl compounds. Attached to the AChE, a process of 'ageing' occurs in which one of the alkyl groups is removed from the phosphate. Once ageing occurs, the AChE cannot be reactivated with oximes. Ageing occurs quickly after dimethyl compound poisoning, with a half-life of 3.7 hours. Seven hours post poisoning, already 75% of the AChE is resistant to reactivation. Ageing occurs more slowly after diethyl compound poisoning, giving more time for administration of oximes—the half-life is about 31 hours. Ageing seems to occur almost immediately in S-alkyl organophosphorus insecticides.

Classification of organophosphorus insecticides

Organophosphorus insecticides can be classified according to:

1 whether they are a pro-poison ('thion') or active ('oxon')
2 their rat oral toxicity (LD_{50}; WHO toxicity class)
3 their chemical structure (diethyl, dimethyl, or S-alkyl according to the alky groups attached to the phosphate)
4 lipid solubility.

Each factor has important implications for human toxicity.

Thion or oxon

Many insecticides are thions—such as parathion, chlorpyrifos, or dimethoate—with a sulphur attached to the phosphate atom (P=S). Each must be converted in the body to the active oxon (P=O)—paraoxon, chlorpyrifos-oxon, omethoate, respectively—by cytochrome P450 enzymes in the gut wall or liver before clinical effects occur. A few insecticides are already in the active oxon form, e.g. profenofos, dichlorvos, and therefore do not need activating. Speed of poisoning onset is partially controlled by the requirement for activation after ingestion.

The WHO classification

The WHO classification is divided, based on rat oral LD_{50}, into the following classes:
- class Ia (extremely hazardous)
- class Ib (highly hazardous)
- class II (moderately hazardous)
- class III (slightly hazardous)
- unclassified (unlikely to cause harm).

(Reproduced from *The WHO Recommended Classification of Pesticides by Hazard*, 2009, with permission from the World Health Organization.)

The majority of organophosphorus insecticides are in classes, Ia, Ib, and II; however, the UN Food and Agriculture Organization has recommended withdrawing all class Ia and Ib organophosphorus insecticides from agricultural use due to their high toxicity. Although class II are safer than class I organophosphorus insecticides, the classification is based upon rat toxicity and occupational use, not self-harm. Ingestion of class II compounds in acts of self-harm is highly dangerous and frequently fatal.

Class I organophosphorus insecticides include parathion, methyl-parathion, monocrotophos, methamidophos, and dichlorvos; the more widely used class II organophosphorus insecticides include chlorpyrifos, dimethoate, diazinon, profenofos, fenthion, and quinalphos.

Chemical structure

Dimethyl and S-alkyl organophosphorus insecticides are relatively resistant to pralidoxime administration—little reactivation of AChE occurs with pralidoxime (Figure 12.1). By contrast, AChE poisoned by diethyl organophosphorus insecticides can be reactivated effectively with oximes. However, the clinical benefit of this treatment is currently unclear (see later in this section).

Inhibition of AChE is often slower with dimethyl organophosphorus insecticides, resulting in a slower onset of severe toxicity and a greater opportunity for reaching healthcare before respiratory arrest occurs. Diethyl organophosphorus insecticides include chlorpyrifos, quinalphos, and parathion. Dimethyl compounds include methyl-parathion, monocrotophos, fenthion, and dimethoate. S-alkyl organophosphorus insecticides include methamidophos and profenofos.

Lipid solubility

Lipid solubility of organophosphorus insecticides determines how long cholinergic features may last or how late they may recur. Fat-soluble organophosphorus insecticides quickly enter the fat which then acts as a sump, slowly releasing the insecticide into the circulation. This results in delayed onset, long drawn out poisoning, and sometimes sudden onset of severe cholinergic features with respiratory arrest in a relatively well patient. Although many organophosphorus insecticides are quite fat-soluble, e.g. parathion and chlorpyrifos, problematic fat-soluble insecticides include fenthion and dichlofenthion.

Syndromes of organophosphorus insecticide poisoning

Initial features are predominantly muscarinic; major features include excess sweating, bronchorrhoea, bronchospasm, bradycardia, and hypotension. Most deaths

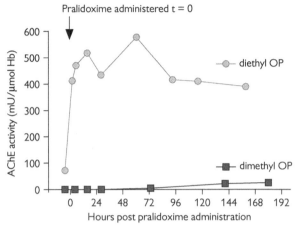

Fig 12.1 Reactivation of red cell AChE after diethyl or dimethyl organophosphorus insecticide poisoning, showing the poor biochemical effect of oximes for the latter.

occur secondary to respiratory failure resulting from loss of central respiratory drive, NMJ failure for the muscles of ventilation, and bronchorrhoea/bronchospasm. Bradycardia and hypotension can be a problem.

Other deaths occur from early complications of acute poisoning rather than the poisoning itself. Some patients develop pulmonary complications after aspirating their gastric contents (insecticide, solvents, gastric acid) with falling level of consciousness. Others will develop hypoxic brain injury following out-of-hospital respiratory arrest. These complications will not respond to the classic antidotes: see later in this section.

Patients severely poisoned by agricultural dimethoate formulations show severe cardiovascular shock, after respiratory failure, that only transiently responds to high dose infusions of vasopressors. This is fatal in the majority of patients presenting with markedly reduced level of consciousness and respiratory failure. Whether other organophosphorus insecticides cause this fatal cardiovascular, rather than respiratory, syndrome is currently unclear.

Many patients develop neuromuscular damage that is revealed as respiratory failure after several days, and after resolution of the cholinergic syndrome (the intermediate syndrome) or as an inability to ventilate as the cholinergic syndrome settles and the level of consciousness rises. This syndrome of neuromuscular dysfunction results in the need for long-term ventilation, often for several weeks, while the NMJ repairs itself. During this time, the patient is at risk of complications of ventilation, including pneumonia and pneumothorax.

Pharmacokinetics and dynamics

Organophosphorus insecticides are absorbed rapidly after ingestion, inhalation, or dermal exposure. There are reports of deaths within 15–30 minutes of ingestion. Low GCS scores, requiring intubation for airway protection, are typical at 30 minutes following parathion exposure.

However, the onset of poisoning may be delayed, due to relatively slow conversion of the thion into the active oxon and due to a slow inhibition of AChE. While parathion is very rapidly activated and very rapidly

inhibits AChE, giving early clinical features, poisoning with dimethoate or fenthion is generally of slower onset due to these issues, as well as modest early reactivation of the AChE.

Fatal dose and case fatality

The fatal dose is variable but will depend on the toxicity of the specific insecticide, concentration of the active compound in the formulation (usually 20–60%), presence and toxicity of co-formulated solvents, speed of onset, availability of healthcare, and person's age.

A fatal dose for the class Ib insecticide parathion is likely to be in the 20–50 mL range; a fatal dose for class II insecticides is probably bigger, in the 50–200 mL range.

Many deaths from class I organophosphorus insecticides occur before hospital, especially where healthcare facilities are distant. Therefore hospital case series likely represent an underestimate. Case fatality is likely to be around 20–40% for these compounds.

Class II insecticides cause slower, less severe toxicity, allowing patients to reach hospital before respiratory arrest occurs. As a result, hospital case series are likely to be more accurate. A recent publication from Sri Lanka has reported case fatalities ranging from 4.8% (95% confidence interval (CI) 1.3–11.7) to 20.6% (95% CI 17.9–23.6) for self-poisoning with the class II organophosphorus insecticides diazinon and dimethoate, respectively.

Clinical features

Key early signs of the acute cholinergic syndrome include constricted pupils (miosis) and excess sweating. Other features include headache, nausea, vomiting, diarrhoea, hypersalivation, abdominal pain, blurred vision, muscle weakness, fasciculations, chest tightness, coughing, bronchospasm, and bronchorrhoea. Cardiovascular signs may include hypotension and sinus tachycardia or bradycardia.

In severe cases, progressive respiratory failure will occur with bradypnoea, abdominal breathing, and dyspnoea in unconscious patients that requires intubation and ventilation. Seizures are uncommon; one reason for their occurrence is hypoxia due to poor airway control.

Features of acute cholinergic toxicity usually resolve over the first few days. However, they may last longer or recur suddenly at a later time point in relatively well patients who have ingested fat-soluble compounds.

Patients may develop NMJ failure over the first few days, with or without cholinergic features. Proximal muscle weakness, perhaps with cranial nerve palsies, may lead to sudden respiratory arrest. Such patients will require long-term ventilatory support.

Days or weeks after the poisoning, the patient may develop a peripheral predominantly motor neuropathy that persists for months. Some recovery usually occurs.

Management

Ensure a clear airway, adequate ventilation, and removal of bronchial secretions. Intubate early if there is risk of respiratory arrest or poorly controlled airway.

Lie the patient in the left lateral position to slow absorption of the pesticide and reduce the risk of aspiration.

Patients with clinically significant hypoxia, bradycardia, and/or hypotension require oxygen and atropine (see later in section) before skin and/or gastric decontamination.

Avoid contaminating yourself! Wear protective clothing.

Prevent further absorption according to the route of exposure:

• Remove to fresh air.
• Remove soiled clothing and wash contaminated skin with soap and water.
• Consider gastric aspiration and gentle lavage if a substantial amount has been ingested within 1 hour. Care should be taken to protect the airway, particularly if a hydrocarbon solvent is involved or if consciousness is depressed. Use an NG tube—aspirate the stomach contents and then lavage the stomach with 3 × 300 mL of fluid at room temperature.

Give oxygen as required; however, reduced oxygen saturations will improve with atropine alone as it treats the bronchorrhoea and bronchospasm.

Monitor pulse, blood pressure, respiratory rate, and cardiac rhythm in symptomatic patients.

If there is bronchorrhoea, bronchospasm, hypoxia, and/or marked hypotension, give atropine (2.0 mg for adults and 0.02 mg/kg for children) urgently by the intravenous route. Further bolus doses of atropine 2 mg in an adult (0.02 mg/kg in children) should be given every 5–10 minutes until the chest is clear, the heart rate is greater than 80/minute, and the blood pressure is adequate.

However, Eddleston et al. (2004) have proposed that in severe organophosphorus insecticide poisoning the dose of atropine should be doubled every 5–10 minutes until clinical improvement (see earlier in section) begins to be seen. Then smaller doses of atropine can be given until the patient is cardiovascularly stable (adequate blood pressure and heart rate) with adequate ventilation (clear lungs to auscultation). This satisfactory condition is termed 'atropinization'. Abedin and colleagues (2012) have recently shown in an RCT that this doubling dose regimen markedly improves clinical outcome.

Once the patient is atropinized, start an infusion of atropine in normal saline. Give about 10–20% of the total dose of atropine required to atropinize the patient every

hour. The patient should then be carefully observed, particularly over the first couple of hours, to ensure that the infusion rate is adequate and not toxic. If inadequate, give bolus doses to regain control; if toxic (see next paragraph), stop the infusion for 30–60 minutes and then restart at a slightly lower rate.

Atropine toxicity (agitation, confusion, urine retention, hyperthermia, ileus, and tachycardia) can make management difficult. Therefore, it is important that the patient is closely monitored and that the dosing of atropine is titrated to the patient's features and response.

There is controversy as to the effectiveness of pralidoxime or obidoxime (not licensed for use in the UK). A recent Cochrane review concluded that there was insufficient evidence to determine whether oximes are beneficial to poisoned patients. Patients requiring atropine should be given pralidoxime 1 g over 5 minutes and then 6 hourly for up to 3 days. Higher doses seem to be associated with an increased risk of complications in patients who are not intubated. An alternative regimen is obidoxime 250 mg as a loading dose over 30 minutes, then 750 mg over the next 24 hours.

Patients receiving pralidoxime or obidoxime should be observed carefully for signs of respiratory arrest. Such patients will need intubation and ventilatory support.

Give diazepam 10–20 mg (0.1–0.3 mg/kg in children) if the patient is agitated.

Patients need to be careful monitored for delayed respiratory failure (the intermediate syndrome). The first signs are a difficulty with flexing the neck against resistance while lying down. At the first sign of mild weakness, ventilatory tidal volumes should be measured regularly (e.g. every 4 hours). Falling tidal volumes will require intubation and mechanical ventilation until recovery occurs.

Further reading

Abedin MJ, Sayeed AA, Basher A, et al. (2012). Open-label randomized clinical trial of atropine bolus injection versus incremental boluses plus infusion for organophosphate poisoning in Bangladesh. *J Med Toxicol*, 8:108–17.

Buckley NA, Eddleston M, Li Y, et al. (2011). Oximes for acute organophosphate pesticide poisoning. *Cochrane Database Syst Rev*, 2:CD005085.

Dawson AH, Eddleston M, Senarathna L, et al. (2010). Acute human lethal toxicity of agricultural pesticides: a prospective cohort study. *PLoS Med*, 7:e1000357.

Eddleston M, Dawson A, Karalliedde L, et al. (2004). Early management after self-poisoning with an organophosphorus or carbamate pesticide – a treatment protocol for junior doctors. *Critical Care*, 8:R391–7.

Eddleston M, Eyer P, Worek F, et al. (2005). Differences between organophosphorus insecticides in human self-poisoning – a prospective cohort study. *Lancet*, 366:1452–9.

Eddleston M, Mohamed F, Davies JOJ, et al. (2006). Respiratory failure in acute organophosphorus pesticide self-poisoning. *Q J Med*, 99:513–22.

Eddleston M, Buckley NA, Eyer P, et al. (2008). Medical management of acute organophosphorus pesticide poisoning. *Lancet*, 371:597–607.

Jayawardane P, Dawson AH, Weerasinghe V, et al. (2008). The spectrum of intermediate syndrome following acute organophosphate poisoning: a prospective cohort study from Sri Lanka. *PLoS Med*, 5:e147.

Carbamates

Background

Carbamates are used as insecticides for garden, medicinal, agricultural and veterinary use. They are formulated as pellets, granules, and liquid formulations. The latter usually contain an organic solvent and a surfactant that aid agricultural use.

There are many carbamates marketed across the world. Examples include: pirimicarb, bendiocarb, fenobucarb, methomyl, carbaryl, and carbosulfan.

Toxicity

Similar to organophosphorus (OP) insecticides, carbamates inhibit the synaptic enzyme acetylcholinesterase (AChE). AChE breaks down acetylcholine, curtailing stimulation at cholinergic synapses. By inhibiting AChE, carbamates therefore cause acetylcholine to accumulate, allowing overstimulation of both muscarinic and nicotinic receptors in the autonomic nervous system, CNS, and NMJ.

Initial features are predominantly muscarinic with major features including excess sweating, bronchorrhoea, bronchospasm, bradycardia, and hypotension. Most deaths occur due to respiratory failure resulting from loss of central respiratory drive, NMJ failure of the muscles of ventilation, and bronchorrhoea/bronchospasm, or alternatively to the complications of the acute respiratory arrest or aspiration (see later in section). A case series from India has recently reported high rates of delayed NMJ failure requiring ventilation in carbamate poisoned patients (Indira 2013).

Unlike OPs, carbamates cause only short-lived inhibition of AChE due to spontaneous reactivation of the carbamylated enzyme; 'ageing' (a state in which OP-inhibited AChE cannot be reactivated from) does not occur. As a result, acute toxicity is usually of shorter duration with carbamate insecticides than with OP insecticides.

However, many deaths occur from complications of acute poisoning rather than the poisoning itself. Some patients develop pulmonary complications after aspirating their gastric contents (insecticide, solvents, gastric acid) as their level of consciousness falls; others will develop hypoxic brain injury following out-of-hospital respiratory arrest. These complications will not respond to the classic antidotes: see later in section.

Pharmacokinetics

Carbamate insecticides are absorbed rapidly after ingestion, inhalation, or dermal exposure. However, their blood–brain barrier penetration is reported to be poor in adults (better in children), hence CNS toxicity is relatively uncommon in adults.

There have been no detailed studies looking at how the chemistry of the individual compounds affects pharmacokinetics (as has been done for OP insecticides) or clinical features. Carbamates do not require a metabolic activation to the active form (unlike many OP insecticides). Onset of features is therefore often rapid.

Fatal dose and case fatality

The fatal dose is variable but will depend on the toxicity of the specific carbamate, concentration of the active compound (usually 3–50%) in the formulation, presence and toxicity of co-formulated solvents, and person's age. Toxicity of the carbamate active ingredients, i.e. the technical grade compound rather than the formulated agricultural product with its solvents and surfactants, is graded using the WHO toxicity classification system also used for OP insecticides (see Organophosphorus insecticides, pp. 298–300).

A recent publication from Sri Lanka has reported case fatalities of 1.0% (95% CI 0.3–2.4) and 10.7% (95% CI 7.7–14.5) for carbofuran and carbosulfan self-poisoning, respectively. This might appear paradoxical since carbofuran has a far higher animal toxicity (rat oral LD_{50} 8 mg/kg; WHO class Ib) than carbosulfan (250 mg/kg; WHO class II). The reason for the lower toxicity is the formulation: carbosulfan is a 25% liquid emulsifiable concentrate while the carbofuran is a 3% wettable powder, reducing the quantity of carbamate that can be easily ingested in an act of self-harm.

Of note, the case fatality for carbosulfan is actually higher than several OP insecticides, despite carbamates having a reputation for being less toxic than OPs.

Clinical features

Key early signs include constricted pupils (miosis) and excess sweating. Other features include headache, nausea, vomiting, diarrhoea, hypersalivation, abdominal pain, blurred vision, muscle weakness, fasciculations, chest tightness, coughing, bronchospasm, and bronchorrhoea. Cardiovascular signs may include hypotension, sinus tachycardia, or bradycardia.

In severe cases, progressive respiratory failure will occur with bradypnoea, abdominal breathing, and dyspnoea in unconscious patients. Seizures are uncommon; one reason for their occurrence is hypoxia due to poor airway control.

Features of acute cholinergic toxicity usually resolve within 24 hours; complications may take much longer to resolve.

Management

Ensure a clear airway, adequate ventilation, and removal of bronchial secretions. Intubate early if there is risk of respiratory arrest or a poorly controlled airway.

Lie the patient in the left lateral position to slow absorption of the pesticide and reduce the risk of aspiration if the patient vomits.

Patients with clinically significant hypoxia, bradycardia, and/or hypotension require oxygen and atropine (see later in section) before skin and/or gastric decontamination.

Avoid contaminating yourself! Wear protective clothing.
Prevent further absorption according to the route of exposure:

• Remove to fresh air.

• Remove soiled clothing and wash contaminated skin with soap and water.

• Consider gastric lavage if a substantial amount has been ingested within 1 hour. Care should be taken to protect the airway, particularly if a hydrocarbon solvent is involved or if consciousness is depressed. Use an NG tube—aspirate the stomach contents and then lavage the stomach with 3 × 300 mL of fluid at room temperature.

Give oxygen as required; however, reduced oxygen saturations will improve with atropine alone as it treats the bronchorrhoea and bronchospasm.

Monitor pulse, blood pressure, respiratory rate, and cardiac rhythm in symptomatic patients.

If there is bronchorrhoea, bronchospasm, hypoxia, and/or marked hypotension, give atropine (2.0 mg for adults and 0.02 mg/kg for children) urgently by the intravenous route. Further bolus doses of atropine 2 mg in an adult (0.02 mg/kg in children) should be given every 5–10 minutes until the chest is clear, the heart rate is greater than 80/minutes, and the blood pressure is adequate.

However, Eddleston et al. (2004) have proposed that in severe carbamate insecticide poisoning the dose of atropine should be doubled every 5–10 minutes until clinical improvement (see earlier in section) starts. Then smaller doses of atropine can be given until the patient is cardiovascularly stable (adequate blood pressure and heart rate) with adequate ventilation (clear lungs to auscultation; 'atropinized'). This doubling-dose approach will markedly speed up the time of the successful atropinization. Abedin and colleagues (2012) have recently shown in an RCT that this doubling dose regimen markedly improves clinical outcome after organophosphorus poisoning. A similar benefit can be expected from carbamate poisoning.

Once the patient is atropinized, start an infusion of atropine in normal saline. Give about 10–20% of the total dose of atropine required to atropinize the patient every hour. The patient should then be carefully observed, particularly over the first couple of hours, to ensure that the infusion rate is adequate and not toxic. If inadequate, give bolus doses to regain control; if toxic, stop the infusion for 30–60 minutes and then restart at a slightly lower rate.

Atropine toxicity (agitation, confusion, urine retention, hyperthermia, ileus, and tachycardia) can make management difficult. Therefore, it is important that the patient is closely monitored and that the dosing of atropine is titrated to the patient's features and response.

There is controversy as to whether pralidoxime increases the toxicity of carbamate poisoning. All available evidence comes from rat studies. There is therefore insufficient evidence either to recommend or to contraindicate its use in severe carbamate poisoning in humans.

Patients need to be careful monitored for delayed respiratory failure (the intermediate syndrome). The first signs are a difficulty with flexing the neck against resistance while lying down. At the first sign of mild weakness, ventilatory tidal volumes should be measured regularly (e.g. every 4 hours). Falling tidal volumes will require intubation and mechanical ventilation until recovery occurs.

Further reading

Abedin MJ, Sayeed AA, Basher A, et al. (2012). Open-label randomized clinical trial of atropine bolus injection versus incremental boluses plus infusion for organophosphate poisoning in Bangladesh. J Med Toxicol, 8:108–17.

Dawson AH, Eddleston M, Senarathna L, et al. (2010) Acute human lethal toxicity of agricultural pesticides: a prospective cohort study. PLoS Med, 7:e1000357.

Eddleston M, Dawson A, Karalliedde L, et al. (2004). Early management after self-poisoning with an organophosphorus or carbamate pesticide – a treatment protocol for junior doctors. Critical Care, 8:R391–7.

Eddleston M, Phillips MR (2004). Self poisoning with pesticides. BMJ, 328:42–4.

Indira M, Andrews MA, Rakesh TP (2013). Incidence, predictors, and outcome of intermediate syndrome in cholinergic insecticide poisoning: a prospective observational cohort study. Clin Toxicol, 51:838–45.

Lifshitz M, Rotenberg M, Sofer S, et al. (1994). Carbamate poisoning and oxime treatment in children: a clinical and laboratory study. Pediatrics, 93:652–5.

Ragoucy-Sengler C, Tracqui A, Chavonnet A, et al. (2000). Aldicarb poisoning. Hum Exp Toxicol, 19:657–62.

Other insecticides: pyrethroids, nicotine, and neonicotinoids

Pyrethroids

Pyrethroids were introduced into agricultural practice in the 1970s; they are also widely used in public health campaigns to combat insect-borne diseases and in the home as ingredients of household insecticides, topical treatments for lice, and veterinary treatments for cats and dogs.

Pyrethrin was first isolated from *Chrysanthemum cinerariaefolium*; however, it was unstable in light and more stable synthetic analogues were therefore developed. These pyrethroids are divided into class I and class II compounds according to their structure, with the latter having an α-cyano group. Pyrethroid insecticides include the class I compounds: allethrin, permethrin; and the class II compounds: cypermethrin, deltamethrin, fenvalerate.

Toxicity

Pyrethroid insecticides predominantly cause their effects by binding to and disrupting voltage-gated sodium channels in insects, delaying their closure and causing repetitive firing of neurons and conduction block. Class II pyrethroids can also block chloride channels, perhaps resulting in seizures, and affect cardiac sodium channels.

Human toxicity is markedly less than insect toxicity because insects have increased sodium channel sensitivity to the insecticides, smaller body size, slow pyrethroid metabolism, and lower body temperature. The reduced sensitivity of human sodium channels has been mapped to a single amino acid polymorphism in the highly conserved intracellular linker sequence between the S4 and S5 transmembrane segments.

Pyrethroids are commonly formulated as powders or low concentration liquids, reducing the likelihood that large amounts of the active ingredient will be ingested.

Deaths are relatively infrequent; in one case series of 573 cases (40% by occupational exposure), seven deaths occurred (1.2%). In another series of 203 cases (the majority (60%) with etofenprox) admitted to Sri Lankan secondary hospitals, two deaths occurred (1.0%). Of 37,397 exposures to pyrethroids reported to the US Toxic Exposure Surveillance System in 2001–2003, only three deaths occurred.

Toxicokinetics

Absorption of pyrethroids via the skin is poor. By contrast, absorption is better after ingestion, the plasma concentration peaking at 3 hours. Elimination is slow due to distribution into fat.

Pyrethroids are metabolized by plasma esterases and cytochrome P450s. They are often therefore formulated with an inhibitor of these enzymes—an organophosphorus or carbamate insecticide, or piperonyl butoxide, respectively—to prolong their activity.

Clinical features

The main effect of pyrethroid poisoning after dermal exposure is paraesthesia, particularly of the face, that may be exacerbated by scratching, water, heat, or sunlight. It comes on over 2 hours, peaks at 6 hours, and generally disappears by 24 hours. Large dermal exposures may result in muscle tremor and/or spasm, pain, and numbness in the affected area. Other features include pruritis, tingling, or burning sensation.

Ingestion results initially in gastrointestinal features, including throat pain, oral ulceration, nausea, vomiting, and abdominal pain. These features are followed by systemic toxicity over the next 2 days including, headache, dizziness, palpitations, chest tightness and blurred vision. The most serious toxicity is coma and seizures. Severe complications include aspiration pneumonitis and pulmonary oedema, likely caused by the solvent co-formulants.

Inhalational exposure may produce symptoms and signs of nasal and pulmonary tract irritation.

Management

Ensure a clear airway, adequate ventilation, and removal of bronchial secretions. Intubate early if there is risk of respiratory arrest or poorly controlled airway.

Lie the patient in the left lateral position to slow absorption of the pesticide.

Avoid contaminating yourself! Wear protective clothing.

Prevent further absorption according to the route of exposure:

• Remove to fresh air.
• Remove soiled clothing and wash contaminated skin with soap and water.
• Consider gastric aspiration and lavage if a substantial amount has been ingested within 1 hour. Care should be taken to protect the airway, particularly if a hydrocarbon solvent is involved or if consciousness is depressed. Use an NG tube—aspirate the stomach contents and then lavage the stomach with 3 × 300 mL of fluid at room temperature.

Give oxygen as required.

Monitor pulse, blood pressure, respiratory rate, and cardiac rhythm in symptomatic patients.

Patients should be carefully monitored for signs of aspiration, respiratory failure, and seizures. Treat symptomatically, using benzodiazepines, phenobarbital, and general anaesthesia for seizures. There is no specific antidote; however, topical application of *dl*-α-tocopherol acetate (vitamin E) may give symptomatic relief.

Patients without symptoms at 6 hours are unlikely to become significantly ill.

Nicotine and neonicotinoid insecticides

These insecticides are agonists of nicotinic acetylcholine receptors, through which they mediate their effects. Nicotine is isolated from the tobacco plant and has been used for centuries as a moderately effective but toxic insecticide. Neonicotinoids are synthetic analogues that were developed in the 1970s–1990s; they have lower acute mammalian toxicity due to increased selectivity for insect receptors. Neonicotinoids are available as liquid and granule formulations.

Neonicotinoid insecticides include: acetamiprid, clothianidin, imidacloprid, nitenpyram, nithiazine, thiacloprid, and thiamethoxam.

Toxicity

Nicotine and neonicotinoid insecticides cause their effects by stimulation of nicotinic acetylcholine receptors in the central nervous system of insects. Human toxicity from nicotine poisoning occurs due their effects on post-synaptic (predominantly α4β2) nicotinic acetylcholine receptors in the central nervous system. Human toxicity is less severe with neonicotinoids than nicotine due to the former's selective toxicity for insects over vertebrates, partly due to a higher affinity for insect than vertebrate receptors, and due to poor CNS penetration.

Two medium-size case series of imidacloprid poisoning have been reported together with many cases reports of imidacloprid poisoning and one of acetamiprid poisoning. Moderate to severe features have been consistent with nicotinic overstimulation; there are also reports of possible muscarinic features.

A retrospective case series reported 70 patients notified to a Poison Control Centre in Taiwan who had been exposed to neonicotinoids (90% imidacloprid). The patients were relatively old (median age: 58 years; range: 2–84 years) and had ingested a median of 75 mL (range: 30–200 mL). Two patents died, five developed aspiration pneumonia, and six developed respiratory failure. In contrast, a prospective study of 68 Sri Lankan patients admitted to hospital reported no deaths, no cases of aspiration pneumonia, and one case of respiratory failure. The milder clinical features in this series may be due to the patients being younger (median age: 28; range: 13–72) and drinking a smaller quantity (median volume: 15 mL (IQR=10–15 mL)).

The pesticide is formulated in the solvent N-methyl-2-pyrrolidone. This compound is irritant to skin and mucous membranes and may be responsible for the GI ulceration and bleeding seen in some patients

Pharmacokinetics

Imidacloprid is rapidly absorbed; distribution and/or elimination appear to be initially slow. Further information on human metabolism is not currently available.

Clinical features

Early signs are predominantly GI and include nausea, vomiting, abdominal pain, and diarrhoea. Headache and dizziness are also common.

Nicotinic features include tachycardia and mydriasis, with seizures and coma in severe toxicity. Excessive sweating has been reported. Respiratory failure occurs, with or without aspiration pneumonia.

GI bleeding may occur

Management

Ensure a clear airway, adequate ventilation, and removal of bronchial secretions. Intubate early if there is risk of respiratory arrest or poorly controlled airway.

Lie the patient in the left lateral position to slow absorption of the pesticide.

Avoid contaminating yourself! Wear protective clothing.

Prevent further absorption according to the route of exposure:

- Remove to fresh air.
- Remove soiled clothing and wash contaminated skin with soap and water.
- Consider gastric aspiration and lavage if a substantial amount has been ingested within 1 hour. Care should be taken to protect the airway, particularly if a hydrocarbon solvent is involved or if consciousness is depressed. Use an NG tube—aspirate the stomach contents and then lavage the stomach with 3 x 300 mL of fluid at room temperature.

Give oxygen as required.

Monitor pulse, blood pressure, respiratory rate, and cardiac rhythm in symptomatic patients.

Patients should be carefully monitored for signs of aspiration, respiratory failure, and seizures. Treat symptomatically. There is no specific antidote.

Due to possible corrosive effects of the solvent, patients with features of upper airway injury should undergo endoscopic assessment of the vocal cords, and the airway should be secured.

Further reading

Bradberry SM, Cage SA, Proudfoot AT, et al. (2005). Poisoning due to pyrethroids. *Toxicol Rev*, 24:93–106.

Dawson AH, Eddleston M, Mohamed F, et al. (2010). A prospective cohort study of the acute human lethal toxicity of agricultural pesticides – implications for improving regulation and reducing global suicide. *PLoS Med*, 7:e1000357.

Soderlund DM (2012). Molecular mechanisms of pyrethroid insecticide neurotoxicity: recent advances. *Arch Toxicol*, 86:165–81.

Imamura T, Yanagawa Y, Nishikawa K, et al. (2010). Two cases of acute poisoning with acetamiprid in humans. *Clin Toxicol*, 48: 851–3.

Mohamed F, Gawarammana I, Robertson TA, et al. (2009). Acute human self-poisoning with imidacloprid compound: a neonicotinoid insecticide. *PLoS One*, 4:e5127.

Phua DH, Lin CC, Wu ML, et al. (2009). Neonicotinoid insecticides: an emerging cause of acute pesticide poisoning. *Clin Toxicol*, 47:336–41.

Tomizawa M, Casida JE (2003). Selective toxicity of neonicotinoids attributable to specificity of insect and mammalian nicotinic receptors. *Annu Rev Entomol*, 48:339–64.

Chlorophenoxy herbicides

Background and uses

Chlorophenoxy (phenoxyacetate) herbicides comprise an aliphatic carboxylic acid moiety attached to a chlorine- or methyl-substituted aromatic ring. Important examples include 2,4-D (2,4-dichlorophenoxyacetic acid) and 4-chloro-2-methylphenoxyacetic acid (MCPA); the formulae for which are shown in Figure 12.2. Chlorophenoxy herbicides typically are formulated as salts or esters and are sometimes coformulated with the hydroxybenzonitrile herbicides ioxynil and/or bromoxynil which generally are more toxic than chlorophenoxy herbicides. 3,6-Dichloro-2-methoxybenzoic acid (dicamba) is not a phenoxyacetate but is an organic acid herbicide and is therefore often considered with the chlorophenoxy compounds. The structures of ioxynil, bromoxynil, and dicamba are shown in Figure 12.3.

Chlorophenoxy herbicides are used for weed control in pastures, cereal crops, and along public rights of way.

Epidemiology

Chlorophenoxy herbicide poisoning is uncommon in the developed world but relatively common in the developing world. For example, 181 patients with MCPA poisoning presented to just three hospitals in Sri Lanka between April 2002 and December 2003. Most serious poisonings are the result of deliberate ingestion of one or more chlorophenoxy herbicides or formulations also containing ioxynil and/or bromoxynil.

Mechanisms of toxicity

The toxicity of chlorophenoxy compounds is exerted principally through the acid form of the pesticide which is derived *in vivo* by dissociation or hydrolysis of the parent ester or salt. Experimental studies indicate the involvement of several mechanisms:

1 Dose-dependent lipid peroxidation-mediated cell membrane damage. This is likely to be important in the mediation of CNS toxicity by damaging the blood–brain barrier and disrupting neuronal membrane transport mechanisms.

2 Interference in cellular metabolic pathways involving acetylcoenzyme A. Chlorophenoxy herbicides are related structurally to acetic acid and are able to form analogues of acetyl-CoA such as 2,4-D-CoA. They can also enter the acetylcholine (ACh) synthetic pathway with the subsequent formation of choline esters (e.g. 2,4-D-ACh) which may act as false cholinergic messengers at muscarinic and nicotinic synapses and effector sites.

3 Uncoupling of oxidative phosphorylation as a consequence of (2) or due to damage to intracellular membranes including those of mitochondria.

4 ATP depletion as a result of (2) and (3). This contributes to the initiation of programmed cell death (apoptosis).

Toxicokinetics

Chlorophenoxy compounds are absorbed rapidly following oral administration in man but dermal and inhalational absorption are limited. Once absorbed, they are extensively bound to serum albumin and have a relatively low volume of distribution (between 0.1 L/kg and 0.2 L/kg for 2,4-D in man). Since these herbicides are acids (the pKa of 2,4-D is 2.73) at physiological pH only a very small percentage is non-ionized and available to penetrate lipid membranes.

Most of an orally administered dose is eliminated unchanged in urine and follows a first-order process, though the renal organic anion secretory system is saturable and if overwhelmed elimination follows Michaelis–Menten kinetics, at least in animals.

Clinical features

Ingestion

Most cases have involved 2,4-D or MCPA. Vomiting is a prominent early feature and may be accompanied by

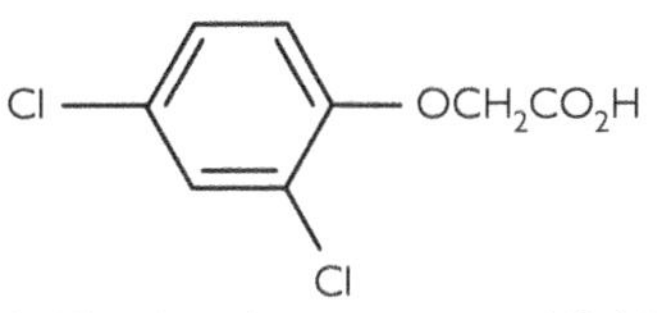

2,4-Dichlorophenoxy acetic acid (2,4-D)

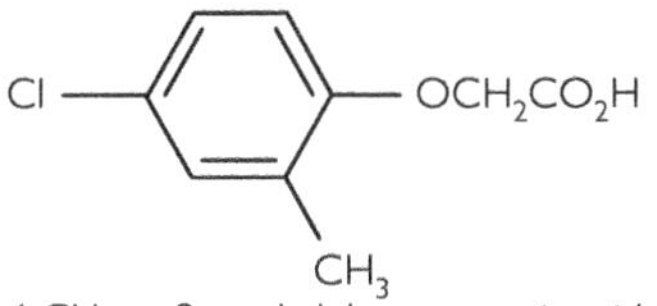

4-Chloro-2-methylphenoxyacetic acid (MCPA)

Fig 12.2 Chemical structures of some chlorophenoxy herbicides.

Bromoxynil

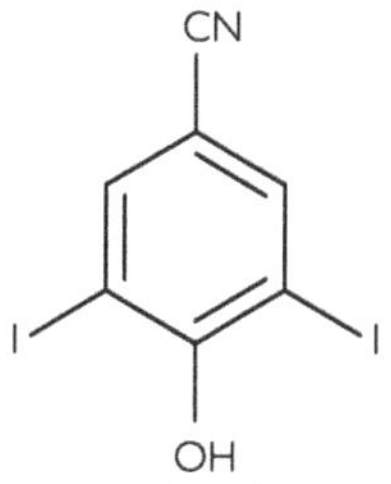

Ioxynil

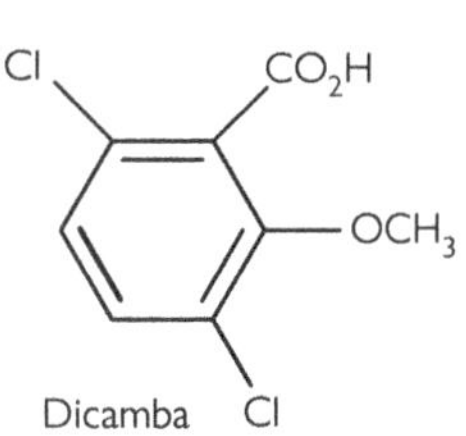

Dicamba

Fig 12.3 Chemical structures of bromoxynil, ioxynil and dicamba.

burning or ulceration in the mouth, abdominal pain, diarrhoea, and occasionally gastrointestinal haemorrhage. Severe corrosive effects are rare and probably due to surfactants/solvents in the formulation. Gastrointestinal fluid loss, vasodilation, and/or direct myocardial toxicity contribute to hypotension, which is common.

In severe cases initial gastrointestinal features are followed by the onset of coma which may be preceded by a period of agitation and confusion. Coma is an almost invariable feature in fatal cases and often lasts several days in those who survive. Hypertonia, hyper-reflexia, clonus, and occasionally extensor plantar responses suggest upper motor neuron damage. Cerebral oedema, miosis, nystagmus, ataxia, alterations in colour vision, memory loss, hallucinations, encephalopathy with triphasic waves on electroencephalography mimicking non-convulsive status epilepticus, and convulsions have also been reported.

Coma is associated frequently with hypoventilation, and occasionally pulmonary oedema. Hypoventilation secondary to CNS depression is the primary cause of hypoxia though respiratory muscle weakness may occur also as part of a generalized myopathy. In such cases there may be limb weakness, or reduced or absent tendon reflexes and increased creatine kinase activity. Aspiration of gastric contents may contribute to pulmonary complications.

Some degree of peripheral neuromuscular damage is common as evidenced by loss of tendon reflexes, muscle twitching, fasciculation, weakness, and/or myotonia. A misdiagnosis of organophosphorus insecticide poisoning may be made as a result of these effects. Neuromuscular effects may persist for several weeks in patients who survive. Peripheral nerve damage with electromyographic evidence of a peripheral neuropathy has been reported rarely.

Other reported features of chlorophenoxy herbicide ingestion include metabolic acidosis, hyperthermia in the absence of infection (possibly reflecting uncoupling of oxidative phosphorylation), renal failure, rhabdomyolysis, increased activities of aspartate and alanine aminotransferase and lactate dehydrogenase activity, thrombocytopenia, haemolytic anaemia, and hypocalcaemia.

Although the prognosis is poor in patients who rapidly became shocked and comatose, full recovery can ensue over weeks to months despite initial severe toxicity and prolonged neuromuscular effects which may mimic the Guillain–Barré syndrome.

Dermal exposure

Skin irritation may occur but since dermal absorption of chlorophenoxy herbicides is poor, systemic toxicity by this route is uncommon.

Inhalation

Gastrointestinal and peripheral neuromuscular symptoms have been reported rarely following occupational exposure which usually involved inhalation alone or in combination with cutaneous exposure.

Management

Most patients require only symptomatic and supportive measures with particular attention to prompt adequate cardiovascular resuscitation and ventilation support. Chlorophenoxy herbicides are adsorbed to activated charcoal and oral administration of 50–100 g to an adult is indicated in patients who have ingested a potentially toxic amount within 1 hour providing the airway is protected.

Measurement of plasma chlorophenoxy herbicide concentrations is available only at specialist laboratories and useful only in cases where diagnostic confirmation is required. Where measured, most cases of severe toxicity have involved total plasma chlorophenoxy concentrations greater than 500 mg/L.

Measures to enhance elimination should be considered in severely poisoned patients. There is some evidence that chlorophenoxy herbicide elimination is increased by urine alkalinization providing a high urine flow and urine pH above 7.5 are maintained.

In addition, chlorophenoxy herbicides are effectively cleared from plasma by haemodialysis.

A recent Cochrane review of the role of urinary alkalinization in acute chlorophenoxy herbicide poisoning concluded 'it is not unreasonable to attempt urinary alkalinization . . . given that toxicity may be prolonged and result in death after 24 hours, few significant adverse effects have been reported from urinary alkalinization, and the potential for this treatment to provide some benefit'. Overall, however, haemodialysis is the preferred means of enhancing chlorophenoxy elimination as it greatly enhances clearance without the need for urine pH manipulation and the administration of substantial volumes of intravenous fluid to compromised patients. The final choice may be dictated by the availability of haemodialysis.

Key points are:
- Serious poisoning only usually follows ingestion.
- Features of gastrointestinal upset predominate.
- Severe poisoning is complicated by coma, convulsions, and neuromuscular involvement.
- Haemodialysis is the treatment of choice for severely poisoned patients.
- Recovery from neuromuscular complications may take weeks to months.

Further reading

Bradberry SM, Watt BE, Proudfoot AT, et al. (2000). Mechanisms of toxicity, clinical features, and management of acute chlorophenoxy herbicide poisoning: a review. J Toxicol Clin Toxicol, 38:111–22.

Roberts DM, Buckley NA (2007). Urinary alkalinisation for acute chlorophenoxy herbicide poisoning. Cochrane Database Syst Rev, 24:CD005488.

Roberts DM, Seneviratne R, Mohammed F, et al. (2005). Intentional self-poisoning with the chlorophenoxy herbicide 4-chloro-2-methylphenoxyacetic acid (MCPA). Ann Emerg Med, 46:275–84.

Paraquat and diquat

Background

Paraquat and diquat are related compounds used as herbicides. Paraquat is the most toxic, and preparations were withdrawn from sale in the European Union in 2005 for amateur use and 2008 for professional application, although products bought before this date may still be available. Paraquat continues to be used in countries with rural economies, as it is a cheap effective agent which leaves no soil residue. Deaths usually result from deliberate ingestion, although skin absorption may result in major toxicity and death if inadequate personal protection is worn, or containers leak. Poisoning and deaths are common in parts of Asia, the Pacific, and Caribbean. A number of techniques have been attempted in order to reduce the risk of paraquat poisoning, including the introduction of a potent emetic into the commercial product and reformulation. Unfortunately these approaches have not resulted in an apparent reduction in the severity of poisoning from paraquat ingestion.

Paraquat

Paraquat is potentially fatal at doses greater than 20 mL of a 20% solution. Death occurs from multi-organ failure, and the time course is dependent on the dose ingested. Large quantities cause coma and death within a few hours, with death from CNS toxicity. Lower doses cause local tissue damage in the GI tract and renal and hepatic failure, and/or pulmonary damage with pulmonary fibrosis causing hypoxia and death.

Mechanisms of toxicity

Once absorbed, paraquat undergoes cyclical oxidation–reduction reactions, and NADPH-dependent reduction of the paraquat anion to a free radical occurs. In the presence of oxygen, this free radical is rapidly oxidized, producing a superoxide anion, which once again regenerates the paraquat anion. This paraquat ion is then available to participate in further oxidation–reduction reactions. The superoxide anion produced contributes to the formation of other toxic species producing cellular damage. These processes are associated with a decrease in NADPH and an inability to maintain levels of NADPH sufficient to maintain cell viability. Paraquat causes multi-organ toxicity as a result of these effects. The organs affected depend on dose ingested. In moderate to severe poisoning paraquat is particularly toxic to the lungs as it is accumulated in the lungs by an energy-dependent diamine transport system found in alveolar epithelial and Clara cells.

Toxicokinetics

Paraquat is rapidly absorbed across the gut by an active process. Bioavailability is about 10%. Peak concentrations occur within 1–2 hours of ingestion. Paraquat is largely eliminated by renal excretion, but as it causes acute kidney injury a major toxic effect this route is only operative for low doses of paraquat. It may be detected in urine as soon as 1 hour after ingestion. Plasma concentrations of paraquat have been shown to predict prognosis, but as there is no clearly identified effective treatment need not be measured other than for forensic or prognostic purposes.

Risk factors

The principal risk factor is the dose ingested and co-ingestion with alcohol therefore tends to increase this dose by altering judgement.

A classification for severity of poisoning and prognosis has been published and is based on dose ingested.

Group 1: mild poisoning following the ingestion, injection, or dermal absorption of less than 20 mg of paraquat ion/kg body weight.

Patients who spit out paraquat before swallowing can develop painful ulceration of the mouth with no systemic features. Those who swallow the toxin are asymptomatic, and may or may not develop vomiting and diarrhoea. Full recovery occurs. There may be a transient fall in the gas transfer factor and vital capacity due to reversible lung damage.

Group 2: moderate to severe poisoning follows the ingestion, injection, or dermal absorption of 20–40 mg of paraquat ion/kg body weight. Vomiting and diarrhoea develop with generalized symptoms indicative of systemic toxicity. Pulmonary fibrosis develops in all cases but recovery may occur. In addition, renal failure, and sometimes, hepatic dysfunction, may supervene. Death occurs in the majority of cases but can be delayed for 2–3 weeks as lung injury worsens.

Group 3: acute fulminant poisoning follows the ingestion, injection or dermal absorption of more than (usually considerably in excess of) 40 mg of paraquat ion/kg body weight. In addition to nausea and vomiting, there is marked ulceration of the oropharynx with multiple organ (cardiac, respiratory, hepatic, renal, adrenal, pancreatic, neurological) failure. In this group the mortality is 100%. Death commonly occurs within 24 hours of exposure and is never delayed for more than 1 week.

Note: provided the herbicide was correctly diluted before application there is little danger from eating crops recently sprayed with paraquat, as it is unstable in the environment and neutralized and detoxified by contact with soil.

Reproduced from *The WHO Recommended Classification of Pesticides by Hazard, 2009*, with permission from the World Health Organization.

Clinical features

Ingestion/systemic toxicity

Nausea and vomiting, with or without diarrhoea, are common together with a burning sensation, soreness, and pain in the mouth, throat, chest, and abdomen (usually epigastric). Ulceration in the mouth (which may be severe), sloughing of the oropharyngeal mucosae, an inability to swallow, dysphagia, and aphonia ensues. Perforation of the oesophagus may result in mediastinitis, surgical emphysema, and pneumothorax.

Within hours of a substantial ingestion generalized weakness, myalgia, giddiness, headache, anorexia, and fever develop. Oliguria or non-oliguric renal failure may supervene due to acute tubular necrosis. Proximal tubular dysfunction (causing proteinuria, microscopic haematuria, glycosuria) is common. Jaundice, hepatomegaly, and central abdominal pain due to pancreatitis occur frequently.

Most patients develop a cough, which may be productive and blood stained. Dyspnoea is a prominent feature and occurs early in those patients who have ingested a substantial amount of paraquat and in these circumstances is due to acute respiratory distress syndrome (ARDS). In less severe cases, the onset of dyspnoea is due to pulmonary fibrosis. Rarely pneumothorax, mediastinitis, pleural effusion and iatrogenic pulmonary oedema, may precipitate dyspnoea.

In addition to a falling gas transfer factor and vital capacity, severely poisoned patients will have a low and falling PO_2 with resultant central cyanosis. Radiological changes do not always parallel the severity of clinical symptoms. Thus, the chest X-ray may be normal in those dying early from multiple organ failure. More usually, patchy infiltration occurs which may progress to an opacification of one or both lung fields.

Except for sinus tachycardia, cardiovascular complications are not usually observed until the terminal phase of intoxication. Then, ventricular tachycardia, intraventricular conduction disturbances, and non-specific T-wave changes occur. Sinus bradycardia, hypotension, and cardiac arrest may supervene. The chest X-ray may show massive cardiomegaly and, at post-mortem, toxic myocarditis is found histologically.

Coma is a common terminal event, though other neurological features such as ataxia and facial paresis are occasionally observed. Convulsions have been reported and may be due to cerebral oedema precipitated by fluid overload.

Adrenal cortical necrosis is often observed particularly in severely poisoned patients with multiple organ failure.

A polymorphonuclear leucocytosis is a frequent finding. A normochromic anaemia and haemolytic anaemia have also been reported. Metabolic acidosis, probably secondary to cardiovascular collapse and hypoxia, is a common complication.

Inhalation
Inhalation of fine spray droplets can cause epistaxis and sore throat.

Dermal and nail exposures
Paraquat, especially in concentrated formulations, has a strong irritant action on various types of epithelia. It will cause erythema, blistering, irritation and ulceration of the skin, and eczematous dermatitis. Diluted paraquat is unlikely to irritate skin unless clothing soaked with spray is worn for prolonged periods. Absorption through broken skin may lead to systemic toxicity.

Concentrated solutions of paraquat may also cause localized discolouration or a transverse band of white discolouration affecting the nail plate. Transverse ridging and furrowing of the nail progressing to gross irregular deformity of the nail plate and loss of nail may also occur. Normal nail growth resumes once exposure has ceased.

Eye exposure
Severe inflammation of the cornea and conjunctiva may develop. The inflammation develops gradually, reaching a maximum after 12–24 hours, and may lead to ulceration of the conjunctiva and cornea with the risk of secondary infection. Although healing may be slow, recovery is usually, though not always, complete.

Investigations
A simple qualitative urine test using sodium dithionite is available. Add 0.1 g sodium dithionite to 10 mL of freshly prepared 1 molar sodium hydroxide solution. Then add 1 mL of this solution to 1 mL of urine. If the solution turns blue within seconds—paraquat is present, the darker the blue the greater the concentration: pale green indicates diquat or a low concentrations of paraquat. This test is not predictive of outcome.

Monograms are available which may be used to estimate prognosis from a blood concentration, but the assay is now very rarely available.

Other investigations that may indicate prognosis and guide fluid management are serum creatinine, a measured creatinine clearance (not estimated glomerular filtration rate), chest X-ray, and blood gases.

Management
Early use of oral activated charcoal or GI lavage has not been shown to be of benefit. Treatment is aimed at symptomatic relief. Fluid loss should be replaced and analgesia provided to alleviate discomfort, for example, from GI ulceration. Antiemetics should be given, though vomiting may be difficult to control. Where possible, supplementary oxygen should be avoided as this may make damage to the lungs worse. Endotracheal intubation may be required if severe oropharyngeal oedema is present. There is no evidence that haemodialysis, haemoperfusion, or immunosuppression improves outcome, despite claims to the contrary. Haemodialysis is appropriate for managing renal failure in mild-to-moderate poisoning. Lung transplant is unlikely to be effective, as the donor lung will take up paraquat.

Diquat
Diquat is a dipyridyl herbicide which is readily absorbed following ingestion. However, unlike paraquat, it does not accumulate in the lungs.

Like paraquat, diquat undergoes cyclical oxidation/reduction reactions. The diquat radical formed is unstable and reacts with oxygen to produce reactive superoxide anions. These contribute to the formation of other toxic species and cellular damage.

Ingestion of diquat may cause severe mucosal damage associated with nausea, vomiting, and abdominal pain. Paralytic ileus may occur with sequestration of fluid in the gut. Nephrotoxicity is common and renal failure may ensue.

Bronchopneumonia may occur, as may ARDS and pulmonary oedema. Unlike paraquat, pulmonary fibrosis does not ensue. Cardiac arrhythmias, conclusions and coma have been described.

Diquat poisoning may be confirmed using a sodium dithionite urine test. Treatment is aimed at symptomatic relief. Fluid loss should be replaced and analgesia provided to alleviate discomfort. Renal failure should be managed conventionally. It should be noted, however, that diquat may interfere with some laboratory estimations of creatinine using the Jaffe method.

Further reading
Bateman DN (2008). New formulation of paraquat: a step forward but in the wrong direction? PLoS Med, 5:e58.

Eddleston M, Wilks MF, Buckley NA (2003). Prospects for treatment of paraquat-induced lung fibrosis with immunosuppressive drugs and the need for better prediction of outcome: a systemic review. Q J Med, 96:809–24.

Gawarammana I, Buckley NA, Mohammed, et al. (2012). A randomised controlled trial of high-dose immunosuppression in paraquat poisoning. J Toxicol Clin Toxicol, 50:278.

Jones GM, Vale JA (2000). Mechanisms of toxicity, clinical features, and management of diquat poisoning: a review. J Toxicol Clin Toxicol, 38:123–8.

Smith LL (1987). Mechanism of paraquat toxicity in lung and its relevance to treatment. Hum Exp Toxicol, 6:31–6.

Senarathna L, Eddleston M, Wilks MF, et al. (2009). Prediction of outcome after paraquat poisoning by measurement of the plasma paraquat concentration. Q J Med, 102:251–9.

Vale JA, Meredith TJ, Buckley BM (1987). Paraquat poisoning: clinical features and immediate general management. Hum Exp Toxicol, 6:41–7.

Glyphosate

Background

Glyphosate-containing herbicides are widely used throughout the world, and in some countries may be the commonest herbicide sold. Usage may be likely to increase as some crops have now been genetically engineered to increase their tolerance to glyphosate.

Glyphosate is active upon contact with the target plant but becomes inactivated by bacterial action once in the soil. Within plants it inhibits an enzyme used in the production of aromatic amino acids, lignins, and flavonoids. However, this enzyme is not found in mammals, thus reducing its toxicity to man.

Glyphosate poisoning is encountered from exposure to pesticides. However, the concentration of glyphosate varies greatly depending upon the formulation. Ready-diluted domestic formulations typically have glyphosate salt concentrations of between 1% and 5%, whilst commercial products require dilution before use and may contain 30–50% glyphosate. Different glyphosate salts occur in different formulations, with the commonest salt encountered being the isopropylamine (IPA) salt.

Glyphosate-containing herbicides contain surfactants to help the pesticide spread over the plant. Different surfactants, in different concentrations, are used in different products. This is important when considering the toxicity of glyphosate-containing pesticides as it is thought that the toxicity due to polyethoxylated amine (POEA) compound surfactants may be greater than that due to the glyphosate itself.

In determining the toxicity of glyphosate herbicides it is therefore important to consider the formulation involved as the toxicity due to the surfactant may be greater than that due to the glyphosate itself. However, case series describing mortality from glyphosate-containing herbicides have ranged between 8% and 16%.

Mechanism of toxicity

Commercial products all contain glyphosate (see figure 12.4) and a surfactant. Within commercial herbicide formulations it appears that the major cause of mammalian toxicity may be due, not to the glyphosate itself, but to other co-ingredients, particularly the surfactants. Data do not strongly support the hypothesis that the presence of the surfactant has a synergistic, rather than an additive effect on toxicity.

Glyphosate

Glyphosate has a low oral and dermal toxicity in mammals. There appears to be little clinical difference between the sodium, ammonium, or IPA salts. It is suggested that its mechanism of action may include uncoupling oxidative phosphorylation although this may in fact be due to surfactants.

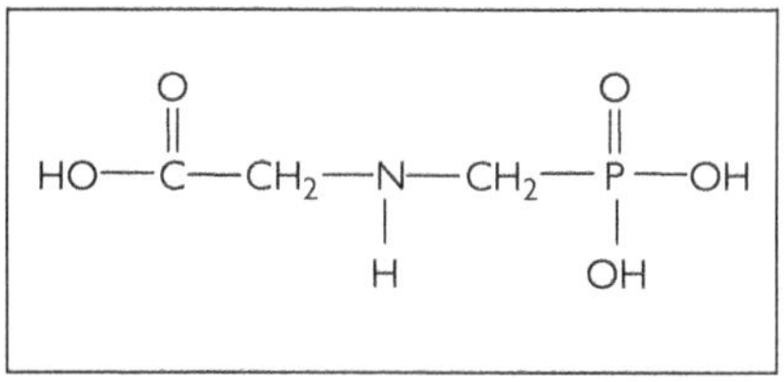

Surfactants

The most commonly encountered surfactants are POEA compounds, consisting of two polyethoxylene groups and a long-chain alkyl group together with a central nitrogen atom. The polyethoxylene chains contribute to the hydrophilic properties whilst the aryl chain is hydrophobic.

The length of each of these chains can be varied, altering the properties of the surfactant. A particular formulation may contain a mix of chain lengths, and different products may contain substantially different chain lengths.

Other surfactants which may be found include alkyl polyoxyphosphate amine, polyethoxylated alkyl etheramine, and alkyl polysaccharides. Domestic products tend to have lower concentrations of glyphosate and are less likely to incorporate the more toxic POEA surfactants

Surfactants interfere with mitochondrial function. They damage the mitochondrial wall and impair energy production. They distribute widely throughout the body and are associated with multiple organ damage.

Toxicokinetics

Glyphosate is poorly, but rapidly absorbed orally, with peak concentrations occurring within 6 hours followed by a prompt decline.

Dermal absorption is poor.

The major route of glyphosate elimination is of the unchanged product in the urine. The elimination half-life is reported to be 3.1 hours.

In one study, ingestion of more than 190 mL (typically of concentrated glyphosate/surfactant formulations) had a specificicity of 86%, but only a sensitivity of only 58% of predicting death. In the same study, a peak glyphosate concentration of 734 mg/L was a good predictor of death.

Clinical features

In a large series of over 600 patients with glyphosate poisoning, the majority of whom had ingested concentrated formulations, 27% remained asymptomatic, 64% developed minor features, and 5.5% developed moderate to severe poisoning. The case fatality rate was 3.2% with a median time to death of 20 hours. Larger ingestions, high concentrations, and older age were all associated with mortality.

Ingestion of small amounts of dilute, domestic products is generally associated only with mild gastrointestinal disturbances including nausea, vomiting, and diarrhoea. More concentrated formulations are corrosive and cause direct damage to the gastrointestinal tract including oesophagitis and gastritis. Vomiting and diarrhoea may be substantial resulting in significant fluid loss.

Respiratory features include breathlessness, tachypnoea, cough, and bronchospasm. Breathlessness can occur due to aspiration pneumonitis and also from the development of non-cardiac pulmonary oedema or ARDS. In severe cases mechanical ventilation may be required.

Following large ingestions more severe features including hypotension, renal and hepatic impairment occur.

Fig 12.4 Chemical structure of glyphosate.

Hypotension may be due both to direct cardiotoxic effects and hypovolaemia due to fluid loss. It is a common feature in more severely poisoned patients. Tachycardia may occur and ECG changes including ST segment changes and AV block have been noted. Hypotension which is resistant to fluid administration and inotropic support is a common feature in fatal cases.

In severe cases convulsions and loss of consciousness occur. Similarly, metabolic acidosis is a common feature in severe cases and should be managed conventionally.

In fatal cases, death typically occurs within the first 3 days, often within the first day. Late fatalities also occur.

Dermal exposure

Dermal exposure can cause irritation although severe skin damage is rare. Some cases of dermatitis have been reported which may be due to preservatives present in some preparations. Substantial systemic toxicity is unlikely to occur following dermal exposure.

Eye exposure

Eye exposure can result in conjunctivitis and corneal injury.

Inhalation

Inhalation of droplets during spraying may result in mouth and throat irritation.

Management

Liquid agent on the skin should be removed and early eye irrigation undertaken if ocular exposure has occurred.

Asymptomatic patients should be observed for at least 4 hours. Symptomatic patients should be observed for at least 24 hours.

Administration of activated charcoal may be considered although there is no evidence to suggest that it adsorbs the surfactant POEA.

In symptomatic patients, blood should be taken to determine the U&Es, creatinine, full blood count, and consideration should be given to blood gas analysis in more severely poisoned patients. A chest X-ray should be considered in patients with respiratory features.

Treatment is largely symptomatic and supportive. Fluid and electrolyte loss from vomiting and diarrhoea can be substantial and should be replaced.

Hypotension should be corrected, initially by fluid resuscitation. In severe cases inotropic support may be required. A case report has suggested that intravenous administration of lipid emulsion may have a role in the treatment of refractory hypotension.

For patients with significant gastrointestinal features early endoscopy should be considered to determine the nature and extent of corrosive damage.

Renal function should be monitored. It may respond to careful fluid management, but in severe cases renal replacement therapy is indicated. It has been suggested that haemodialysis may have a role to play in enhancing removal of glyphosate in severe cases.

Further reading

Bradberry SM, Proudfoot AT, Vale JA (2004). Glyphosate poisoning. *Toxicol Rev*, 23:159–67.

Lee HL, Chen KW, Chi CH, *et al.* Clinical presentations and prognostic factors of a glyphosate-surfactant herbicide intoxication: a review of 131 cases. *Acad Emerg Med.*7:906–10.

Moon JM, Chun BJ (2010). Predicting acute complicated glyphosate intoxication in the emergency department. *Clin Toxicol*, 48:718–24.

Roberts DM, Buckley NA, Mohamed F, *et al.* (2010). A prospective observational study of the clinical toxicology of glyphosate-containing herbicides in adults with acute self-poisoning. *Clin Toxicol*, 48:129–36.

Coumarin rodenticides

Background and uses

Warfarin and coumatetralyl are derivatives of 4-hydroxycoumarin and were introduced as rodenticides in the 1940s. Widespread warfarin use led to the emergence of rats resistant to it and 'second-generation' anticoagulant rodenticides were developed. These super-warfarins or long-acting coumarins include brodifacoum, bromadiolone, difenacoum, flocoumafen, and the indanedione derivatives chlorophacinone and diphacinone and will be the focus of this article. Superwarfarins differ structurally from warfarin in that they possess a polycyclic hydrocarbon side chain that renders them more potent and prolongs their duration of action. While warfarin-based baits must be eaten daily for several days to be lethal, a single feed of a long-acting one is usually all that is required.

Commercial formulations include cereal-based baits (loose grain, blocks, or pellets), pastes, powders, and wax blocks typically impregnated with 0.0025% long-acting rodenticides. Concentrates containing up to 0.25% are also available for professional use.

Most exposures to coumarin rodenticides are accidental ingestions by children aged less than 6 years. This rarely results in symptoms or altered coagulation. In contrast, deliberate ingestion of larger quantities by adults is potentially much more serious and fatal haemorrhage may occur.

Brodifacoum has caused clotting abnormalities in drug users who have laced illicit drugs with it in the belief that it potentiates euphoria.

While ingestion is by far the most common route of exposure, inhalation and dermal absorption have also resulted in haemorrhage.

Mechanisms of toxicity

The anticoagulant action of long-acting coumarin rodenticides results from inhibition of vitamin K_1-2,3 epoxide reductase and reduced synthesis of clotting factors II, VII, IX, and X. There is no anticoagulant effect until existing stores of vitamin K and clotting factors are depleted. Thus, although an anticoagulant effect is usually apparent by 24 hours, the peak effect may not be achieved until 2 or 3 days later.

The greater potency and duration of action of long-acting anticoagulant rodenticides compared to warfarin is attributed to a combination of their greater affinity for vitamin K_1-2,3-epoxide reductase, accumulation in the liver and long biological half-lives due to entero-hepatic circulation and high lipid solubility.

Toxicokinetics

Anticoagulant rodenticides can be absorbed via the gastrointestinal tract, the respiratory tract, and skin. They accumulate rapidly in the liver until the microsomal binding sites are saturated. There is evidence that difenacoum undergoes substantial hepatic degradation though other second-generation anticoagulants such as brodifacoum and flocoumafen are excreted predominantly unchanged.

Second-generation anticoagulants are thought to be subject to entero-hepatic circulation which prolongs their already lengthy elimination half-lives. They have a two-compartment model of elimination with initial plasma half-lives of 1–6 days and terminal half-lives of 7–60 days.

Clinical features

The amounts of long-acting coumarins ingested accidentally by young children are almost always small and the vast majority develop no symptoms.

Significant coagulopathy usually results from ingestion of large amounts and, rarely, from skin contamination, inhalation or a combination of both. Bleeding unprovoked by trauma is likely to become apparent within 1–3 days.

Spontaneous haemorrhage may occur in virtually any organ following significant exposure (Table 12.1) and many patients will bleed from more than one site. Common sites are the skin, nose, and gums. The single most frequent and most dramatic presentation in both sexes is frank haematuria, usually associated with renal angle, flank, or abdominal pain. Abnormal reproductive tract bleeding is not uncommon in females.

The greatest threat to life is posed by significant accumulation of blood at critical anatomical locations. Most deaths are due to bleeding into the confined space of the skull.

Gastrointestinal bleeding secondary to anticoagulant rodenticides seldom seems to be of sufficient magnitude to pose a risk to life but the speed of onset of spontaneous haemorrhage occasionally results in hypovolaemic shock. In most cases, however, it is less acute and the patient presents with anaemia.

Management

Initial assessment

Most patients will not require treatment after exposure to rodenticide baits, particularly children who have

Table 12.1 Potential haemorrhage sites and lesions after anticoagulant rodenticide poisoning

System	Site/lesion
Skin	Ecchymosis
	Haematoma
Musculoskeletal	Muscle haematoma
	Compartment syndrome
	Haemarthrosis
Respiratory	Epistaxis
	Haemoptysis
	Lung haemorrhage
	Haemothorax
	Mediastinal haematoma
Renal	Haematuria (macroscopic)
	Hydroureter/hydronephrosis
	Obstructive nephropathy
	Renal parenchymal haemorrhage
	Ureteric haematoma
Gastrointestinal	Gum haemorrhage
	Pharyngeal haematoma
	Sub-ungual haematoma
	Haematemesis
	Melaena
	Rectal bleeding
	Intra-abdominal bleeding
Reproductive	Abnormal uterine bleeding
Central nervous system	Subarachnoid haemorrhage
	Intracerebral haemorrhage
	Intracranial subdural haemorrhage
	Pontine and cerebellar infarction
	Hemisphere infarction
	Spinal subdural haemorrhage
Eyes	Conjunctival bleeding

ingested very small amounts (<1 mg of the active ingredient). These cases need not be referred to hospital. Pregnant patients with unintentional small exposures should be reviewed by their obstetrician but need not be referred to hospital immediately.

Patients with haemorrhagic features require urgent assessment as do those in whom exposure is due to suspected self-harm, abuse, misuse, or potentially malicious administration of anticoagulant rodenticides, and those chronically exposed.

The possibility of surreptitious ingestion of oral anticoagulants should be considered in all cases of unexplained bleeding with a prolonged INR.

Reducing absorption

Activated charcoal binds warfarin and second-generation coumarins and 50–100 g for an adult should be given to all patients presenting within 1 hour of deliberate ingestion.

Monitoring

Any patient who has accidentally ingested 1 mg or more of active ingredient and is asymptomatic should have their prothrombin time or INR measured at 48–72 hours after the incident. Administration of vitamin K prior to evaluation of the degree of anticoagulation is not recommended.

Patients taking anticoagulants therapeutically who ingest any amount of an anticoagulant rodenticide should have their prothrombin time or INR measured on presentation and again at 48–72 hours after ingestion. Management depends on the result; if within the target range, no further action is indicated.

Patients who require reversal of coagulopathy after exposure to long-acting formulations should have their INR measured for 2 weeks after cessation of treatment. Failure to do so may result in recurrence of anticoagulation and risk haemorrhage being missed.

If bleeding has occurred, the haemoglobin concentration and haematocrit should be measured to assess the severity of blood loss.

Administration of phytomenadione (vitamin K_1)

Intravenous phytomenadione results in a more rapid INR reduction than the subcutaneous route or oral routes. Oral treatment should only be considered if a safe parenteral preparation is unavailable.

Treatment with phytomenadione may be required for several weeks if a long-acting anticoagulant has been ingested. Insufficient doses of vitamin K or patient failure to comply with medication are potential reasons for treatment failure.

Intravenous administration of phytomenadione has occasionally caused severe reactions resembling hypersensitivity or anaphylaxis. Symptoms have included facial flushing, sweating, chest constriction or pain, dyspnoea, cyanosis, and cardiovascular collapse; fatalities have been reported. These reactions are thought to be due to polyethoxylated castor oil present as a surfactant in some parenteral formulations and have been associated generally with a rapid rate of infusion.

Patients not receiving long-term anticoagulant therapy

Risk of bleeding

It is important to reverse rapidly anticoagulation in patients who have no clinical indication to be at this increased risk of haemorrhage. The specific management will depend on whether active bleeding is present.

Active bleeding

If active bleeding occurs, prothrombin complex concentrate (which contains factors II, VII, IX, and X) 25–50 units/kg should be given over 30 minutes. If prothrombin complex concentrate is not available, fresh frozen plasma 15 mL/kg can be used, though this preparation usually does not revert the INR to normal unless large volumes are given. Recombinant activated factor VII is not recommended for emergency anticoagulation reversal. Whenever plasma or prothrombin complex concentrate are given, phytomenadione 10–20 mg intravenously (250 micrograms/kg body weight for a child) should be given by slow intravenous infusion because the half-lives of the vitamin K-dependent clotting factors found in plasma or prothrombin complex concentrate are short and, without vitamin K, patients continue to synthesize dysfunctional clotting proteins for some time after anticoagulant exposure ('rebound anticoagulation').

No active bleeding

If there is no active bleeding and the INR is 4.0 or less, treatment with phytomenadione is not required. If there is no bleeding or only minor bleeding and the INR is 4.0 or higher, phytomenadione 10 mg by slow intravenous injection (250–300 micrograms/kg body weight for a child) should be administered. An alternative is oral phytomenadione 10 mg, though this may be less effective than intravenous vitamin K.

Patients receiving long-term anticoagulant therapy

Active bleeding

If active bleeding occurs in a patient who is being prescribed an anticoagulant, the drug should be discontinued and one of the treatments previously outlined should be instituted.

No active bleeding

If the INR is 8.0 or greater and there is no active bleeding or only minor bleeding, stop warfarin (restart when the INR ≤5.0), give phytomenadione 0.5–1.0 mg by slow intravenous injection (12.5–25 micrograms/kg for a child) and repeat the dose if the INR is 8.0 or higher 12–24 hours later.

If the INR is 6.0–8.0 and there is no active bleeding or only minor bleeding, warfarin should be discontinued and restarted when the INR is 5.0 or lower.

Note: large doses of phytomenadione may completely reverse the effects of warfarin with devastating clinical consequences and make it difficult to re-establish anticoagulation.

Increasing elimination

In patients with severe poisoning who have ingested a long-acting formulation, oral colestyramine 4 g three times daily for an adult should be considered in order to shorten the plasma half-life of the rodenticide. Preliminary data suggest that the elimination of brodifacoum may also be increased by multiple-dose oral activated charcoal.

Further reading

Caravati EM, Erdman AR, Scharman EJ, et al. (2007). Long-acting anticoagulant rodenticide poisoning: an evidence-based consensus guideline for out-of-hospital management. Clin Toxicol, 45:1–22.

Aluminium phosphide and phosphine

Background

Aluminium phosphide is used to kill insects and rodents, often found in association with grain stores. It is frequently used as pellets, each weighing around 3 g. On contact with moisture, or if swallowed on contact with the acid contents of the stomach, it reacts to liberate gaseous phosphine which produces toxicity. Clinical effects are therefore seen following ingestion, or by inhalation of phosphine gas liberated from aluminium phosphide reaction with moisture in the environment. Typically, deliberate self-poisoning follows ingestion of aluminium phosphide whilst accidental exposures occur most often following inhalation of phosphine gas, often in a confined space, for example, a ship's hold or a grain silo.

Aluminium phosphide

In some parts of the world pesticides are a major contributor to deliberate self-harm. In parts of India, aluminium phosphide is the commonest pesticide used for this purpose. This contrasts with the pattern of poisoning seen in the United Kingdom where ingestion of aluminium phosphide is uncommon. There is a high case fatality ratio. When fatalities occur, they occur early following ingestion, with one case series reporting 55% dying within 12 hours and over 90% within the first day.

Mechanisms of toxicity

The toxicity of aluminium phosphide is thought primarily to be due to the release of phosphine upon contact with water or acid in the stomach.

$$AlP + 3H_2O \rightarrow Al(OH)_3 + PH_3$$
$$AlP + 3H^+ \rightarrow Al^{3+} + PH_3$$

The phosphine released is then absorbed. This process can occur rapidly and clinical features typically occur soon after ingestion.

Several different mechanisms of action have been proposed for the toxicity of the aluminium phosphide.

Local corrosive damage occurs to the upper gastrointestinal tract. This can produce oesophagitis, gastritis, and haematemesis, with subsequent stricture formation in survivors.

Systemic absorption of phosphine produces subsequent toxic effects. A major effect is on mitochondrial activity, which is decreased following phosphine exposure impairing aerobic respiration. This effect is likely to be due to a variety of mechanisms, although inhibition of cytochrome C oxidase is no longer thought to be the major cause of mitochondrial impairment.

Free radical formation plays a part in the toxicity as phosphine reacts to form hydroxyl radicals. Phosphine also inhibits catalase and peroxidase and this decreases free radical scavenging thereby worsening free radical-induced lipid peroxidation and cellular damage.

In addition to damage due to phosphine, aluminium may also contribute to the toxicity.

Although decreases in cholinesterase activity have been noted, this is not thought to play a major part in the toxicity.

Toxicokinetics

Phosphine is formed rapidly following ingestion although data on its kinetics in man are scarce. Higher blood concentrations have been detected in fatal cases and in more serious cases of poisoning than in those with less severe clinical features. Phosphine reacts irreversibly *in vitro* with haemoglobin to form a hemichrome, a methaemoglobin-derived compound, and may also produce Heinz bodies.

The mechanisms by which aluminium phosphide and phosphine are eliminated are not fully elucidated. Both phosphide and phosphate are eliminated via the kidneys and phosphine gas may be excreted via the lungs.

Clinical features

The onset of clinical features is rapid.

Early features may be non-specific and include nausea and vomiting. Chest and epigastric pain occur and may be due to local corrosive effects.

Local corrosive effects cause oesophagitis, gastritis, and may result in haematemesis. Oesophageal strictures may develop and oesophago-tracheal fistula has been reported.

Hypotension may develop rapidly and is associated with decreased cardiac output and hypokinesis. Venous pressure may become raised. Damage to myocytes occurs and is associated with elevated cardiac enzymes. ECG changes, particularly of the ST segment and T waves are common. Both atrial and ventricular arrhythmias are common and bradycardias have also been described.

Pulmonary oedema is common and may occur within a few hours of ingestion. The oedema may occur due to both cardiac failure and to a direct effect on the lungs producing exudates rich in protein. ARDS has been described.

Hypokalaemia is common and acute kidney injury can occur. Hypoglycaemia may also be found due to a failure of gluconeogenesis and glycogenolysis. Raised transaminases associated with hepatic congestion are found commonly. Metabolic acidosis, sometimes accompanied by a compensatory respiratory alkalosis, is found. A low arterial pH is associated with a poor prognosis and may have prognostic significance. Haemolysis has been described rarely and appears to be more common in patients with glucose-6-phosphate dehydrogenase deficiency. Methaemoglobinaemia, Heinz body formation, and disseminated intravascular coagulation have also been described.

Management

Staff safety is important. This is particularly important in first responders in confined spaces, and rescue personnel must have appropriate respiratory protection.

Consideration should be given to decontamination as phosphine gas might arise from the reaction of residual, uningested, aluminium phosphide with moisture or water in the environment. There is a theoretical hazard from phosphine eliminated via the respiratory tract or from vomited fluids. However, in many cases in developing countries, staff without special protective equipment have managed patients uneventfully. While in developed countries emergency departments have sometimes been closed due to concern about possible effects on other patients and staff, this often seems an over-reaction to what is usually a minimal hazard unless the patient has pellets on their person.

Symptomatic cases should be admitted to hospital urgently. Patients who are asymptomatic should be observed for at least 12 hours before discharge and should be advised to return if they develop symptoms subsequently.

Blood should be taken for glucose, electrolytes, calcium, magnesium, phosphate, creatinine, transaminases, cardiac enzymes, full blood count, and blood gases including methaemoglobin.

Electrolyte imbalances and hypoglycaemia should be addressed carefully and hypotension addressed.

Magnesium has been suggested as a treatment for ventricular arrhythmias and as prophylactic therapy in patients with hypotension. However, trial data are inconclusive with some studies showing benefit and others not. Similarly, there are some data suggesting that the use of hyper-insulinaemia euglycaemic therapy (HIET) may be of benefit.

Pulmonary oedema may require treatment using assisted ventilation and positive end-expiratory pressure. Acidosis may respond to fluid replacement. If not, consideration should be given to administration of sodium bicarbonate. Methaemoglobinaemia should be treated if necessary, but may be resistant to therapy.

It should be recognized that many patients presenting following ingestion of aluminium phosphide will die, despite optimum treatment. Particular care should therefore be given to the palliation of symptoms.

In order to maintain staff safety, consideration of the possibility of ongoing phosphine generation in the stomach should be considered if post-mortem examinations are to be considered.

Phosphine

Phosphine has the chemical formula PH_3. Synonyms include hydrogen phosphide, phosphorus trihydride, and phosphorus hydride.

It is a colourless and odourless gas. However, impure forms have unpleasant odours, sometimes described as fishy or resembling garlic. It is available commercially in cylinders, in which it may also be combined with carbon dioxide.

It is generated by the reaction of metal phosphides (e.g. aluminium, zinc, magnesium, or calcium phosphide) and water. It may also be generated during the illegal manufacture of methamphetamine.

Poisoning with phosphine occurs via inhalation, either from an environment where metal phosphides have been in contact with water, or from direct exposure to the commercially available product. Commonly, exposure occurs either accidentally, or occupationally, where aluminium phosphide has been used as a pesticide; the metal phosphide reacting with moisture in the environment to produce phosphine. Exposure typically may occur in confined spaces, for example, the hold of a grain ship being fumigated.

Mechanism of toxicity
Phosphine is highly toxic via inhalation. It is estimated that as little as 100–190 parts per million (ppm) of phosphine

inhaled for between half an hour to an hour causes serious poisoning whilst 300–600 ppm inhaled over the same time period could be fatal.

Local irritant effects on the eyes, skin, and respiratory tract may occur. Systemic effects are due to absorption of phosphine and are predominantly similar to those following ingestion of aluminium phosphide (as previously discussed).

Toxicokinetics
Toxicokinetic data are sparse. However, the rapidity of the onset of symptoms and the early development of systemic effects indicate that it is rapidly absorbed through the lungs. It is metabolized to hypophosphite, phosphate, and phosphite.

Clinical features
The onset of clinical features is rapid.

Inhalation
Inhalation is associated with irritation of the respiratory tract including the mucus membranes of the mouth and throat. Chest tightness, pain, breathlessness, and cough develop.

Eye exposure
Eye exposure causes irritation and blurred vision whilst dermal exposure has been reported to cause irritation, sweating and paraesthesia.

Systemic features
Systemic features due to absorption of phosphine are similar to those encountered following aluminium phosphide poisoning (as previously discussed). In particular, patients are at risk of developing cardiac failure and arrhythmia and pulmonary oedema. Nausea and vomiting are very common and may be accompanied by diarrhoea.

Management
Staff safety is important and rescuers should not enter an area where phosphine is present without wearing appropriate breathing apparatus. In the unlikely event that liquid agent is encountered this should be decontaminated.

Local damage to the skin and eyes should be treated conventionally.

Systemic features due to absorbed phosphine should be treated as for ingestion of aluminium phosphide (as previously discussed).

Further reading
Nath NS, Bhattacharya I, Tuck AG, et al. (2011). Mechanisms of phosphine toxicity. J Toxicol, 2011:494168.

Proudfoot AT (2009). Aluminium and zinc phosphide poisoning. Clin Toxicol, 47:89–100.

Poisoning due to fungi, plants, and animals

Poisonous fungi

Background

Most fungi are not toxic, but several species (around 100 worldwide) can produce clinical toxicity. Exposures to potentially toxic fungi tend to occur in two main scenarios. Young children, who normally eat only small quantities of raw material, and consumption by adults of larger quantities, often foraged. Misidentification in the latter situation may result in accidental ingestion of a poisonous species and the production of a range of clinical features some of which can be associated with serious sequelae. Some fungal toxins are denatured by heat, but others are not, so it is important to understand the precise nature of the ingestion.

In assessing toxic risk it is useful to have information from a mycologist. It may be helpful to take photographs of any uncooked specimens for transmission for identification by smartphone or e-mail. Information on a number of aspects will also be useful, including the following:

- At what time were the mushrooms eaten?
- When was the onset of symptoms after the ingestion?
- Was more than one kind of mushroom ingested?
- Are all persons who ate the mushroom ill?
- Are persons in the group who ate none of the mushroom ill?
- Was the mushroom eaten raw or cooked?
- If cooked, how and how long were they cooked (i.e. sautéed, fried, soup, stew, etc.)?
- Was any alcohol consumed with a meal?
- Were the mushrooms eaten at more than one meal? If so, were they reheated?
- Were specimens with old or wormy fruit-bodies gathered?
- How were the mushrooms stored and transported between collection and preparation?
- What was the condition of the mushrooms at the time of preparation? Were they cleaned before being put into the basket? (Note: important identifying features may be destroyed during cleaning.)
- Were the mushrooms put in plastic bags (and did they become slimy)?
- What was it growing on (i.e. wood, soil, etc.)?
- In a wild area or a cultivated area?
- What kind of tree(s) was it growing near?
- What time of year was the mushroom collected?

It is convenient to divide fungi according to the clinical syndromes they produce. The common species and their toxidromes are outlined in Table 13.1.

Fungi producing gastrointestinal features

GI features occur commonly in poisoning with fungi. Several species causing serious toxicity to other organs can also cause GI features. It is important therefore to monitor closely all patients with GI features after ingestion of fungi for clinical and biochemical signs of toxicity affecting other organ systems. Baseline biochemistry is of value in identifying and monitoring future changes. A few of the fungi in the following list are toxic when raw, whereas others can cause symptoms despite having been cooked.

Those fungi generally associated only with GI features include:

- *Agaricus placomyces, A. semotus,* and *A. xanthodermus* (Yellow Stainer)
- *Boletus* species such as the Lurid Bolete (*B. luridus*), the Devil's Bolete (*B. satanus*), *B. legaliae* and *B. rhodopurpureus*
- *Chlorophyllum molybdites* (False- or Green-spored Parasol of North America)
- *Coprinus* species such as *Hygrophoropsis aurantiaca* (False Chanterelle)
- *Entoloma sinuatum* (Livid Entoloma)
- *Lactarius helvus* (Fenugreek Milkcap), *L. torminosus* (Wooly Mikcap)
- *Mycena pura* (Lilac Bonnet)
- *Omphalotus illudens*
- *Pholiota squarrosa* (Shaggy Scalycap)
- *Russula emetica* (Sickener), *R. nobilis* (Beechwood Sickener)
- *Scleroderma citrinum* (Common Earth-Ball)
- *Stropharia aeruginosa* (Verdigris Agaric)
- *Tricholoma sulphureum* (Sulphur Knight), and *T. saponaceum* (Soapy Knight).

Clinical features

Early onset (normally within 3 hours) of nausea, vomiting, diarrhoea, and abdominal pain, normally resolving within 24 hours.

The Common Ink Cap (*Coprinus atramentarius*) can produce an 'antabuse'-like reaction caused by the toxin, coprine (or a metabolite of coprine), inhibiting aldehyde metabolism after alcohol ingestion. This may last for up to 5 days. The Club-footed Clitocybe (*Ampulloclitocybe clavipes*) can cause similar symptoms, but does not contain coprine.

Management

This is generally supportive and symptomatic. Appropriate management of fluid balance is needed. Identification of the causative mushroom will assist in reassuring all involved.

Fungi producing hepatotoxic features

Certain fungi contain cyclopeptides (e.g. amatoxins, phallotoxins, and virotoxins) that are potent hepato-toxins, producing fatty degeneration and centrilobular necrosis. Such fungi include the Amanita species *Amanita phalloides* (Death Cap) and *A. virosa* (Destroying Angel). Several *Lepiota* species contain amatoxins, including *Lepiota brunneoincarnata* (Deadly Dapperling), as well as some *Galerina* species, such as *Galerina marginata*.

Clinical features

A latent period of 5–24 hours is followed by GI toxicity (e.g. nausea, profuse vomiting, cramping abdominal pain and watery diarrhoea hypotension, tachycardia, lactic acidosis and metabolic acidosis, electrolyte abnormalities and renal toxicity). This may be followed temporarily by an apparent recovery period before signs of liver damage may appear after 2–6 days, sometimes progressing to severe jaundice, liver and kidney failure, and death.

The shorter the interval between ingestion and onset of diarrhoea, the worse the prognosis. An interval of less than 8 hours after ingestion appears to indicate poor prognosis.

Table 13.1 Common fungi and their toxidromes

Toxin	Responsible species include:	Timing of symptom onset	Summary of symptoms
Amatoxin	Amanita phalloides Amanita virosa	5–24 hours	**Latent phase:** a duration of <8 hours is associated with poor outcome
		5–24 hours post ingestion. Duration: 1–2 days	**Phase 1**: sudden onset abdominal pain and watery diarrhoea, vomiting, and thirst
		Duration: 12–36 hours	**Phase 2**: phase of 'well-being' in which GI symptoms abate; however, liver and renal function may deteriorate. In severe cases this period may not occur
		2–6 days post ingestion	**Phase 3**: hepatic and renal failure, hypoglycaemia, seizures, coma, and death
Coprine	Coprinus atramentarius	20 minutes–2 hours after ethanol consumption Can occur up to 5 days after mushroom consumption	Disulfiram-like reaction in presence of ethanol. Features include flushing of the face, neck, and chest, metallic taste, nausea, vomiting, tachycardia, headache, anxiety, and hypotension. Toxicity does not develop unless ethanol is consumed.
GI toxins	Many species	30 minutes–3 hours	Nausea, vomiting, diarrhoea, and abdominal pain, normally resolving within 24 hours
Gyromitrin	Gyromitra esculenta	2–24 hours (mostly 5–15 hours) post ingestion	**Phase 1**: bloating followed by abdominal cramps, vomiting and watery diarrhoea (which may persist), headache and lethargy/weakness
		36–48 hours post ingestion	**Phase 2**: seizures, coma, liver toxicity with jaundice, intravascular haemolysis and methaemoglobinaemia, renal failure, and respiratory failure
Immune mechanism (unknown toxin)	Paxillus involutus		Haemolytic anaemia, particularly in patients who have previously ingested the fungus
Muscarine	Inocybe spp. Clitocybe rivulosa, Omphalotus olearius	15–300 minutes post ingestion	Cholinergic features including increased secretions (sweating, salivation, lachrymation) miosis, blurred vision, abdominal pain, watery stools, and asthmatic wheezing. Bradycardia and hypotension in severe cases
Muscimol (and ibotenic acid which is converted to muscimol)	Amanita gemmata Amanita muscaria Amanita pantherina	30–120 minutes. Duration: c.12 hours	Drowsiness, confusion, ataxia, euphoria, fluctuating conscious level, delirium, visual or auditory hallucinations, hyper-reflexia, myoclonus, seizures, coma
Orellanine	Cortinarius spp.	36 hours–17 days post-ingestion	**Latent phase:** the shorter the latent phase, the more severe the toxicity. If >6 days, long-term effects are unlikely; if <2–4 days, renal failure may be irreversible
		Duration: around 7 days	**Pre-renal phase:** anorexia, nausea and vomiting, headache, chills, sweats (without pyrexia), thirst. and polyuria
		7–21 days	**Renal phase** (50–70% cases): loin pain, anuria, renal dysfunction and renal failure
Psilocybin	Psilocybe cyanescens Psilocybe semilanceata	30–240 minutes	Nausea, vomiting, abdominal pain, flushing of the face and neck, tachycardia, dilated pupils, impaired judgment, euphoria, ataxia, drowsiness (progressing to sleep)

This GI phase may last for 1–2 days, before a transient improvement occurs for 12–36 hours.

Later feature: hepatic central lobular necrosis occurs after 2–6 days resulting in jaundice and liver failure, the complications of which include coma, hypoglycaemia, disseminated intravascular coagulation, and haemorrhage. Hypoglycaemia may also occur earlier, from direct insulin-releasing effects of the toxins on the pancreas. Acute tubular necrosis leads to renal failure. Tachycardia, hypotension which may be severe, hypocalcaemia, cardiomyopathy, muscle twitching, and convulsions may also occur.

Management
Treat symptomatically with fluid replacement and correction of acidosis. In some areas of the world specific tests for amatoxins are available to confirm diagnosis, but not in the UK.

Observe asymptomatic patients for a minimum of 24 hours if ingestion of *Amanita phalloides* is thought likely (beware latent period). It is very important to verify the type of mushroom, if possible by a mycologist.

Treatment with multiple doses of oral activated charcoal is of theoretical benefit because amatoxins are excreted in bile and activated charcoal is likely to interrupt entero-hepatic circulation. However, there are no controlled trials which demonstrate benefit and use is often precluded by severe vomiting. Nevertheless, provided the patient is not vomiting and the airway can be protected, multiple-dose activated charcoal should be considered.

Check U&Es, creatinine, full blood count, and LFTs. Consider checking arterial blood gases in symptomatic patients. Ensure adequate hydration and monitor urine output. If the patient has deranged LFTs, check prothrombin time, which is the single most useful prognostic test of liver failure.

Early convulsions or coma may be due to hypoglycaemia so monitor plasma glucose concentrations.

Correct hypoglycaemia and treat convulsions conventionally. Single brief convulsions do not require treatment.

Penicillin reduces the uptake of amatoxins into the liver in experimental models and benzylpenicillin has been used in the treatment of poisoning. Doses of 300 mg/kg/day (0.5 million units/kg/day) as a continuous infusion for 2–3 days from the day of ingestion, with close monitoring of renal function, have been suggested. NB Giving IV benzylpenicillin too rapidly may cause convulsions. Penicillin allergy should be excluded. The evidence base for this, and other specific treatments is poor. Renal and hepatic damage is managed conventionally, and liver transplantation has been required occasionally.

The following are of no confirmed benefit: constant duodenal aspiration to prevent enterohepatic circulation of amatoxins; intravenous N-acetylcysteine; early plasmapheresis, haemodialysis or haemoperfusion for removal of circulating amatoxins; silibinin; and thioctic acid.

Fungi producing nephrotoxic features

The Deadly Webcap (Cortinarius rubellus), Fool's webcap (C. orellanus), and some other Cortinarius species contain a range of toxins, including orellanine, a nephrotoxin which can cause interstitial nephritis and acute tubular necrosis after a latent period of 7–21 days. Two north-western US species, Smith's Amanita (Amanita smithiana) and the Abrupt-bulbed Lepidella (A. abrupta) and also A. proxima (in Spain) and A. pseudoporphyria (in Japan) have also been associated with acute kidney injury after 6–24 hours, probably as a result of an acute tubulopathy. It has been suggested that 2-amino-4,5-hexadienoic acid may be the responsible toxin.

Clinical features

In Cortinarius poisoning features are delayed and occur in three phases:

- The latent phase lasts for at least 36 hours, but rarely up to 17 days, post ingestion. The shorter the latent phase, the more severe the toxicity. A latent phase of more than 6 days suggests long-term effects are unlikely, while less than 2–4 days suggests that renal failure may be irreversible.
- The pre-renal phase is predominantly gastrointestinal and lasts for around 7 days. Nausea, vomiting, diarrhoea, abdominal pain, anorexia, and headache are common. A burning sensation in the mouth causes intense thirst, polyuria, and polydipsia. Other features include chills, shivering, sweating, muscle and loin pains, liver damage, paraesthesiae, fatigue, tinnitus, and seizures.

- The renal phase: usually occurs after 7–21 days (occasionally earlier). 50–70% of patients develop some renal involvement, 10–15% are likely to develop chronic renal failure. The main pathology is interstitial nephritis with leucocyturia, proteinuria, haematuria; oliguria occurs initially followed by anuria.

Damage may be reversible with renal function recovering slowly over 3–4 weeks in mild cases or several months in more severe cases. An initial recovery of renal function may not be sustained, and permanent renal damage can occur.

Management

Symptomatic and supportive. Dialysis may sometimes be required, and renal transplantation has been performed in some cases of chronic renal failure associated with Cortinarius poisoning.

Fungi producing haematological features

The Brown Roll-rim (Paxillus involutus) may cause haemolytic anaemia by an immune mechanism, (involving IgG) particularly in patients who have previously ingested the fungus.

Clinical features

Severe haemolysis and shock may result in acute kidney injury in affected individuals.

Management

Plasma exchange has been used to remove possible immune complexes, and the renal failure is treated conventionally.

Fungi producing toxicity to muscles

Ingestion of Tricholoma equestre (Yellow Knight) also known as T. flavovirens and of Russula subnigricans (the Blackening Russula found in China and North America) have been associated with rhabdomyolysis occurring 24–72 hours later.

Clinical features

Nausea (without vomiting) and muscle pain (especially of the quadriceps), and/or weakness may be accompanied by features of acute myocarditis and hyperthermia.

Management

There are no specific antidotes and management is symptomatic.

Fungi producing cholinergic (muscarinic) features

This toxidrome is produced by the cholinomimetic, muscarine which is present in several fungi, including Clitocybe rivulosa, (False Champignon or Fool's Funnel), Inocybe, and Omphalotus olearius (Jack-o-Lantern).

Clinical features

Symptoms occur early, often between 15 minutes and 5 hours after ingestion, and reflect the effects of muscarine. These include: increased perspiration, salivation, lachrymation, vomiting, abdominal pain, diarrhoea, urgency of micturition, flushing, bradycardia, hypotension, constricted pupils, and blurred vision.

Management

Supportive and symptomatic. Atropine may be required if peripheral cholinergic features are troublesome.

Fungi producing neuropsychiatric features

The Jewelled Deathcap (*Amanita gemmata*), Fly Agaric (*Amanita muscaria*), and Panther cap (*Amanita pantherina*) contain ibotenic acid (a glutamate receptor agonist), and muscimol (a GABA$_A$ receptor antagonist). *Psilocybe* species such as the Bluing Psilocybe (*Psilocybe cyanescens*) and the Liberty Cap (*P. semilancealata*) ('Magic mushrooms') contain the hallucinogenic agents psilocybin and psilocin. These fungi are often picked and ingested for these psychoactive effects as agents of misuse. As the quantity of toxin varies with season, variety, and age of the fungus fruiting parts, effects may be unpredictable, and in some cases prolonged.

Clinical features

Amanita gemmata, *A. muscaria*, and *A. pantherina* ingestion may result in the early onset (30–120 minutes) of GI symptoms (not always prominent), which may be accompanied by somnolence or agitation, with visual and/or auditory hallucinations. Bradycardia and pyrexia have also been reported. CNS effects usually peak around 2–3 hours post ingestion and usually wear off within 12 hours but may be followed by a deep sleep. Drowsiness may persist for 24 hours. A residual headache may last for days. Retrograde amnesia is a frequent result of poisoning. Delirium, hyper-reflexia, myoclonus, seizures (more commonly in children), and coma have also been noted in more severe poisoning.

Psilocybe cyanescens may also be associated with visual and/or auditory hallucinations that may persist for several days. Physical effects include nausea, vomiting, abdominal pain, flushing of the face and neck, tachycardia, dilated pupils, diastolic hypertension, and drowsiness. Rhabdomyolysis leading to renal failure, arrhythmias, and myocardial infarction have been reported. Methaemoglobinaemia and abnormal LFTs have sometimes been reported after IV abuse of fungal extracts. CNS effects are common initial symptoms including dizziness, confusion, euphoria and ataxia (i.e. resembling alcohol intoxication), myoclonus, hyperkinesia, and seizures. Neuropsychiatric effects vary from restless over-activity with lack of cooperation and aggressiveness to withdrawn, uncommunicative staring. Perceptual abnormalities such as visual hallucinations, distorted body image, sounds, and tactile sensation may occur. Ability to judge heights and distances may be grossly impaired. These effects occasionally persist for some days.

Management

Agitation in adults may necessitate benzodiazepine administration (NB it is normally better to manage agitation without sedation in children). Benzodiazepines may also be needed to treat convulsions. Atropine is not recommended, since it is thought to increase the adverse effects of ibotenic acid. In patients with more severe features, such as hallucinations or psychosis, an antipsychotic such as haloperidol may be required.

Fungi producing neurological features

Gyromitra esculenta (False Morel) contains gyromitrin, which is hydrolysed in the body to monomethylhydrazine (MMH) an inhibitor of GABA synthesis, which may cause convulsions and methaemoglobinaemia. Further MMH metabolism can lead to hepatic damage.

A rare toxidrome consisting of delayed onset of decreased visual acuity, somnolence, weakness, and reduced motor tone and activity occurring 24 hours after the ingestion of *Hapalopilus rutilans* (Purple-Dye Polypore) mushrooms has been attributed to the toxic effects of polyporic acid, a dihydrorotate dehydrogenase inhibitor. There may be associated hepatic and renal dysfunction.

Clinical features

In poisoning with *Gyromitra esculenta*, GI symptoms (occurring after 2–24 hours) include bloating, abdominal cramps, vomiting, and watery diarrhoea. Headache and lethargy/weakness, tremor, nystagmus, ataxia, slurred speech, mydriasis, delirium, coma and convulsions may also occur. Later features include liver toxicity with jaundice, intravascular haemolysis and methaemoglobinaemia, renal failure, and respiratory failure.

Management

Treatment of *Gyromitra esculenta* poisoning is supportive and symptomatic. Intravenous pyridoxine may be considered in treating convulsions and possibly also to reduce the risk of, or treat, established hepatic damage. Methylene blue may be indicated if methaemoglobinaemia occurs. Management of poisoning with *Hapalopilus rutilansis* is also symptomatic and supportive, although repeated-dose activated charcoal has been advocated.

Further reading

Diaz JH (2005). Syndromic diagnosis and management of confirmed mushroom poisonings. *Crit Care Med*, 33:427–36.

Fungi of Europe: <http://en.wikipedia.org/w/index.php?title=Category:Fungi_of_Europe&pageuntil=Dacryonaema#mw-pages>.

Kibby G (1997). *An illustrated Guide to Mushrooms and other Fungi of Britain and Northern Europe*. London: Parkgate Books Ltd.

Levine M, Ruha A-M, Graeme K, *et al.* (2011). Toxicology in the ICU Part 3: natural toxins. *Chest*, 140:1357–70.

UK Mushrooms: <https://sites.google.com/site/scottishfungi/eating-fungi/identifying-fungi-to-eat/toxic-fungi>.

Common plant poisonings

Background

Most accidental ingestions of plant material by small children do not result in more than minor symptoms; however, deliberate ingestion of some plants can cause serious features or even death. All patients who have deliberately ingested toxic plants need referral for psycho-social assessment as well as medical treatment. In some cases collecting wild plants for food has resulted in ingestion of misidentified plants and this can also cause problems.

When contacting a poisons centre about a plant poisoning it is preferable to have the Latin name of the plant, as many common names can refer to more than one plant, e.g. laurel, oleander. Poisons centres do not generally attempt to identify plants over the telephone. If identification is required then botanic gardens or garden centres may be able to help and photographs of the plant may aid identification.

In the UK plant poisonings represent less than 1% of enquiries to poisons centres. Table 13.2 shows the most common plant accesses on TOXBASE® in 2011.

In considering plants and their toxic hazard it may be useful to classify them in various groups depending on their properties. These include either their toxic hazard, low or high, or their mechanism of causing symptoms. This section includes both approaches and provides illustrative examples. Low-toxicity plants are grouped in Box 13.1. Some plants are only available at certain times of the year and cause seasonal exposures (Box 13.2).

Plants of low toxicity

- *Lilium* spp. (stargazer lilies, oriental lilies, Easter lilies)—this includes most of the lilies bought in supermarkets but not lily of the valley, peace lily, calla lily which belong to other families. NB *Lilium* species are extremely toxic to cats.
- *Saintpaulia ionanthe* (African violet) is considered to be of very low toxicity but may cause dermatitis.
- *Sorbus aucuparia* (rowan, mountain ash) contains parasorbic acid, which is an irritant. The cooked berries are said to be edible. Ingestion of raw berries may cause mild GI upset.

Table 13.2 Most common TOXBASE® plant accesses in 2011 (total 2011 product accesses >1.3 million)

Plant	Accesses
Capsicum (chillies)	526
Amaryllidaceae (daffodil)	512
Saintpaulia ionantha (African violet)	495
Taxus baccata (yew)	495
Laburnum anagyroides	427
Lily (supermarket type e.g. Asiatic, Oriental)	360
Atropa belladonna (deadly nightshade)	349
Valeriana officinalis (valerian)	312
Digitalis purpurea (foxglove)	305
Laurus nobilis (laurel, bay tree)	287

Data from TOXBASE®, 2011, National Poisons Information Service.

Box 13.1 Plants of low toxicity—may cause irritation and mild GI upset

- African violet (*Saintpaulia ionantha*)
- Carnation (*Dianthus*)
- Christmas cactus (*Schlumbergera bridgesii*)
- Dandelion (*Taraxacum officinale*)
- Daisy (*Bellis perennis*)
- Fuschia (*Fuchsia* spp.)
- Geranium (*Pelargonium* spp.)
- Hawthorn (*Crataegus* spp.)—may cause thorn injury
- Honeysuckle (*Lonicera* spp.)
- Marigold (*Calendula officinalis*)
- Nasturtium (*Tropaeolum majus*)
- Pansy (*Viola tricolor*)
- Petunia (*Solanacae*)
- Primrose (*Primula vulgaris*)
- Rose (*Rosa* spp.)—may cause thorn injury
- Rowan (*Sorbus aucuparia*)
- Snapdragon (*Antirrhinum majus*)
- Spider plant (*Chlorophytum comosum*)
- Violet (*Viola tricolor*).

- *Valeriana officionalis* (valerian) is considered to be of low toxicity and is used extensively in herbal preparations. Ingestion may cause drowsiness.

Plants which cause irritation

- *Aesculus hippocastanum* (horse chestnuts, conkers) contain aesculin and ingestion of large quantities is likely to cause GI upset. Allergic reactions have been reported.
- *Capsicum* species (chilli peppers) contain capsaicin which is severely irritating to respiratory tract, causing a burning sensation to mucous membranes, eyes, and skin. Inhalation may cause eye irritation, bronchospasm, and pulmonary oedema. Cold water or vegetable oil may give some relief for skin irritation.
- *Euphorbia* spp., e.g. *Euphorbia helioscopia* (sun spurge), which contains diterpene esters in the sap is very irritant to eyes and skin. Although *Euphorbia pulcherrima* (poinsettia) was formerly thought to be toxic no serious cases have been reported recently and it is probably less irritating than other members of the *Euphorbia* spp.
- *Laurus nobilis* (laurel, bay tree, sweet bay), is an irritant and is unlikely to cause more than GI upset, if ingested. However, bay leaves used in cooking and accidentally ingested have occasionally lodged in the GI tract, requiring surgical removal.

Generally ingestion of the above plants and those mentioned in Box 13.1 require only symptomatic treatment. Wash contaminated skin well with soap and water.

Toxicodendron spp, *Rhus* spp. (poison ivy, poison sumac, poison oak). All parts of the plant contain urushiol. This plant is generally found in North and Central America but since the onset of symptoms may be delayed patients may report symptoms after returning from holiday. Contact can be direct with damaged plants, indirect with clothing or shoes, or even from smoke from burning plants. Allergic contact dermatitis results in symptoms (redness, pruritus and bullae in severe cases) within 24–48 hours and lasting up to 2 weeks. Washing is only effective within 10 minutes of contact. For moderate cases calamine lotion, cold compresses, and topical corticosteroids may help. In more severe cases systemic corticosteroids should be given early and oral antihistamines may be useful.

Oxalate containing plants include:

- *Amaryllidacae* spp. (daffodil, narcissus)—dermatitis from handling the bulbs; severe nausea and vomiting from eating raw or cooked bulbs (mistaken for onions) may last 3–4 hours. Treatment is symptomatic with an antiemetic if required.
- *Rheum raponticum* (rhubarb)—causes dermatitis; ingestion of large amounts of the leaves (cooked or uncooked) has resulted in corrosive features. The systemic features of oxalate toxicity are unlikely, but include hypocalcaemia, tetany, convulsions, renal and hepatic damage, and death.
- *Spathiphyllum* spp. (peace lily), *Zantedeschia aethiopica* (calla lily, altar lily), *Monstera deliciosa* (swiss cheese plant), *Arum maculatum* (lords and ladies), and *Dieffenbachia* (leopard lily) all cause severe irritation of the buccal mucosa with a painful burning sensation and hypersalivation with a risk of obstruction of the airway if oedema occurs. Cold drinks or ice cream may be helpful.

Box 13.2 Seasonal plant exposures

- Christmas trees (evergreen coniferous trees)—skin contact is reported to cause dermatitis; ingestion may cause irritation. Symptomatic treatment.
- *Euphorbia pulcherrima* (poinsettia) is less irritating than other members of the *Euphorbia* family. May cause mild GI upset if ingested. Symptomatic treatment.
- *Hedera* spp. (ivy; do not confuse with the American plant poison ivy *Toxicodendron radicans*) causes burning in the mouth, GI upset, and allergic reactions. Symptomatic treatment.
- *Ilex aquifolium* (holly)—while all parts of the plant are potentially toxic ingestion of a few berries is only likely to result in mild GI upset and drowsiness. Symptomatic treatment.
- *Schlumbergera bridgesii* (Christmas cactus) considered to be of low toxicity.
- *Viscum album* (mistletoe; *Phoradendron flavescens* in the USA which has similar effects) contains viscotoxins and lectins. Ingestion of three to four berries in a child may cause mild GI symptoms and only symptomatic treatment is required. Deliberate ingestion of very large quantities of plant material or of mistletoe extract may cause local irritation and hepatitis. Parenteral administration is potentially much more toxic and may result in convulsions, coma, and bradycardia which should be managed conventionally.

Plants that cause photosensitization

Hypericum perforatum (St John's wort) is of low toxicity if ingested. Over-the-counter tablets are used to treat mild depression. Ingestion of large quantities of the plant (but not skin contact) can cause photodermatitis, i.e. dermatitis which develops after subsequent exposure to the sun, which should be managed conventionally.

Skin contact with *Heracleum mantegazzianum* (giant hogweed) results in dermatitis and photosensitization after exposure to sunlight, resulting in erythema, burn-like lesions, and large fluid filled blisters developing over 24–48 hours. All patients even if asymptomatic should be protected by covering the skin or wearing sun-block for at least 48 hours after exposure. Itching may be relieved with tepid baths, cool compresses, calamine lotion, steroid creams, and oral antihistamines. Patients with severe dermatitis should be reviewed by a burns specialist. Hyperpigmentation may occur and does not require treatment but skin may be sensitized for years and sun screen should be used. Ingestion may cause irritation, hypersalivation, GI upset, and also photosensitization. For ingestion manage symptomatically and advise to avoid going out in the sun for at least 12 hours.

Plants that contain cyanogenic glycosides

A number of plants contain cyanogenic glycosides and can potentially cause cyanide poisoning in large quantity e.g. members of the *Prunus* family (*Prunus armeniaca* (apricot); *Prunus dulcis x. amara* (bitter almonds); *Prunus laurocerasus* (ornamental cherry, cherry laurel); *Prunus spinosa* (blackthorn, sloe)—may also cause thorn injury, see 'Plant thorn injury' later in this section). In these cases accidental ingestion of small quantities (e.g. one or two apricot kernels ingested by a child) is unlikely to cause toxicity but may cause obstruction. Apricot kernels contain amygdalin and extracts have been falsely claimed to be a cancer cure (laetrile), and this use has occasionally resulted in cyanide toxicity. Early features may include dizziness and drowsiness leading in severe cases to coma, cardiovascular collapse, respiratory depression, and pulmonary oedema. See Cyanide, pp. 229–231, for further information on cyanide.

Cotoneaster spp. also contain cyanogenic glycosides but in low concentrations and ingestion of berries does not usually causes more than GI upset. Only symptomatic treatment is required.

Pyracantha spp. (firethorn) contain cyanogenic glycosides in low concentrations and ingestion of berries does not usually cause more than GI upset requiring symptomatic treatment. Injury from plant thorns may result in local irritation, erythema, pain, and swelling—see 'Plant thorn injury' later in this section.

Sambucus nigra (elder) does contain cyanogenic glycosides but the flowers and ripe cooked berries are not toxic. Ingestion of raw berries and other parts of the tree may cause weakness, dizziness and numbness. In severe cases consider cyanide toxicity (see Cyanide, pp. 229–231).

Toxic plants

Abrus precatorius (jequirity beans, rosary peas) are used in jewellery due to their bright colour and in Ayurvedic medicine. They contain abrin which is highly toxic. A single seed may pass through, but if chewed, ground, or pierced (as in a necklace) it is potentially fatal. All cases should be managed in hospital and should be discussed with a poisons centre. Initial features are gastrointestinal followed by neurological and in severe cases multiorgan failure occurs resulting in death up to 4 days after ingestion. Treatment of hypotension, ECG abnormalities, convulsions, and metabolic acidosis may be required.

Aconitum napellus (aconite, monkshood, wolf's bane) is probably the most toxic of UK plants and contains aconitine, a potassium efflux channel blocker. All parts of the plant are toxic and ingestion causes nausea, vomiting, diarrhoea, paraesthesia, tachyarrhythmias, convulsions, coma, and death. Serious cases should be discussed with a poisons centre. Cardiac resuscitation may be required and conventional management for hypotension, bradycardia, and arrhythmias. If unresponsive, intravenous lipid emulsion may be tried.

Atropa belladonna (deadly nightshade) contains hyoscyamine (atropine) and scopolamine (hyoscine). Ingestion can cause anticholinergic effects and may require management of hypotension, convulsions, and delirium (see sections in Chapter 3, pp. 63–94).

Colchicum autumnale (Autumn crocus) and *Gloriosa superba* (flame lily, glory lily) both contain colchicine especially in the corms. All patients should be referred to hospital. Features after ingestion may be delayed for 6 hours and can last 7 days or more. Initial features include severe GI upset, hypotension, and cardiogenic shock. Later features after 24 hours may include bone marrow suppression leading to sepsis, acute respiratory distress syndrome, renal failure, DIC, and direct cardiotoxic effects. Management will require treatment of hypotension, hyperthermia, and convulsions. Death is usually the result of intractable hypotension and asystole. For more information see Colchicine, pp. 164–165.

Cicuta virosa (cowbane, water hemlock) contains cicutoxin, a potent, non-competitive GABA receptor antagonist. All parts of the plant are toxic, especially the roots. Features usually start within 1 hour of ingestion but can be delayed for 10 hours and may last up to 4 days. Poisoning is characterized by severe convulsions. There may also be cardiac features and neurological complications. Intensive supportive treatment will be required with management of convulsions, hypotension/hypertension, bradycardia, agitation, hyperthermia, metabolic acidosis, and rhabdomyolysis.

Conium maculatum (hemlock) contains toxic alkaloids including coniine and all parts of the plant are toxic. Initial features develop within 15 minutes–3 hours after ingestion and include irritation, and tachycardia followed by bradycardia, and muscular paralysis leading to respiratory failure. Rhabdomyolysis and convulsions may also occur. Treatment may require management of hypotension, bradycardia, convulsions, and rhabdomyolysis. Death has occurred within 2 hours of ingestion.

Digitalis purpurea (foxglove) contains cardiac glycosides and causes poisoning similar to digoxin (see Digoxin, pp. 142–145). All patients should be referred to hospital. Initial features within 6 hours include GI features and later marked bradycardia and arrhythmias which may require treatment with digoxin-specific antibodies. Management of hypo/hyperkalaemia, metabolic acidosis, hypotension, and cardiac arrhythmias may be required. Note when requesting a digoxin concentration it is important to specify that it is due to plant material since methods vary. Similar features occur with *Nerium oleander* (pink oleander), *Thevetia peruviana* (yellow oleander), *Convollaria majalis* (lily of the valley), and *Drimia maritime*

(sea squill) which also contain cardiac glycosides. In serious cases where considering the use of digoxin-specific antibodies consult a poisons centre for dosage.

Laburnum anagyroides is generally considered to be toxic but few serious poisonings have occurred in recent years. While all parts of this tree are potentially toxic (especially the pods and seeds) it contains cytosine which is an emetic and this may limit toxicity. Common effects are nausea, vomiting, and abdominal pain and if these do not develop within about an hour subsequent toxicity is unlikely. In more severe cases there may be convulsions and cardiac effects which should be managed conventionally. Clinical effects may last up to 48 hours.

Ricinus communis (castor oil plant, castor beans) contains ricin in the seeds (see Ricin and abrin, pp. 345–346). Swallowing the beans whole may not cause problems but fatalities have occurred after chewing and swallowing beans. All patients should be referred to hospital. However, ricin is less toxic by ingestion than by inhalation or injection. Contact with the beans may also cause allergic reactions. GI upset usually occurs within a few hours of ingestion followed by drowsiness, confusion, convulsions, intravascular haemolysis, metabolic acidosis, and ECG abnormalities. Allergic reactions have been reported following inhalation and skin contact with castor bean dust. Note that the plant *Fatsia japonica* is also known as the castor oil plant but is much less toxic and is expected to cause only mild GI upset.

Taxus baccata (yew) contains taxane alkaloids (used clinically as cytotoxics). All parts of the plant are toxic with the exception of the fleshy red part of the berry. Ingestion of the whole berry or the fleshy red part of the berry is unlikely to cause more than nausea and vomiting. Chewing the berries or seeds or ingestion of other parts of the tree can result in hypotension, bradycardia, cardiac arrhythmias, respiratory depression, convulsions, coma, and death. Cardiac monitoring and pacing may be required.

Plants that may be abused

Cannabis sativa and *Cannabis indica* both contain tetrahydrocannabinol. Adults are unlikely to require treatment after ingestion or smoking but agitation may be controlled with diazepam or haloperidol. Children who have accidentally ingested cannabis may develop coma and all children should be observed for 6 hours after ingestion. Advice of a paediatrician should be sought in serious cases.

Catha edulis Forsk (khat) contains cathinone, norpseudoephedrine, norephedrine, sympathomimetic alkaloids, and tannins. Khat is commonly used in African and Middle Eastern countries for its mildly euphoric properties. Leaves are chewed and the liquid swallowed giving effects lasting 20 minutes to several hours. Euphoria is followed by irritability, depression, anorexia, and insomnia. A variety of side effects may occur from single and chronic use and management of agitation, hypo- or hypertension, tachycardia, and hyperthermia may be required. Note that a drug of abuse screen will be positive for amfetamines.

Datura stramonium (jimson weed, thorn-apple) contains atropine, scopolamine, and hyoscyamine, especially in the seed pods and is abused for its hallucinogenic potential. Features after ingestion are those of anticholinergics (see The anticholinergic syndrome, pp. 83–84). *Brugmansia* spp. (angel's trumpet) contains scopolamine, hyoscyamine, and atropine, and produces similar effects.

Ephedra spp. (Ma Haung) are used in herbal preparations for asthma and fevers, in dietary supplements, and in some herbal ecstasy tablets. Sympathomimetic features (see The stimulant syndrome, pp. 87–88) are expected and substance dependence has developed.

Myristica fragrans (nutmeg) is abused for its hallucinogenic features (reported from one to three nutmegs or 5–20 g of ground nutmeg). Symptoms appear within 1–8 hours of ingestion and may last at least 36 hours. There may be GI, cardiovascular, and CNS effects and management of agitation and hypertension may be required.

Lophophora williamsii (peyote cactus) contains mescaline and is abused for its hallucinogenic effects which are similar to LSD (see Psychedelic agents, pp. 192–193). GI effects occur within 30–60 minutes and hallucinogenic effects in 1–2 hours lasting 12–18 hours. Management of agitation, hypertension, hyperthermia, and rhabdomyolysis may be required.

Ipomoea purpurea (morning glory) seeds contain an indole alkaloid similar to LSD. Clinical features including restlessness and heightened awareness, auditory and visual hallucinations, disorientation, anxiety, violent behaviour, and flashbacks. Agitation should be managed with diazepam or haloperidol (see Delirium (acute confusional state) pp. 89–90).

Herbal products

Licensed herbal products are unlikely to cause toxicity. Some herbal products have been banned in the UK (<http://www.mhra.gov.uk/Howweregulate/Medicines/Herbalmedicinesregulation/Prohibitedor restrictedherbalingredients/index.htm>), e.g. *Aristolochia* spp. (renal failure and cancers), *Piper methysticum* (kava kava) permitted for external application—hepatic failure and acute dystonic reactions reported after oral use.

Chinese herbal medicine and Ayurvedic medicine are becoming more popular in the West and medicines brought from developing countries or over the Internet may contain pharmaceuticals, disallowed herbals, and heavy metals.

Other sources of plant poisoning

Honey

There have been reports of poisoning from honey where the bees have collected nectar from poisonous plants but this has not been reported in the UK. The plants involved include those containing:

- Pyrrolizidine alkaloids (e.g. *Senecio jacobaea*, ragwort). Poisoning with these is more common in animals. Toxicity is more likely following chronic ingestion. Liver function tests should be checked.

- Grayanotoxins (e.g. *Rhodendron* spp., azalea) which are sodium channel agonists. Ingestion of the flowers, decoctions of the plant, or honey from bees that fed on the plants has lead features such as nausea, vomiting, dizziness, hypotension, and cardiac complications which may required treatment with atropine.

Plant thorn injury

Plant thorn injury may occur from hairs or thorns from, for example, cacti, rose bushes, blackthorn, etc. Damage may be mechanical with intense pain and a histamine-like reaction. Thorns should be removed completely, otherwise secondary infection and ulceration may develop over days or weeks, which may require topical steroids and antibiotics.

Essential plant oils

These are used in aromatherapy and the pure oils (undiluted) are highly toxic. Doses of up to 10 mL clove oil have caused serious toxicity in children, Symptoms start within 30 minutes–4 hours and all children and adults should be observed for at least 6 hours after ingestion. Hypoglycaemia, metabolic acidosis, convulsions, and liver and renal failure may occur in severe cases. Aspiration may cause pneumonitis. Splashes in the eye may cause severe irritation and corneal damage (Essential oils, pp. 234–235).

Red kidney beans

Red kidney beans contain a phytohaemagglutinin, which is destroyed on adequate cooking. Ingestion of raw or partially cooked beans causes acute gastroenteritis within 1–2 hours, and lasting 3–4 hours.

Where to get advice

Plants may be identified by Botanic Gardens or a local garden centre. Advice on management may be obtained from a poisons centre (or public health advice call centre if appropriate) or TOXBASE® (if registered).

Further reading

Chan TY (2009). Aconite poisoning. *Clin Toxicol*, 47:279–85.

Dauncey EA (2010). *Poisonous Plants – A Guide for Parents and Childcare Providers*. London: The Royal Botanic Gardens.

Frohne D, Pfänder H (2005). *Poisonous Plants: A Handbook for Pharmacists, Doctors, Toxicologists, Biologists and Veterinarians*, 2nd edition. London: Manson Publishing.

Jansen SA, Kleerekooper I, Hofman ZL, et al. (2012). Grayanotoxin poisoning: 'mad honey disease' and beyond. *Cardiovasc Toxicol*, 2:208–15.

Krenzelok EP, Mrvos R (2011). Friends and foes in the plant world: a profile of plant ingestions and fatalities. *Clin Toxicol*, 49:142–9.

Schep LJ, Slaughter RJ, Becket G, et al. (2009). Poisoning due to water hemlock. *Clin Toxicol*, 47:270–8.

The Royal Botanic Gardens (2000). *Poisonous Plants and Fungi in Britain and Ireland*. CD-ROM. London: The Royal Botanic Gardens.

Venomous animals—spiders and scorpions

Background

Venomous snakes are the single most important group of toxin-producing animals worldwide; however, venomous arthropods have a significant impact on human health, particularly in the tropics and subtropics. Fortunately only small subsets of known spider and scorpion species are proven causes of harm to human health, but this small subset can cause major and sometimes lethal envenoming. In Europe scorpions and spider envenomation is most commonly from 'pets'. Occasionally returning travellers present with later features, particularly from spider bite.

Spiders

Spiders, like scorpions, are obligate predators, and virtually all species possess paired fangs and venom glands. Most spiders are too small to bite effectively and envenom, even if their venom was toxic to humans. There are a very small number of exceptions, spiders that contain toxins in their venom that targets humans and causes medically significant effects. These represent only a tiny fraction of the huge diversity of spider species. Spiders are, with very few exceptions, members of one of two major groups (suborders); Mygalomorphae (the more 'primitive' spiders), and Araneomorphae (most other spiders). Species capable of harming humans are found in both these groups.

Epidemiology of spider bites

There are few reliable studies of the incidence of spider bites to humans. In the UK these are from 'pets' or rarely on imported products. In Australia, spider bite calls are the commonest call to poison centres (~5000 per annum), and widow spider bite is common, with around 1000 cases a year receiving antivenom. Conversely, the far more dangerous funnel web spiders cause few bites.

In parts of South America recluse spiders are a common problem. In North America, widow spiders and, to a lesser extent, recluse spiders cause medically significant bites, but such bites are uncommon and are largely restricted to southern and eastern USA. In Africa, notably southern Africa, widow spiders and recluse spiders are medically important.

Spider venom

Spider venoms capable of harming humans fall into the same two broad groupings as scorpion venoms: excitatory neurotoxins and locally necrotic cytotoxins.

Neuroexcitatory spider venoms

The structure of spider neuroexcitatory venoms varies, but the effects are similar, and the target is a nerve cell membrane ion channel. The most potent spider toxin against humans is the atracotoxin group from funnel web spiders. These are low-molecular-weight toxins (around 4–5 kD) targeting potassium channels. Widow spider toxins (latrotoxins) are far larger (around 130 kD).

Cytotoxic spider venoms

Only recluse spiders (*Loxosceles* spp.) are clearly associated with local necrosis in humans. The component of most importance is a sphingomyelinase-D that causes both direct tissue damage, and indirect damage by attracting neutrophils which then also cause tissue damage.

Clinical effect of spider venoms

Medically significant spider bites are either neuroexcitatory or cytotoxic. Other spiders can bite humans and cause temporary local pain, but no significant local or systemic effects.

Neuroexcitatory envenoming

Neuroexcitatory envenoming produces a range of clinical presentations, depending on the type of spider venom. It is more distinctive than seen with scorpion stings.

Australian funnel web spiders (genera *Atrax* and *Hadronyche*, found in eastern Australia) are the most dangerous of all spiders and without adequate treatment envenoming can cause death, even in adults. Because of large fangs, local bite-site pain is common, increased by the spider 'hanging on', and the acidity of the venom. When systemic envenoming occurs it develops rapidly, within minutes to an hour. Patients bitten by a funnel web spider symptom-free for 4 hours have not been effectively envenomed. First symptoms of systemic envenoming can occur from 5 minutes post bite, commencing with peri-oral tingling and sometimes tongue fasciculation. This rapidly progresses, in significant cases, to one or more of: headache, nausea, profuse sweating, lacrimation, salivation, piloerection, hypertension, tachycardia. In the most severe cases there may be rapid progression to: pulmonary oedema, hypoxia, intracranial hypertension, coma. In severely envenomed untreated patients the pulmonary oedema phase is often fatal, but if survived, then progresses through generalized muscle fasciculation to hypotension, bradycardia, cardiac arrhythmia, to terminal cardiac arrest. Specific antivenom changes the clinical picture as it effectively reverses envenoming. The rate and severity of envenoming from funnel webs varies between species.

Bites by the closely related mouse spiders (genus: *Missulena*) rarely cause problems, but when significant envenoming does occur it is similar to funnel web spiders.

Widow spiders (genus: *Latrodectus*) occur almost worldwide and the syndrome of envenoming, latrodectism, is sufficiently uniform to be considered a single entity. Other related theriid spiders (family: *Theriidae*) can cause milder forms of latrodectism; e.g. cupboard spiders (genus: *Steatoda*). Classic widow spider bite causes only minor bite-site pain. In significant cases increasing pain develops in the bite area about 15–45 minutes (or more) post bite, with associated local erythema, sometimes local central blanching, and local profuse sweating. Over a variable time period the pain can track centrally, sometimes causing severe regional pain, associated with profuse sweating in some cases, tender and/or enlarged draining lymph nodes. Nausea, malaise, and hypertension also occur. In the most severe cases the pain can be excruciating, come in waves, involve much of the body, with profuse sweating, and occasionally severe hypertension. This systemic pain can mimic myocardial infarction, or an acute abdomen. Without treatment the pain and other features may persist beyond 1 week. Irrespective of bite site, if inadequately treated pain may devolve to burning pain in the soles of both feet and severe pain and profuse sweating of both legs below the knee. Death directly from envenoming is unlikely; rarely pulmonary oedema occurs. Debilitation secondary to envenoming may cause secondary fatal illness, particularly in children, the elderly, or infirm.

Banana spiders (genus: *Phoneutria*) cause phoneutrism which is a common toxinological cause of hospital attendance in parts of Central and South America, notably Brazil. Phoneutrism is similar to latrodectism, with sometimes severe pain and sweating, but is generally less severe. In young males priapism is a common envenoming effect, unlike latrodectism, where it occurs only rarely. Envenoming resolves over hours to days and is rarely fatal. Risks increase in the very young, old, and infirm, in whom antivenom is recommended.

Cytotoxic envenoming
Recluse (brown recluse, violin) spiders (genus: *Loxosceles*) have a wide global distribution, but are not native to all areas. These are the only spiders proven to regularly cause skin damage, with a toxin that induces damage (sphingomyelinase-D). The bite occurs most often at night, may be felt, but often goes unnoticed. Local symptoms may take more than 12 hours to develop, starting as local discomfort and redness, progressing over hours to days to a classic target lesion of central blue-black skin, surrounded by blanched skin, and an outer ring of erythema. There may pain, sometimes severe. In some there is blister or bleb formation. As the lesion develops the patient may develop a concurrent systemic illness, with fever. Full-thickness skin necrosis of large areas can occur, with skip lesions. In most cases the concern is the local tissue injury; cutaneous loxoscelism. In a minority systemic effects can be prominent, severe, or even lethal; viscerocutaneous loxoscelism. The latter can include intravascular haemolysis, thrombocytopenia, DIC, renal failure, or multi-organ failure. When first described (in Chile) mortality rate was 30%. Venom-induced local necrosis results, this may be exacerbated by secondary infection. Venom-induced skin necrosis is difficult to treat and slow to heal, potentially taking months to resolve. It is clear that many alleged loxoscelism cases are due to other causes, e.g. infection.

Diagnosis of spider bite
Diagnosis of spider bite often relies on recognizing a distinctive pattern of envenoming, both local and systemic. An actual spider will be seen in a minority of cases.

There are no clear diagnostic tests and no venom detection kits. Blood tests are diagnostically unhelpful. In widow spider bite creatine kinase may rise, but is neither diagnostic nor influences treatment. In recluse spider bite it is, conversely, important to undertake serial blood tests to ensure viscerocutaneous loxoscelism is not missed, including: full blood count, renal and liver function, and coagulation studies. Necrotic skin lesions should also be swabbed for culture/sensitivity.

Treatment of spider bite
The approach varies with spider. Most bites are from species of no medical significance, not requiring treatment. For medically important species, only a minority develop significant envenoming. A few species cause rapid and life-threatening envenoming and where they occur (e.g. Australia) the first aim of treatment is to ensure any at-risk case is urgently assessed and managed. This has resulted in a triage algorithm in Australia that separates out bites by 'big black spiders', which might be funnel webs, from all other spider bites.

Treating neuroexcitatory envenoming
Depending on the type of spider, antivenom may be: the mainstay of treatment (Australian funnel web spiders); a common treatment used in all significantly symptomatic cases (widow spider bite in Australia); or a treatment

reserved for high-risk severe cases (banana spiders, widow spiders in many regions). The only other currently accepted treatments for neuroexcitatory spider envenoming are secondary or symptomatic, but clear evidence on best practice is generally absent.

For Australian funnel web spider bite all possible (i.e. bite by unidentified 'big black spider' within known range) and definite funnel web bites: urgently transport to hospital, urgently triage and assess, and observe for 4 hours post bite. If no evidence of significant envenoming occurs, safely discharge. If envenoming consistent with funnel web spiders develops, specific antivenom should be given IV and expert clinical toxinologist consultation sought regarding the dose and need for further doses.

For patients presenting with either a clear history of widow spider bite in Australia (red back spider), or an envenoming syndrome consistent with latrodectism, patients should seek medical help only if symptomatic, because envenoming generally is not rapidly progressive, and many cases never develop effects. If significant envenoming develops patients are offered specific red back spider antivenom IM, or IV (IV two vials). Antivenom seems effective and safe. In most other regions with widow spider antivenom available, it is only used in severe cases in high-risk patients (young, elderly, infirm). This reflects concern about the risk of fatal ADRs to antivenom treating a non-fatal illness. This approach is controversial. The Australian antivenom has been used in clinical studies in North America, and used successfully to treat severe bites by the related cupboard (*Steatoda* spp.) spiders.

In Brazil, bites by banana spiders are managed by an escalating protocol. For most cases treatment is symptomatic, using analgesia, often local anaesthetic injection. In the minority developing severe envenoming, IV antivenom is considered.

For other spiders reassurance or symptomatic care is warranted.

Treating cytotoxic envenoming
Treating cytotoxic spider bite is controversial. Since diagnosis and treatment is delayed more than 24 hours post bite, and cellular damage has occurred, antivenom is unlikely to reverse this. Steroids, dapsone, and surgery are of no benefit. Treatment should be symptomatic, recovery may be long and incomplete.

Prevention of spider bite
In areas with potentially lethal spiders, simple modification of human behaviour may reduce the risk of bites.

Scorpions
Scorpions are obligate predators with a venom delivery apparatus in their 'tail' (the telson), but have pincer-like 'claws'. One group have large powerful 'claws', though their sting may cause pain this is generally not a threat to life. The other group have evolved more potent venom. Many are small and slightly built, and are the scorpions of most threat to human health. Nearly all the dangerous scorpions fall within a single grouping, family Buthidae. Within this group there are more similarities than differences in the clinical pattern of envenoming caused to humans.

Epidemiology of scorpion sting
In some parts of the World, scorpion sting is of greater medical impact than snakebite. Examples include Mexico, North Africa, and parts of the Middle East. However, not all scorpion sting hot-spots are in arid regions; thus

scorpion stings are important in parts of Brazil including urban environments.

In Mexico, scorpion stings (annual hospital presentation rates approaching 300,000) are far more than for snakebite. It is likely that a similar or higher number of cases occur across North Africa and the Middle East. Though it receives less attention than snakebite, in parts of SW USA medically significant scorpion sting may also be comparatively common, compared to snakebite. The most recent global estimate is more than 1 million stings per year with about 3000 fatalities.

Scorpion venom

Much research has been focused on venoms (especially ion channel toxins) of medically significant scorpions. Detailed exposition on this topic is beyond the scope of this section. There is little information on *Hemiscorpius lepturus* venom, but so far no sphingomyelinase-D toxin, which is found in recluse spider venom, has been identified despite the strong similarity in envenoming between these two disparate arthropods. Studies suggest metalloproteinase activity of venom may be involved in necrosis. Though apparently not significant in human envenoming, a calcium channel neurotoxin (hemicalcin) has been isolated.

Clinical effects of scorpion stings

The clinical pattern of scorpion sting envenoming can be divided into two classes; neuroexcitatory, as caused by nearly every medically significant scorpion species, all within family Buthidae, and cytotoxic, caused by a very limited group of scorpions in family Hemiscorpiidae (formerly family Scorpionidae).

Neuroexcitatory scorpion envenoming

The vast majority of medically significant scorpions, and scorpion stings, fall into this category. Some major genera/species are shown in Table 13.3. This form of envenoming has a distinctive pattern, with initial severe pain at the sting site, rapidly followed by progressive systemic envenoming with gross excitation of portions of the nervous system, sometimes described as 'catecholamine-storm-like', resulting in peripheral autonomic effects (increased sweating, salivation), hypertension, tachy- or bradycardia, cardiac dysfunction, pulmonary oedema, nystagmus, coma. Gastrointestinal symptoms/signs are common. Cardiac problems include acute myocarditis and cardiac failure; myocardial perfusion abnormalities are documented, for *Tityus* spp. stings in Brazil. Transitory myocardial ischaemia has been postulated as contributory to cardiac problems in scorpion envenoming, possibly secondary to the catecholamine storm. Severity is greater in children who are at risk of a lethal outcome; adults generally have non-lethal envenoming. The emphasis of clinical features varies between scorpions within this group. For instance, rotary nystagmus and ocular movement abnormalities are prominent in stings by *Centruroides* spp. scorpions in SW USA and parts of Mexico. A study in Tunisia reported on cases in ICU, with 62% pulmonary oedema, 21% cardiogenic shock, 39% elevated blood sugar, 80% leucocytosis, 74% GI tract signs, and there was a 7.5% mortality rate. In this study poor prognosis was associated with age less than 5 years, fever greater than 38.5° C, and the presence of pulmonary oedema, leucocytosis higher than $25 \times 10^3/mm^3$, and GCS less than 8. The effects of scorpion sting in pregnancy are poorly documented, but antepartum fetal death is reported. There are rare reports of cerebral infarction following scorpion sting, notably in India, possibly due to severe hypertension, or coagulopathy.

Table 13.3 Some medically important scorpion groups

Scientific name	Distribution	Clinical effects
Family Buthidae		
Leiurus quinquestriatus + other *Leiurus* spp. (common name— yellow scorpion)	North Africa to Middle East	Neuroexcitatory envenoming
Androctonus spp.	North Africa to Middle East	Neuroexcitatory envenoming
Buthus spp.	Mediterranean region	Neuroexcitatory envenoming
Centruroides spp.	North and Central America	Neuroexcitatory envenoming
Tityus spp.	South America	Neuroexcitatory envenoming
Parabuthus spp.	Southern Africa	Neuroexcitatory envenoming
Mesobuthus spp.	Middle East to India	Neuroexcitatory envenoming
Family Hemiscorpiidae		
Hemiscorpius lepturus	SW Iran	Moderate to severe local necrosis + in some cases systemic organ damage

Cytotoxic scorpion envenoming

This form of envenoming is rare amongst scorpions, principally in a scorpion restricted to SW Iran (Khuzestan), *Hemiscorpius lepturus*. A few related species cause less severe cytotoxic envenoming. *H. lepturus*, though not the most frequent cause of stings in Iran (12%), cause the majority of fatal stings (95%) and predominate during winter. 95% of *H. lepturus* stings affect the skin, with indurated purpuric changes, oedema and necrosis (47%), and bullous reactions (19%). The initial sting may cause only minor discomfort, unlike other scorpion stings, but as necrosis develops, pain can become severe. Necrotic ulcers develop over several days with cellulitis, bullae, or blue-black skin discolouration, and may take months to heal. Necrosis is less common in young children than in older children and adults, but young children are more likely to develop severe systemic effects, including intravascular haemolysis, cardiac toxicity and arrest, CNS problems, and renal failure. Non-specific systemic symptoms (in order of frequency) include malaise, dry mouth, dizziness, nausea, thirst, headache, fever, vomiting, anorexia, tachycardia, hypotension, sweating, vertigo, restlessness, haemolysis, and haematuria.

Diagnosis

In most cases of scorpion sting (neuroexcitatory species) the diagnosis will be obvious: the patient will have had severe local pain from the time of the sting and often have seen the scorpion. In cases where none was seen, sudden onset of severe local pain consistent with a scorpion sting, in a setting where stings are possible, and the subsequent effects consistent with scorpion envenoming, point to the diagnosis. However, snakebite, centipede, or spider bite may also need to be considered in this scenario. There are no diagnostic laboratory tests in neuroexcitatory scorpion envenoming.

Treatment of scorpion envenoming
Though controversial, specific antidote therapy using appropriate antivenom is the mainstay of managing major scorpion envenoming in most regions where antivenom is available. Some areas use a clinical score for assessing severity of scorpion stings but utility of this score system is uncertain.

Treating neuroexcitatory scorpion envenoming
The major risk group in neuroexcitatory scorpion envenoming is children. Efficacy of antivenom remains unclear. Some maintain antivenom is ineffective citing it cannot: target key venom effects; be given soon enough to be effective; there are other more effective safer therapies. Clinicians in countries such as Mexico who use scorpion antivenom claim dramatic reductions in fatality rate in children; 86.5% reduction in mortality in one study. A recent study of antivenom versus placebo in the US reported that antivenom was clearly effective.

Experience in Saudi Arabia and Brazil indicates that one problem with antivenom use may have been under-dosing and an inappropriate route (IM), while higher doses given IV appear effective. IV is the preferred route for scorpion antivenom.

Antivenom is not available in all areas so other treatments should be considered. In India, prazosin is used to manage cardiac toxicity following *Mesobuthus* spp. envenoming. However, two recent Indian studies indicate that antivenom is more effective than prazosin alone. Prazosin should be reserved for cases developing severe hypertension and pulmonary oedema, as an adjunct to antivenom. Where antivenom is not available prazosin is preferable to dobutamine as first-line therapy. Addition of dobutamine in severe cases with left ventricular failure may be beneficial. Captopril has also been suggested and used in India.

A novel treatment, but not available for human use, is monoclonal bispecific antibody against selected toxins.

Treating cytotoxic scorpion envenoming
This type of envenoming is essentially restricted to SW Iran, where a local polyvalent antivenom, covering several Iranian scorpions, is used, but not documented by clinical trials. However, given the delayed presentation of *H. lepturus* stings, so delayed antivenom therapy, there are reasons to doubt effectiveness. At present it would seem reasonable to use antivenom at the earliest opportunity, at least two vials, IV (not IM as the manufacturer suggests).

Prevention of scorpion stings
Given the frequency and importance of scorpion stings in some regions, with associated costs to the health system, prevention is a worthwhile exercise. Thus in areas where rural workers are at risk of stings, such as corn pickers in Mexico, use of gloves can dramatically reduce sting incidence.

Venomous ticks
There is a vast array of ticks and mites, many of which can bite humans, and a number are vectors for disease. A few produce salivary toxins that can envenom humans, causing progressive flaccid paralysis. Only these latter will be considered here.

Epidemiology of tick envenoming
Tick paralysis is well documented in Australia, North America, and southern Africa. Paralysis cases are largely restricted to the known range of these ticks in eastern Australia. Children are at highest risk. In North America the incidence of tick paralysis does not appear to closely track the distribution of these ticks.

Tick venom
Australian paralysis tick venom has been well studied and a presynaptic neurotoxin has been identified.

Clinical effects of tick venom
Most bites do not result in envenoming. Paralysis occurs when a mature female tick attaches to the skin and commences feeding; these are easily overlooked. It may be several days before paralytic symptoms develop. Most commonly these commence as an ascending flaccid paralysis first manifest as ataxia, but potentially progressing to complete paralysis; progression varies from hours to days. Effects may be local, e.g. an apparent Bell's palsy if the tick is attached near the facial nerve.

For North American ticks, once the tick is removed, paralysis declines, but for Australian ticks the paralysis may progress for up to 48 hours post removal.

Diagnosis of tick envenoming
There are no definitive diagnostic tests for tick paralysis, though clearly finding a tick in a patient with progressive paralysis is strongly suggestive. If no tick is found, other paralytic bites and Guillain–Barré syndrome should also be considered.

Treatment of tick envenoming
Tick paralysis requires supportive and secondary treatment; no specific antidote (antivenom) is available. All ticks are located and removed, using specific tick-removal devices; it is important not to squeeze the engorged body or leave mouth-parts behind. If paralysis is severe then respiratory support may be required for a period of hours to a few days. In Australia it is essential that a patient with partial tick paralysis be observed for 2 days post tick removal. This is not required in North America. Where appropriate, check for evidence of tick borne diseases such as Lyme disease.

Prevention of tick envenoming
Preventing tick paralysis essentially consists of limiting opportunities for ticks to attack, e.g. ensuring clothing minimizes exposure and possibly the use of pesticides.

Further reading
Chippaux J-P, Goyffon M (2008). Epidemiology of scorpionism: a global appraisal. *Acta Tropica*, 107:71–9.

Daly F, White J (2005). Widow and related *Latrodectus* spiders. In: Brent J, Wallace K, Burkhart K (eds) *Critical Care Toxicology*, pp. 1187–94. Philadelphia, PA: Elsevier Mosby.

Isbister GK, White J (2004). Clinical consequences of spider bites: recent advances in our understanding. *Toxicon*, 43(5):477–92.

Miller MK, Whyte IM, White J, et al. (1999). Clinical features and management of *Hadronyche* envenomation in man. *Toxicon* 38:409–27.

White J (1995). Clinical toxicology of tick bites. In: Meier J, White J (eds), *Clinical Toxicology of Animal Venoms and Poisons*, pp. 191–203. Boca Raton, FL: CRC Press.

White J, Cardoso JL, Fan HW (1995). Clinical toxicology of spider bites. In: Meier J, White J (eds), *Clinical Toxicology of Animal Venoms and Poisons*, pp. 259–329. Boca Raton, FL: CRC Press.

Marine envenoming

Background
Venomous marine creatures cause envenoming with a specialized venom apparatus. Specialized glands produce venom which is injected, or applied to another organism. Most marine creatures cause 'stings' rather than 'bites'. Marine stings are rare, except in some coastal regions. The most important are jellyfish, which sting by skin-contact with their tentacles, and venomous fish which have spines that cause penetrating injuries. Less common are stings from sea urchins, sponges, and sea snakes.

Jellyfish stings
There are more than 100 medically important jellyfish (cnidariae) around the world. In general, jellyfish stings cause similar types of stings.

Mechanism of injury
Jellyfish have millions of stinging cells (nematocysts), mainly on the tentacles. Each stinging cell contains a small amount of venom and a coiled harpoon-like mechanism to inject it. Physical or chemical stimuli trigger the cell to fire off and inject venom.

Epidemiology
Excepting a few species of jellyfish such as *Physalia physalis*, the type of jellyfish that sting is dependent on the geographic location. Local expertise will be required in more severe cases.

Overview of jellyfish stings
There are two major clinical syndromes that result from jellyfish stings—linear or tentacle-like stings and Irukandji-like stings. The majority of stings are the former with variations in severity and range of effects.

Linear/tentacle-like stings
Stings typically cause immediate pain that lasts minutes to hours, associated with a linear erythematous or urticarial eruption. Systemic effects are rare, usually non-specific symptoms such as nausea, vomiting, and headache.

Irukandji-like stings
Symptoms are usually delayed 20–30 minutes after the sting. There is minimal local pain and erythema, but severe generalized pain, abdominal, back, chest, and muscular, commonly associated with nausea, vomiting, headache, and hypertension. Myocardial injury and pulmonary oedema occur rarely.

Specific jellyfish
Physalia species
Physalia species are widespread, the commonest jellyfish stings worldwide, causing thousands of stings in North America and Australia and are referred to as Portuguese man-o-war, Pacific man-o-war, or blue bottles. Few cases present to hospital. *Physalia* stings cause immediate localized and intense pain, lasting 1 or more hours. There are linear erythematous marks at the sting site lasting 1–2 days. Systemic effects are rare. Delayed localized bullous reactions can occur but scarring is rare.

Treatment
Tentacles should be removed by washing them off with seawater or by hand. Hot water immersion (45° C) for 20 minutes is the recommended treatment for local pain. Test the water temperature first. Alternatively use a hot shower or a constant flow of hot water. Vinegar may increase the pain and is not recommended. Rarely analgesia, or local dressings for skin reactions are required.

Chironex fleckeri (box jellyfish)
Chironex fleckeri from northern Australia is often referred to as the most venomous creature in the world. Over 70 deaths have resulted from stings, mostly in children.

C. fleckeri have a box shape with multiple long tentacles on each corner. Most stings are minor, similar but more severe than other jellyfish. Potentially life-threatening adult stings are associated with several metres of skin contact; just over 1 metre resulted in the death of a child.

Immediate local pain is associated with linear erythematous eruptions, 'whip-like' marks. Stings are often multiple causing severe and longer lasting pain. Local necrosis can occur, rarely resulting in permanent scarring. Delayed papular urticarial reactions occur along the sting sites in about half to two-thirds of cases. Severe envenoming is characterized by cardiovascular collapse and potentially death within 20–30 minutes.

Treatment
In severe envenoming pre-hospital first aid and resuscitation are essential. Survival depends on early cardiopulmonary resuscitation. First aid (tentacle removal by hand or seawater, and the sting sites covered in vinegar) should occur simultaneously with basic life support. Vinegar stops further nematocyst discharge and prevents severe envenoming, but not pain.

Minor stings require simple analgesia, initially with ice packs. The utility of hot water immersion for *C. fleckeri* stings remains uncertain. Treat severe pain with oral or parenteral opioids. Most stings do not require local treatment except if there is necrosis, which requires local dressings. Systemic envenoming develops rapidly with an hour. Treat cardiovascular collapse as for any cardiac arrest, with cardiopulmonary resuscitation and advanced life support; consider intravenous antivenom and magnesium.

There is increasing evidence box jellyfish antivenom is unlikely to be effective in human envenoming, thus only consider its use in patients with severe envenoming.

Irukandji syndrome
Irukandji syndrome, first reported in northern Australia, is now recognized in most parts of Australia and in other parts of the world. Irukandji syndrome refers to the constellation of clinical effects that was first reported for *Carukia barnesi*. It is characterized by the delayed onset of generalized pain and systemic effects, with minimal local effects at the time of the sting. One death is reported in Irukandji syndrome.

There are normally minimal local effects and in many cases no evidence of a sting. After 20–30 minutes severe generalized abdominal, back, chest, and muscular pain develops, associated with systemic symptoms (nausea, vomiting, and diaphoresis), anxiety, agitation, tachycardia, and hypertension. Cardiac toxicity occurs in severe cases. ST segment depression and T wave changes on the ECG and elevated troponin indicate myocardial injury. Rarely cardiogenic pulmonary oedema occurs.

Treatment
The majority of stung patients require hospital treatment for severe pain, often associated with other systemic symptoms. Titrated intravenous opiates, morphine or fentanyl, with antiemetics should be given. Benzodiazepines may be used for anxiety and agitation.

An ECG and troponin should be done in all patients. If patients are pain free with a normal ECG and troponin they can be discharged after 6 hours. If there is cardiac involvement continue monitoring. Admit to critical care unit if patients are unstable or there is evidence of acute pulmonary oedema. Standard supportive care is appropriate.

Other jellyfish stings
There are many other species of jellyfish that cause medically important stings; clinicians need to be aware of jellyfish in their local region. In most cases the jellyfish will not be identified and treatment is based on history of, and clinical effects consistent with, a jellyfish sting. Most jellyfish cause local immediate pain and linear eruptions, and in the vast majority of cases the effects are minor and similar to *Physalia* stings. Systemic effects are rare.

Hydrozoa
- Feather hydroids are the most numerous of the hydrozoa group and are plume-like animals that cause minor effects—painful itching and urticaria.
- *Millepora* or fire corals cause minor effects.
- *Gonionemus* spp. occur in both Russia and Japan and are reported to cause an Irukandji-like envenoming syndrome.
- *Olindias* spp. occur in South America and cause effects similar to *Physalia*.

Scyphozoa
- Hair jellyfish (*Cyanea* spp.) occur in open or colder waters. The tentacles can break off and still cause stings. Stings to the eye or cornea are reported.
- *Catastylus* spp. (blubber jellyfish) common jellyfish that rarely cause stings
- *Chrysaora quinquecirrha* (sea nettle) occur in the Americas, Japan, and the Philippines. The best known is *C. quinquecirrha*, common in the Chesapeake Bay. Clinical effects are as for *Physalia*.
- Mauve stinger (*Pelagia* spp.) are reported in the Mediterranean and Australia and cause minor effects such as local pain and urticaria.
- *Linuche unguiculata* (thimble jellyfish) larvae occur in the Atlantic and can cause a vesicular pruritic dermatitis that lasts days and resolves spontaneously. Often referred to incorrectly as 'sea lice' it usually occurs in areas covered by bathing suits.

Cubozoa (other box jellyfish)
- Hawaiian box jellyfish (*Carybdea alata*) cause large numbers of stings in Hawaii. Clinical effects are similar to *Physalia* but may be more severe. Hot water immersion is reported to be effective for pain.
- *Chiropsalmus quadrigatus* is reported to have caused deaths in the Philippines and Japan, but there is limited information.
- *Chiropsalmus quadrumanus* is found along the Atlantic coast of the USA and generally causes minor effects. One unusual death in a child has been reported.
- Jimble and other box jellyfish (*Chiropsalmus bronzeii*) occur in Australia and cause minor effects.

Anthozoa
This is the largest group of jellyfish and includes sea anemones. Anemones generally cause very mild effects but can cause local pain associated with local erythema.

Treatment for other jellyfish
Treatment is similar to *Physalia*, but there is less evidence for topical treatments and geographical variation in treatment approaches. In all cases the tentacles should be removed by washing with sea water or removing by hand. Hot water immersion is likely to be effective and has not been tested for jellyfish other than *Physalia*. Vinegar is not recommended because it may increase the pain. Hospital treatment is only required for severe local effects or systemic envenoming.

Penetrating venomous marine injuries
The other major type of marine envenoming is from penetrating marine injuries which includes venomous fish stings, stingray injuries, and sea urchin injuries.

Mechanism of injury
Penetrating marine injuries occur when a spine that is usually covered by a sheath ruptures as the spine penetrates the skin. In most cases there is venom between the spine and sheath which is injected as the spine enters the skin. Spines come from fish, stingray tail spines, and sea urchin spines; the latter does not have a sheath.

Venomous fish
Worldwide the important venomous fish include catfish, stonefish, bullrout, lesser and greater weever fish, and the scorpion fish group (e.g. lionfish, zebra fish). Venomous fish are found throughout coastal waters and fresh water.

Clinical effects
The predominant symptom is localized pain due to the puncture wound, but severity varies based on size of the puncture and amount of venom injected. More severe and persistent pain occurs with stonefish, bullrout, weever fish, or marine catfish where large amounts of venom may be injected. Bleeding is usually minimal but there may be significant swelling and oedema. The spines rarely remain in the wound but small amounts of foreign material can. Secondary infection is a risk; systemic effects are likely to be secondary to severe pain.

Stingray
Fresh water and marine stingrays occur throughout the world. Most injuries occur when people tread on stingrays in shallow water; rarely severe thoraco-abdominal trauma occurs when divers swim too close to them.

Clinical effects
In general, stingray injuries cause more trauma than other venomous fish due to their size, including severe local pain and bleeding. The pain may be more severe due to venom, and local necrosis may occur in some cases. Secondary infection is a risk, particularly in larger wounds.

Sea urchins
Sea urchins occur worldwide and most injuries occur when they are trodden on or occasionally when they are picked up. Most spines are non-venomous and the type of spines range from chalk-like to strong thorn-like material. Crown-of-thorns sea stars in the Indo-Pacific region may cause similar injuries.

Clinical effects

Sea urchin spine injuries rarely cause severe pain. Multiple retained spines are the major problem. These can be difficult to remove and cause persistent pain.

Treatment of penetrating marine injuries

First aid

The wound site should be washed and pressure applied if significant bleeding. Immerse the wound site in hot water (45° C) for up to 90 minutes if this improves the pain. Use an unaffected limb to check the temperature first, since excess heat can cause burns.

Analgesia

Oral or parenteral analgesia can be given, e.g. a combination of ibuprofen (200–400 mg) and paracetamol (1 g) initially and oxycodone (5–10 mg) can be added. Treat severe pain with titrated intravenous opiates. Local or regional infiltration of anaesthetic may be useful, particularly for exploring and cleaning larger wound sites.

Wound management

Good wound management is essential in all cases, including generous irrigation and removing any foreign material. Radiography or ultrasound assists in identifying foreign bodies; essential with sea urchin injuries as multiple retained spines are common. Larger wounds are best left open for delayed primary closure. Stingray injuries may require surgical exploration and debridement. Treat rare thoracic or abdominal injuries with stingray initially as major trauma. Surgical involvement is essential for wounds into joints or sterile body cavities. Sea urchin spines are problematic, because they can be difficult to find and remove. Spines near the surface should be removed and the patient reviewed regularly until symptoms resolve, and if not have surgical review.

Wound infection and antibiotics

Although rare, an important complication of penetrating marine injuries is secondary infection. These include *Vibrio* spp. (marine environment) and *Aeromonas* spp. (fresh water) which can be associated with significant morbidity and mortality. All penetrating marine injuries should be followed up over the first week rather than using prophylactic antibiotics, particularly in uncomplicated wounds. Skin infections with normal flora can also occur and tetanus status should be reviewed and updated. Manage infections conventionally.

The role of prophylactic antibiotics is controversial. Treatment should rather focus on good wound care and follow up so that infection can be treated early.

Antivenom

An antivenom is available for stonefish stings. It should be used in cases not responsive to analgesia, or if there is evidence of systemic envenoming. Antivenom should be given intravenously as a 1:10 dilution over 15 minutes. The dose is one vial, in both children and adults.

Sponges

Of the thousands of sponge species only a few are medically important. Some produce toxic secretions, e.g. the fire sponges (*Tedania* spp.) and *Neofibularia* spp.

Clinical effects

Contact injuries with sponges are uncommon, often referred to as stinging sponge dermatitis. Most are minor injuries including local tingling, transient pain, itchiness, and numbness. Pain may develop in the hours after the sting and persist for a number of days. Fire sponges can cause delayed effects 2–3 weeks after contact, with painful swelling and erythema, followed by desquamation.

Treatment

First aid includes washing the sting site. Analgesia may be required and symptoms can be treated with antihistamines. Effects resolve over days to weeks irrespective of treatment.

Blue-ringed octopus

The Australian blue-ringed octopus (*Hapalochlaena* spp.) saliva contains tetrodotoxin. Bites have caused deaths. The clinical effects are similar to tetrotodotoxin (TTX) poisoning (see later in this section). Most cases cause bite marks and local pain and systemic TTX envenoming with paralysis is rare. Treatment is supportive and mechanical ventilation may be required. The recommended first aid is a pressure bandage with immobilization.

Cone snails

Cone snails are univalve creatures found in the Indo-Pacific region. They sting by projecting a harpoon-like apparatus and inject a neurotoxic venom. Stings are exceedingly rare, only if the snail is handled. There is usually local pain, followed by local numbness, rapidly spreading in severe envenoming. Partial and complete paralysis has been reported, including respiratory failure. Treatment is supportive; a pressure bandage can be used for first aid.

Sea snake envenoming

Sea snakes are closely related to Australian elapids and occur in tropical parts of the Pacific and Indian Oceans. The most important species is the beaked sea snake (*Enhydrina schistosa*), which caused numerous fatalities in Southeast Asia when net fishing was common. The bite is generally painless, and it may initially go unnoticed. Systemic symptoms develop over 1–4 hours and depend on whether there is predominantly myotoxic or neurotoxic effects. There may be decreased mobility secondary to pain or paralysis. The creatine kinase will increase and may be diagnostic in some cases. Rhabdomyolysis will develop in severe cases and can be complicated by acute kidney injury. Some sea snake bites have been reported to cause predominantly neurotoxicity, with an ascending flaccid or spastic paralysis.

First aid is the same as Australian elapids (see Common venomous snakes, pp. 332–333).

Marine poisoning

Marine poisoning occurs when marine creatures that contain toxic substances are ingested. The most common and important marine poisoning is ciguatera resulting from eating some types of reef fish. Other marine poisoning includes TTX, shellfish poisoning, and scombroid.

Ciguatera

Ciguatera is the commonest marine poisoning and is endemic to regions of the Indo-Pacific and Caribbean. However, it can occur anywhere in the world with increased transport of fish. Ciguatera is due to accumulated toxins in tropical reef fish. Numerous fish have been implicated, such as moray eels, bass, Spanish mackerel, various cod species, emperors, and coral trout. Unfortunately there is no way to determine if a fish can cause ciguatera, including the appearance and taste of the fish.

Clinical effects

Ciguatera in the Indo-Pacific region is characterized by the combination of gastrointestinal and neurological effects, compared to the Caribbean where gastrointestinal effects predominate. Gastrointestinal effects (vomiting, diarrhoea, and abdominal cramping) usually occur first within hours of ingestion and last about 12–24 hours. Neurological effects are the characteristic features of ciguatera and are delayed, developing during the initial 24 hours. The predominant neurological effect is a sensory polyneuropathy:

- cold allodynia: often referred to as a heat reversal and is an unpleasant sensation when touching cold objects
- distal and perioral paraesthesia
- numbness.

Other effects are pruritis, arthralgia, and myalgia. Subacute and chronic forms are poorly defined with numerous non-specific symptoms. The diagnosis is made if there is both a history of eating fish known to cause ciguatera and gastrointestinal and neurological effects.

Treatment

There is no specific treatment for ciguatera. Management consists of supportive care and symptomatic relief. There is no evidence to support the use of mannitol and intravenous fluids should be administered for dehydration. Numerous medications have been suggested for acute and chronic symptoms with only anecdotal evidence to support their use. Non-steroidal anti-inflammatories appear to be beneficial for acute symptoms. Tricyclic antidepressants, gabapentin, and calcium antagonists, have been used for chronic symptoms with variable success.

Tetrodotoxin poisoning

TTX poisoning is rare and potentially lethal, and occurs most commonly from ingestion of puffer fish (e.g. fugu poisoning in Japan) and related fish. TTX is a sodium channel blocker that causes nerve conduction failure which manifests as paralysis.

Clinical effects

TTX poisoning manifests as a sensorimotor neuropathy which may be associated with mild gastrointestinal effects. Poisoning develops over hours and more rapidly with severe cases. Neurological effects include:

- perioral paraesthesia and numbness
- ataxia
- progressive distal to proximal muscle weakness.

Severe poisoning is characterized by respiratory muscle paralysis and rarely cardiovascular toxicity (bradycardia, arrhythmias and hypotension).

Treatment

No antidote exists for TTX poisoning. Treatment consists of supportive care, including early and often prehospital institution of airway and breathing support in severe cases. Severe poisoning will usually require mechanical ventilation for 2–5 days.

Shellfish poisoning

Shellfish poisoning is due to toxins that accumulate, in contrast to the more common viral and bacterial illnesses resulting from shellfish ingestion. There are four types of shellfish poisoning:

- Diarrhoetic shellfish poisoning: similar to infectious gastroenteritis and requires supportive and symptomatic treatment.
- Paralytic shellfish poisoning: similar to TTX poisoning, but results from other potent sodium channel blockers such as saxitoxin.
- Neurotoxic shellfish poisoning: causes neuroexcitatory effects, sometimes similar to ciguatera.
- Encephalopathic shellfish poisoning: due to domoic acid and only ever reported once as an outbreak.

Scombroid

Scombroid poisoning occurs from ingestion of fish containing high concentrations of histamine and is similar to an acute allergic reaction. It results from the spoilage of fish after it has been caught, during storage or transport. Commonly implicated fish are from the Scombridae family—tuna, kingfish, mackerel, and wahoo.

Clinical effects

The clinical effects differ from an acute allergic reaction because they result from direct release of histamine. Scombroid develops in the first few hours of ingestion and lasts up to 6 hours. The major effects are:

- skin effects: diffuse erythema, urticaria, flushing and itch.
- gastrointestinal effects: nausea, vomiting, diarrhoea and abdominal cramps
- hypotension
- respiratory effects: wheeze, bronchospasm are rare.

The diagnosis is clinical although it can be confirmed by the detection of high concentrations of histamine in the fish.

Treatment

Treatment includes intravenous fluids for hypotension or dehydration, and antihistamines (H_1- and H_2-receptor antagonists). Epinephrine is rarely used except in severe poisoning.

Further reading

Isbister GK (2001). Venomous fish stings in tropical northern Australia. *Am J Emerg Med*, 19:561–5.

Isbister GK (2004). Marine envenomation and poisoning. In: Dart RC (ed), *Medical Toxicology*, 3rd edition, pp. 1621–44. Philadelphia, PA: Lippincott Williams & Wilkins.

Isbister GK, Hooper JN (2005). Clinical effects of stings by sponges of the genus *Tedania* and a review of sponge stings worldwide. *Toxicon*, 46:782–5.

Isbister GK, Kiernan MC (2005). Neurotoxic marine poisoning. *Lancet Neurology*, 4:219–28.

Isbister GK (2010). Trauma and envenomation from marine fauna. In: Tintinalli JE, Stapczynski JS, Cline DM, et al. (eds), *Tintinalli's Emergency Medicine: A Comprehensive Study Guide*, 7th edition, pp. 1358–1366. New York: McGraw-Hill.

Loten C, Stokes B, Worsley D, et al. (2006). A randomised controlled trial of hot water (45 degrees C) immersion versus ice packs for pain relief in bluebottle stings. *Med J Aust*, 18:329–33.

Williamson JA, Fenner PJ, Burnett JW, et al. (1996). *Venomous and Poisonous Marine Animals*. Sydney: University of New South Wales Press.

Common venomous snakes

Medically important snakes

Snakebite is an important cause of death in rural agricul-tural communities worldwide. In India alone, about 50,000 people die of snakebite each year. Most parts of the world, including the Indian and Pacific Oceans, have venomous snakes. The medically important groups are elapids, vipers, pit-vipers, burrowing asps, and some back-fanged colubrid snakes. In Europe, bites by captive exotic snakes may be more serious than those by indigenous species.

Europe

- Vipers only: in UK, Scandinavia, Benelux countries and Poland, the adder *Vipera berus* is the only venomous species.

Africa and the Middle East

- Elapids: cobras and spitting cobras (*Naja*), mambas (*Dendroaspis*)
- Vipers: saw-scaled vipers (*Echis*), puff adders (*Bitis*), desert horned-vipers (*Cerastes*)
- Burrowing asps: (*Atractaspis*)
- Back-fanged colubrid: boomslang (*Dispholidus*), twig snake (*Thelotornis*).

Asia

- Elapids: cobras (*Naja*) and kraits (*Bungarus*)
- Vipers: Russell's vipers (*Daboia*), saw-scaled vipers (*Echis*)
- Pit-vipers: Malayan pit viper (*Calloselasma rhodostoma*), green tree vipers (*Cryptelytrops*), habus (*Protobothrops*), and mamushis (*Gloydius*)
- Back-fanged colubrids: red-necked keel back and yam-akagashi (*Rhabdophis*).

Australia, New Guinea, Eastern Indonesian Islands

- Elapids only: taipans (*Oxyuranus*), black snakes (*Pseudechis*), brown snakes (*Pseudonaja*), tiger snakes (*Notechis*), death adders (*Acanthophis*).

Americas

- Elapids: coral snakes (*Micrurus*)
- Pit-vipers: lance-heads—*Bothrops*), moccasins (*Agkistrodon*), bushmasters—*Lachesis*), rattlesnakes (*Crotalus* and *Sistrurus*).

Indian and Pacific Oceans

- Elapids: sea snakes (*Enhydrina, Hydrophis, Astrotia* etc.).

Clinical features

Snakebite envenoming usually causes local pain and swell-ing, regional tender lymphadenopathy, malaise, nausea, vomiting, and other gastrointestinal symptoms. The fol-lowing are the main clinical syndromes of envenoming:

Adder —(Vipera berus) and other European Vipera species

- Local pain and paraesthesiae, swelling, bruising, inflammation, lymphangitic lines and tender regional lymphadenopathy
- Hypotension (early, late, transient, recurrent or sus-tained with or without shock)
- Other anaphylactic features—urticaria, angio-oedema, bronchospasm, gastrointestinal symptoms
- Myocardial abnormalities (ECG arrhythmias, T wave/ST segment changes)
- Spontaneous systemic gastrointestinal bleeding and consumption coagulopathy.

Elapids

- Descending paralysis, starting with ptosis and external ophthalmoplegia
- Local swelling and regional tender lymphadenopathy
- Asian cobras and African spitting cobras: local swelling, blistering, and necrosis
- Asian kraits: painless bites inflicted on sleepers, minimal local swelling, delayed descending paralysis
- Australasian elapids: descending paralysis, spontaneous systemic bleeding and consumption coagulopathy (some-times shock (hypotension), rhabdomyolysis, microangi-opathic haemolysis (MAH), acute kidney injury (AKI))
- sea snakes: minimal local swelling and pain, descending paralysis, rhabdomyolysis.

Vipers and pit vipers

- Local swelling, bruising, blistering, necrosis, regional tender lymphadenopathy
- Shock (hypotension)
- Spontaneous systemic bleeding and consumption coagulopathy
- AKI
- With some species: descending paralysis, rhabdomyoly-sis, MAH.

Burrowing asps

- Local swelling, blistering, necrosis
- Middle Eastern species (e.g. *Atractaspis engaddensis* in Israel): shock, cardiac conduction abnormalities, angina pectoris.

Back-fanged colubrids

- Minimal local swelling
- Delayed spontaneous systemic bleeding and consump-tion coagulopathy
- MAH, AKI.

Laboratory

Useful investigations include:

- Blood count—neutrophil leucocytosis, (initial) haemo-concentration from increased permeability, (later) anaemia from bleeding
- Blood film – schistocytes (MAH)
- Blood coagulation—20-minute whole blood clotting test (20 WBCT), prothrombin time (or INR), activated Partial thromboplastin time, fibrinogen concentration (consumption coagulopathy), fibrin degradation prod-ucts or D-dimer (increased fibrinolysis), thrombocyto-penia (DIC or MAH)
- Blood biochemistry—creatine kinase and transami-nases (muscle/tissue damage), potassium, urea, and creatinine (AKI)
- Urine 'sticks' testing: blood/haemoglobin/myoglobin; microscopy—erythrocytes, casts.

Management of snake bite

First-aid treatment

Reassure the terrified victim. Do not interfere with the bite site in any way. Remove rings, bracelets, and tight clothing from the bitten limb.

In bites from non-European snakes immobilize the body, especially the bitten part. Consider using pressure immo-bilization or pressure pad (see later in section). Then:

- arrange transport to medical care as quickly, safely, passively, and comfortably as possible
- treat pain with paracetamol or codeine tablets (avoid aspirin and NSAIDs)
- do not attempt to catch or kill the snake. If already dead, bring it safely—do not touch.
- avoid useless and potentially harmful traditional remedies (incisions, ligatures, ice packs, instillation of chemicals or herbs, 'snake stones', etc.).

Pressure immobilization and pressure pad: these methods delay systemic absorption of lethal venom toxins by compressing lymphatics and veins draining the bite site, using pressures of 50–70 mmHg to avoid the unacceptable dangers of arterial occlusion. *They are not necessary for UK bites* from *Vipera berus*.

Pressure immobilization: elasticated bandages (10–15 cm wide, 4.5 metres long) are bound firmly around the entire bitten limb (but not so tightly as to occlude peripheral pulses), starting around the fingers or toes and continuing proximally up to the axilla or groin.

Pressure pad: a pad of rubber or folded fabric (5 cm square and 2–3 cm thick) is bound directly over the bite site using a non-elastic bandage.

Hospital treatment

Specific treatment with antivenom: antivenoms (hyperimmune animal serum immunoglobulins) are the only specific antidotes. Monovalent antivenoms neutralize the venom of only one species. Polyvalent antivenoms neutralize venoms of selected important venomous species of a particular region.

Indications for antivenom treatment worldwide are any of the following:

- spontaneous systemic bleeding (see earlier in section)
- consumption coagulopathy
- shock: low or falling blood pressure or cardiac arrhythmia
- descending paralysis
- black or dark brown urine (haemoglobinuria from haemolysis or myoglobinuria from rhabdomyolysis)
- local swelling involving more than half the bitten limb.

Mild local swelling alone is not an indication for antivenom.

Antivenom is administered by slow IV injection (2 mL per minute) or IV infusion diluted in about 5 mL/kg body weight over about 30–60 minutes. Initial dosage depends on the type of antivenom, species of snake, and severity of symptoms. A second dose is justified if, after 1–2 hours, life-threatening bleeding or shock have not resolved or paralysis has intensified, or if, after 6 hours, the blood remains incoagulable.

Early anaphylactic and pyrogenic antivenom reactions occur within 2 hours of starting treatment. They can be prevented with SC epinephrine (0.25 mL of 0.1% solution). Treatment is with IM epinephrine (adult dose 0.5 mL of 0.1% solution) given into the lateral thigh, followed by IV hydrocortisone and a histamine H_1 blocker (e.g. chlorphenamine). Asthmatic reactions require an inhaled bronchodilator.

Late serum sickness reactions (urticaria, arthralgia and joint swellings, fever, lymphadenopathy, etc.) occur after 5–14 days. Treatment is with a 5-day course of oral prednisolone and/or histamine H_1 blocker.

Supportive treatment

Hypovolaemic shock

Massive external bleeding or leakage of blood and tissue fluid into a swollen limb may leave the patient with an inadequate circulating volume so that the blood pressure falls. Plasma expanders such as 0.9% saline may be needed.

Respiratory failure from bulbar and respiratory muscle paralysis

This requires endotracheal intubation and assisted ventilation. Neuromuscular block from elapid postsynaptic toxins (cobras and Australasian death adders) may respond to the 'Tensilon test' (atropine and edrophonium). Anticholinesterase treatment can be continued with atropine and neostigmine.

Acute kidney injury

Clinical and biochemical evidence of AKI indicates the need for dialysis.

Wound infection

Wound infection introduced by the snake's fangs or by ill-advised tampering with the bite site presents as local inflammation or abscess treated by aspiration and antibiotics such as co-amoxiclav or chloramphenicol. A tetanus toxoid booster is indicated.

Surgical complications

Necrotic tissue should be debrided and the area grafted. Fasciotomy to relieve suspected compartment syndrome is commonly practised but rarely indicated. It can be considered after normal haemostasis has been restored with antivenom and raised intracompartmental pressure has been confirmed by direct measurement with a pressure transducer.

Spitting cobra eye injuries

Spitting elapids (cobras and ringkals) can spray venom from the tips of their fangs into an aggressor's eyes, causing painful conjunctivitis and risking corneal ulceration and blindness.

First aid

First aid is urgent irrigation with generous volumes of water under a tap. Topical 1% epinephrine or local anaesthetic eye drops (caution!) relieve the pain. Exclude corneal abrasion (slit lamp) or give prophylactic antibiotic eye ointment. Topical antivenom or corticosteroid should not be used.

Further reading

Australia Toxinology. <http://www.toxinology.com/>.

Mackessy SP (ed) (2010). *Handbook of Venoms and Toxins of Reptiles*. Boca Raton, FL: CRC Press.

Meier J, White J (eds) (1995). *Handbook of Clinical Toxicology of Animal Venoms and Poisons*. Boca Raton, FL: CRC Press.

Munich AntiVenom INdex (MAVIN) Poison Centre Munich: antivenoms holdings in Europe <http://www.toxinfo.org/antivenoms/>.

Sutherland SK, Tibballs J (2001). *Australian Animal Toxins. The Creatures, their Toxins and Care of the Poisoned Patient*, 2nd edition. Melbourne: Oxford University Press.

Vapaguide <http://www.vapaguide.info/cgi-bin/WebObjects/vapaGuide.woa/wa/getContent?type=page&id=1>.

Warrell DA (2010). *Guidelines for the Management of Snake-Bites*. New Delhi: WHO Regional Office for South-East Asia. <http://apps.searo.who.int/PDS_DOCS/B4508.pdf>.

Weinstein, SA, Warrell, DA, White J, et al. (2011). '*Venomous*' Bites from Non-Venomous Snakes: A Critical Analysis of Risk and Management of Bites From Snakes of the Artificial Family, Colubridae. Philadelphia, PA: Elsevier.

WHO. *Guidelines for the Prevention and Clinical Management of Snakebite in Africa*. <http://www.afro.who.int/en/clusters-a-programmes/hss/essential-medicines/highlights/2358-whoafro-issues-guidelines-for-the-prevention-and-clinical-management-of-snakebite-in-africa.html>.

WHO. *Venomous snake distribution (and other key details)*. <http://www.who.int/bloodproducts/snake_antivenoms/en/>.

Chemical warfare agents

Principles of triage

Background

Prioritizing patient care in mass casualty incidents, which will typically involve more patients than first responders, is essential. Triage means to sort and must therefore be implemented upon arrival of the first-on-scene responder units. In most countries, including the UK, this would involve police, fire and rescue, and ambulance/paramedic units.

An area in which a chemical release has occurred may be considered as different zones, reflecting potential hazard to responders (see also Outline of chemical incident management, pp. 338–341):
- Red zone; often highly dangerous, requiring full personal protective equipment (PPE) in responders. Casualties contaminated.
- Warm zone; area for decontamination, less hazardous but responders require some PPE.
- Cold zone; clean casualties PPE often not required by clinicians.

The degree and type of PPE is dependent on the agent involved, chemical, biological, radiation, or nuclear (CBRN) (see later in section).

The aim of triage in the hot zone is to identify casualties requiring immediate treatment prior to delivering them to more definitive medical care, but still ensuring that the most good is done for the most patients. In many chemical incidents, whether deliberate release or accidental, treatment cannot be postponed until after decontamination and casualties must be assessed and treated before they are moved, or they may not survive. Although the basis of triage can be easily taught and is quickly understood, in a mass casualty situation in a toxic atmosphere with the pressing need to identify those for whom care may be futile, triage should only be carried out by experienced and trained teams/individuals who are able to balance the demands of the environment and the scarcity of resources against the need to identify those who can be saved and those who can not.

However, it should be noted that patients exposed to chemical weapons or toxic industrial chemicals that produce delayed symptoms (e.g. mustard gas, phosgene) may be misprioritized using any immediate triage system. The system should therefore be dynamic enough to be used on a continuous basis and patients should be reassessed frequently throughout the incident and afterwards. It is also common for people to deny their injuries and allow others to receive care first. This can be a problem with family members and the experienced triager must be aware of this. The other complicating factor, particularly in a deliberate release, is that the incident is effectively a crime scene and that all victims are potential sources of evidence and this should be collected and preserved. However, this must not be at the expense of immediate lifesaving treatment/intervention. It may also be that in a deliberate act the perpetrator(s) may also be victims and may have weapons as well as injuries. Police on the scene will be familiar with this and also the possibility of secondary devices, if relevant, and will have protocols in place to deal with these events.

Triage categories

There are numerous triage systems in use and being trialled in the world including: SALT; Simple Triage and Rapid Treatment (START); Jump START; Homebush; triage sieve (see later in section); Pediatric Triage Tape (PTT); CareFlite; Sacco Triage Method (STM); Military Triage; and CESIRA.

It is outside the scope of this article to discuss them all and so the system in the UK will be outlined here.

Historically, there have been two parallel triage systems in use in the UK: the 'P' system and the 'T' system. The T system is described in Table 14.1. The only patients needing treatment are priority 1 (T1) (those needing emergency treatment to survive) and priority 2 (T2), those who are less injured but who require urgent extrication.

However the first act/instruction is likely to be to ask all patients who are able to move, to do so to a designated area and are all therefore classed as category T3 (see 'Triage sieve').

- *T1 casualties* have life-, limb-, or sight-threatening injuries. Immediate treatment before decontamination is essential.
- *T2 casualties* have serious injuries that require treatment within 2 hours. They are unable to walk. Medical intervention is urgent for T1/T2 casualties and cannot be delayed until after decontamination.
- *T3 casualties* are those whose injuries can safely wait for up to 4 hours before treatment. They are able to walk. Priority 3 (T3) casualties can self-extract from the scene, and in a chemical incident are likely to do so.
- *T4—expectant casualty*. In a toxic/CBRN mass casualty environment there is the very real possibility of having to institute the expectant category. This category is not used in all countries and in all triage systems. This is not something to be taken lightly and requires an experienced physician to undertake. This is not a role a paramedic can be given as their lack of medical expertise and diagnostic skills would render this unacceptable. T4 casualties are expectant: they will die despite aggressive medical intervention. This priority classification should not be used lightly. Its appropriate use, however, is essential to ensure the optimal outcome for the many over the few when resources are limited. Using resources to treat T4 patients would jeopardize the potential survival of other casualties. However, it does not mean that all treatment (analgesia and fluids) is withheld.

It is important to recognize death and to label bodies as dead. This prevents repeated assessment, unnecessary interventions, and resources wasted on rescue attempts.

Triage sieve

The triage sieve can be used at the scene and involves a rapid assessment:

Table 14.1 Triage categories

Category	Description	Colour
T1	Immediate treatment	Red
T2	Urgent treatment	Yellow
T3	Delayed treatment	Green
T4	Expectant	Blue
Dead	Dead	Black/white

1 Can the patient walk?
   Yes: *T3 (green)*
   No: *THEN go to 2.*
2 Is the patient breathing?
   No, even after opening airway: *dead (black/white)*
   Yes, after opening airway: *T1 (red)*

   Yes, without resuscitation: What is the respiratory rate?

   <10 or >30/minute: *T1 (red)*

   10–30/minute: *THEN go to 3*

3 What is the pulse rate (or capillary refill time (CRT))?

   <40 or >120 (or CRT >2 seconds): *T1 (red)*.

   Between 40 and 120 (or CRT <2 seconds): *T2 (yellow)*.

   Modified sieve systems are available for use in children (e.g. PTT).

Triage in a toxic environment

Triage in a chemical environment is additionally difficult because of extrinsic and intrinsic factors, in particular the need to be able to work in the dark, hampered by a toxic atmosphere and in PPE.

Level A PPE denotes fully encapsulated suit, with over-gloves and overboots integrated into the suit. Respiratory protection is a self-contained breathing apparatus. Level A protection is required for entry into an unknown hazardous environment.

Level B PPE denotes a hooded suit, double gloves, over-boots, and a self-contained breathing apparatus, and may be used for decontamination procedures for an unknown substance and for entry into hot zones where the agent is not caustic.

Level C PPE is similar to level B, but uses an air-purifying respirator instead of a self-contained breathing apparatus. Level C PPE can be used only after the hazardous substance has been identified, and upon verification of adequate oxygen in the environment.

These constraints mean that the usual triage sieve will most likely be impossible to perform, as a first responder cannot assess circulation whilst in full PPE. Thus triage in a toxic environment may only be possible by assessing two signs: signs of life and symptoms of toxicity.

There are two triage systems used. One for triage in the hot zone is fast, basic, and crude. It is aimed at identifying the critically ill casualty and those who are alive. This is to minimize the time spent in a hostile environment and to safe those that can be saved. It is being adopted internationally.

The second system is a modification of the triage sieve and is used in the warm zone. It is more refined and more discriminating. It is used to identify patients requiring the emergency medical team and those who need decontamination and in what order.

Toxic triage—triage in the hot zone

Can the patient walk?
Yes: *T3 (green)*

No:
Is the patient conscious?
Yes: *T2 (yellow)*
No: signs of life?
Yes: *T1 (red)*
No: expectant or dead

Toxic triage—triage in the warm zone
Can the patient walk?
Yes: *T3 (green)*
No:
Is the airway patent?
No: *dead (black/white)*
Yes: breathing <10 or >30/minute
Yes: *T1 (red)*
No: *T2 (yellow)*

Further reading

Benson M, Koenig KL, Schultz CH (1996). Disaster triage: START, then SAVE—a new method of dynamic triage for victims of a catastrophic earthquake. *Prehosp Disaster Med*, 11:117–24.

Cone DC, MacMillan DS, Parwani V, et al. (2008). Pilot test of a proposed chemical/biological/radiation/nuclear-capable mass casualty triage system. *Prehosp Emerg Care*, 12:236–40.

Cone DC, Serra J, Burns K, et al. (2009). Pilot test of the SALT mass casualty triage system. *Prehosp Emerg Care*, 13:536–40.

Coule P, Dallas C, James J, et al. (eds) (2003). *Basic Disaster Life Support (BDLS) Provider Manual*. Chicago, IL: American Medical Association.

Garner A, Lee A, Harrison K, et al. (2001). Comparative analysis of multiplecasualty incident triage algorithms. *Ann Emerg Med*, 38:541–8.

Hines S, Payne A, Edmondson J, et al. (2005). Bombs under London. The EMS response plan that worked. *JEMS*, 30:58–67.

Hodgetts T, Hall J, Maconochie I, et al. (1998). Paediatric triage tape. *Prehosp Immed Care*, 2:155–9. <http://www.dmphp.org/cgi/reprint/2/Supplement_1/S25>.

Kerby JD, MacLennan PA, Burton JN, et al. (2007). Agreement between prehospital and emergency department Glasgow coma scores. *J Trauma*, 63:1026–31.

Lerner EB, Cone DC, Weinstein ES, et al. (2008). Mass casualty triage: an evaluation of the data and development of a proposed national guideline. *Disaster Med Public Health Preparedness*, 2(Suppl 1):S25–S34.

Nocera A, Garner A (1999). An Australian mass casualty incident triage system for the future based upon triage mistakes of the past: the Homebush triage standard. *Aust NZ J Surg*, 69:603–8.

Reilly MJ, Markenson DS (2010). *Health Care Emergency Management: Principles and Practice*. Sudbury, MA: Jones and Bartlett Publishers, Inc.

Romig L (2008). The JumpSTART Pediatric MCI Triage Tool. <http://www.jumpstarttriage.com/JumpSTART_and_MCI_Triage.php>.

Wiseman DB, Ellenbogen R, Shaffrey CI (2002). Triage for the neurosurgeon. *Neurosurg Focus*, 12:E5.

Outline of chemical incident management

Background

Chemical incidents include events in which there is release to the environment of chemicals with potential to cause harm to human health. In the context of this section the focus will be on deliberate release and the use of chemical warfare agents. It must be remembered that the vast majority of chemical incidents worldwide are accidental in nature and there will be no overt intent of deliberate release. There also needs to be a distinction between acute and chronic releases. This section will concentrate on acute immediate release of chemicals; although there are many examples of chronic release into the environment, e.g. arsenic into the water supply in Bangladesh that has occurred over many years and continues to be a major public health problem. That type of chronic release incident will not be considered here.

There are a significant number of acute incidents in any year in any country—chemical spillages, non-domestic fires, release of chemicals into the air, soil, or water systems, all of which potentially lead to the exposure of substantial numbers of people. Few lead to direct health effects either in the short or long term but all require careful and coordinated management by health protection professionals and the emergency services.

There are many publications on the public health planning and response to chemical incidents in the context of industrial, transportation, or other releases and readers are directed elsewhere for information on those as the focus here is on chemical weapon release. The deliberate use of chemical weapons has been limited in the past but have been used to great effect both from acute health effects to economic and social disruption and historical examples include:

- contamination of water supplies with chemicals (biologicals including animal and human carcasses were also used) in ancient times, e.g. in 600 BC the Assyrians used ergot and the ancient Chinese warriors used arsenic
- World War I—chlorine, sulphur mustard and phosgene
- World War II—soman
- Iran/Iraq War—mustards, tabun, cyanide
- Tokyo subway attack 1995—sarin.

There is a continued threat particularly in areas of conflict and this has been recently highlighted in Libya and Syria

Definitions

The definition of a chemical incident is not universal and many different agencies have their own descriptions. A non-exhaustive list is given here:

- An acute event in which there is, or could be, exposure of the public to chemical substances which cause, or have the potential to cause ill health. (Health Protection Agency (UK) 2007.)
- A public health chemical incident that resulted in actual or potential exposure to a chemical substance or its hazardous by-products that caused, or had the potential to cause, ill health. Incidents that occurred on industrial premises and only resulted in exposure to employees are excluded. (WHO 2005.)
- Chemical incident: an uncontrolled release of a chemical from its containment that either threatens to, or does, expose people to a chemical hazard (IPCS 1999, Public Health and Chemical Incidents: Guidance for National and Regional Policy Makers in the Public/Environmental Health Roles). Such an incident could occur accidentally, for example a chemical spill or deliberately, for example, the use of sarin on a public transport system. In both cases the release of the chemical or chemicals is usually obvious.
- Acute public health chemical incident: a public health chemical incident where the exposure dose is rising or is likely to rise rapidly and where rapid public health measures may limit the exposure. (WHO Key definitions 2012.)
- Chemical emergency: a chemical incident that has passed the control capability of one emergency service. (WHO Key definitions 2012.)
- A chemical emergency occurs when a hazardous chemical has been released and the release has the potential for harming people's health. Chemical releases can be unintentional, as in the case of an industrial accident, or intentional, as in the case of a terrorist attack. (CDC 2012.)

As can be seen, with a diversity of views categorization can be a problem and individual countries and states must agree on their own definition, either from the list or self-formulated.

Planning and preparedness

Integrated response

The planning process for chemical incidents should make no distinction between possible chemical weapons and other chemicals of concern, e.g. toxic industrial chemicals. It should begin with a local community hazard analysis and risk assessment. This will vary depending where you are both in the world and locally. The most important early flag will be whether the population at risk is near to an industrial complex and therefore there is likely to be a higher risk of release of chemicals into the environment compared to a rural, country area.

The following is focused on what the current arrangements are in the UK but with a more generic approach to suit other countries. The results of the community hazard analysis and risk assessment will inform public safety officials and emergency response agencies to develop appropriate response plans and conduct relevant training exercises. There has been a large amount of effort and money spent on this type of planning in the recent past accelerated after the 9/11 tragedy in 2001 in the USA. These response plans will depend on where you are situated and should have been developed for the area you are situated.

Monitoring and detection equipment on frontline first responder vehicles can expedite the identification of unknown agents. It is likely, however, that a specialist team (e.g. HAZMAT in the USA and Fire & Rescue Service Detection, Identification and Monitoring (DIM) teams in the UK) will often be required to assist the identification process and remediation of threats posed by the agent(s). It may not be possible in the immediate phase of the incident for the first responders to definitively identify the agent(s) released and so they may have to proceed with initial activities to protect the public. It is important that initial assessments are made using readily available information such as the signs and symptoms of initially affected victims. This clearly impacts on the training of suitable first responder personal so they are skilled in such assessments.

Large-scale incidents (such as the Tokyo sarin incident) may overwhelm local responders and therefore plans should be in place to integrate mutual aid from multiple sources such as fire and rescue teams, police, and industrial sites. The planning process should clearly identify how these other teams will be notified and activated and then integrated, if needed, into the local response. These arrangements should be exercised on a regular basis

Specialty teams

In some situations, specialty assistance may need to be requested and this will depend on what each country's arrangements are. In the UK there is an integrated response to the management of chemical, nuclear, and biological incidents and on-scene support would include:

* police
* fire and rescue
* ambulance including paramedic support
* Health Protection Agency.

And others may be drafted in, including Ministry of Defence, Coastguard, etc. Each country and state should be aware of its own arrangements.

Response protocols

First responder directors with accident and emergency/trauma centre facilities should develop protocols specifying what medications, including antidotes, should be administered to chemical incident patients and how chemical-related burns should be managed. In the UK the National Ambulance Resilience Unit (NARU) was established in 2011 to help strengthen the UK national resilience and improve patient outcomes in a variety of challenging pre-hospital environments. Within that framework the frontline delivery of such care would be through a specialist part of the ambulance service named HART (Hazardous Area Response Team) in England and Wales and the Special Operations Response Teams (SORT) in Scotland. In the USA it is usually through the HAZMAT teams but can vary from state to state. The planning process should also address ambulatory, non-ambulatory, and special needs patient decontamination procedures. In the UK there is currently a debate as to the best type of decontamination procedures and the details are beyond the scope of this section. A protocol that is consistent with local and wider regulations should be established determining whether emergency medical personnel are permitted to administer antidotes etc. HART trained staff are trained in a variety of scenarios including: IRU—Incident Response Unit, USAR—Urban Search and Rescue, IWO—Inland Water Operations and TMO—Tactical Medicine Operations. Interested readers are directed to the website in the 'Further reading'. Amongst the skill set for the HART team members are the ability to provide toxic triage in the hot zone (see Principles of triage, pp. 336–337), deliver catastrophic haemorrhage control (tourniquets/compression dressings), give nerve agent antidotes (via combo-pens), gain interosseous (IO) access, assist ventilation via bag, valve mask (BVM) + CBRNE filter and give oxygen (via multiple delivery system where necessary). Similar teams operate in other countries and jurisdictions.

Chemical agents

Type of attack/release

A chemical weapon release is in essence no different to an industrial chemical release except it is likely to be intentional and targeted but is still likely to involve a vapour or a liquid. The type and absolute volume (which can be particularly difficult to estimate) of the chemical released are two of the most important factors in determining the scale of the likely casualties. The terrain, urban or rural, affects the likely event. A deliberate release is more likely in an urban conurbation, a sports stadium or transport hub. Prevailing weather conditions, particularly humidity, the wind velocity, and direction are also key to understanding the outcome of a release. Examples of simple scenarios are given as follows:

1 A vapour cloud releases into a fast moving wind would be quickly dissipated and would probably only lead to a small number of casualties close to the release site.
2 An agent released in an indoor area (e.g. Tokyo underground release in 1995 of sarin) will lead to greater numbers of casualties near to the release and subsequently as the agent disperses throughout the system.

The awareness that a chemical weapon has been released or may be involved will help save lives and mitigate the risk to both the public and first responders. Historically we have not been as efficient as we could be in the area. The Tokyo sarin release, for instance, is an example of a mass casualty event where the causative agent took some time (hours) to be detected and confirmed. However with the rapid advances in technology, particularly in detection equipment in the last decade, hopefully an attack similar to the Tokyo event will be evaluated far more rapidly. Ensuring that PPE of the correct specification, is available with rapid deployment, and is used properly by all personnel working in the hot zone (and warm zone if the dynamic risk assessment deems necessary) is vital to aid in the prevention of additional morbidity and mortality (see also Principles of triage, pp. 336–337). This aspect of response should be trained for by exercises on a regular basis.

Initial first responder units should attempt to identify the release point(s) to attempt to prevent further dissemination. If it is a liquid release appropriate bunding (both temporary and semi-permanent) and containment procedures should be implemented to prevent additional environmental harm. However, the protection of the public and the rapid intervention to save further injury and death *must* take precedence over environmental concerns in the short term. A dynamic risk assessment for environmental issues should run in parallel with the health risk assessment.

A covert release requires first responders to identify patterns of illness (toxidromes). Recognition of toxidromes with knowledge of indications for antidotes and their limitations for treating is crucial for the acute care of poisoned patients to maximize the recognition that an attack has taken place. Other clues may be helpful, e.g. death or behaviour changes in animals in the area where casualties have been found. It is important that first responders (including police, fire and rescue, HART teams) and healthcare workers in secondary admitting centres have a high level of suspicion when dealing with unusual events and casualties.

Properties

Chemical agent properties and effects on humans vary considerably (see subsequent sections of this chapter and also Chapter 9, pp. 205–264). Most chemical agents are liquids; the exceptions are the toxic gases, which include chlorine, phosgene and ammonia (Chapter 9, pp. 205–264), and solid riot control agents (see Riot control agents, pp. 352–354) dispersed as a fine powder or aerosol (suspended liquid). Depending on the nature of the release and prevailing environmental conditions, chemical agents may be present in the environment as liquids, aerosols, or vapour. Aerosolized droplets will also evaporate (the time dependant on the temperature and other factors) leaving agent liquid and agent vapour (see also Nerve agents, pp. 342–344).

Liquid agents may be disseminated by:

• force, e.g. exploding munitions
• mechanical spraying
• addition to water supplies, e.g. rivers, reservoirs, etc.
• evaporation
• non-explosive breach of pressurized and non-pressurized containers (valve failure, rupture, or intentional release).

Gaseous agents may be disseminated and immediately dispersed by:

• mechanical spraying
• explosive breach of pressurized containers (e.g. munitions detonation on side of chlorine tanker)
• non-explosive breach of pressurized containers (valve release, mechanical rupture).

Solid agents may be disseminated by mechanical means as outlined in Riot control agents, pp. 352–354, or simply left at an event scene.

Identifying the incident/agent

Responders entering an area where there are multiple casualties from an unknown substance must approach cautiously wearing appropriate PPE (set by whichever agency has set the standard operating procedures) and self-contained breathing apparatus (SCBA). They must recognize that contamination risk can come from liquid on the ground, near objects, and/or vapour produced when the liquid evaporates (off-gassing).

Patient diagnosis will often first be made from clinical signs and symptoms but may not exhibit the classical signs expected of the chemical involved in the attack. It is therefore likely that multiple effects over a number of casualties would be needed to make a diagnosis and this will lead to a dynamic situation that will change rapidly during the first phase of the event. Chemical agent detectors may be available but there may be a delay in deployment by first responders or false readings that may mislead.

• Rapid loss of consciousness, convulsions, severe shortness of breath and death nerve agents (see Nerve agents, pp. 342–344), or cyanide and hydrogen sulphide (see Chapter 9, pp. 205–264).
• Shortness of breath can be an early sign of a number of agents including chlorine and riot control agents as well as the others just listed.
• Eye and nose irritation can be a sign of exposure to chlorine, riot control agents, hydrogen sulphide, and high levels of phosgene.
• Rhinorrhoea and miosis are likely to be caused by nerve agents.

Upper airway irritation with the listed agents will tend to diminish over time but will get worse after exposure to sulphur mustard agents (see Sulphur mustard, p. 349).

Rapid detection equipment

Chemical agent detection in combination with clinical awareness are clearly the vital response elements in any incident. It is beyond the scope of this section to give a detailed thesis of rapid detection equipment and readers are advised to look elsewhere for more details; however, an overview will be given here. The most rapid form of detection is visual observations at the scene and how the casualties are presenting and in some cases agent identification will be based solely on the signs and symptoms of the victims. This may be best illustrated by the Tokyo subway attack in 1995. Knowledge of the incident area is also a useful tool in risk-based assessments.

Detection equipment should be deployed and used as rapidly as possible with properly trained and protected first responders. *No single system will detect all chemical agents*, even allowing for the rapid technological advances in detection currently happening, so multiple complementary systems may be required to provide a definitive answer and this may be some time (hours or even days) after the event has started. Clearly the signs and symptoms of the casualties would be a useful tool with detection equipment to aid identification of the agent.

Detection equipment

The following is a non-exhaustive list of common and available detection devices/equipment, although this is a rapidly expanding field and numerous companies offer solutions to detect unknown chemicals. The examples given here do not imply they are the best in their respective fields:

• Chemical detector paper, e.g. M-8, M-9—colour change in the presence of liquid nerve or blister agents.
• Chemical agent detector kits, e.g. M256, M18A3—these are old and virtually obsolete as vapour detectors as they use various ampoules and colour charts and are time consuming to set up and difficult to interpret and have been superseded by direct reading instruments.
• Chemical agent monitor (CAM)—vapour detector for personnel and equipment and distinguish between nerve and mustard agents. It is a useful tool to be used during decontamination but has major flaws with false positives to some solvents and once alarmed it tend to have a long reset delay time.
• Detection tubes, e.g. Dräger™, Kitagawa™, Gastec™—a series of tubes that detect chemical agents and toxic industrial chemicals (TICs) and use a combination of colour change and direct reading technologies. Dräger™ tubes are available for over 500 gases and vapours and are especially sensitive for toxic industrial chemicals. Tubes are available for cyanide, lewisite, mustard and nerve agents (amongst others).
• Gas chromatography mass spectrometry (GC/MS) portable detectors, e.g. Smiths Detection GUARDION™, Inficon HAPSITE ER™—GC/MS is considered the 'gold standard' for chemical identification coupling gas chromatography and mass spectrometry to identify single or multiple substances within complex samples and therefore can identify chemicals and mixture analysis system for volatile and semi-volatile organic compounds in complex gases, vapours liquids, and solids. Additionally, it can identify trace compounds that can go undetected by other technologies.

- Fourier-Transform Infrared Spectroscopy (FT-IR), e.g. Smiths Detection HazMatID 360™, Bruker Optics Mobile-IR™—portable devices using FT-IR and an extensive on-board spectral library to rapidly identify solid and liquid chemicals based on their distinct molecular fingerprint usually within a few minutes providing the chemical is present in the on-board library.
- Raman spectrometer e.g. Smiths Detection RespondeR RCI™, PerkinElmer® Raman IdentiCheck™, Thermo Scientific's TruScan RM™—these portable devices use Raman spectrometry technology and can give fast, accurate detection and identification of unknown chemicals, including white powders, explosives, nerve and blister agents, narcotics, and common toxic industrial chemicals.
- Differential mobility spectrometry (DMS) e.g. Chemring Detection Systems JUNO®—these are relatively new hand-held chemical detectors using DMS where ions are subjected to different field strengths for different amounts of time. These units are capable of detecting, identifying, quantifying, and alerting the user to the presence of some chemical vapours.

Sampling and collecting

It will be necessary to collect samples of the agent for definitive analysis and identification in the laboratory. It will also be necessary to collect and analyse biological specimens from casualties including blood, urine, etc.

Zones of operation

A detailed review of this important aspect of chemical incident response is beyond the scope of this section and readers are recommended to use alternative resource specific for their areas. However an overview of the general concepts will be discussed (see also Principles of triage, pp. 336–337).

There are three zones in a chemical incident and these should ideally be sited upwind and uphill from the previous zone:

- Hot (exclusion) zone—this is the most dangerous area and surrounds the central incident point—only personnel with appropriate PPE should enter. Casualties should be located and transferred to the warm zone for decontamination; however, immediate lifesaving medical care (i.e. airway and haemorrhage control) can be performed and antidote treatment could be considered (this is an area of intense debate as to whether any treatment should be attempted in the hot zone and is for local agencies to agree their policy on this).
- Warm zone—upwind and uphill from hot zone where victims will be treated (usually to medically stabilize but may also include antidotes) and decontaminated by suitably trained staff wearing appropriate PPE. A triage point should be established in the warm zone (although this should be a dynamic process).
- Cold zone—upwind and uphill from warm zone and the prime purpose is to provide medical care and prepare casualties for transport on to secondary care facilities (hospitals etc.). This will be scenario dependant and will also be fluid depending on availability of trained personnel and local emergency planning considerations.

Security

The site security and control will usually be the responsibility of the police/law enforcement agencies but may also be handed over to the military depending on local arrangements and the nature of the incident.

The key point to focus on is to prepare and exercise for chemical incident management in your area and make sure all personnel allocated tasks are both *competent* and are *aware* that specific tasks have been allocated to them. Much better to practise and exercise and get it wrong at that stage than to get it wrong during a real event.

Further reading

Crawford IWF, Mackway-Jones K, Russell DR, *et al.* (2004). Planning for chemical incidents by implementing a Delphi based consensus study. *Emerg Med J,* 21:20–3.

DeAtley J (ed) (2003). *Jane's Mass Casualty Handbook: Pre-hospital Emergency Preparedness and Response.* Chicago, IL: Jane's Information Group.

Dwyer A, Eldridge J, Kernan M (eds) (2003). *Jane's Chem-Bio Handbook,* 2nd edition. Chicago, IL: Jane's Information Group.

Health Protection Agency (2008). *CBRN Incidents: A Guide to Clinical Management and Health Protection, V4.* <http://www.hpa.org.uk/Topics/EmergencyResponse/CBRNAndDeliberateRelease/CBRNIncidentsAGuideToClinicalManagementAndHealthProtec/>

Nerve agents

Background

Although available, nerve agents were not used in World War II, but were employed by Iraq against that country's own Kurdish population. Nerve agents were released on an unprotected civilian population in Japan on 11 occasions in 1994–1995.

Two classes of nerve agent are recognized: G and V. Tabun (NATO designation GA), sarin (GB), and soman (GD) were synthesized in Germany in 1936, 1938, and 1944 respectively. GE and GF were synthesized subsequently. The V agents were introduced later

and are exemplified by VX, synthesized in the 1950s. The G agents are both dermal and respiratory hazards, whereas the V agents, unless aerosolized, are contact poisons.

Mechanisms of toxicity

The organophosphorus nerve agents are chemically related to organophosphorus insecticides and have a similar mechanism of toxicity (Figure 14.1), but their mammalian acute toxicity is considerably greater, particularly via the dermal route.

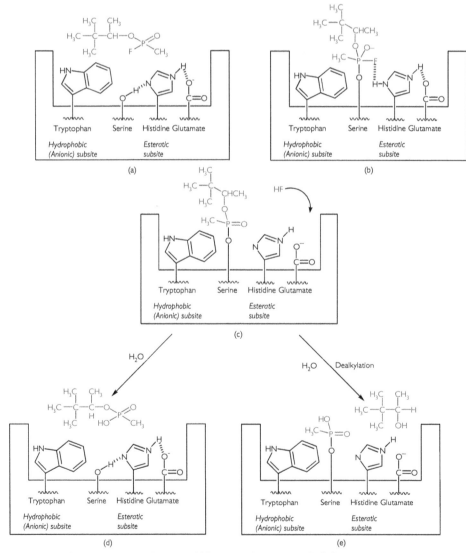

Fig 14.1 Reaction of soman with acetylcholinesterase (a) Soman and the active site of AChE shown together, but not having undergone any reaction. (b) Soman combined with AChE to form an inhibitor–enzyme intermediate. (c) The leaving group (F) has been lost, leaving a complex of soman with AChE. (d) The ester link in the phosphonylated AChE has been hydrolysed, the enzyme has reactivated and an alkylphosphate has been formed. (e) The link between the large pinacolyl group and phosphorus has been cleaved with the formation of a stable monoalkyl–phosphonylated complex with AChE and pinacolyl alcohol. This process is known as aging. Reproduced from Springer, *Toxicological Reviews*, 25, 2006, pp. 297–323, 'The role of oximes in the treatment of nerve agent poisoning in civilian casualties', Marrs TC et al., with kind permission from Springer Science+Business Media B.V.

Nerve agents phosphonylate the serine hydroxyl group in the active site of the enzyme acetylcholinesterase (AChE). This results in accumulation of acetylcholine (ACh), which in turn leads to enhancement and prolongation of cholinergic effects and depolarization blockade. The rate of spontaneous reactivation of AChE is variable, which partly accounts for differences in acute toxicity between the nerve agents.

With soman in particular, an additional reaction occurs termed 'aging'. This involves monodealkylation of the inhibited enzyme, which is then resistant to spontaneous reactivation by oximes (e.g. pralidoxime). Monodealkylation occurs to some extent with all dialkylphosphonylated AChE complexes, but is generally of clinical importance only in relation to the treatment of soman poisoning, in which it is a serious problem.

The approximate aging half-lives of human AChE inhibited by soman, sarin, and tabun are 1.3 minutes, 3 hours, and 13 hours respectively. With soman, therefore, aging is so fast that no clinically relevant spontaneous reactivation of AChE is possible before it has occurred, and recovery of function depends on resynthesis of the enzyme. As a consequence, it is important that an oxime is administered as soon as possible after exposure to soman, to enable some reactivation of AChE before all the enzyme becomes aged.

Aging occurs more slowly and reactivation relatively rapidly with nerve agents other than soman, but early oxime administration is still clinically important in patients poisoned with these agents. Reactivation of tabun-inhibited acetylcholinesterase is slow or non-existent; this is not due to aging but its unique chemical structure.

Clinical features

The diagnosis of nerve agent poisoning is based on the patient's history, clinical presentation, and laboratory tests. In a patient with a positive history, characteristic symptoms, and depressed erythrocyte AChE activity, the diagnosis is not difficult to make. Unfortunately, the history may be unobtainable and the clinical features may not be recognized as such by those clinicians who have no personal experience of diagnosing cholinergic crisis as a result of nerve agent poisoning. Only the number of casualties may prompt consideration of the diagnosis.

Miosis, which may be painful and last for several days, occurs rapidly following ocular exposure to a nerve agent and appears to be a very sensitive index of exposure. (Miosis may also occur as a systemic feature, though more usually it follows direct exposure.) Ciliary muscle spasm may impair accommodation and conjunctival injection and eye pain may occur.

Contact with liquid nerve agent may produce localized sweating and fasciculation, which may spread to involve whole muscle groups. Chest tightness, rhinorrhoea, and increased salivation occur within seconds/minutes of inhalation of a nerve agent. In contrast, ingestion of food or water contaminated with nerve agent may cause abdominal pain, nausea, vomiting, diarrhoea, and involuntary defecation, though the onset of symptoms may be delayed.

Systemic nerve agent poisoning may follow inhalation, ingestion, or dermal exposure, though the onset of systemic toxicity is slower by the latter route. Abdominal pain, nausea and vomiting, involuntary micturition and defecation, muscle weakness and fasciculation, tremor, restlessness, ataxia, and convulsions may follow dermal exposure, inhalation, or ingestion of a nerve agent. Bradycardia, hypotension, tachycardia, and hypertension

may occur, dependent on whether muscarinic or nicotinic effects predominate. If exposure is substantial, death may occur from respiratory failure within minutes, whereas mild or moderately exposed individuals usually recover completely, though persistent electroencephalogram (EEG) abnormalities have been reported in those severely exposed.

Forty-nine subjects were exposed by inhalation to tabun. Effects included miosis, retrobulbar pain, engorgement of vessels in the eye, blurred vision, frontal headache, rhinorrhoea, nausea, and vomiting and chest tightness. The effects were at their maximal 24–48 hours after exposure.

Some 600 people (including 95 rescuers) were exposed by inhalation to sarin released in a residential area of the Japanese city of Matsumoto in June 1994 as a result of a terrorist attack. Fifty-eight residents were admitted to hospital and seven died.

In March 1995 a terrorist attack occurred in the Tokyo subway system during the morning rush hour. Eleven plastic bags each containing 600 mL impure sarin (n-hexane and N,N-diethylaniline were also present) were placed on the floor of subway trains and one station and eight bags were ruptured using umbrellas with sharpened tips so that sarin, which is liquid under temperate conditions, could evaporate. Over 5000 'casualties' sought medical attention of whom 984 were moderately poisoned and 54 were severely poisoned; 12 died. However, a substantial number of those presenting (some 4000) had no signs of nerve agent poisoning and 4973 individuals were seen on day one and sent home.

Management

The general principles of management include maintaining vital body functions, undertaking adequate clinical monitoring, minimizing further absorption of the nerve agent and using atropine, oxime, and diazepam optimally.

Patients who are moderately or severely poisoned, as shown, for example, by drowsiness, coma, hypotension, severe bronchorrhoea, and marked muscle fasciculation, require treatment in a critical care unit as soon as possible as further deterioration may occur and mechanical ventilation may be required.

Bronchorrhoea requires prompt relief with intravenous atropine (see later in section) and supplemental oxygen should be given to maintain PaO_2 greater than 10 kPa (75 mmHg). If these measures fail, the patient should be intubated, and assisted ventilation (with positive end-expiratory pressure) instituted.

In severely poisoned patients who are hypotensive, it may be necessary not only to expand plasma volume by giving colloid but also to use an inotrope, such as dobutamine 2.5–10 micrograms/kg/minute (paediatric dose 2–20 micrograms/kg/minute), or dopamine 2–5 micrograms/kg/minute (paediatric dose 3–20 micrograms/kg/minute).

Frequent or prolonged convulsions should be controlled with intravenous diazepam 10–20 mg (0.1–0.3 mg/kg body weight in children) or lorazepam 4 mg (0.1 mg/kg in children).

Careful attention must be given to fluid and electrolyte balance and adjustments to infusion fluids made as necessary. Heart rate, blood pressure, ECG, and arterial blood gases should be monitored routinely. Cardiac arrhythmias should be treated conventionally and hypoxia must be considered as a possible aetiology.

Skin decontamination

If exposure is dermal, skin decontamination should be carried out by removing all contaminated clothing and washing affected skin thoroughly with soap and cold water, including exposed areas (e.g. hands, arms, face, neck, and hair), after resuscitation and stabilization of the casualty. This should be done without care-givers themselves being contaminated and casualties becoming hypothermic. However, given the circumstances of likely exposure and the number of casualties, decontamination may be difficult to achieve in practice after a deliberate release. The removal and appropriate storage of contaminated clothing may be all that can be done. It is essential that decontamination does not lead to delays in the administration of antidotes to those who are severely poisoned. If exposure is by inhalation, skin decontamination is unnecessary.

Atropine and oximes

Atropine competes with ACh and other muscarinic agonists for a common binding site on the muscarinic receptor, thus effectively antagonizing the actions of ACh at muscarinic receptor sites. If bronchorrhoea develops, atropine 2 mg in an adult (20 microgram/kg in a child) should be administered intravenously every 5–10 minutes until secretions are minimal and the patient is atropinized (dry skin and sinus tachycardia). In severe cases, very large doses of atropine may be required.

With the possible exception of the treatment of cyclosarin and soman poisoning, when HI-6 (not yet generally available) might be preferred, a review of the available experimental evidence suggests that there are no clinically important differences between pralidoxime, obidoxime, and HI-6 in the treatment of nerve agent poisoning.

An oxime, for example, pralidoxime chloride, should be administered parenterally in a dose of 30 mg/kg every 4 hours to patients with systemic features who require atropine. Alternatively, an infusion of pralidoxime mesilate (8–10 mg/kg/hour) may be given, the infusion rate depending on the severity. The duration of oxime treatment depends on the presence of features, the clinical response, and the red blood cell AChE activity. It is recommended that an oxime should be administered for as long as atropine is indicated. In most individuals, this will be less than 48 hours.

Diazepam

Intravenous diazepam 10–20 mg (1–5 mg in children) is useful in controlling apprehension, agitation, fasciculation, and convulsions. The dose may be repeated as required. In some experimental studies, addition of diazepam to an atropine and oxime regimen further increased survival.

Ocular pain

Severe eye pain from ciliary spasm may be relieved by atropine sulfate or homatropine hydrobromide eye drops, but as these drugs cause blurred vision they should not be used unless the pain is severe.

Treatment of casualties outside hospital

Healthcare workers should put on adequate self-protection before decontaminating casualties, because secondary contamination from casualties has been reported. If available, pressure-demand, self-contained breathing apparatus should be used in contaminated areas. Casualties should be moved to hospital as soon as possible.

Casualties should receive antidotal treatment as soon as possible after exposure. This is of particular importance in poisoning with soman, because of the very rapid ageing of the soman–enzyme complex. Casualties who develop rhinorrhoea and bronchorrhoea should be administered atropine as a matter of urgency, and whichever oxime is available. This can be achieved most conveniently by the use of an autoinjector.

Further reading

Marrs TC (2004). The role of diazepam in the treatment of nerve agent poisoning in a civilian population. *Toxicol Rev*, 23:145–57.

Marrs TC, Rice P, Vale JA (2006). The role of oximes in the treatment of nerve agent poisoning in civilian casualties. *Toxicol Rev*, 25:297–323.

Murata K, Araki S, Yokoyama K, et al. (1997). Asymptomatic sequelae to acute sarin poisoning in the central and autonomic nervous system 6 months after the Tokyo subway attack. *J Neurol*, 244:601–6.

Nozaki H, Hori S, Shinozawa Y, et al. (1997). Relationship between pupil size and acetylcholinesterase activity in patients exposed to sarin vapor. *Intensive Care Med*, 23:1005–7.

Okudera H, Morita H, Iwashita T, et al. (1997). Unexpected nerve gas exposure in the city of Matsumoto: report of rescue activity in the first sarin gas terrorism. *Am J Emerg Med*, 15:527–8.

Okumura T, Takasu N, Ishimatsu S, et al. (1996). Report on 640 victims of the Tokyo subway sarin attack. *Ann Emerg Med*, 28:129–35.

Sekijima Y, Morita H, Yanagisawa N (1997). Follow-up of sarin poisoning in Matsumoto. *Ann Intern Med*, 127:1042.

Sidell FR (1974). Soman and sarin: clinical manifestations and treatment of accidental poisoning by organophosphates. *J Toxicol Clin Toxicol*, 7:1–17.

Sidell FR (1992). Clinical considerations in nerve agent intoxication. In: Somani SM (ed), *Chemical Warfare Agents*, pp. 155–94. San Diego, CA: Academic Press.

Vale JA, Rice P, Marrs TC (2007). Managing civilian casualties affected by nerve agents. In: Marrs TC, Maynard RL, Sidell FR (eds), *Chemical Warfare Agents: Toxicology and Treatment*, 2nd edition, pp. 249–60. Chichester: John Wiley & Sons.

Ricin and abrin

Ricin (CAS 9009-86-3)

Source, structure, and potential use as a chemical weapon

Ricin is a globular glycoprotein derived from the beans of the castor oil plant, *Ricinus communis*. It can be extracted easily from whole beans or from the waste 'mash' remaining after castor oil extraction. The toxin is inactivated by heating for 10 minutes at 80° C.

Ricin toxin comprises an A chain (or RTA) and a B chain (or RTB), linked by a single disulphide bond. The A chain confers cellular toxicity, whereas the B chain is essential for cell binding.

The suitability of ricin as a chemical weapon derives from its extreme toxicity to mammalian cells and the fact that the source is naturally occurring and relatively easily prepared. However, use of ricin to cause mass casualties would require either aerosolization by means of a dispersal device or its addition to food or beverages as a contaminant.

By inhalation or injection, the lethal dose of ricin in man is estimated to be 5–10 micrograms/kg but it is approximately 1000-fold less toxic by ingestion. Ricin is not absorbed through intact skin.

Mechanisms of toxicity

Ricin binds to cell surface carbohydrates containing terminal N-acetyl galactosamine or β-1,4-linked galactose residues. In addition, ricin contains a large number of mannose residues by which it can bind to the limited number of cell lines that bear mannose receptors. Among these are cells of the reticuloendothelial system, which are particularly susceptible to ricin toxicity. Once internalized, the A chain inhibits protein synthesis by cleaving a specific glycosidic bond within the 60S subunit of ribosomal RNA and protein synthesis is halted. Subsequent to protein synthesis termination, a process of programmed cell death (apoptosis) ensues via an independent mechanism.

Many of the features seen in skin poisoning can be explained by ricin-induced endothelial cell damage, which leads to fluid and protein leakage and tissue oedema, causing the so-called 'vascular leak syndrome'.

Clinical features

Ingestion

Most cases of ricin poisoning involve eating castor beans. Beans swallowed whole may pass through the gastrointestinal tract intact, whereas chewing facilitates ricin release.

Vomiting, diarrhoea, and abdominal pain typically occur within a few hours of ricin ingestion. Gastrointestinal fluid and electrolyte loss may be substantial and complicated by haematemesis or melaena, hypovolaemic shock, and multi-organ failure.

Some degree of transient liver damage is likely in all but the mildest cases with increased hepatic transaminase and lactate dehydrogenase activities. There may also be a metabolic acidosis, leucocytosis, hyperglycaemia or hypoglycaemia, hypophosphataemia, and increased creatine kinase activity.

Inhalation

Non-human primates exposed to ricin by the inhalation route develop a fibrinopurulent necrotizing pneumonia, typically after a dose-dependent delay of 8–24 hours. Non-pulmonary effects have not been reported.

Parental administration

Among the small number of reports of parenteral ricin administration, the best known is the assassination of the Bulgarian dissident Georgi Markov, who died 3 days after being stabbed with an umbrella believed to be loaded with a ricin-containing pellet. Fatigue, nausea, vomiting, and fever developed over 24 hours followed by widespread necrotic lymphadenopathy and tissue necrosis at the injection site. Preterminal complications included gastrointestinal haemorrhage, hypovolaemic shock, and renal failure.

A 53-year-old man who injected part of 13 chewed castor beans into his thigh with suicidal intent developed necrotic cellulitis complicated by *Enterococcus faecalis* infection requiring emergency surgical debridement, but recovered after 3 months of hospitalization.

A 20-year-old man was admitted to hospital 36 hours after injecting castor bean extract subcutaneously. He complained of nausea, weakness, dizziness, chest and abdominal pain, and myalgia with paraesthesiae of the extremities. Hypotension, anuria, and a metabolic acidosis were noted on examination and fresh blood was present in the rectum, possibly related to the development of a bleeding diathesis. Hepatorenal and cardiorespiratory failure then developed and the patient died 18 hours after admission following an asystolic arrest.

Topical exposure

Both type I and type IV allergic responses have been reported following dermal exposure to castor bean dust. A 21-year-old woman had an anaphylactic-type response after a castor bean from her necklace disintegrated in her fingers. She immediately developed sneezing, rhinitis, and periorbital oedema with facial urticarial and erythema, requiring subcutaneous epinephrine. However, ricin is only one of several allergenic proteins in castor beans.

Ricin is severely irritating to the eye. In animal studies, pseudomembranous conjunctivitis occurred following application of ricin solutions in concentrations of 1:1000–1:10,000.

Diagnosis

Prompt diagnosis of exposure to ricin is crucial because the effectiveness of treatment with neutralizing antibodies is dependent on administration before ricin is internalized. A highly sensitive immunochromatographic test is now available that can detect ricin at a concentration of 1 ng/mL and can be read with the naked eye. Detection of antiricin antibodies could aid diagnosis in those who survive for 2–3 weeks but will not be detected in those who die soon after exposure.

Management

Current management is primarily symptomatic and supportive, though both vaccination (prophylaxis) and antitoxin antibody administration (therapeutic) as $F(ab)_2$ fragments are in advanced stages of development.

Patients who receive prompt symptomatic and supportive care following castor bean ingestion are likely to survive, with a fatality rate for treated patients of approximately 2%. In fatal cases, death usually occurs on the third day or later and is due to multi-organ failure. The most common findings at autopsy are ulceration of the mucosa of the stomach and small intestine, necrosis of mesenteric lymph nodes, hepatic necrosis, and nephritis.

Abrin (CAS 1393-62-0)

Source, structure, and potential use as a chemical weapon

Abrin is a plant toxin, which is closely related to ricin in its structure and chemical properties. It is obtained from the seeds of *Abrus precatorius* (commonly known as jequirity bean or rosary pea), a tropical vine cultivated as an ornamental plant in many locations. Jequirity beans are usually scarlet with a black spot at one end (though less common different coloured varieties exist) and measure approximately 3×8 mm. Like ricin, abrin is a type 2 ribosome inactivating protein with A and B chains linked by a disulphide bond. At least theoretically, the similarity of abrin to ricin gives it similar potential as a bioterrorism agent.

Mechanisms of toxicity

The mechanism of ribosome inactivation by abrin is essentially identical to ricin, except that *in vitro* studies suggest abrin is an even more potent toxin than ricin in this regard.

Clinical features

Features following substantial abrin ingestion have usually been very similar in nature and time course to those described for ricin, with initial gastrointestinal manifestations, followed in severe cases by neurological features and organ failure.

Management

The principles of management of abrin poisoning are similar to those for ricin poisoning.

Further reading

Bradberry SM, Lord JM, Rice P, et al. (2007). Ricin and abrin poisoning. In: Marrs TC, Maynard RL, Sidell FR (eds), *Chemical Warfare Agents: Toxicology and Treatment*. 2nd edition, pp. 613–31. Chichester: John Wiley & Sons.

Bradberry SM, Dickers KJ, Rice P, et al. (2003). Ricin poisoning. *Toxicol Rev*, 22:65–70.

Challoner KR, McCarron MM (1990). Castor bean intoxication. *Ann Emerg Med*, 19:1177–83.

Crompton R, Gall D (1980). Georgi Markov—death in a pellet. *Med Leg J*, 48:51–62.

Fernando C (2001). Poisoning due to Abrus precatorius (jequirity bean). *Anaesthesia*, 56:1178–80.

Griffiths GD, Phillips GJ, Holley J (2007). Inhalation toxicology of ricin preparations: animal models, prophylactic and therapeutic approaches to protection. *Inhal Toxicol*, 19:873–87.

Griffiths GD, Lindsay CD, Upshall DG (1994). Examination of the toxicity of several protein toxins of plant origin using bovine pulmonary endothelial cells. *Toxicology*, 90:11–27.

Guglielmo-Viret V, Splettstoesser W, Thrullier P (2007). An immunochromatographic test for the diagnosis of ricin inhalational poisoning. *Clin Toxicol*, 45:505–11.

Hughes JN, Lindsay CD, Griffiths GD (1996). Morphology of ricin and abrin exposed endothelial cells is consistent with apoptotic cell death. *Hum Exp Toxicol*, 15:443–51.

Lord MJ, Jolliffe NA, Marsden CJ, et al. (2003). Ricin: mechanisms of cytotoxicity. *Toxicol Rev*, 22:53–64.

Metz G, Böcher D, Metz J (2001). IgE-mediated allergy to castor bean dust in a landscape gardener. *Contact Derm*, 44:367.

Passeron T, Mantoux F, Lacour J-P, et al. (2004). Infectious and toxic cellulitis due to suicide attempt by subcutaneous injection of ricin. *Br J Dermatol*, 150:154.

Pillay VV, Bhagyanathan PV, Krishnaprasad R, et al. (2005). Poisoning due to white seed variety of Abrus precatorius. *J Assoc Physicians India*, 53:317–19.

Poli MA, Chad R, Huebner KD, et al. (2007). Ricin. In: Dembek ZF (ed), *Medical Aspects of Biological Warfare*, pp. 4149–58. Washington, DC: Office of the Surgeon General, United States Army.

Sahoo R, Hamide A, Amalnath SD, et al. (2008). Acute demyelinating encephalitis due to Abrus precatorius poisoning –complete recovery after steroid therapy. *Clin Toxicol*, 46:1071–3.

Sikriwal D, Batra JK (2010). Ribosome inactivating proteins and apoptosis. *Plant Cell Monographs*, 18:167–89.

Subrahmanyan D, Mathew J, Raj M (2008). An unusual manifestation of Abrus precatorius poisoning: a report of two cases. *Clin Toxicol*, 46:173–5.

Targosz D, Winnik L, Szkolnicka B (2002). Suicidal poisoning with castor bean (Ricinus communis) extract injected subcutaneously—case report. *J Toxicol Clin Toxicol*, 40:398.

Wilhelmsen C, Pitt L (1993). Lesions of acute inhaled lethal ricin intoxication in rhesus monkeys. *Vet Pathol*, 30:482.

Sulphur mustard

Background
Sulphur mustard (CAS 505-60-2) is an oily, colourless-to-brown liquid at room temperature. By the end of World War I, extensive use of sulphur mustard had resulted in 400,000 casualties, although the mortality was only 3%. More recently, well-founded allegations of the use of mustard by Iraq against Iran (1984–1987) were made; numerous Iranian casualties arrived for hospital treatment in several Western European countries.

Mechanisms of toxicity
Sulphur mustard is a bifunctional alkylating agent capable of forming covalent linkages with nucleophilic groups in the cell and cross-linking complementary strands of DNA, as well as binding various important enzyme systems and structural proteins.

Clinical features
Dermal exposure
Sulphur mustard causes a chemical burn. The naturally moist areas of the body (e.g. genitalia, perineal region, groin, lower back, axillae) are often the most severely affected. Erythema develops within a few hours of exposure. Vesication is not usually seen until the second day and subsequently progresses for several more days. Necrosis is complete 4–6 days after exposure, and separation of necrotic slough then begins. The accompanying oedema and erythema may persist. Scab formation begins within 7 days. By 16–20 days, separation of slough is complete and re-epithelialization begins. Complete healing may take 3–8 weeks, and the patient is often left with depigmented areas surrounded by zones of hyperpigmentation. Those with severe burns may require weeks of hospital care followed by lengthy convalescence.

In cases where dermal exposure has been high, a leucocytosis develops initially, followed by leukopenia and aplastic anaemia over a period of 7–10 days.

Inhalation
Rhinorrhoea, coughing, epistaxis, inflammation, and ulceration of the palate, nasopharynx, oropharynx, and larynx are the main features after vapour exposure.

Ophthalmic exposure
A marked conjunctivitis, local oedema, including oedema of the eyelids, blepharospasm, and lacrimation are the classical signs of eye exposure; miosis, photophobia, and severe eye pain result. Early corneal changes leading to corneal necrosis are observed with vapour causing less damage than liquid exposure. Conjunctival necrosis, together with iritis and iridocyclitis, were seen in severe cases during World War I.

Management
The current clinical management is essentially that for a thermal burn:
- For areas of erythema and minor blistering, bland lotions such as calamine are useful. Topical bacteriostatic agents such as 1% silver sulfadiazine (Flamazine™) cream were used on Iranian casualties to reduce the incidence of secondary infection once the blisters had ruptured.
- Moderately severe pain and itching are common problems once blisters have developed and may be managed by the use of mild analgesics, antihistamines, and small doses of diazepam. Occasionally, some patients experience severe pain and these may require narcotic analgesics such as morphine. Carbamazepine is reported to have proved valuable in alleviating pain in one patient, and its use allowed the withdrawal of narcotic analgesics.
- Dilute topical steroids have proved beneficial in relieving irritation and reducing the attendant oedema at exposed sites. However, their use appeared to have little or no effect on the subsequent rate of healing of the lesions.
- Fluid replacement is calculated in the same way as for a thermal burn although unlike a thermal burn, large amounts of fluid loss will only occur once the blisters have formed, rather than in the first 24 hours.

Although the time to healing may be long, the evidence suggests that the eventual scar is softer and more pliable than that seen in thermal injuries. Wound contracture does not appear to be a major problem.

The techniques of mechanical dermabrasion and 'lasablation' represent notable advances in the management of chemical agent burns. In addition to their use in a military context, it seems likely that such procedures would similarly benefit the management of civilian chemical and thermal injuries to the skin.

Granulocyte-colony stimulating factor (G-CSF) and other growth factors should be considered in cases showing evidence of bone marrow suppression.

Ophthalmic exposure
Early decontamination following eye exposure is very important; thereafter, expert ophthalmic assessment is mandatory.

Further reading
Evison D, Brown RFR, Rice P (2006). The treatment of sulphur mustard burns with laser debridement. *J Plast Reconstr Aesthet Surg*, 59:1087–93.

Hendrickx A, Hendrickx B (1990). Management of war gas casualties. *Lancet*, 336:1248.

Maynard RL (2007). Mustard gas. In: Marrs TC, Maynard RL, Sidell FR (eds), *Chemical Warfare Agents: Toxicology and Treatment*, 2nd edition, pp. 375–407. Chichester: John Wiley & Sons.

Mellor SG, Rice P, Cooper GJ (1991). Vesicant burns. *Br J Plast Surg*, 44:434–7.

Newman-Taylor AJ (1991). Experience with mustard gas casualties. *Lancet*, 337:242.

Rice P, Brown RF, Lam DG, et al. (2000). Dermabrasion – a novel concept in the surgical management of sulphur mustard injuries. *Burns*, 26:34–40.

Rice P (2003). Sulphur mustard injuries of the skin: pathophysiology and management. *Toxicol Rev*, 22:111–18.

Rice P (2007). Sulphur mustard injuries of the skin: pathophysiology and clinical management of chemical burns. In: Marrs TC, Maynard RL, Sidell FR (eds), *Chemical Warfare Agents: Toxicology and Treatment*, 2nd edition, pp. 423–42. Chichester: John Wiley & Sons.

Treleaven JG (2007). The normal bone marrow and management of toxin-induced stem cell failure. In: Marrs TC, Maynard RL, Sidell FR (eds), *Chemical warfare agents: toxicology and treatment*, pp. 443–66. Chichester: John Wiley & Sons.

Vogt RF, Dannenberg AM, Schofield BH, et al. (1984). The pathogenesis of skin lesions caused by sulphur mustard. *Fund Appl Toxicol*, 4:S71–S83.

Willems JL (1989). Clinical management of mustard gas casualties. *Ann Med Mil Belg*, 3:1–61.

Botulinum toxin

Background

Botulism describes flaccid paralysis following exposure to botulinum toxin. Botulinum toxin is a neurotoxin synthesized by anaerobic Gram-positive *Clostridium* bacilli. At least four genetic bacterial species have been identified that can produce seven different toxins capable of producing the clinical features of botulism. These include *Cl. botulinum* (toxin types A, B, D, and E); *Cl. baratii* (toxin types C and F), *Cl. butyricum* (toxin types E and C), and *Cl. argentine* (toxin type G). Toxin types C and D do not appear to affect humans.

Clostridium bacilli capable of producing botulinum toxin are ubiquitous in soil throughout all regions of the world. All subtypes are able to form spores under anaerobic conditions that are capable of remaining dormant for long periods and are highly resistant to extremes of temperature.

Consequently, botulism is classically associated with food poisoning from poorly processed fish, meat, and vegetables. The development and marketing of botulinum toxin for the treatment of localized spastic muscle contracture and as a cosmetic aid has also resulted in case reports of iatrogenic botulism. It may also be useful in the treatment of severe persistent migraine headache.

This section shall focus on botulinum toxin as a potential biological weapon, however, the clinical features and management are also applicable to the conventional routes of exposure.

The threat

Botulinum toxin has a claim to be the most toxic substance known. This has bought it to the attention of those who seek to weaponize microbial toxins. The case fatality rates vary according to the toxin type but typically range from 7–18%. These rates are, however, from individuals following episodes of food poisoning and those who recovered often required long periods of respiratory support. The development of botulism in a large number of individuals following a deliberate release of botulinum toxin would be likely to tax most healthcare systems.

Potential routes of exposure include:

- oral administration from either the deliberate contamination of food supplies with the toxin or the sabotage of food production facilities to increase the likelihood of spore formation
- inhalation of aerosolized toxin following delivery by either explosive munitions or a spray system
- direct inoculation of the toxin would be impractical for mass delivery but could in theory be used to target individuals.

The toxic potential of food deliberately contaminated by *Cl. botulinum* was demonstrated by the Japanese biological warfare group (Pingfan Unit 731), which was believed to have experimented on prisoners of war during the occupation of Manchuria (1931–1945) using bacteria obtained from local soil samples.

To date there have been no confirmed reports of botulinum toxin being successfully deployed by a sovereign nation during a war-like act. Following the end of World War II several nations are believed to have attempted to develop botulinum toxin as a biological weapon including both the former USSR and the USA. Iraq declared after the First Gulf War (1990–1991) that it had prepared munitions containing approximately 10,000 L of botulinum toxin.

The potential for aerosolized botulinum toxin to cause disease in humans was reported following symptoms of botulism in German veterinary professionals disposing of animal carcases in 1962. It has been estimated that aerosolized botulinum toxin has the potential to kill or incapacitate 10% of the exposed population half a kilometre down-wind of a single point source.

A non-state actor, the Aum Shinrikyo cult, attempted to covertly disperse aerosolized botulinum toxin in several location in Japan, in the 1990s, without causing a single recorded case of botulism, suggesting that effective dissemination of the toxin might require significant research and development.

Pathophysiology

Botulinum toxin is formed from a single polypeptide chain than undergoes post-translational cleavage to form a light chain (LC) of approximately 50 KDa and a heavy chain (HC) of approximately 100 KDa jointed by a disulphide chain. The tertiary structure of the toxin has been resolved by X-ray crystallography: the HC wraps around the LC in a 'belt-like' loop and appears to chaperone LC unfolding.

The HC facilitates the entry of the LC into the acetylcholine secreting motor neurons that synapse with the motor-end plate of the neuromuscular junction. The carboxyl terminus of the HC is capable of binding to glycophospholipid motifs on the neuronal membrane. The amine terminus then allows the translocation of the LC across the neuron membrane by a pH-dependent endocytosis. The LC is a zinc metalloprotease that disrupts the trafficking and secretion of acetylcholine-containing vesicles. The enzyme substrate is very specific for each toxin type. Toxins A, C, and E each cleave a different peptide bond on the presynaptic membrane protein, synaptasome associated protein (SNAP). Toxins B, D, F, and G each cleave a different peptide bond of the vesicle associated membrane protein (VAMP)/synaptobrevin-2 complex.

Toxicology

The lethal dose of botulinum toxin in humans is not known precisely. An approximate LD_{50} (human) for botulinum toxin type A is dependent on the route of exposure (Table 14.2).

Botulinum toxin is capable of crossing mucosal membranes. It is thought that it is unlikely to be able to penetrate intact skin effectively. The toxin is then spread haematogenously to all peripheral acetylcholine nerve terminal endings including the pre-neurons of autonomic ganglia, parasympathetic post-ganglionic neurons and motor neurons that synapse with neuromuscular junctions. Botulinum toxin does not readily penetrate the blood–brain barrier due to its large molecular weight of approximately 150 KDa.

Clinical features

The majority of clinic experience of botulism comes from food poisoning. It is expected that inhalation of aerosolized botulinum toxin would produce similar symptoms. Oral ingestion of botulinum toxin typically

Table 14.2 Route of exposure of botulinum, and estimated human LD_{50}

Route of exposure	Dose LD_{50} (micrograms/kg)
Intravenous	0.001
Inhalation	0.01
Intramuscular	0.1
Oral	1

produces gastrointestinal symptoms of colicky abdominal pains, vomiting and occasionally diarrhoea within 12–36 hours of exposure, although a delayed in onset might be expected post-inhalation.

Neurological features usually start with bulbar signs (dysphagia, dysarthria, dysphonia, and diminished gag reflex) and ophthalmological signs (diplopia, dilated pupils, and ptosis). Autonomic anticholinergic features of dry mouth, postural hypotension, paralytic ileus, and urinary retention may occur. These features are then followed by a symmetrical, descending, flaccid paralysis. Diaphragmatic paralysis may result in acute respiratory failure. Sensory examination would be expected normal and no features of central nervous system involvement should be present, such as ataxia or upper motor reflexes. Patients would be expected to be afebrile.

The differential diagnosis for individual cases would include myasthenia gravis, Miller Fisher syndrome, atypical Guillain–Barré syndrome or tick paralysis. The presence of several cases should, however, suggest the diagnosis of botulism.

Investigations

The administration of botulinum antitoxin should *not* be delayed pending confirmatory investigations.

Routine biochemical, haematological, and CSF investigation would be expected to be normal. Serum samples (5 mL) and a stool sample in anaerobic medium should be obtained in all suspected cases. Care should be taken in handling samples due to the risk of exposure to the toxin. In the United Kingdom the Health Protection Agency should be contacted for advice for the most appropriate laboratory to send samples:

Foodborne Pathogens Reference Unit
PHE Colindale
61 Colindale Avenue
London
NW9 5EQ
Tel: 020 8200 4400
Fax: 020 8200 8264

In isolated cases it would be also be appropriate to investigate the differential diagnosis by requesting acetylcholine-receptor antibodies, anti-GQ1b antibodies, electromyography, and nerve conduction studies.

Management

Decontamination

In the event of a release of aerosolized toxin suspected cases will require decontamination by removing clothes using soap and low-pressure water. First responders and those involved in decontamination require full PPE. Once an individual has been decontaminated there is no risk of sustained person-to-person transmission. Biological fluids from suspected cases should, however, be handled with care since they may contain the toxin.

Antitoxin

Patients with clinical features require a rapid assessment of their respiratory and cardiovascular systems and urgent administration of the antitoxin. Respiratory and/or circulation inadequacies should be with supportive treatment. These systems require continuous monitoring due to the risk of sudden failure. A trivalent antitoxin effective against botulinum toxin types A, B, and E is available in the United Kingdom. Holding centres can be located by contacting poisons information services, e.g. the National Poisons Information Service in the UK. Administration of the antitoxin carries a risk of hypersensitivity reactions, especially in individuals allergic to horses. Anaphylaxis should be treated in the standard way with epinephrine, antihistamines, and corticosteroids. There is also a risk of serum sickness 1–2 weeks after exposure to the antitoxin, which should be treated with antihistamines and corticosteroids.

Vaccination

At present there is no vaccine available. A vaccine for individuals in occupations at high risk of botulism was withdrawn in 2011 by the Centers for Disease Control and Prevention, USA. Several experimental vaccines are currently being developed

Prognosis

Botulism is a notifiable disease in the UK and doctors attending suspected cases should notify the Proper Officer (usually the local consultant in communicable disease control). The antitoxin neutralizes the toxin and can limit the extent of neurological injury but cannot reverse the effects. Functional recovery therefore requires regeneration of neurones. This is a slow process and can take from 5–10 weeks. This may entail a prolonged intensive care admission if ventilation is required. Symptoms of lethargy and weakness may also persist for months to years post exposure.

Further reading

Arnon SS, Schechter R, Inglesby TV, *et al.*; Working Group on Civilian Biodefense (2001). Botulinum toxin as a biological weapon: medical and public health management. *JAMA*, 285:1059–70.

Bossi P, Van Loock F, Tegnell A, *et al.* (2004), BICHAT guidelines for the management of botulism and bioterrorism-related botulism. *Euro Surveill*, 9(12). <http://www.eurosurveillance.org/ViewArticle.aspx?ArticleId=499>.

Organic arsenicals

Background

A number of organic arsenicals have been developed historically as potential chemical warfare agents due to their ability to cause irritation or blistering (vesicant action) of the skin and respiratory tract. Some also produce vomiting as a prominent clinical feature and have been considered as riot control agents.

Each of these compounds contains an $AsCl_2$ group, which is responsible for their main clinical effects. The most well-known chemical in the group is Lewisite, although there are no confirmed reports of its use as a chemical warfare agent. In addition to their official chemical names, they have also become known by familiar names, sometimes covering a number of different compounds.

There are two main types.

Vesicants

- Lewisite (CAS 541-25-3)
- The 'Dicks':
  - ethyl dichlorarsine (CAS 598-14-1)
  - methyl dichlorarsine (CAS 593-89-5)
  - phenyl dichlorarsine (CAS 696-28-6).

Irritants

- Diphenyl chlorarsine (DA) (CAS 712-48-1)
- Diphenyl cyanarsine (DC) (CAS 23525-22-6)
- Diphenylamine chlorarsine (DM, Adamsite) (CAS 578-94-9).

Vesicants

Lewisite can be considered as a typical example of this class. Symptoms and management of other vesicants is as for Lewisite.

Lewisite: 2-chlorovinyl dichlorarsine (ClCH=CHAsCl₂)

Pure Lewisite is said to be an odourless and colourless liquid, although impure forms have a dark colour and smell of geraniums. It has a boiling point of 190° C and a freezing point variously quoted between −18° C and 0° C. Mixtures of Lewisite and sulphur mustard were prepared in order to decrease the freezing point of mustard and increase its utility; the Lewisite acting as an antifreeze.

Lewisite hydrolyses readily in water to produce an oxide which is also a vesicant, in strong alkalis.

Toxicity

The mechanism of action is not clearly understood but is thought to be due to the ability of arsenic to inhibit the activity of enzymes that contain sulfhydryl groups: both systemic and local effects occur. Enzyme inhibition prevents formation of acetyl coenzyme-A from pyruvate, leading to cell death, necrosis, and skin blistering. Exposure to large amounts can be fatal. About 30 drops (2.6 g) applied to skin and not washed off would be expected to produce a fatal outcome in an average man while vesication is caused by 14 micrograms of liquid. It is estimated that 0.3 mL of Lewisite left on the skin would be expected to cause systemic illness while 1.4 mL may produce death in humans in 3 hours to 5 days. It is absorbed by the skin within 3–5 minutes. Those with thinner skin could be more susceptible to exposure, for example, the elderly or young.

Severe ocular lesions can be produced by doses as low as 0.1 mg or exposure to saturated vapour for 8 seconds at 23° C.

Clinical features

Dermal exposure

Immediate pain, a burning sensation, and local oedema can occur depending on the concentration. Rapid absorption is accompanied by deep, aching pain within a few minutes. Erythema develops within 15–30 minutes. Vesication may be delayed; blisters are often well developed after 12 hours and cover the whole erythematous area over 4 days. Pain lessens after 2 or 3 days.

Itching and irritation occur regardless of the development of blisters. Systemic features may develop.

Ingestion

Ingestion of contaminated food or water is possible, though Lewisite is poorly soluble in water.

Immediate pain, burning sensation, and local oedema occur in the mouth and throat. Rapid absorption is accompanied by deep, aching pain within a few minutes. Erythema develops within 15–30 minutes. Vesication may be delayed although blisters are often well developed within 12 hours and may progress to cover the effected areas over the next few days. Pain lessens after 2 or 3 days.

Absorption through the gut may produce systemic effects.

Inhalation

Immediate irritation, coughing, sneezing, lacrimation, rhinorrhoea, and vomiting occur. Hoarseness, barky cough, and sinus pain may also be present.

In severe cases necrosis of the epithelium, accompanied by pseudomembrane formation occurs. This pseudomembrane can become detached and cause bronchial obstruction.

Pulmonary oedema may be delayed and fatal respiratory failure may occur.

Absorption may produce systemic effects.

Management

- Decontaminate the patient. Irrigation with DMSA solution applied 30 minutes after exposure was shown to have a protective effect against skin damage from Lewisite but should not replace early irrigation with water.
- Skin lesions should be managed as thermal burns. Do not de-roof intact blisters initially as this can increase the risk of infection. Consult a burns expert. Dermabrasion and laser therapy may increase the rate of healing.
- Manage cardiovascular and respiratory effects conventionally.
- Consider the need for chelation therapy with DMPS or DMSA in patients who have systemic symptoms, have elevated urine arsenic concentrations, have large areas of dermal burns and/or were contaminated over greater than 5% of their body surface area with Lewisite.
- Treat eye contamination as for other chemical burns. Remove contact lenses if present and immediately irrigate the affected eye thoroughly with water or 0.9% saline for at least 10–15 minutes. Continue until the conjunctival sac pH is normal (7.5–8.0). Retest after 20 minutes and use further irrigation if necessary.
  - Irrigation with a chelation agent such as DMSA has been shown to have a protective effect, but should not be replaced by early irrigation with water.

- Repeated instillation of local anaesthetics (e.g. tetracaine) may reduce discomfort and help more thorough decontamination. Cover an anaesthetized eye to protect from traumatic injury.

The 'Dicks'

The blistering agents ethyl dichlorarsine, methyl dichlorarsine and phenyl dichlorarsine are sometimes known as the 'Dicks.' These three chemicals are all liquids at room temperature. They produce initial irritation of the eyes, skin and respiratory tract with subsequent blister formation.

Ethyl dichlorarsine (Dick) $C_2H_5AsCl_2$

Is a low boiling point liquid. It was used during World War I as a chemical warfare agent. It produces irritation of the eyes and nasal passages at very low concentrations. Exposure of the skin produces early irritation with later blister formation.

Methyl dichlorarsine (methyl Dick) CH_3AsCl_2

Is a colourless liquid with a melting point of $-55°$ C and boiling point of $133°$ C.

Phenyl dichlorarsine (phenyl Dick) $C_6H_5AsCl_2$

Is a colourless liquid with a melting point of $-20°$ C and a boiling point of $252°$ C although impure forms have a brown colour. It was used during World War I as a chemical warfare agent.

Irritants

The irritant agents diphenyl chlorarsine (DA), diphenyl cyanarsine (DC), and diphenylaminochlorarsine (DM, Adamsite) are sometimes known as vomiting agents. They are all solids at room temperature and are insoluble in water.

They are distributed mainly as aerosols and the prime route of absorption is therefore via the respiratory tract though they may also be absorbed via other routes.

Adamsite was first used during World War I in 1917. More recently, in 2003, letters containing Adamsite were sent to a number of embassies, causing hospitalization of police and postal workers with skin irritation, eye irritation, and breathing difficulties.

Features

Features may be delayed for several minutes during which exposure will continue. Therefore significant exposure may have occurred before the victim is removed from the source.

Initial symptoms typically involve the upper respiratory tract, including irritation of the nasal mucosa and sinuses, irritation of the nasal mucosa, burning of the throat, violent and uncontrollable sneezing and coughing, and acute pain and tightness in the chest. Exposure will also cause eye irritation, lachrymation, blepharospasm, and injected conjunctivae. Exposure of the skin to high concentrations results in erythema, pruritus and vesication.

Systemic effects may last from 30 minutes to several hours. These include severe headache, nausea, persistent vomiting, diarrhoea and abdominal cramps. Minor effects may persist for 24 hours or longer.

Severe lung and airway damage were seen in one fatal case following exposure in an enclosed environment.

The onset of symptoms is said to be slower than with some other substances used as riot control agents, e.g. CS (see also Riot control agents pp. 352–354). Due to the slower onset of symptoms, the need to move away from a source of exposure or put on a respirator may not be appreciated before a significant dose has been absorbed. The presence of vomiting may be an incitement to remove a respirator and therefore increase exposure.

The lowest concentration of Adamsite that causes irritation of the throat and respiratory tract is 0.38 and 0.5 mg/m^3 respectively. The initial features described following exposure to diphenylalanine chlorarsine (DM, Adamsite) are those of a burning sensation and pain in the eyes, nose, throat, and respiratory tract, followed by coughing, sneezing, lachrymation, and salivation. Headache, abdominal cramps, vomiting, and diarrhoea may subsequently occur.

Management

Management involves decontamination, as for Lewisite, and symptomatic treatment.

Since these compounds contain arsenic it may, as with Lewisite, be appropriate to use chelation systemically in more severe cases.

Further reading

Departments of The Army, The Navy, and The Air Force (1996). *Nato Handbook on the Medical Aspects of NBC Defensive Operations. A Med P-6 (B)*. <http://www.fas.org/irp/doddir/army/fm8-9.pdf>.

Marrs TC, Maynard RL, Sidell F (eds) (2007). *Chemical Warfare Agents: Toxicology and Treatment*, 2nd edition. Chichester: John Wiley & Sons.

Owens EJ, McNamara BP, Weimer JT, et al. (1967). *The Toxicology of DM*. Edgewood Arsenal Technical Report 4108. Edgewood Arsenal, MD: Department of the Army Edgewood Arsenal.

Sidell FR. (1997). Riot control agents. In: Sidell FR, Takafuji ET and Franz DR (eds), *Medical Aspects of Chemical and Biological Warfare*, pp. 307–24. Washington, DC: Office of the Surgeon General. <http://www.globalsecurity.org/wmd/library/report/1997/cwbw/Ch12.pdf>

Riot control agents

Background

Riot control agents which can be sometimes referred to as 'tear gas' or lacrymators, are chemical compounds that temporarily affect function by having a direct effect on individuals leading to irritation to the eyes, mouth, throat, lungs, and skin. Several different compounds are considered to be riot control agents:

- chlorobenzylidenemalononitrile (CS)
- chloroacetophenone (CN)
- dibenzoxazepine (CR)
- pepper spray (OC)/pelargonic acid vanillylamide (PAVA) (synthetic OC)
- combinations of various agents.

Others that have been used historically will not be considered here—*chloropicrin* (PS) and *bromobenzylcyanide* (CA).

They are used worldwide for crowd control, the most common being CS, by police and military, delivered by various spray devices, frangible (i.e. readily broken up on contact) projectiles, shells, and grenades. In some countries individuals use them for personal protection (e.g. pepper spray in the USA). The military, and elite police units wishing to test the speed and ability of personnel to use their gas masks, and also assess whether individual officers have resilience and can cope with unprotected exposure, use CS. It will also give them an understanding of the effects on individuals.

These agents are liquids or solids (e.g. powder) and could be released in the air as fine droplets or particles (e.g. CN and CS). When released into the air exposure will be through skin contact, eye contact, or inhalation. The extent of poisoning depends on the same factors as chemical exposures in general i.e. dose (amount), the location of exposure (indoors vs outdoors), how the person was exposed, and the length of time of the exposure.

Mode of action

Riot control agents work by causing irritation to the area of contact (e.g. eyes, skin, nose) within seconds of exposure. The effects of exposure are usually short-lived (15–30 minutes) after the person has been removed from the source and decontaminated. Details for individual agents are given as follows.

Chlorobenzylidenemalononitrile (CS) (CAS 2698-41-1)

Commonly used by police forces worldwide (including UK and Republic of Ireland). It was synthesized in 1928 by Corson and Stoughton (hence CS), but CS did not replace CN in general use until 1959 following development at Porton Down in England. Mace™ is sometimes a mixture of pepper spray and CS (see later in section). It is a white solid at room temperature. It is typically dissolved in an organic solvent such as methyl isobutyl ketone (MIBK), in order to be used as an aerosol or microparticulate cloud. In the UK, police forces use a 5% w/v CS gas spray with MIBK and nitrogen as a propellant. It has a melting point 95–96° C and a boiling point of 310–315° C. CS is soluble in acetone, dioxane, methylene chloride, ethyl acetate, and benzene.

Mode of action

CS is a potent sensory irritant particularly to the mucous membranes of the eyes, nose, mouth, and throat.

Marked toxicity would only be expected after exposure to a high concentration within a confined space for a prolonged time. Symptoms should resolve 15–30 minutes after removal from exposure, as CS breaks down rapidly in the body, although erythema may persist for an hour or longer. Patients with bronchial asthma or COPD may have their respiratory disease aggravated by exposure to CS. Secondary contamination with CS powder can occur. In spite of its extensive use, sometimes in a confined space, there have been no verified human fatalities following CS exposure.

CS is an 'SN2 alkylating agent' (S = substitution; N = nucleophilic). A nucleophile is a reactive chemical species that has spare electrons available to donate to a chemical bond. The nucleophiles most often implicated in reactions with CS are sulfhydryl (-SH) groups on enzymes and co-enzymes. A carbon atom of the CS molecule forms a bond with the nucleophile and in so doing the bond between the carbon and chlorine atoms of CS is broken. The result is inhibition of sulfhydryl-containing enzymes, such as lactic dehydrogenase. CS also reacts rapidly with the disulfhydryl form of thioctic acid (α-lipoic acid), a coenzyme of the pyruvate decarboxylase system, resulting in inhibition of pyruvic decarboxylase and tissue injury and necrosis. Exposure to CS causes bradykinin release. CS also activates a specialized cation selective channel (TRPA1—transient receptor potential A1 channel) that mediates mechanical, thermal, and pain-related inflammatory signals. All these effects are transient, however, as the enzymes affected are rapidly reactivated when CS is metabolized.

The cyano groups of CS are unlikely to cause systemic cyanide toxicity since a 1-minute exposure to an intolerable concentration (10 mg/m^3) produces less cyanide than two inhalations of a cigarette. Clinically significant concentrations of free cyanide do not appear in the plasma.

On contact with water in mucous membranes, CS hydrolyses to 2-chlorobenzaldehyde and malononitrile. 2-Chlorobenzaldehyde is metabolized to 2-chlorohippuric acid and 2-chlorobenzoic acid, which are excreted in urine. Malononitrile is metabolized to thiocyanate. The half-lives of CS and the metabolites 2-chlorobenzaldehyde and 2-chlorobenzylmalononitrile are in the region of 5–10 seconds.

Chloroacetophenone (CN) (CAS 532-27-4)

CN was used widely until CS replaced it in 1959. However, CN is still employed in various countries in riot control and peacekeeping operations, as grenade-generated smoke, in projectile cartridges, and as an incapacitant solution. A 1% solution was introduced in 1965 for self-defence (Mace™; methyl chloroacetophenone) but this formulation of Mace™ is now legal in few countries. Most Mace™ sold currently contains pepper spray alone or pepper spray and CS.

Mode of action

CN is a white solid at room temperature. It is typically dissolved in solvents such as kerosene and 1,1,1-trichloroethane in order to produce an aerosol or microparticulate cloud. It has a melting point of 59° C and a boiling point of 244–245° C.

It is the most toxic of the riot control agents and is 3–10 times more toxic (lower LCt_{50}) than CS. Several deaths have been attributed to CN exposure, especially to grenade-generated smoke and in confined spaces. At post-mortem, necrosis of the laryngeal, tracheal, and bronchial epithelium with pseudomembrane formation, bronchiolar epithelial desquamation, and pulmonary oedema were observed. CN is a 'SN2 alkylating agent' (see earlier in section). The nucleophiles most likely to react with CN are sulfhydryl (-SH) groups (as for CS). CN also activates TRPA1 (see as for CS).

Dibenzoxazepine (CR) (CAS 257-07-8)

First introduced in 1962 it is the parent compound of the antipsychotic drug, loxapine.

Mode of action

CR is a pale yellow solid at room temperature and is highly stable. It has a melting point of 71–72° C and a boiling point of 335° C. It is soluble in acetone, benzene, dichloromethane and alcohols and its vapour is 6.7 times heavier than air. It is usually formulated as a 0.1% solution in 80:20 w/v mix of propylene glycol and water. It is less toxic than CN or CS. Substantial toxicity is only expected after exposure to a high concentration within a confined space for a prolonged time though injection of the conjunctival vessels and erythema may persist for several hours. There are no reports of sensitization, vesication, severe skin, eye or lung effects, or long lasting exposure-related problems.

CR activates TRPA1 (see for CS). Aerosols of CR are rapidly absorbed from the respiratory tract and it may also be absorbed from the gastrointestinal tract and cornea. It is oxidized to a lactam derivative that is then metabolized further, undergoes entero-hepatic recirculation, and renal excretion and the plasma half-life after inhalation is about 5 minutes.

Pepper spray (OC)/pelargonic acid vanillylamide (PAVA) (synthetic OC) (CAS 404-86-4 (capsaicin)/CAS 2444-46-4 (PAVA))

Oleoresin capsicum (OC) is the extract from the dried ripe fruits of Capsicum annuum and Capsicum frutescens, which consists of several different capsaicinoids (alkaloids), the most potent of which is capsaicin. Pepper spray is a reddish brown liquid. Depending on the brand, pepper spray may contain water, alcohols, or organic solvents as liquid carriers and nitrogen, carbon dioxide, and/or halogenated hydrocarbons as propellants. One of the most significant developments in recent years has been an increase in the usage of PAVA ($C_{17}H_{27}NO_3$), a synthetic version of OC that is more potent than the natural product and less variable in its potency. It is used widely by law enforcement organizations in North America and some European countries, including police forces in the UK who now use both CS and PAVA sprays and the US military is also investigating its use.

Mode of action

Pepper spray causes rapid incapacitation due to severe ocular pain/discomfort, excess lacrimation, blepharospasm, bronchoconstriction, severe coughing and sneezing, shortness of breath, and burning sensation of the skin. Since the capsaicinoid content of extracts varies widely amongst manufacturers from 1.2–12.6%, the effects associated with pepper spray exposure may vary by as much as 30-fold among brands. PAVA is a much more consistent performer due to the ability to regulate the concentration and is usually used as a 0.3% solution

of PAVA in 50% aqueous ethanol. Pepper spray is thought to have contributed directly to the death of one prisoner in the USA with pre-existing bronchiolitis.

Capsaicin stimulates specific receptors (TRPVR1 receptors) on a subset of sensory neurons triggering release of neuropeptides, neurogenic inflammation, and the sensation of pain. Transient stimulation of sensory neurons is followed by a prolonged refractory state, resulting in loss of responsiveness to further application of capsaicinoids. Skin absorption of capsaicin is low but is absorbed readily from the gastrointestinal tract in rats. Capsaicin is distributed widely; it is broken down to non-active metabolites in the liver

As well as the symptoms already described the following effects can occur with OC/PAVA exposure:

Eye exposure

Severe discomfort, pain, lacrimation, blepharospasm, involuntary or reflex closing of the eyelids, redness, conjunctival inflammation, loss of blink reflex, and corneal abrasions. Severe conjunctival chemosis and symblepharon with conjunctival necrosis and epithelial defects, which healed within 2 weeks, have been reported.

Inhalation

Significant airway irritation, coughing, wheeze, rhinorrhoea, sneezing, dyspnoea, shortness of breath, retrosternal discomfort, bronchoconstriction, bronchospasm, subglottic oedema, and pulmonary oedema. Pneumomediastinum, pneumopericardium, respiratory failure, and severe hypotension have been reported.

Health effects

Immediate signs and symptoms of exposure to a riot control agent

Individuals may experience some or all of the following symptoms immediately after exposure:

Respiratory signs and symptoms

- Cough
- Hoarseness
- Chest tightness
- Sensation of suffocation
- Dyspnoea
- Tachypnoea
- Wheezing
- Hypoxemia
- Cyanosis
- Non-cardiogenic pulmonary oedema.

Skin and mucous membranes

- Redness, pain, and blistering of exposed skin
- Pruritus, scaling, erythema, and blistering of the skin may occur
- Burn injury to exposed skin (following prolonged contact, especially in association with wet skin or clothing)
- Rarely, allergic contact dermatitis, leucoderma, initiation or exacerbation of seborrhoeic dermatitis and aggravation of rosacea can occur
- Eye: lacrimation, ocular irritation and redness, blurred vision, corneal burns
- Oropharynx: oral burns and irritation, sore throat, hoarseness, dysphagia, salivation
- Nose: rhinorrhoea, burning, irritation, oedema.

However it must be noted that the actual clinical presentation of tear gas exposure might be more variable than the syndrome described here. It should also be noted that the listed effects are very non-specific and other causes should be in the differential diagnosis unless the history dictates that a riot control agent has been used. The differential diagnosis should include exposure to:

- ammonia
- phosgene
- chlorine
- sulphuric acid
- hydrogen chloride
- sodium azide
- hydrogen sulphide
- nickel carbonyl.

Most of these chemicals are discussed in detail in Chapter 9, pp. 205–264.

Prolonged or exposure to a large dose of riot control agent, especially in a closed setting, may cause:

- blindness
- glaucoma
- cataracts
- immediate death due to severe chemical burns to the throat and lungs (very rare)
- respiratory failure possibly resulting in death
- reactive airways dysfunction syndrome (RADS).

Exposure during pregnancy

There are very limited preclinical and human data available concerning acute exposure to CS gas in pregnancy, and no available data for CR gas, CN gas, or pepper sprays. Available data on CS gas used for crowd control do not indicate an association with adverse effects on the fetus.

Management

Primary responders should wear appropriate PPE. Secondary care staff should not need to wear protective equipment other than routine precautions against secondary contamination with vomit and body fluids.

Remove from site of exposure, particularly if in a confined space. The agent should disperse in fresh air in a few minutes. Hospital treatment is rarely needed because spontaneous recovery occurs rapidly (within 15–30 minutes) after the end of exposure unless exposure has been extensive.

If features persist for longer than 30 minutes after the end of exposure:

- Move the patient away from other casualties to a clean atmosphere.
- Remove all contaminated clothing and seal in plastic bags. Disposable rubber gloves should be used when handling contaminated clothes.

- Wash exposed skin with soap and water only if symptoms persist (with OC/PAVA vegetable oil may help).
- Remove contact lenses. Hard ones may be washed and re-used in the future; soft ones should be discarded.
- If eye irritation persists, irrigate the eyes with room-temperature water or normal saline for at least 15 minutes. The eyes should then be examined by a slit-lamp and fluorescein eye drops. Refer to an ophthalmologist if eye symptoms persist.
- Local anaesthetics such as tetracaine have been found to relieve symptoms (especially with OC/PAVA).
- Patients with features of severe poisoning, particularly respiratory complications, should be admitted to hospital and managed appropriately.
- Manage skin burns conventionally.
- Other measures as indicated by the patient's clinical condition.

Patients should be advised on discharge to seek medical attention if symptoms subsequently develop.

If symptoms go away soon after a person is removed from exposure to riot control agents, long-term health effects are unlikely to occur.

Further reading

Anderson PJ, Lau GS, Taylor WR, et al. (1996). Acute effects of the potent lacrimator o-chlorobenzylidene malonitrile (CS) tear gas. *Hum Exp Toxicol*, 15:461–5.

Ballantyne B (2007). Riot control agents in military operations, civil disturbance control and potential terrorist activities, with particular reference to peripheral chemosensory irritants. In: Marrs TC, Maynard RL, Sidell FR (eds), *Chemical Warfare Agents: Toxicology and Treatment*, 2nd edition, pp. 543–612. Chichester: John Wiley & Sons.

Blain PG (2003). Tear gases and irritant incapacitants. 1-chloroacetophenone, 2-chlorobenzylidene malononitrile and dibenz[b,f]-1,4-oxazepine. *Toxicol Rev*, 22:103–10.

Brone B, Peeters PJ, Marrannes R, et al. (2008). Tear gasses CN, CR, and CS are potent activators of the human TRPA1 receptor. *Toxicol Appl Pharmacol*, 231:150–6.

Committees on Toxicity, MaCoCiFCPatE, Department of Health (1999). *Statement on 2-Chlorobenzylidene Malonitrile (CS) and CS Spray*. London: The Department of Health.

Hill AR, Silverberg NB, Mayorga D, et al. (2000). Medical hazards of the tear gas CS—a case of persistent, multisystem, hypersensitivity reaction and review of the literature. *Medicine*, 79:234–40.

Hu H, Christiani D (1992). Reactive airways dysfunction after exposure to tear gas. *Lancet*, 339:1535.

Karagama YG, Newton JR, Newbegin CJ (2003). Short-term and long-term physical effects of exposure to CS spray. *J R Soc Med*, 96:172–4.

Olajos EJ, Salem H (2001). Riot control agents: pharmacology, toxicology, biochemistry and chemistry. *J Appl Toxicol*, 21: 355–91.

Varma S, Holt PJ (2001). Severe cutaneous reaction to CS gas. *Clin Exp Dermatol*, 26:248–50.

Centrally acting incapacitating agents

Background

Incapacitating chemical agents are distinguished from lethal chemical agents in that there is a wide margin between the dose at which they cause physical and/or mental incapacity and the dose at which they cause death.

Several sovereign states, most notably the USA, have previously developed incapacitating chemical agents, presumably to give field commanders a non-lethal capability in order to overcome an opposing force with minimal loss of life and collateral damage.

The Chemical Weapons Convention (CWC) prohibits the development, manufacture, and stockpiling of any toxic chemical that has been weaponized with an intent to cause incapacity. The CWC defines a toxic chemical as: 'Any chemical which through its chemical action on life processes can cause death, temporary incapacitation or permanent harm to humans or animals' (Article II.2).

The CWC does however make provision for the manufacture and use of riot control agents, which the CWC define as: 'Any chemical not listed in a Schedule, which can produce rapidly in humans sensory irritation or disabling physical effects which disappear within a short time following termination of exposure' (Article II.7).

This definition has been criticized by several member states in that some temporary incapacitating agents, such as BZ (quinuclidinyl benzilate) are controlled under Schedule 2A of the convention whilst the status of other chemical entities remains ambiguous.

BZ, 3-quinuclidinyl benzilate (CAS 62869-69-6)

3-Quinuclidinyl benzilate, referred to by its NATO classification BZ, is a glycolic acid ester with potent central anticholinergic effects that is capable of producing a delirium of several days' duration following exposure to a single dose.

The threat

The USA developed a BZ capability during the 1970s. The programme was abandoned, apparently because of concerns that exposure to BZ might increase the irrationality of an opposing force. BZ may still remain attractive to those with intent to demonstrate or cause disruption, particularly non-state actors. Central incapacitating agents may also be deployed against an individual in order to undermine their credibility and effectiveness due to the prolonged neuropsychological features following exposure.

Toxicology

BZ forms a stable white crystalline powder under standard conditions that can be administered effectively through either inhalation, ingestion or a parental route. Percutaneous absorption of BZ is, however, limited and, in addition, BZ is only slightly soluble in water. Weaponized BZ would therefore be likely to be disseminated as an aerosolized fine solid. An optimum particle size of 0.6–0.8 micrometres is required for effective inhalation.

BZ antagonizes muscarinic receptors of the peripheral and central nervous system. The incapacitating dose (IC_{50}) of BZ is approximately 6 micrograms/kg in humans, whilst the median lethal dose (LD_{50}) is estimated to be around 200 micrograms/kg. Clearance occurs through hepatic metabolism and renal elimination.

Detection

BZ can be detected by (field) GC-MS or by HPLC although hospitals can not undertake the assay routinely. Clinical suspicion of exposure is very important, and consideration to the use of this agent may be triggered by the presence of a number of individuals who present with similar features, including those of 'classical' antocholinergic toxicity, who have been in the same place at the same time. In effect, initially, 'man becomes the detector'.

Clinical features

The duration of action of BZ is greater than atropine and its effects can be detected up to 96 hours post-exposure to a signal dose. An accumulative effect following multiple exposures can also occur, further prolonging the duration and potency of the clinical features.

Post exposure to a typical dose within the IC_{50} range the following clinical effects can be expected:

- 1–4 hours: peripheral anticholinergic effects such as tachycardia, dry mouth, and vomiting. Central anticholinergic effects such as sedation, confusion, and ataxia.
- 4–12 hours: limited capability, sedation, and onset of hallucinations that may vary from entertaining to terrifying.
- 12–96 hours: profound delirium with increased activity and unpredictable behaviour followed by gradual recovery.

Management

All patients potentially exposed to aerosolized BZ will require decontamination. Any contaminated clothing should be disposed of in a manner to prevent exposure to rescuers.

- The majority of patients are likely to require supportive treatment only. Those capable of walking may require firm restraint to prevent secondary injury.
- Heat injury is a recognized complication of BZ exposure due to the anticholinergic effects of reduced sweating and decreased oral intake. Oral fluids should be encouraged and parental fluids considered if the casualty is unable to drink. Clothing should be removed if the ambient temperature is greater than 25° C. Active cooling should be initiated if core body temperature rises above 39° C.
- Urinary retention may also be anticipated from the anticholinergic action of BZ. Bladder distension and urine output should be monitored. Acute urinary retention may be both painful and distressing for the patient. Urinary catheterization may be required to relieve urinary symptoms, and may also contribute to decreasing agitation.
- Physostigmine (not licensed for use in the UK), a carbamate that reversibly inhibits cholinesterases, should be considered for patients with serious cardiovascular and/or neurological features of BZ toxicity. Physostigmine appears to be superior to benzodiazepines in treating the delirium associated with BZ and may also reduce the cardiovascular features. An initial, slow, intravenous loading dose of 1 mg per 20 kg of body weight should be given and repeated every 15 minutes until the heart rate is below 100 beats per minute and the mental effects clear. A maintenance dose of 2–5 mg of physostigmine should then be administered every 1–2 hours. If resources are available

administration via a syringe pump will avoid potentially toxic peaks and troughs of the antidote. The required dose should be titrated against the cardiovascular and CNS symptoms and the dose tapered as the effects of BZ diminish.

- Central and peripheral acetylcholinesterase can also be reversibly inhibited by 7-methoxytacrine (7-MTHA– not licensed for use in the UK) and its derivatives, and may be an alternative to physostigmine. Peripherally acting cholinesterase inhibitors, such as neostigmine, pyridostigmine, and pilocarpine, are ineffective against BZ poisoning.

Dimethylheptylpyran (DMHP) (CAS 32904-22-6)

The threat

The cannabinol analogue dimethylheptylpyran, hereafter known as DMPH, is believed to have been developed by the USA as an incapacitating agent. Several open-source reports describe that the effects of DMPH and its isomers were assessed on human participants. It is not clear whether DMHP or any of its derivatives has been weaponized by state or non-state actors.

Toxicology

DMHP appears to predominantly be an agonist of the cannabinoid 1 (CB_1) receptor. At a dose of 0.5 mg/70 kg of body mass DMPH induces postural hypotension, ataxia, diplopia, and psychomotor retardation in humans. At a dose of 2 mg/70 kg body mass a tachycardia, hypothermia, and decreased visual acuity are observed. CNS effects appear to be minimal in humans.

The lethal dose of DMHP is not known in humans. In mice the LD_{50} is 63 mg/kg compared with a minimal effective dose of 0.075 mg/kg, suggesting a safety factor of 840. In dogs a dose of 0.05 mg/kg induces tranquillity, whilst the LD_{50} is 10 mg/kg. Canine mortality is increased

in the presence of CNS stimulates such as amfetamine, caffeine, and cocaine. Hypothermia is also associated with an increase risk

In common with other Δ9-tetracannabinoids analogues, DMHP has a relatively long half-life of approximately 39 hours (range of 19–57 hours). DMHP can undergo acetylation and is also eliminated unmetabolized in the faeces and urine.

Management

There is no consensus for the treatment of acute DMHP toxicity. From first principles, supportive treatment of hypotension by positioning the casualty head down with a fluid challenge would seem sensible. If hypotension is not corrected by fluids then the use of pressor agents such as norepinephrine or phenylephirine could be considered. Core body temperature should be maintained. The long- term sequelae of DMHP exposure is not well described in humans.

Further reading

Burns MJ, Linden CH, Graudins A, et al. (2000). A comparison of physostigmine and benzodiazepines for the treatment of anticholinergic poisoning. Ann Emerg Med, 35(4):374–81.

Departments of The Army, The Navy, and The Air Force (1996). Nato Handbook on the Medical Aspects of NBC Defensive Operations. A Med P-6 (B). <http://www.fas.org/irp/doddir/army/fm8-9.pdf>.

Hilliard CJ (2000). Endocannabinoids and vascular function. J Pharmacol Exp Ther, 294(1):27–32.

Toxicology and Environmental Health Hazards Committee; National Research Council Staff (2000). Possible Long-Term Health Effects of Short-Term Exposure to Chemical Agents: Vol. 2: Final Report —Current Health Status of Test Subjects. Washington, DC: National Academies Press.

World Health Organization (2004). Public Health Response to Biological and Chemical Weapons: WHO Guidance, 2nd edition. Geneva: WHO.

Principles of radiation toxicology

Outline to radiation biology as applied to poisoning

What is radiation?
We are constantly exposed to background radiation as a part of our natural environment; natural sources include cosmic rays and radiation arising from minerals in the ground.

Radiation may be ionizing or non-ionizing. The difference relates to the ability of the radiation to eject an electron from its orbit around the nucleus. This overview concentrates on ionizing radiation.

Ionizing radiation may be subdivided into:

- particles
- electromagnetic radiation.

It may arise as part of a natural radioactive decay process or may be man-made.

The primary effect ionizing radiation causes is electrical, producing a charged molecule or ion when it passes through a substance, e.g. air, human tissue, etc. This charged molecule or ion may then undergo a chemical interaction inducing a biological change. In turn, this biological change (e.g. altered DNA) may, or may not, produce a subsequent change of biological importance, e.g. cancer.

The biological effects of ionizing radiation depend upon the ability of the radiation to interact with biological tissues and the susceptibility of the tissue that is exposed. The effects depend on the type of radiation, the dose, and the rate of exposure. It also depends upon the tissues that are exposed, as some are more radiosensitive than others, e.g. bone marrow and gonads.

Types of radiation
Low-frequency electromagnetic waves, e.g. radiowaves, do not have sufficient energy to eject electrons from their orbit and do not cause ionization, although they may cause localized heating (e.g. from very close proximity to radar installations). Electromagnetic waves with higher energy (e.g. X-rays and gamma-rays) produce ionization.

Radioactive particles include alpha particles (helium nuclei and beta particles (fast moving electrons), both of which can produce ionization. Protons may be produced in particle accelerators. However, the ability of each type of radiation differs and this needs to be considered when assessing 'dose'.

Radioactive particles are emitted from the unstable nuclei of radioactive atoms. This results in the production of a new element—a radiation decay product. As the radioactive decay takes place energy is released. Additional energy released not contained in an ejected particle may be released as a gamma wave.

Alpha (α) particles
Alpha particles are heavy particles with a mass of four and a positive charge of two (i.e. a helium nucleus ^4_2He). They interact readily with other matter, losing energy as they do so. An α particle will travel only a few centimetres in air and less than 100 μm in tissue. They do not penetrate the stratum corneum and do not represent an important hazard if the source remains outside the body. However, if inhaled or ingested, they interact readily with tissue presenting a significant hazard (see examples in Alpha sources, pp. 363–366).

Beta (β) particles
Beta particles are formed when a neutron disintegrates into a proton and an electron, thus forming a different element. The electron subsequently ejected from the nucleus is called a β particle. They are fast moving and carry a single negative or positive charge. The maximum energy of each β particle depends upon the difference in mass between the original and the new nucleus. β particles do not lose their energy as rapidly as α particles (see examples in Beta sources, pp. 367–370).

Gamma (γ) rays
The ejection of a β particle may be accompanied by a γ ray. β particles do not lose their energy as rapidly as α particles. When a radioactive particle is released from a nucleus not all the energy released may be transferred to the particle and the nucleus may remain in an excited state. The excess energy is released as γ rays and is identical to X-rays except that they result from radioactive decay. γ rays are capable of penetrating several metres through air or several centimetres through biological tissues (see examples in Gamma rays and X-rays, pp. 371–374).

Protons
Particle accelerators may produce protons. They are able to penetrate tissues fairly readily. They have a mass of one and a single positive charge.

X-rays
X-rays are part of the continuous spectrum of electromagnetic waves. They have neither mass nor charge (see examples in Gamma rays and X rays, pp. 371–374).

Radioactivity and its effects
Terms used to describe radiation

Activity
Describes the rate at which radioactive decay occurs. 1 radioactive decay per second = 1 Becquerel (1 Bq).

Dose
Dose is a general term sometimes used to describe quantity of ionizing radiation. The dose of radiation is measured by its ability to transfer energy into a given material. The unit of dose is the Gray (Gy), which corresponds to 1 Joule of energy per kilogram of material ($1J.Kg^{-1}$).

Equivalent dose
The ability of different types of radiation to cause biological damage varies. For example, the same dose of gamma rays and alpha particles has different biological effects. So, 'dose equivalent' is used when considering biological effects.

To normalize the effects of different types of radiation a weighting factor is used. This weighting factor reflects the dose of radiation that will produce the same biological endpoint.

The equivalent dose is reported in Sieverts (Sv). The equivalent dose is equal to the dose multiplied by the radiation weighting factor: H = DW
  Where H = equivalent dose
  D = absorbed dose
  W = weighting factor.
  For electrons (β) and gamma rays W = 1
  For alpha particles W = 20

Biological effects
The susceptibility of different tissues to radiation damage varies. Fast multiplying tissues are particularly sensitive, for example, the bone marrow and gastrointestinal tract.

Effective dose
A tissue-weighting factor expresses the relative sensitivities of particular organs. The effective dose for each tissue is equal to the equivalent dose multiplied by the tissue weighting factor. The International Commission on Radiological Protection (ICRP) continually monitors and reviews tissue weighting factors and the most recent assessments are shown in Table 15.1. Note there are orders of magnitude differences, i.e. brain c.f. colon.

Half-life (t½)
The time for the activity to decline by half.

Mass number
The number of protons plus neutrons in the nucleus of an atom.

Atomic number
The number of protons in the nucleus of an atom.

Biological effects
The effects of radiation upon the body depend upon:
- amount of radiation
- type of radiation
- rate of exposure
- area exposed
- radiosensitivity of organ.

Radiation may cause both acute and chronic effects.

At low doses the chance of a biological effect increases with dose. A person may, or may not, develop effects. The chance (risk) of an effect occurring increases with dose. These are known as stochastic effects.

At high doses a person will develop effects and these become predictable, rather than a matter of chance. Their severity increases with dose. These are known as deterministic effects.

Acute clinical effects of radiation
Acute exposure to high dose of radiation can cause:
- acute radiation syndrome (ARS)
- localized radiation injury.

The effects are related to the equivalent dose, with fast multiplying tissues (e.g. bone marrow and gastrointestinal tract) being particularly sensitive. See Table 15.2, which summarizes ARS.

ARS can occur when the body has been exposed to substantial doses of ionizing radiation. The effects may occur either from exposure to an external source of radiation, contact with a radioactive source, or absorption of a source into the body. The effects caused will vary according to the amount and type of radiation, the rate of exposure, and the part of the body exposed.

ARS normally has four phases:
1 prodromal
2 latent
3 manifest illness
4 recovery or death.

Typically the patient will have a prodromal phase characterized by nausea, vomiting, and fatigue. There follows a latent phase before characteristic features of illness develop, which is then followed by either recovery or death.

It is convenient to think of the acute radiation syndrome as comprising:
- haemopoietic syndrome
- gastrointestinal syndrome
- CNS syndrome.

Other syndromes (e.g. pulmonary and cutaneous) are also described. The rate of onset of symptoms, the duration of the latent phase, and the likelihood of death depend upon the dose and the availability of treatment.

Whole-body doses of 1–2 Gy will result in nausea and vomiting, a decrease in the white cell count, and an increased risk of developing cancer. Larger doses (3–6 Gy) will produce earlier vomiting and diarrhoea

Table 15.1 Weighting factors for different organs used in dosimetry calculations

Organs	Tissue weighting factors		
	ICRP 30(1979)	ICRP 60(1991)	ICRP 103(2008)
Gonads	0.25	0.20	0.08
Red bone marrow	0.12	0.12	0.12
Colon	–	0.12	0.12
Lung	0.12	0.12	0.12
Stomach	–	0.12	0.12
Breasts	0.15	0.05	0.12
Bladder	–	0.05	0.04
Liver	–	0.05	0.04
Oesophagus	–	0.05	0.04
Thyroid	0.03	0.05	0.04
Skin	-	0.01	0.01
Bone surface	0.03	0.01	0.01
Salivary glands	–	–	0.01
Brain	–	–	0.01
Remainder of body	0.30	0.05	0.12

Table 15.2 Acute clinical effects of radiation

Approx. dose (Gy)	Manifestation of illness	Prognosis without therapy
0.5–1.0	Slight decrease in blood cell counts	Almost certain survival
1–2	Early signs of bone marrow damage	Highly probable survival (>90%)
2.0–3.5	Moderate to severe bone marrow damage	Probable survival
3.5–5.5	Severe bone marrow damage; slight GI damage	Death within 3.5–6 weeks (50% of victims)
5.5–7.5	Pancytopenia and moderate GI damage	Death probable within 2–3 weeks
7.5–10.0	Marked GI and bone marrow damage, hypotension	Death probable within 1–2.5 weeks
10–20	Severe GI damage, pneumonitis, altered mental status, cognitive dysfunction.	Death certain within 5–12 days
20–30	Cerebrovascular collapse, fever, shock	Death certain within 2–5 days

followed by a latent phase and subsequent gastrointestinal damage and some deaths. Untreated, the estimated average lethal dose at 2 months is around 3–4 Gy.

Haemopoietic syndrome

The haemopoietic system is particularly sensitive to the effects of radiation, but this does not often occur with doses less than 1 Gy. An initial increase in the white cell count is followed by granulocytopenia that predisposes to infection. Lymphocytes are the most sensitive marker of exposure and the rate of fall may be used to estimate exposure and prognosis. Similarly thrombocytopenia occurs and may lead to bleeding, though typically the platelet count falls more slowly than the white cell count.

Gastrointestinal syndrome

Radiation damages the intestinal mucosa. This results in nausea, vomiting, abdominal pain, and diarrhoea. Patients are at an increased risk of infection from gastrointestinal organisms. At high doses, features may occur within hours.

Neurological syndrome

Neurological features of acute radiation syndrome include radiation-induced encephalopathy and myelopathy. Encephalopathy is characterized by nausea, vomiting, and drowsiness, thought to be a result of raised intracranial pressure. It may occur within days or weeks. Myelopathy may present with transient paraesthesia or may be delayed, manifesting as permanent paralysis or sensory changes.

Local effects

Local exposure can cause tissue destruction and necrosis. Recovery may be hampered by damage of blood vessels and local ischaemia. Should surgery be required it should be undertaken early if exposure to more than 1 Gy has occurred, or delayed until after bone marrow recovery has taken place.

Late effects

Acute exposure to radiation may result in an increased risk of cancers developing later in life. This may result in anxiety regarding effects on health later in life. Acute stress around the time of exposure is to be expected and may persist to become a post-traumatic stress disorder.

Treatment

It is beyond the scope of this section to give detailed treatment options; however, the reader is directed to the 'Further reading' and subsequent sections in this chapter.

Symptom relief, for example, the use of 5-HT$_3$ receptor-blocking antiemetics is important. Infection control (e.g. reverse barrier nursing) and treatment (antibiotics, antifungals etc.) is important, as is the use of transfusion support and granulocyte colony stimulating factors for the treatment of bone marrow depression. Fluid replacement is necessary, as loss through the gastrointestinal tract or via bleeding may be substantial.

Intensive treatment may allow casualties to survive doses 1–2 Gy higher than otherwise would occur. Dose estimation may help inform the most appropriate treatment for a particular individual, as in some cases palliation of symptoms will be the most important intervention (see also Biological dosimetry for the clinician, pp. 361–362).

Further reading

Armed Forces Radiobiology Research Institute (AFRRI) (2013). *Medical Management of Radiation Casualties*, online 4th edition. <http://www.usuhs.edu/afrri/outreach/pdf/4edmmrchandbook.pdf>.

Jarrett DG, Sedlak RG, Dickerson WE, et al. (2007). Medical management of radiation injuries— current US status. *Radiat Meas*, 42:1063–74.

Radiation Emergency Medical Treatment website: <http://www.remm.nlm.gov/>.

Radiation Emergency Assistance Center/Training Site (REAC/TS). (2013). *The Medical Aspects of Radiation Incidents*. <http://orise.orau.gov/files/reacts/medical-aspects-of-radiation-incidents.pdf>.

United Nations Scientific Committee on the Effects of Atomic Radiation (2008). *Sources and Effects of Ionizing Radiation. UNSCEAR 2008 Report to the General Assembly with Scientific Annexes*. New York: UNSCEAR.

Waselenko JK, MacVittie TJ, et al. (2004). Medical management of the acute radiation syndrome: recommendations of the Strategic National Stockpile Radiation Working Group. *Ann Intern Med*, 140:1037–51.

Biological dosimetry for the clinician

Background

Biodosimetry is the use of the individual's biological response as an indicator of radiation dose. There is no single test or assay available to give a fast, reliable, and robust indication of whole-body radiation dose in either single casualty or mass casualty scenarios. Cytogenetic biodosimetry is considered to be the gold standard for determination of whole-body radiation dose. It is beyond the scope of this section to give a detailed treatise of biodosimetry but an overview is outlined and interested readers are directed to further reading.

Summary of biodosimetry parameters

It is important to realize that there will be an immediate need for triage of single or mass casualties within the first few hours of an incident or exposure. This will then be followed by a more considered approach to the casualty/casualties over the following 24–72 hours using more biological indicators as they become available. Not all proposed biodosimetry indicators would be available at all treatment sites. Biodosimetry is not intended to replace, but can be used as an additional resource for, dose assessments that would include early health physics dose estimation and formal dose reconstruction.

Triage

There has been considerable work performed on this subject particularly by the USA, France, and Germany and the consensus as outlined in NCRP Commentary No. 19 (2005) and the following are indicated as a multi-parameter triage tool as the current best estimate of a casualty's absorbed dose:

- time to emesis
- lymphocyte kinetics and neutrophil/lymphocyte ratio (N/L)
- other biodosimetry and biochemical indicators.

Examples of doses and findings are given in Table 15.3. This should also be read in relation to Triage, monitoring, treatment for management of the public in the event of a radiation release, pp. 376–377.

It should be noted that if emesis occurs in the first 1–2 hours, provided it is not psychogenic, it is a particularly serious sign. In addition, if the absolute lymphocyte count drops to below 50% of baseline then it indicates a potentially lethal situation. Conversely if time to emesis is more than 8–10 hours then the dose is likely to be below 1 Gy and not a priority casualty.

For externally irradiated patients without trauma, patients receiving a high whole-body dose can be distinguished from those with a dose less than 1 Gy using two criteria: the N/L ratio and whether emesis has occurred. A triage score, T, is assigned as follows:

$$T = N/L + E,$$

where E = 0 if no emesis; E = 2 if emesis.

In a normal, healthy human population, the N/L ratio has been found to be approximately 2.21. For a time longer than 4 hours post event, T is significantly elevated for a dose greater than 1 Gy. A cut-point of 3.7 has been chosen to maximize sensitivity and specificity. If T is greater than 3.7, the patient should be referred for further evaluation. This technique is useful for times up to 2 weeks post event. An excellent on-line tool exists to aid clinicians in the early dose assessment of radiation casualties using biological indicators and can be found at: <http://www.remm.nlm.gov/ars_wbd.htm>.

Current biodosimetry recommendations include:

- signs and symptoms
- radioactivity assessment
- haematology
- personal and area dosimetry
- cytogenetics (dicentrics)
- electron spin resonance (ESR)-based dose assessment
- serum amylase activity, C-reactive protein (CRP), FLT-3 ligand, citrulline, blood protein assays.

Cytogenetics

Cytogenetic biodosimetry has been used for decades to estimate dose on the basis of radiation-induced chromosome aberrations in circulating lymphocytes and the classical assay looks at dicentric chromosomes. It is of most value in recent whole-body acute radiation exposures. Dicentric chromosomes are formed when broken segments of two irradiated chromosomes are misrepaired forming a chromosome with two centromeres. The number of dicentric chromosomes correlates well with the absorbed dose. As the background level of dicentric chromosomes in lymphocytes in normal subjects is low, the assay has a high sensitivity, with a threshold whole-body dose of 0.1–0.2 Gy (based on analysis of 1000 cells), and it shows strong dose dependence up to 5 Gy for acute photon exposures. The reproducibility, relative specificity of dicentric aberrations to radiation, and its sensitivity to doses below acute medical significance have allowed the assay to become the gold standard in radiation biodosimetry. However, the standard method of scoring 500–1000 metaphase spreads requires about 4–5 days, including timely transport to the laboratory, processing and scoring the sample, and providing a dose estimate. Most scorers will therefore be able to evaluate no more than approximately 300 metaphase cells per day.

Other methods that can be used include cytokinesis-block micronucleus, chromosomal translocations, and premature chromosomal condensation assays. Readers are directed to cytogenetics books for further information on these methods. However, it is worth discussing premature chromosomal condensation (PCC) assays in further detail.

Table 15.3 Multiple parameter biodosimetry

Parameter	Dose (Gy)		
	0	4	>6
% Emesis	–	72	90–100
Median onset of emesis (hours)	–	1.7	1.0
Absolute lymphocyte count; % of normal in first 24 hours	100	60	<47
Relative ↑ relative to day 1	1	10	>15
Dicentrics per 50 metaphases	0.05–0.1	35	–

Premature chromosomal condensation

One limitation of assays requiring lymphocyte stimulation (dicentrics) is that cells receiving higher radiation doses also experience cell cycle delay and may not reach mitosis. This can result in a large underestimation of the absorbed dose. Chromosomes, however, can be forced to condense prematurely and the PCC techniques exploit this. The PCC assay enables direct observation of chromosome damage and earlier than is possible when cells must be stimulated to mitosis. The assay's lower limit of detection is not as low as that of dicentric chromosome assay. It is sensitive to doses higher than detectable with the dicentric chromosome aberration assay and can be used in suspected doses of greater than 3.5 Gy. Your local cytogenetics laboratory will be able to advise you of the utility of this method.

Electron spin resonance (ESR)

ESR or electron paramagnetic resonance (EPR) spectroscopy is a technique for studying chemical species that have one or more unpaired electrons, such as organic and inorganic free radicals or inorganic complexes possessing a transition metal ion. The basic physical concepts of ESR are analogous to those of nuclear magnetic resonance (NMR), but it is electron spins that are excited instead of spins of atomic nuclei. Because most stable molecules have all their electrons paired, the ESR technique is less widely used than NMR. However, this limitation to paramagnetic species also means that the ESR technique is one of great specificity, since ordinary chemical solvents and matrices do not give rise to ESR spectra. Exposure of humans to ionizing radiation results in radiation-induced changes that can be measured and, depending on the absorbed dose, quantified. The use of ESR for biodosimetry is based on the capability of the technique to provide specific and sensitive measurement of unpaired electrons in solid tissue, which are created in proportion to the absorbed dose. The lifetimes of these electrons are very short (nanoseconds) in aqueous systems such as most biological tissues but can be extremely stable in non-aqueous media, including teeth, bone, fingernails, and hair. ESR has been used for *in vitro* analyses of exfoliated teeth to measure doses in populations from Japan and the former Soviet Union. The effectiveness of ESR has been well demonstrated but may not be locally available.

Initial biological parameters

It is important, as already outlined, to attempt to gain as much information as quickly as possible to aid in dose estimation and medical management of radiation casualties. The key tests are as follows:

1 Full blood count with white cell differential and absolute lymphocyte count. This will need to be repeated every 6 hours in order to evaluate lymphocyte kinetics and to calculate the neutrophil/lymphocyte ratio.

2 Serum amylase (baseline and again after 24 hours): a dose-dependent increase in amylase is expected after 24 hours in the event of significant radiation exposure.

Other biological parameters that may be available

- Blood FLT-3 ligand levels are a marker for hematopoietic damage and the FL c FLT-3 ligand concentration in the blood will increase with the severity of bone marrow aplasia. This is therefore a reflection of increasing radiation dose and the levels appear to be proportional to received whole-body radiation dose.

- Blood citrulline is a marker of gastrointestinal damage and is inversely proportional to gastrointestinal damage and in the context of a significant radiation dose a decreasing level may indicate impending or actual gastrointestinal syndrome (see Outline to radiation biology as applied to poisoning, pp. 358–360).

- Interleukin-6 (IL-6) appears to be a useful marker that is increased in serum at higher radiation doses (>9 Gy) and shows promise for future evaluation. Serum IL-6 levels were maximal at 12 hours after irradiation in a mouse model.

- Granulocyte colony-stimulating factor (G-CSF), although a mainstay of treatment in high-dose exposures leading to acute radiation syndrome can be used as a quantitative marker which is increased at higher radiation doses. Maximal levels of G-CSF were observed in peripheral blood of mice 8 hours after irradiation.

- CRP seems to increase with dose and shows promise to discriminate between minimally and heavily exposed patients. There is a significant correlation between the presence of acute mucositis and CRP level in a recent study.

- Cytogenetic studies with over-dispersion index to evaluate for partial body radiation exposure show promise and may be available in the future.

Further reading

Armed Forces Radiobiology Research Institute (AFRRI). Biodosimetry tools website: <http://www.usuhs.mil/afrri/outreach/biodostools.htm>.

Bolognesi, C, Balia, C., Roggieri, P, et al. (2011). Micronucleus test for radiation biodosimetry in mass casualty events: evaluation of visual and automated scoring. *Radiat Meas* **46**:169–75.

Center for High-Throughput Minimally-Invasive Radiation Biodosimetry website: <http://www.cmcr.columbia.edu/>.

Radiation Emergency Assistance Center/Training Site (REAC/TS). (2013). *The Medical Aspects of Radiation Incidents.* <http://orise.orau.gov/files/reacts/medical-aspects-of-radiation-incidents.pdf>.

Radiation Emergency Medical Treatment website: <http://www.remm.nlm.gov/>.

Alpha sources

Background

The alpha (α) particle is a completely ionized helium nucleus and therefore has no orbital electrons. It consists of two neutrons and two protons, is massive (approximately 8000 times as massive as an electron), and carries a strong, double-positive charge. Therefore, it is directly ionizing. These positively charged particles are emitted by certain radionuclides with a substantial amount of uniquely defined and discrete energy (typically 5 mega electron volts (eV) or higher).

α decay only occurs in very heavy elements, i.e. atomic number (Z) greater than 83, such as uranium, thorium, and radium. The nuclei of these atoms are very 'neutron rich' (i.e. have significantly more neutrons in their nucleus than protons), which makes emission of the α particle possible. After an atom ejects an α particle, a new parent atom is formed which has two less neutrons and two less protons. Thus, when ^{238}Uranium (Z=92) decays by α emission, ^{234}Thorium is created (Z=90).

Decay may be represented as:

$$^A_Z X \rightarrow {}^{A-4}_{Z-2} Y + {}^4_2 He$$

e.g. $^{238}_{92}U \rightarrow {}^{234}_{90}Th + {}^4_2He$

α particles, being relatively heavy, and having a 2+ electrical charge, are less penetrating than X-rays, gamma rays, and beta radiation, and can be stopped by a single sheet of paper (see Beta sources, pp. 367–370 and Gamma sources and X-rays, pp. 371–374). α particles interact strongly with atomic electrons because of their strong positive charge. They exert coulombic forces on the electrons over great distances (on the scale of atoms), ripping electrons from their orbits as they pass by. Because α particles interact so strongly with atomic electrons, they have a short range. They travel in a straight line, deposit all their energy quickly, and are what is known as a densely ionizing radiation.

The average amount of energy lost per unit path of the charged particles (α particles and electrons) during their passage through matter is termed linear energy transfer (LET). Radiations with LET above approximately 10 keV (10,000 eV) μm^{-1} are considered high-LET radiations (e.g. α particles, protons liberated by neutron interactions, and heavy ions). Because these radiations have such a high rate of energy loss, they do not penetrate very far into tissue. Depending upon their energy, they may traverse only a few cells. Those radiations with a LET less than approximately 10 keV μm^{-1} are considered low-LET radiations. The high-LET α particle will lose all of its kinetic energy in penetrating only a few tens of micrometres in any material, including tissue. However, because they release all their energy quickly and locally this can lead to significant tissue damage if α particles are ingested or inhaled. If internal contamination with radionuclides is suspected, early investigation is important and is discussed in detail in Treatment of internal contamination with radionuclides, (pp. 378–379).

As a basic rule of thumb the longer the t½ of these isotopes the lower the specific activity.

Specific examples

Pure alpha emitters

Pure α emitters are rare and the most important ones to consider are ^{241}Americium, ^{239}Plutonium, ^{210}Polonium, ^{232}Thorium and ^{235}Uranium. With ^{210}Po being the most hazardous.

^{241}Americium

- t½—458 years
- Biological t½—200 years
- Radiation energy (MeV)—5.5
- Specific activity (GBq/g)—129.5
- Major exposure pathways—inhalation and ingestion
- Focal accumulation—lung, liver, bone, and bone marrow
- Treatment—diethylenetriamine penta-acetate (DTPA).

Americium does not occur naturally but is produced artificially by successive neutron capture reactions by plutonium isotopes. ^{241}Am was first produced in 1944 in a nuclear reactor at the University of Chicago and is the most common isotope, a decay product of ^{241}Pu. The most common use of americium is in smoke detectors. These detectors rely on the α particle associated with the decay of ^{241}Am to ionize the air in a gap between two electrodes, causing a very small electrical current to flow between the electrodes. When smoke enters the space between the electrodes, the α radiation is absorbed by the soot particles, the current is interrupted, and the alarm is sounded. α particles from smoke detectors do not themselves pose a health hazard, as they are absorbed in a few centimetres of air or by the structure of the detector. Americium is also used as a portable source for gamma radiography, for crystal research, and as target material in nuclear reactors or particle accelerators to produce even heavier elements. A common neutron source is composed of ^{241}Am and beryllium (Be).

Atmospheric testing of nuclear weapons generated most environmental americium. Accidents and other releases from weapons production facilities have caused localized contamination. Americium oxide is the most common form in the environment. Americium is typically quite insoluble, although a small fraction can become soluble through chemical and biological processes. It adheres very strongly to soil, with americium concentrations associated with sandy soil particles estimated to be 1900 times higher than in interstitial water (the water in the pore spaces between the soil particles); it binds more tightly to loam and clay soils so those concentration ratios are even higher.

Americium can be present in areas that contain waste from the processing of irradiated nuclear fuel.

There are two principal routes by which ^{241}Am can be a hazard:

- ingestion
- inhalation.

Gastrointestinal absorption from food or water is a likely source of internally deposited americium in the general population. After ingestion or inhalation, most americium is excreted from the body within a few days and never enters the bloodstream; only about 0.05% of ingested americium is absorbed into the blood. After leaving the intestine or lung, about 10% clears the body. The remainder from the bloodstream deposits in the liver and skeleton where it remains, with biological retention t½ of about 20 and 50 years, respectively. This deposition is dependent on the age of the individual, with fractional uptake in the liver increasing with age. Americium in the skeleton is deposited uniformly on cortical and trabecular surfaces of bones and slowly redistributes throughout the volume of mineral bone over time. Because americium is taken up in the body much more readily if inhaled rather than ingested, both exposure routes can be important. It is in the liver and bone that the deposited americium's α radiation may eventually cause cancer as a stochastic process but there is little chance of deterministic early effects due to its relatively low activity compared to something like ^{210}Po (see later in this section).

Management

If internal contamination is suspected (see also Treatment of internal contamination with radionuclides, pp. 378–379), the treatment of choice is to use the chelating agent DTPA, either the calcium or the zinc salt. This can be used either intravenously, nebulized, or as a solution for wound irrigation. For current advice on doses seek expert advice or see: <http://www.remm.nlm.gov/int_contamination.htm#blockingagents_2>.

^{239}Plutonium

- t½—2.2×10^4 years
- Biological t½—bone 50 years; liver 20 years; gonads permanent
- Radiation energy (MeV)—5.1
- Specific activity (GBq/g)—2.33
- Major exposure pathways—inhalation, contaminated wounds, and ingestion
- Focal accumulation—lung, liver, bone, bone marrow, and gonads
- Treatment—DTPA.

As ^{239}Pu will undergo a fission chain reaction if enough of it is concentrated in a critical mass, it is used in nuclear weapons and can be used as a fuel for some nuclear power plants. It is a by-product of the fission process in nuclear reactors. When operating a typical nuclear reactor contains within its uranium fuel load there is a significant amount of plutonium, with ^{239}Pu being the most common isotope. It is created when non-fissionable ^{238}U absorbs a neutron released by the fission process. Through neutron capture, ^{239}Pu becomes ^{240}Pu (and then subsequently ^{241}Pu). When fission bombs are detonated (as in nuclear tests), highly radioactive fission by-products are released into the atmosphere and spread over a wide area. Radioactive fallout in the form of fine particulate matter is particularly dangerous because it can be ingested. Both ^{238}U and ^{239}Pu are found in the environment from weapons testing fallout.

There are three principal routes by which plutonium can be a hazard:

- ingestion
- contamination of open wounds
- inhalation.

Ingestion is not a significant hazard, because plutonium is poorly absorbed systemically from the gastrointestinal tract, and is normally expelled from the body before it can do harm.

Contamination of wounds has rarely occurred, although thousands of people have worked with plutonium.

The main threat comes from inhalation. While it is very difficult to create airborne dispersion of a heavy metal like plutonium, certain forms, including the insoluble plutonium oxide at particle size less than 10 μm are a hazard.

If inhaled, much of the material is immediately exhaled or is expelled by mucous flow from the bronchial tract into the gastrointestinal tract, as with any particulate matter. Some, however, will be trapped and readily transferred, first to the blood or lymph system and later to the liver, bone marrow, gonads, and bones. It is here that the deposited plutonium's α radiation may eventually cause cancer as a stochastic process but there is little chance of deterministic early effects due to its relatively low activity compared to something like ^{210}Po (see later in this section). Plutonium is toxic if ingested but the problems associated with the toxicity of plutonium are no different in type from those presented by a whole range of heavy metals.

Management

If internal contamination is suspected (see Treatment of internal contamination with radionuclides, pp. 378–379) the treatment of choice is to use the chelating agents DTPA or desferrioxamine (DFO) can be used as in iron poisoning (see Iron poisoning, pp. 166–167).

There is some evidence that using both DTPA and DFO in combination may have added efficacy.

^{210}Polonium

- t½—138.4 days
- Biological t½—bone 60 days
- Radiation energy (MeV)—5.3
- Specific activity (TBq/g)—166
- Major exposure pathways—inhalation, skin, and ingestion
- Focal accumulation—lung mucosa, liver, bone marrow, spleen, lymph nodes, and kidneys
- Treatment—gastric lavage, British anti-Lewisite (BAL), DMSA, D-penicillamine.

Polonium is a silvery-grey, soft, volatile, radioactive metallic element naturally occurring in the environment at extremely low levels. In addition ^{210}Po can be produced by chemical processing of uranium ores or minerals, although uranium ores only contain less than 0.1 mg ^{210}Po per tonne. As ^{210}Po is present in the earth's crust in small amounts, direct root uptake by plants is generally small but it can be deposited on broad-leaved vegetables. Deposition from the atmosphere onto tobacco leaves results in elevated concentrations of ^{210}Po in tobacco smoke. There are normally small amounts of ^{210}Po in the human body. ^{210}Po is manufactured artificially by irradiating stable bismuth (^{209}Bi) with thermal neutrons to form radioactive ^{210}Bi, which decays into ^{210}Po. Polonium can be made in small (mg) amounts by this procedure in nuclear reactors. Only about 100 g of ^{210}Po are produced each year worldwide. ^{210}Po is used in neutron sources (where it is mixed or alloyed with beryllium). When contained in substances such as gold foil, which prevent the α radiation from escaping, it can be used in devices that eliminate the static electricity in machinery caused by processes such as paper rolling, manufacturing sheet plastics, and spinning synthetic fibres. Brushes containing ^{210}Po are used to remove accumulated dust from photographic films and camera lenses.

^{210}Po emits so many α particles each second that the thermal energy released from 1g = 120–140 watts, and the metal will self-heat—0.5g will spontaneously reach a temperature of 500° C and have a blue glow. It has been used as a lightweight heat source to power thermoelectric cells in satellites. A ^{210}Po heat source was used in each of the Lunokhod Rovers, deployed on the surface of the Moon, to keep their internal components warm during the lunar nights. ^{210}Po was vital to the Manhattan Project as a neutron source to initiate a chain reaction. Initiators made of ^{210}Po and beryllium were located at the centre of the fissile cores of early atomic weapons.

There are two principal routes by which ^{210}Po can be a hazard:

• ingestion
• inhalation.

Po is a probable human carcinogen with severe radiotoxicity due to high-energy α particle decay. It is very dangerous to handle. Interest in the clinical toxicology of ^{210}Po has been stimulated by the poisoning of Alexander Litvinenko in 2006 when prior to that it was thought that internal contamination with radiation sources, e.g. α emitters, did not cause acute radiation syndrome (ARS). Ingested ^{210}Po is concentrated initially in red blood cells and then the liver, kidneys, spleen, bone marrow, gastrointestinal tract, and gonads. After chronic exposure, highest activities are found in bone and teeth. ^{210}Po is excreted in urine, bile, sweat, and (possibly) breath and is also deposited in hair. After ingestion, unabsorbed ^{210}Po is present in the faeces. In the absence of medical treatment, the fatal oral dose is probably in the order of 10–30 micrograms. If the absorbed dose is sufficiently large (e.g. >0.7 Gy), ^{210}Po causes ARS.

The diagnosis of ^{210}Po poisoning is established by the presence of ^{210}Po in urine and faeces and the exclusion of other possible causes.

Management
Gastric aspiration or lavage may be useful if performed soon after ingestion. Chelation therapy is also likely to be beneficial. Dimercaprol (BAL) may be used as an IM injection; D-penicillamine orally is an alternative but has a narrow therapeutic index and its use is associated with high risk of toxicity; meso 2, 3-dimercaptosuccinic acid (DMSA) orally can be used as for lead poisoning (see Lead, pp. 276–277).

Animal studies have indicated that the following drugs may be of benefit but may not be available:

• 2,3-dimercapto-1-propanesulfonic acid
• N,N´-dihydroxyethylethelene-diamine-N,N´-bis-dithiocarbamate.

Conclusion
Internal contamination with ^{210}Po can cause ARS, which should be considered in patients presenting initially with unexplained emesis, followed later by bone marrow failure and hair loss.

^{232}Thorium

• t½– 1.41×10^{10} years
• Biological t½—bone 22 years; liver/total body 2 years
• Radiation energy (MeV)—4
• Specific activity (kBq/g)—407
• Major exposure pathways—inhalation and ingestion
• Focal accumulation—bone
• Treatment—DTPA.

Thorium is a radioactive element that occurs naturally in low concentrations (10 ppm) in the earth's crust. It is about three times as abundant as uranium and about as abundant as lead or molybdenum. In its pure form it is a silvery-white heavy metal that is about as dense as lead

that is pyrophoric in powdered form. When heated in air, thorium turnings ignite and burn brightly with a white light. In nature, almost all thorium is ^{232}Th; however, its low specific activity means it is not highly radioactive, but it is present in soil and ores in equilibrium with ^{228}Radium which is much more active.

The chief commercial source is monazite sands in the USA, Brazil, India, Australia, and South Africa. The concentration of thorium oxide in monazite sands is about 3–10%. Thorium is also found in the minerals thorite (thorium silicate) and thorianite (mixed thorium and uranium oxides). The principal use is in the manufacture of incandescent gas mantles (Welsbach mantle) for portable gas lanterns. These mantles contain thorium oxide with about 1% cerium oxide and other ingredients, and they glow with a bright light when heated in a gas flame. Thorium is an important alloying element in magnesium and is used to coat tungsten wire for components of electronic equipment. It can also be added to ceramics to make them more heat resistant, as well as to refractive glass to allow for smaller and more accurate camera lenses. It is used in welding rods and electric bulb filaments. It can also be used as a fuel in nuclear reactors. While ^{232}Th itself is not fissile, it transforms into the fissile isotope ^{233}U following absorption of a neutron.

There are two principal routes by which ^{232}Th can be a hazard:

• ingestion
• inhalation.

Most thorium that is inhaled or ingested is excreted within a few days and only a small fraction (0.02–0.05%) is absorbed. Gastrointestinal absorption from food or water is the principal source of internally deposited thorium in the general population. 70% deposits in endosteal surfaces of mineral bone, 4% in the liver, and 16% is uniformly distributed to the rest of the body. Most of the remaining 10% is directly excreted. Rapid absorption following inhalation is seen. The main health concern for environmental exposures is bone cancer.

Most of the human data for thorium exposure comes from diagnostic studies. Colloidal ^{232}Th dioxide (Thorotrast) was as an IV radiographic contrast medium used between 1928 and 1955. The epidemiological data suggests a link with liver and gall bladder tumours. Some evidence of increased incidence of lung, pancreatic, and hematopoietic cancers was found in workers occupationally exposed to thorium via inhalation. However, these workers were also exposed to several other toxic agents.

Management
If internal contamination is suspected (see Treatment of internal contamination with radionuclides, pp. 378–379) the treatment of choice is to use the chelating agent, DTPA.

^{235}Uranium

• t½– 7.1×10^{8} years
• Biological t½—15 days
• Radiation energy (MeV)—4.68
• Specific activity (kBq/g)—814
• Major exposure pathway—ingestion
• Focal accumulation—kidneys and bone
• Treatment—sodium bicarbonate.

Uranium occurs naturally in low concentrations in soil, rock, surface water, and groundwater. It is the heaviest naturally occurring element (Z = 92). In its pure form it is a silver-coloured heavy metal that is nearly twice as dense as lead. In nature, uranium exists as several isotopes: primarily ^{238}U (99.27%), ^{235}U (0.72%) and a very small amount of ^{234}U (0.0055% by mass). In its natural state, uranium occurs as an oxide ore, U_3O_8. The environmental transport of uranium is strongly influenced by its chemical form. It is one of the more mobile radioactive metals and can move down through soil with percolating water to underlying groundwater. It preferentially adheres to soil particles, with a soil concentration typically about 35 times higher than that in the interstitial water and concentration ratios are usually much higher for clay soils. It can bioconcentrate in certain food crops and in terrestrial and aquatic organisms.

Uranium has been mined in the southwest USA, Canada, Australia, parts of Europe, the former Soviet Union, Namibia, South Africa, Niger, and elsewhere. It is a contaminant at many nuclear energy sites and other facilities that used natural uranium, including mining, milling, and production facilities.

For many years, uranium was used to colour ceramic glazes, producing colours that ranged from orange to lemon yellow. It was also used for tinting in early photography. The radioactive properties of uranium were not recognized until 1896, and its potential for use as an energy source was not realized until the middle of the 20th century. In nuclear reactors, uranium serves as both a source of neutrons (via the fission process) and a target material for producing plutonium—^{239}Pu is produced when ^{238}U absorbs a neutron. Currently, its primary use is as fuel in nuclear power reactors to generate electricity. Uranium is also used in small nuclear reactors to produce isotopes for medical and industrial purposes around the world. Natural uranium must be enriched in the isotope ^{235}U for use as a nuclear fuel in light-water reactors, and this enrichment has generally been achieved by gaseous diffusion techniques. Highly enriched uranium is a primary component of certain nuclear weapons. A by-product of the enrichment process is depleted uranium, i.e. uranium depleted in the isotope ^{235}U.

There are two principal routes by which ^{235}U can be a hazard:

- ingestion
- inhalation.

Gastrointestinal absorption from food or water is the main source of internally deposited uranium in the general population. After ingestion, most uranium is excreted within a few days. The small fraction (0.2–5%) that is absorbed into the bloodstream is deposited preferentially in bone (22%) and kidneys (12%), with the rest being distributed throughout the body (12%) and excreted. Most of what goes to the kidneys is excreted within a few days in urine, while that deposited in bone can remain for many years. After inhalation, generally only a small fraction penetrates to the lung's alveolar region, where it can remain for years and from which it can also enter the bloodstream. The major health concern is kidney damage caused by the chemical toxicity of soluble uranium compounds *not* the radioactive properties. That effect can be reversible depending on the level of exposure. A second concern is for uranium deposited in bone, which can lead to bone cancer as a result of the ionizing radiation associated with its radioactive decay products.

Management

Sodium bicarbonate, either IV or orally may be used to alkalinize the urine, and therefore potentially enhance excretion of uranium.

Other alpha emitters

Other important isotopes that emit α particles include:

- ^{252}Californium—α and gamma
- ^{226}Radium—α, β, and gamma.

Further reading

Harrison J, Leggett R, Lloyd D, et al. (2007). Polonium-210 as a Poison. *J Radiol Prot*, 27(1):17–40.

Jefferson RD, Goans RE, Blain PG, et al. (2009). Diagnosis and treatment of polonium poisoning. *Clin Toxicol*, 47(5):379–92.

National Council on Radiological Protection & Measurements (NCRP) (2008). *Management of Persons Contaminated with Radionuclides, Volumes I and II. Report No. 161*. Bethesda, MD: NCRP.

Radiation Emergency Assistance Center/Training Site (REAC/TS). (2013). *The Medical Aspects of Radiation Incidents*. <http://orise.orau.gov/files/reacts/medical-aspects-of-radiation-incidents.pdf>.

Radiation Emergency Medical Treatment website: <http://www.remm.nlm.gov/>.

Scott BR (2007). Health risk evaluations for ingestion exposure of humans to polonium-210. *Dose Response*, 5:94–122.

Tochner ZA, Glatstein E (2008). Radiation bioterrorism (Internal Contaminant Radionuclides: properties and treatment (Table 216-1)). In: Fauci AS, Longo DL, Kasper DL, et al. (eds), *Harrison's Principles of Internal Medicine*, 17th edition, pp. 1358–64. New York: McGraw Hill.

Beta sources

Background

Beta (β) particles are identical to electrons but, like α particles, they are ejected from a nucleus when the nucleus rearranges itself into a more stable configuration. β decay occurs when a nucleus has too many neutrons, i.e. it is proton deficient and it transforms a neutron into a proton plus an electron known as a beta minus particle and a neutrino (ν). The total energy released is shared between the electron and the neutrino. The neutrino has no mass or charge. The mass number remains unchanged. The decay may be described as:

$$n \rightarrow p + e- + \nu$$

This may also be represented as:

$$^{A}_{Z}X \rightarrow {}^{A}_{Z+1}Y + e^{-} + \nu$$

e.g. $^{131}_{53}I \rightarrow {}^{131}_{54}Xe + e^{-} + \nu$

The daughter product is a different element to the parent as it has an atomic number increased by 1. β particles are emitted with a continuous energy spectrum ranging from zero to a maximum value depending on the radionuclide. The average energy of the beta particle is $E = E_{max}/3$. β-particles have only a very short range in tissue before being absorbed. Some β-emitting radionuclides may leave the daughter nucleus in an excited energy state and the stable state is reached by the immediate emission of one or more gamma rays, e.g. ^{131}I.

β particles, similar to α particles, possess the ability to excite or ionize atoms or both. The method of ionization, however, is somewhat different from the ionization of α particles. An α particle attracts an orbital electron and thus creates an ion pair. The β particle repels the orbital electron from its energy shell to create an ion pair. Each ion pair produced by the β particle represents a loss of energy by the β particle. These processes of excitation and ionization continue until the β particle loses all its kinetic energy. If these β particles are ejected with enough energy, they can travel through the medium, causing additional ionization. β particles, with their smaller mass, higher velocity, and single charge, deposit their energy over a much greater range than α particles of comparable energy. Since its mass is equal to that of an electron, a large deflection can occur with each interaction, resulting in many path changes or scattering. β particles can only penetrate a few millimetres of tissue. β particle ranges are considerably greater than those of α particles. Unlike the interaction of α particles with matter, the path of β particles through matter is not in a straight line. While β particles may only penetrate a short distance into a medium, their mean path length (the average distance that a β particle would travel in a medium if its path were straightened out) can be quite long. In addition to a difference in range when compared with α particles, there is also a significant difference in the pattern of energy deposition. If the β-emitting material is on the surface of the skin, the resulting beta irradiation causes damage to *the epithelial basal stratum*. The lesion is similar to a superficial thermal burn. However, if the isotope is incorporated internally, the β radiation can cause much more significant damage. The damage will be in spheres of tissue around each fragment or source of radioactive material. The total damage is a function of the number of incorporated sources, the activity, and distribution of the radionuclides within the body. The distribution pattern is determined by the chemical nature of the compound containing the radioisotope. The density of energy deposited is much less for β irradiation than for α, and as a result, the target cells may be damaged rather than killed outright. Damaged cells may be of greater significance to the total organism than killed cells, particularly if they become malignant or otherwise malfunction. Killed cells are replaced quickly in most tissues with any degree of reserve capacity and do not cause significant overall clinical effects unless the individual cells involved are highly critical or the fraction of cells killed in a given organ is large.

Beta plus or positron decay

This occurs when a nucleus has too many protons, i.e. it is neutron deficient and it transforms a proton into a neutron plus a positron (β+), and a neutrino. The mass number remains unchanged:

$$P \rightarrow n + e^{+} + \nu$$

This may also be represented as:

$$^{A}_{Z}X \rightarrow {}^{A}_{Z-1}Y + e^{+} + \nu$$

e.g. $^{18}_{9}F \rightarrow {}^{18}_{8}O + e^{+} + \nu$

Like β particles, positrons are emitted in a continuous spectrum up to a maximum energy.

The important and recognizable feature of positron decay is annihilation radiation. A positron will lose its kinetic energy through ionization and excitations by collision with electrons in a similar fashion to a β particle. A positron cannot exist at rest, and therefore when it has expended all its kinetic energy it combines with an electron and their mass is converted into energy in the form of two 0.511 MeV gamma-rays 180° apart. For this form of decay to occur, a minimum energy of 1.022 MeV is required, any excess energy being given to the positron.

If internal contamination with radionuclides is suspected, early investigation is important and this is discussed in detail in Treatment of internal contamination with radionuclides, pp. 378–379.

As a basic rule of thumb, the longer the $t\frac{1}{2}$ of these isotopes, the lower the specific activity.

Specific examples

Pure beta emitters

Pure β emitters, as α emitters, are rare and will have other decay modes, e.g. gamma, however the most important predominantly β emitters to consider are ^{32}Phosphorous, ^{90}Strontium, ^{3}Tritium, and ^{90}Yttrium.

^{32}Phosphorous

- $t\frac{1}{2}$– 14.3 days
- Biological $t\frac{1}{2}$– approximately 3 years
- Radiation energy (MeV)—1.71 (max.)
- Specific activity (PBq/g)—10.545
- Major exposure pathways—inhalation, skin, and ingestion
- Focal accumulation—rapidly replicating cells, bone, and bone marrow
- Treatment—hydration and phosphate drugs.

There are three allotropic forms of elemental phosphorus: white, red, and black phosphorus. All have specific toxicological problems and are not discussed here (for discussion see Phosphorus, pp. 284–285). The following is only concerning the radioactive isotope ^{32}P. It is used in university research, medicine, biochemistry, and molecular biology to label biological molecules. Many radioisotopes are used as tracers in nuclear medicine, including ^{32}P. It is of particular use in the identification of malignant tumours as cancerous cells have a tendency to accumulate phosphate more than normal cells. The β radiation emitted by ^{32}P can be used for therapeutic as well as diagnostic purposes and ^{32}P-chromic phosphate has been explored as a possible chemotherapy agent to treat disseminated ovarian cancer. ^{32}P finds use for analysing metabolic pathways in pulse chase experiments where a culture of cells is treated for a short time with a ^{32}P-containing substrate. DNA contains a large quantity of phosphorus in the phosphodiester linkages between bases in the oligonucleotide chain. DNA can therefore be tracked by replacing the phosphorus with ^{32}P. This technique is extensively used in Southern blot analysis of DNA. ^{32}P is used in plant sciences for tracking a plant's uptake of fertilizer from the roots to the leaves. The ^{32}P-labelled fertilizer is given to the plant hydroponically or via water in the soil and the usage of the phosphorus can be mapped from the emitted β radiation.

Due to its high specific activity it can be a very hazardous substance. Plexiglas®, lucite, acrylic, plastic, or wood will act as a shield. The β particles from ^{32}P can travel up to 6.1m in air and 0.8cm in tissue whereas 1cm of Plexiglas® will shield completely. For high-activity sources, it may be desirable to add lead shielding outside the Plexiglas®® shielding to shield against penetrating bremsstrahlung X-rays. The use of lead foil or sheets alone will lead to penetrating bremsstrahlung X-rays.

There are three principal routes by which ^{32}P can be a hazard:

• ingestion
• inhalation
• skin absorption.

High-energy β particles pose an external (skin and lens of the eye) dose hazard, as well as a potential internal hazard. A high local skin dose can be received if contamination was allowed to remain on the skin or gloves. After ingestion or inhalation, most ^{32}P is excreted in the urine and this can be a useful tool in detection of internal contamination. The ^{32}P that remains in the body can accumulate in the bones, bone marrow, and all rapidly replicating cells, e.g. liver. There is a potential long-term cancer risk but the main aim of early treatment is to stop local burns and internal local gastrointestinal or respiratory tract damage.

Management

If internal contamination is suspected (see also Treatment of internal contamination with radionuclides, pp. 378–379), the treatment of choice is to use hydration therapy and phosphate binders.

Phosphate binders include:

• sodium glycerophosphate
• sodium phosphate
• potassium phosphate
• aluminium hydroxide
• aluminium carbonate.

Also consider use of IV calcium carbonate, which competes for bone binding sites.

^{90}Strontium

• t½—28 years
• Biological t½—49 years
• Radiation energy (MeV)—0.2
• Specific activity (TBq/g)—5.18

• Major exposure pathways—inhalation and ingestion
• Focal accumulation—bone
• Treatment—calcium gluconate, and barium sulfate (strontium lactate and strontium gluconate).

Strontium is a soft, silver-grey metal that occurs in nature as four stable isotopes. Sixteen major radioactive isotopes of strontium exist, but only ^{90}Sr has a t½ sufficiently long to warrant health concerns and it is present in surface soil around the world as a result of fallout from past atmospheric nuclear weapons tests. ^{90}Sr decays to ^{90}Yttrium (see later in this section) by emitting a β particle, and ^{90}Y decays by emitting a more energetic β particle with a t½ of 64 hours to ^{90}Zirconium. The main health concerns for ^{90}Sr are related to the energetic β particle from ^{90}Y. ^{90}Sr is produced by nuclear fission. When an atom of ^{235}U (or other fissile nuclide) fissions, it generally splits asymmetrically into two large fragments—fission products with mass numbers in the range of about 90 and 140—and two or three neutrons. ^{90}Sr is such a fission product, and it is produced with a yield of about 6% therefore six atoms of ^{90}Sr are produced per 100 fissions. ^{90}Sr is a major nuclide in spent nuclear fuel, high-level radioactive wastes resulting from processing spent nuclear fuel, and radioactive wastes associated with the operation of reactors and fuel reprocessing plants.

Strontium has a variety of commercial and research uses. It has been used in optical materials, and it produces the red flame colour of pyrotechnic devices such as fireworks and signal flares. It has also been used as an oxygen eliminator in electron tubes and to produce glass for colour television tubes. In addition, ^{90}Sr has been used as an isotopic energy source in various research applications, including in radiothermal generators to produce electricity for devices to power remote weather stations, navigational buoys, and satellites.

There are two principal routes by which plutonium can be a hazard:

• ingestion
• inhalation.

Strontium can be taken into the body by eating food, drinking water, or breathing air. Gastrointestinal absorption from food or water is the principal source of internally deposited strontium in the general population. On average, 30–40% of ingested strontium is absorbed into the bloodstream. The amount absorbed tends to decrease with age, and is higher (about 60%) in children in their first year of life. Adults on fasting and low-calcium diets can also increase intestinal absorption to these levels, as the body views strontium as a replacement for calcium. Strontium behaves similarly to calcium, although it is not homeostatically controlled, but living organisms generally use and retain it less effectively. For adults, about 31% of the activity entering the plasma from the gastrointestinal tract is retained by bone surfaces; the remainder goes to soft tissues or is excreted in urine and faeces. Much of the activity initially deposited on bone surfaces is returned to plasma within a few days. About 8% of the ingested activity remains in the body after 30 days, and this decreases to about 4% after 1 year. This activity is mainly in the skeleton as it concentrates in bone surfaces and bone marrow. Bone tumours, leukaemia, and tumours of the soft tissue surrounding bones are the main health concern. These tumours are associated with the β particles emitted during the radioactive decay of ^{90}Sr and ^{90}Y.

Management

If internal contamination is suspected (see also Treatment of internal contamination with radionuclides, pp. 378–379) the treatment of choice is to use the following:For inhalation:

- calcium gluconate competes for bone binding sites and is given IV
- barium sulfate blocks intestinal absorption and is given orally.

For ingestion:

- aluminium hydroxide blocks intestinal absorption and is given orally
- barium sulfate blocks intestinal absorption and is given orally
- sodium alginate blocks intestinal absorption and is given orally
- calcium phosphate increases excretion and is given orally.

Additional treatment may include stable strontium compounds to compete with the ^{90}Sr, e.g. strontium lactate or strontium gluconate.

^{3}Tritium

- t½—12.5 years
- Biological t½—12 days
- Radiation energy (MeV)—0.0057
- Specific activity (TBq/g)—363
- Major exposure pathways—inhalation, skin, and ingestion
- Focal accumulation—whole body
- Treatment—fluid diuresis.

Tritium (T or ^{3}H) is the only radioactive isotope of hydrogen but comprises only 10–16% of natural hydrogen and is produced as a result of the interaction of cosmic radiation with gases in the upper atmosphere. The most common forms of tritium are tritium gas and tritium oxide, also called 'tritiated water'. In tritiated water, a tritium atom replaces one of the hydrogen atoms so the chemical form is HTO rather than H_2O. The chemical properties of tritium are the same as hydrogen. It decays by emitting a β particle to produce ^{3}Helium (^{3}He). Tritium has a relatively high specific activity and is generated by both natural and artificial processes. After being produced in the atmosphere, it is readily incorporated into water and enters the natural hydrological cycle. Tritium is also produced as a fission product in nuclear weapons tests and in nuclear power reactors, with a yield of about 0.01%. There is approximately five times as much artificially produced ^{3}H released into the atmosphere than naturally occurring particularly from previous nuclear weapons tests. Each year a large commercial nuclear power reactor produces about 700 TBq of tritium (this equates to 2 g), which is generally incorporated in the nuclear fuel and cladding. ^{3}H is produced by neutron absorption of a ^{6}Lithium (^{6}Li) atom. The ^{6}Li atom, with three protons and three neutrons, and the absorbed neutron combine to form a ^{7}Li atom with three protons and four neutrons, which instantaneously splits to form an atom of tritium (one proton and two neutrons) and an atom of ^{4}He (two protons and two neutrons).

^{3}H is used as a component in nuclear weapons to boost the yield of both fission and thermonuclear warheads and is also used as a tracer in biological and environmental studies, and as an agent in luminous paints, e.g. building exit signs, airport runway lights, and watch dials.

The form of most concern, HTO, is generally indistinguishable from normal water and can move rapidly through the environment in the same manner as water.

There are three principal routes by which ^{3}H can be a hazard:

- ingestion
- inhalation
- skin.

^{3}H can be taken into the body by drinking water, eating food, or breathing air. It can also be taken in through the skin. Nearly all (99%) inhaled tritium oxide can be taken into the body from the lungs, and circulating blood then distributes it to all tissues. Ingested HTO is also almost completely absorbed, moving quickly from the gastrointestinal tract to the bloodstream. Within minutes it is found in varying concentrations in body fluids, organs, and other tissues. Skin absorption of airborne HTO can also be a significant route of uptake, especially under conditions of high humidity. For someone immersed in a cloud of airborne tritium oxide (HTO), the uptake by absorption through the skin would be about half that associated with inhalation. No matter how it is taken into the body, tritium is uniformly distributed through all biological fluids within 1–2 hours. The biological t½ of ^{3}H is the same as water. It will incorporate into easily exchanged hydrogen sites in organic molecules. The health hazard of tritium is associated with cell damage caused by the ionizing radiation that results from radioactive decay, with the potential for subsequent cancer induction. It is unlikely to pose an immediate deterministic health impact.

The diagnosis of ^{3}H poisoning is established by the presence of ^{3}H in urine and the exclusion of other possible causes.

Management

(See also Treatment of internal contamination with radionuclides, pp. 378–379.)

Fluid diuresis is the treatment of choice to enhance excretion and needs to be >3–4 L per day.

^{90}Yttrium

- t½—64 hours
- Biological t½—N/A
- Radiation energy (MeV)—0.94
- Specific activity (PBq/g)—19.9
- Major exposure pathways—inhalation and ingestion
- Focal accumulation—bone
- Treatment—DTPA.

The yttrium isotope ^{90}Y is directly linked to ^{90}Sr exposure as ^{90}Sr decays to ^{90}Y by β decay and ^{90}Y decays by emitting a more energetic β particle (~4000 times more active) with a much shorter t½ of 64 hours to ^{90}Zirconium. The main health concerns for ^{90}Sr are related to the energetic β particle from ^{90}Y (see earlier in this section). There are two principal routes by which ^{90}Y can be a hazard:

- ingestion
- inhalation.

Yttrium resembles strontium (see earlier in this section).

Management

If internal contamination is suspected (see also Treatment of internal contamination with radionuclides, pp. 378–379), the treatment of choice is to use the chelating agent DTPA, either the calcium or the zinc salt. The zinc salt can be used intravenously. For current advice on doses seek expert advice or see:<http://www.remm.nlm.gov/int_contamination.htm#blockingagents_2>.

Further reading

Harrison J, Leggett R, Lloyd D, *et al.* (2007). Polonium-210 as a Poison. *J Radiol Prot*, 27(1):17–40.

Jefferson RD, Goans RE, Blain PG, *et al.* (2009). Diagnosis and treatment of polonium poisoning. *Clin Toxicol*, 47(5):379–92.

National Council on Radiological Protection & Measurements (NCRP) (2008). *Management of Persons Contaminated with Radionuclides, Volumes I and II.* Report No. 161. Bethesda, MD: NCRP.

Radiation Emergency Assistance Center/Training Site (REAC/TS). (2013). *The Medical Aspects of Radiation Incidents.* <http://orise.orau.gov/files/reacts/medical-aspects-of-radiation-incidents.pdf>.

Radiation Emergency Medical Treatment website: <http://www.remm.nlm.gov/>.

Scott BR (2007). Health risk evaluations for ingestion exposure of humans to polonium-210. *Dose Response*, 5:94–122.

Tochner ZA, Glatstein E (2008). Radiation bioterrorism (Internal Contaminant Radionuclides: properties and treatment (Table 216-1)). In: Fauci AS, Longo DL, Kasper DL, *et al.* (eds), *Harrison's Principles of Internal Medicine*, 17th edition, pp. 1358–64. New York: McGraw Hill.

Gamma sources and X-rays

Background

Heat waves, radio waves, infrared light, visible light, ultraviolet light, X-rays and gamma (γ)-rays are all forms of electromagnetic (EM) radiation. They differ only in frequency and wavelength. Longer wavelength, lower-frequency waves (heat and radio) have less energy than the shorter wavelength, higher-frequency waves (X- and γ-rays). Not all EM radiation is ionizing. Only the high-frequency portion of the EM spectrum, which includes X-rays and γ-rays are ionizing. γ radiation is described as consisting of photons of energy. These photons of energy can be thought to be analyzing to α or β particles. However, the photons have no mass but are quanta of energy transmitted in the form of a wave motion. Other examples of this class of radiation are radio waves and visible light. The amount of energy in each quantum is related to the wave-length of the radiation. The energy is inversely proportional to the wavelength, i.e. the shorter the wavelength, the higher the energy. X-rays and γ-rays have exactly the same properties—they differ only in their origin. X-rays come from the atomic structure outside the nucleus and are produced by excitation and ionization of electrons in the atom whereas γ-rays are produced from excess energy in the nucleus of the atom.

Gamma and X-rays are EM indirectly ionizing radiation because they are electrically neutral (as are all EM radiations), and do not interact with atomic electrons through coulombic forces (as do α and β particles).

The release of energy as an α-ray may be as a part of another decay process. For example, the emission of γ-rays from ^{60}Cobalt follows a β decay (see later in this section).

γ-ray emission represents a mechanism for an excited nucleus to release energy. When energy is added to the nucleus, but not enough to cause particle emission, the nucleus may merely be raised to another energy state. Both the protons and the neutrons have their own set of discrete energy levels to which either nucleon can be raised if sufficient energy is supplied to the nucleus. A nucleus is in its ground state when all of its lower energy levels are filled. When an excited state of the nucleus occurs, the nucleus instantaneously returns to ground state and releases energy corresponding to the energy differential. This energy release is known as γ radiation. As γ radiation deposits its energy over longer distances than α or β radiation, γ radiation can cause damage from external exposure.

There are three major mechanisms by which γ- and X-rays interact with matter:

- *Photoelectric effect* is where a γ photon interacts with and transfers all of its energy to an orbiting electron, ejecting that electron from the atom.
- *Compton scattering* is an interaction in which an incident γ photon loses enough energy to an orbital electron to cause its ejection, with the remainder of the original photon's energy being emitted as a new, lower-energy γ photon with an emission direction different from that of the incident γ photon.
- *Pair production* is the interaction in the vicinity of the Coulomb force of the nucleus, the energy of the incident photon is spontaneously converted into the mass

of an electron-positron pair. The electron of the pair, frequently referred to as the secondary electron, is densely ionizing. The positron has a very short lifetime. It combines in 10^{-8} seconds with a free electron (annihilation reaction).

- Characteristic X-rays are produced when an electron is removed from one of the inner shells of an atom, an electron from an outer shell promptly moves in to fill the vacancy, and energy is released in the process. The energy may appear as a photon of electromagnetic radiation.

γ-rays are the most penetrating type of radiation and can travel many metres in air and many centimetres in tissue. Because γ-rays (and X-rays) can travel through the body, they are sometimes referred to simply as 'penetrating radiation'. β particles, γ-rays constitute both an internal and external hazard.

Specific examples

Gamma emitters

Pure γ emitters, as α and β emitters, are rare and will have other decay modes, e.g. β, however the most important predominantly γ emitters to consider are ^{137}Caesium, ^{60}Cobalt, ^{131}Iodine, ^{192}Iridium, and ^{226}Radium. Exposure to all these isotopes for long enough will lead to local radiation injuries and ultimately acute radiation syndrome. The treatments listed here correspond with each isotope for internal contamination (see also Treatment of internal contamination with radionuclides, pp. 378–379).

^{137}Caesium

- Half-life—30 years
- Biological t½—approximately 70 days
- Radiation energy β (MeV)—0.19
- Specific activity (TBq/g)—3.3
- Major exposure pathways—inhalation and ingestion
- Focal accumulation—renal excretion
- Treatment—Prussian blue.

Caesium is a soft, silvery white-grey metal that occurs in nature as ^{133}Cs. The natural source yielding the greatest quantity of caesium is the rare mineral pollucite. There are 11 major radioactive isotopes of caesium. Only three have t½ long enough to cause concern: ^{134}Cs, ^{135}Cs, ^{137}Cs. Each of these isotopes decays by emitting a β particle, and their t½ range from about 2 years to 2 million years. The t½ of the other caesium isotopes are less than 2 weeks. Of these three, the isotope of most concern is ^{137}Cs. ^{137}Cs has a radioactive t½ of about 30 years and decays by β decay either to stable ^{137}Barium or a meta-stable form of barium (^{137}mBa). The meta-stable isotope (^{137}mBa) is rapidly converted to stable ^{137}Ba (t½ of about 2 minutes) accompanied by γ-ray emission whose energy is 0.662 MeV. The specific activity of ^{137}mBa is over 6 million times more active than ^{137}Cs (19,980 PBq/g). It is this decay product that makes ^{137}Cs an external hazard (that is, a hazard without being taken into the body). The three radioactive caesium isotopes identified previously are produced by nuclear fission with ^{135}Cs and ^{137}Cs being produced with relatively high yields of about 7% and 6%, respectively. That is, about seven atoms of ^{135}Cs and six atoms of ^{137}Cs are produced per 100 fissions. ^{137}Cs is a major radionuclide in spent nuclear fuel, high-level radioactive wastes resulting from the processing of spent nuclear fuel, and radioactive wastes associated with the operation of nuclear reactors and fuel reprocessing plants.

Caesium metal is used in photoelectric cells and various optical instruments, and caesium compounds are used in the production of glass and ceramics. ^{137}Cs is also used in brachytherapy to treat various types of cancer. Brachytherapy is a method of radiation treatment in which sealed sources are used to deliver a radiation dose at a distance of up to a few centimetres by surface, intracavitary, or interstitial application.

There are two principal routes by which caesium can be a hazard in addition to penetrating external γ radiation:

• ingestion
• inhalation.

Caesium can be taken into the body by eating food, drinking water, or breathing air. After being taken in, caesium behaves like potassium and distributes uniformly throughout the body. Gastrointestinal absorption from food or water is the principal source of internally deposited caesium in the general population. Essentially all caesium that is ingested is absorbed into the bloodstream through the intestines. Caesium tends to concentrate in muscles because of their relatively large mass. Like potassium, caesium is excreted from the body fairly quickly. In an adult, 10% is excreted with a biological t½ of 2 days, and the rest leaves the body with a biological t½ of 110 days. Clearance from the body is somewhat quicker for children and adolescents. This means that if someone is exposed to radioactive caesium and the source of exposure is removed, much of the caesium will readily clear the body along the normal pathways for potassium excretion within several months. While in the body, ^{137}Cs poses a health hazard from both β and γ radiation, and the main health concern is associated with the increased likelihood for inducing cancer although if the dose is high enough, ingested soluble ^{137}CsCl has led to deaths from ARS. The most famous incident of this type was the incident in Goiânia, Brazil in September 1987 and is fully discussed by the IAEA (see 'Further reading' at the end of this section).

Management
If internal contamination is suspected (see Treatment of internal contamination with radionuclides, pp. 378–379), the treatment of choice is to use Prussian blue, insoluble, for known or suspected internal contamination with radioactive Cs and/or radioactive or non-radioactive thallium. It acts by ion exchange and inhibits enterohepatic recirculation in the gastrointestinal tract.

^{60}Cobalt

• Half-life—5.26 years
• Biological t½—9.5 days
• Radiation energy β (MeV)—0.097
• Specific activity (TBq/g)—40.7
• Major exposure pathways—inhalation and ingestion
• Focal accumulation—liver
• Treatment—DMSA or DTPA.

Cobalt is a hard, silvery-white metal that occurs in nature as ^{59}Cobalt (^{59}Co) and is a constituent of the minerals cobaltite, smaltite, erythrite, and other ores, and it is usually found in association with nickel, silver, lead, copper, and iron. It is similar to iron and nickel in its physical properties.

There are nine major radioactive cobalt isotopes. Of these, only ^{57}Co and ^{60}Co have t½ long enough to cause concern. The t½ of all other isotopes are less than 80 days. ^{60}Co is the isotope of most concern and decays with a t½ of 5.3 years by emitting a β particle with two energetic γ-rays; the combined energy of these two γ-rays is 2.5 MeV and makes this isotope an external hazard.

^{60}Co is produced by neutron activation of components in nuclear reactors; it can also be produced in a particle accelerator. A number of reactor components are made of various alloys of steel that contain chromium, manganese, nickel, iron, and cobalt, and these elements can absorb neutrons to produce radioactive isotopes, including ^{60}Co. It is in spent nuclear fuel (as a component of the fuel hardware) and in the radioactive wastes associated with nuclear reactors and fuel reprocessing plants.

High-energy γ-rays emitted during the radioactive decay of ^{60}Co can be used to detect flaws in metal components and in brachytherapy to treat various types of cancer.

There are two principal routes by which plutonium can be a hazard:

• ingestion
• inhalation.

Cobalt can be taken into the body by eating food, drinking water, or breathing air. Gastrointestinal absorption from food or water is the principal source of internally deposited cobalt in the general population. Estimates of the gastrointestinal absorption of cobalt range from 5–30%, depending on the chemical form and amount ingested; 10% is a typical value for adults and 30% for children. Cobalt is an essential element found in most body tissues, with the highest concentration in the liver. Vitamin B_{12} is a cobalt-containing essential vitamin. 50% of cobalt that reaches the blood is excreted immediately, mainly in urine; 5% deposits in the liver, and the remaining 45% deposits evenly in other tissues of the body. Of the cobalt that deposits in the liver and other tissues, 60% leaves the body with a biological t½ of 6 days and 20% clears with a biological t½ of 60 days; the last 20% is retained much longer, with a biological t½ of 800 days. Inhaled cobalt oxide moves from the lung to body tissues quite readily. While in the body, ^{60}Co poses a health hazard from both β and γ radiation, and the main health concern is associated with the increased likelihood for inducing cancer. The radiological accident in San Salvador in 1989 is probably the most significant worldwide and has been extensively studied and reported on—see 'Further reading'.

Management
If internal contamination is suspected (see Treatment of internal contamination with radionuclides, pp. 378–379) the treatment of choice is to use a chelating agent. Options include:

• DMSA given orally
• DTPA, either the calcium or the zinc salt.

The latter can be used either intravenously, nebulized, or as a solution for wound irrigation. For current advice on doses seek expert advice or see: <http://www.remm.nlm.gov/int_contamination.htm#blockingagents_2>.

^{131}Iodine

• Half-life—8.1 days
• Biological t½—138 days

- Radiation energy (MeV)—0.19
- Specific activity (PBq/g)—4.8
- Major exposure pathways—inhalation, skin and ingestion
- Focal accumulation—thyroid
- Treatment—potassium iodate/potassium iodine.

Iodine is a bluish-black, lustrous solid that mainly occurs in nature as stable ^{127}Iodine. Iodine exhibits some metal-like properties and is only slightly soluble in water. It occurs in nature as iodide ions, and it is in this form that it is taken into our bodies. Of the 14 major radioactive isotopes of iodine, only ^{131}I is of health concern. Radioactive isotopes of iodine are produced by nuclear fission and the yield of ^{131}I is close to 3%. It can also be present in spent nuclear fuel, high-level radioactive wastes resulting from processing spent nuclear fuel, and radioactive wastes associated with the operation of nuclear reactors and fuel reprocessing plants.

^{131}I is used for a number of medical procedures, including monitoring and tracing the flow of thyroxin from the thyroid. With its short t½ of 8 days, it is essentially gone in less than 3 months.

There are three principal routes by which ^{131}I can be a hazard:

- ingestion
- inhalation
- skin.

The human body contains 10–20 mg of iodine, of which more than 90% is contained in the thyroid gland. Iodine can be taken into the body by eating food, drinking water, or breathing air. It is a constituent of thyroid hormone and as such is a required element for humans. Iodine is readily taken into the bloodstream from both the lungs and the gastrointestinal tract (essentially 100%) after inhalation and ingestion. Upon entering the bloodstream, 30% is deposited in the thyroid, 20% is quickly excreted in faeces, and the remainder is eliminated from the body within a short time. Clearance from the thyroid is age dependent, with biological t½ ranging from 11 days in infants to 23 days in a 5-year-old child and 80 days in adults.

Iodine is an essential component of the human diet, and lack of dietary iodine is a cause of goitre. Elemental iodine (I_2) can be toxic, and its vapour irritates the eyes and lungs. While iodine is generally a health hazard only if it is taken into the body in substantial doses, ^{131}I emits fairly high-energy β particles and a number of γ-rays. The γ-rays are of sufficient energy to be measured outside the body if deposited in tissue such as the thyroid. Because iodine selectively deposits in the thyroid, the primary health hazard for iodine is thyroid tumours resulting from ionizing radiation emitted by ^{131}I. Hypothyroidism is also a risk, with special consequences in infants and children

Historically, the major exposure pathway has been ingestion of milk from cows grazing on iodine-contaminated crops. The major incident was the Chernobyl accident in 1986 and has been extensively studied and reported on—see 'Further reading'. Other pathways include ingestion of fruits and vegetables and inhalation.

Management
Administration of non-radioactive potassium iodide (KI) such as potassium iodate or potassium iodine, or other iodine substances orally blocks the thyroid from accumulating radioactive iodine, thereby minimizing subsequent risks. KI is most effective if given a few hours before exposure, but it is also effective if given within several hours after exposure.

^{192}Iridium
- Half-life—74 days
- Biological t½—50 days
- Radiation energy β (MeV)—0.22
- Specific activity (TBq/g)—340
- Major exposure pathways—external only likely
- Focal accumulation—various
- Treatment—DTPA.

Iridium is a silvery white metal with highly coloured salts. It is twice as dense as lead, and occurs in nature as two stable isotopes, ^{193}Ir and ^{191}Ir. Of the 15 major radioactive iridium isotopes, only three have t½ longer than a month and could cause potential health issues - ^{192}Ir, ^{192m}Ir and ^{194m}Ir. Of these three radioactive isotopes, ^{192}Ir is of most concern based on general availability; it is used in a number of industrial and medical applications and is readily available. ^{192}Ir is produced by neutron activation of iridium metal, usually in nuclear reactors. The strength of a ^{192}Ir source is related to the amount of neutron irradiation. Natural iridium contains 37% ^{191}Ir, and when this isotope absorbs a neutron it produces ^{192}Ir. When ^{192}Ir decays by either β decay or electron capture it gives off a γ-rays of 0.82 MeV energy.

Iridium is used as an alloying agent with a number of other metals to produce composites that are extremely hard and have good corrosion resistance. Its principal use is as a hardening agent in platinum alloys. Iridium is used for high-temperature applications, including in crucibles and thermocouples and as electrodes in spark plugs for severe operating conditions, such as those experienced by jet engine igniters. ^{192}Ir is used industrially as a radiotracer in the oil industry and in gamma radiography to identify flaws in metal castings and welded joints. These radiographic sources are constructed of metal discs or pellets in a welded stainless steel capsule, and their activity levels can be very high and this makes them a significant hazard for local radiation burns and potentially acute radiation sickness. ^{192}Ir is also used medically in brachytherapy to treat various types of cancer used especially in the head and breast. They are produced in wire form and are introduced through a catheter to the target area. After being left in place for the time required to deliver the desired dose, the implant wire is removed. This procedure is very effective at providing localized radiation to the tumour site while minimizing the patient's whole-body dose.

Iridium can be taken into the body by eating food, drinking water, or breathing air but its main hazard is external γ exposure. This has been seen in a number of accidents the most famous being at the Yanango Hydroelectric Power Plant, Peru in February 1999, when a welder picked up an ^{192}Ir industrial radiography source and put it in his pocket for several hours—see 'Further reading'. Gastrointestinal absorption from food or water is the likely source of internally deposited iridium in the general population. After ingestion or inhalation, most iridium is excreted from the body and never enters the bloodstream; only about 1% of the amount taken into the body by ingestion is absorbed into the blood. 20% of the iridium that reaches the blood is excreted immediately, 20% deposits in the liver, 4% deposits in the kidney, 2% deposits in the spleen, and the remaining 54% is evenly distributed among other organs and tissues of the body. Of the iridium that deposits in any organ or tissue, 20% leaves the body with a biological t½ of 8 days and 80% clears with a biological t½ of 200 days. Inhaled iridium compounds appear to clear the lungs quite rapidly.

Management
If internal contamination is suspected (see also Treatment of internal contamination with radionuclides, pp. 378–379) the treatment of choice is to use the chelating agent DTPA.

Further reading

Radiation Emergency Assistance Center/Training Site (REAC/TS). (2013). *The Medical Aspects of Radiation Incidents*. <http://orise.orau.gov/files/reacts/medical-aspects-of-radiation-incidents.pdf>.

Radiation Emergency Medical Treatment website: <http://www.remm.nlm.gov/>.

The Chernobyl Project: <http://www-ns.iaea.org/projects/chernobyl.asp>.

The ^{60}Co radiological accident in San Salvador: <http://www-pub.iaea.org/MTCD/publications/PDF/Pub847_web.pdf>.

The ^{137}Cs radiation incident in Goiania: <http://www-pub.iaea.org/mtcd/publications/pdf/pub815_web.pdf>.

The radiological accident in Yanango, Peru: <http://www-pub.iaea.org/MTCD/publications/PDF/Pub1101_web.pdf>.

Neutron radiation

Background

The neutron is an indirectly ionizing particle. It is indirectly ionizing because it does not carry an electrical charge. Ionization is caused by charged particles, which are produced during collisions with atomic nuclei. The neutron is an uncharged particle with a mass slightly greater than that of the proton, approximately equal to the sum of the masses of a proton and an electron and is a normal constituent of atoms except hydrogen.

Neutrons give up their energy through a variety of interactions dependant on the neutron energy. Neutrons are usually split into three energy groups:

- fast
- intermediate
- thermal.

Neutrons are very penetrating and will travel large distances even in dense media, e.g. lead, although they will be slowed down by water (see later in section).

In fission, a heavier unstable nucleus divides or splits into two or more lighter nuclei, with a release of substantial amounts of energy. For example, when a thermal neutron is absorbed by a ^{235}U nucleus, it becomes ^{236}U and either emits a γ-ray or undergoes fission. On average, the ^{236}U nucleus will split into two smaller parts called fission fragments (FF), release two or three free neutrons, γ-rays and a tremendous amount of energy. The nuclear potential energy released in the fission process originates from the binding energy of the nucleus. Splitting a uranium atom also releases neutrons, which act like microscopically small bullets. Neutrons are about one-fourth the size of α particles and have almost 2000 times the mass of an electron. If there are other fissionable atoms nearby (e.g. ^{235}U, ^{239}Pu) these neutron projectiles may strike them, causing them to split and to release more neutrons. This is a *chain reaction*. It takes place spontaneously when fissionable material is sufficiently concentrated, i.e. forms a critical mass. In a typical atomic bomb, the fission is very rapid. In a nuclear reactor, water, gas, or the control rods function to slow down and absorb neutrons and control the chain reaction.

Since neutrons are electrically neutral they interact with matter by either collisions with or absorption by an atomic nucleus. Collisions with atomic nuclei slow down—or thermalize—a neutron so it may undergo nuclear capture. In nuclear capture, the incident neutron is actually absorbed into the nucleus. This can make the nucleus unstable and, therefore, radioactive. An unstable nucleus will shed its excess energy through radioactive decay and will emit particulate radiation and/or γ-rays. Nuclear capture is how objects, people, soil, etc., become radioactive after a nuclear detonation.

Neutron activation is responsible for some of the delayed radiation from a nuclear detonation. In this process, an atom absorbs a neutron, placing the original atom in an 'excited state', which means that the atom has excess energy. Atoms in this condition are unstable, and the primary mechanism by which they return to a stable condition is through the emission of nuclear radiation, usually in the form of or accompanied by a γ-ray (see Gamma sources and X-rays, pp. 371–374).

$$_0n^1 + {}^A_ZX \rightarrow {}^{A+1}_ZX + \gamma$$

$$_0n^1 + {}_{27}Co^{59} \rightarrow {}_{27}Co^{60} + \gamma\ 1.3\ MeV$$

In the equations given, an isotope of cobalt, ^{59}Co, absorbs a neutron and becomes ^{60}Co, which is unstable and achieves stability through the emission of a 1.3 MeV γ-ray. Various biological materials have been used or suggested for measurements in connection with accidental exposure to neutrons. ^{32}P activity in body hair has been employed in the evaluation of exposures to neutrons. Both blood and whole-body measurements of ^{24}Na activity are also important in the more accurate assessment of absorbed dose. This has been used in the criticality accident in Tokaimura, Japan, in 1999—see 'Further reading' at the end of this section. A large number of neutrons escape the area of an explosion without interacting with the fuel; they then cause activation of the materials in the soil immediately beneath the burst. This area is known as the induced area. Not all neutron releases will be after an explosion, i.e. in a criticality event. A criticality is when during a fission process the neutron production rate equals the neutron loss rate to absorption or leakage. A nuclear reactor is 'critical' when it is operating.

Specific examples

Neutron emitters

Pure neutron emitters, as α, β, and γ emitters, are rare and will have other decay modes e.g. α; however the most important predominantly neutron emitter to consider is $^{244}Curium$. Exposure to neutrons leads to health effects due to the other decay modes α, β, X-rays, and γ-rays, rather than neutrons per se (see earlier in this section).

$^{244}Curium$

- t½—18 years
- Biological t½:
  - liver 20 years
  - bone 50 years
- Radiation energy:
  - α (MeV)—5.8
  - β (MeV)—0.086
  - γ (MeV)—0.0017
- Specific activity (TBq/g)—3
- Major exposure pathways—inhalation and ingestion
- Focal accumulation—liver and bone
- Treatment—DTPA.

Management

If internal contamination is suspected (see Treatment of internal contamination with radionuclides, pp. 378–379) the treatment of choice is to use DTPA, either the calcium or the zinc salt which can be used intravenously. For current advice on doses seek expert advice or see: <http://www.remm.nlm.gov/int_contamination.htm#blockingagents_2>.

Further reading

Radiation Emergency Assistance Center/Training Site (REAC/TS). (2013). *The Medical Aspects of Radiation Incidents*. <http://orise.orau.gov/files/reacts/medical-aspects-of-radiation-incidents.pdf>.

Radiation Emergency Medical Treatment website: <http://www.remm.nlm.gov/>.

The nuclear fuel processing facility accident at Tokaimura, Japan, 1999: <http://www-pub.iaea.org/MTCD/publications/PDF/TOAC_web.pdf>.

Triage, monitoring, treatment for management of the public in the event of a radiation release

Background

Victims of radiation events require prompt treatment for medical and surgical conditions and initial evaluation for radiation exposure. Since radiation-related illness requires hours to days to become clinically evident, hospital emergency personnel should triage victims of such incidents using the traditional medical and trauma categories T1–T4 (see Biological dosimetry for the clinician, pp. 361–362). The treating physician will stabilize trauma and attempt a credible evaluation of the extent of radiation injury. Many considerations in public triage will depend on the number of patients relative to the amount of supplies. Patients should be medically stabilized and then assessed for radiation injury based on clinical symptoms, dose, isotope (if known), and whether there is internal contamination. Resource limitations may necessitate some differences in care in the event of mass casualties. The 'golden hour' (the first hour after a traumatic event) has been widely recognized by trauma surgeons to be an hour of opportunity in which the lives of severely injured people may be saved if they are rapidly triaged by first-response personnel to definitive treatment. Patients in shock or near shock can die if not treated within the golden hour. In a terrorist event involving a radioactive dispersal device (RDD) or an improvised nuclear event (IND), the presence of radiation issues must not interfere with rapid triage and removal of trauma victims from the field of injury.

Contamination issues

Some patients involved in a radiation event may be externally contaminated. Removing contaminated clothing will eliminate 80–90% of external contamination and soap and water should be the first approach to removing remaining radioactive material. Irrigation of contaminated wounds is readily performed using a saline jet under mild pressure. Ambient radiation levels from contaminated wounds rarely exceed a few tens of μSv/hour and hospital personnel should be reassured that their dose will be insignificant or minimal. In the analysis of external irradiation events, simple health physics dose estimates are generally sufficient for medical decision-making. If the patient has significant facial contamination, strong consideration should be given for 24-hour urine and faecal bioassay and treatment for internal contamination.

History of radiation accidents

Radiation events have historically fallen into certain major categories:

• Low-dose incidents with the patient showing essentially no signs or symptoms.
• Higher dose, acute whole-body or partial-body incidents with significant systemic signs and symptoms associated with the acute radiation syndrome (ARS) or the cutaneous syndrome.
• Local radiation injury (cutaneous syndrome) arising primarily from lost high-level radiation sources and involving a regional portion of the body, often the hands.
• Inhalation or ingestion of radioactive material, often without systemic signs and symptoms. In a terrorism event, it is certainly possible to have trauma in addition

to the scenarios. Trauma plus radiation injury is called combined injury and is currently an active field of research. After medical and surgical stabilization of the patient, it is prudent to consult medical staff experienced in the management of radiation victims.

In order for the treating physician to provide proper treatment for the victim of a radiation terrorism event, it is helpful to be able to diagnose the radiation accident in a timely manner. However, physicians generally do not have experience with major radiation syndromes and therefore often do not include radiation injury in the differential diagnosis of common radiation-induced prodromal symptoms (nausea, vomiting, and diarrhoea). If acute radiation injury is not a consideration, then rarely will the diagnosis be correctly made, at least in a timely manner. Analysis of the recent history of radiation medicine shows many cases of delayed diagnosis.

Issues in early diagnosis of radiation injury

In the particular case of high-level radiation accidents, it is evident that victims will have improved survival if the proper diagnosis is made early post-accident and if definitive medical treatment is available. In order to evaluate the magnitude of such an accident, it is important for the radiation physicist, physician, and radiobiologist to work closely together and to evaluate many variables. These include the initial patient medical history and physical examination, the timing of prodromal signs and symptoms of ARS (nausea, vomiting, diarrhoea, transient incapacitation, hypotension, and other signs and symptoms suggestive of high-level exposure). Many radiation accidents have come about because of a loose source in the public domain or accidents in the hospital setting. If the source term is known, a time and motion study near the source can give a rough order-of-magnitude of the incident.

Early in the patient work-up, an initial full blood count with differential should be obtained and repeated every 6–8 hours as indicated to monitor the lymphocyte and neutrophil count. Blood for biodosimetry (dicentrics, rings, premature chromosome condensation techniques) may also be obtained at this time for dose determination (see also Biological dosimetry for the clinician, pp. 361–362). The time to emesis and lymphocyte depletion kinetics have also proven to be early information useful to evaluate the approximate magnitude of dose.

Clues in the medical history that might point toward radiation injury include the following:

• Finding an unknown metallic object.
• Working with fluorescence spectroscopy, industrial radiography, etc.
• Family history of several family members or close friends with skin lesions and a history of nausea, vomiting, and fatigue.
• Radiation injury should be considered in the patient's differential diagnosis if he/she presents with a work history suggestive of recent accidents (e.g. working in a scrap metal yard).
• A history of nausea, vomiting, and fatigue, especially if accompanied by observations of skin erythema, and not explainable by other causes.

• In the physical examination, observation of skin lesions and a history of desquamation and erythema could be strongly suspicious of radiation injury if not explained by thermal burns, insect bites or allergy. In addition, epilation or petechial or gingival bleeding with a history of nausea and vomiting 2–4 weeks previously should be suspicious.

Early triage markers for radiation injury in a mass casualty event

If there been a civil disturbance from a radiation-related improvised explosive device (IED) or improvised weapon, then many people could have high γ dose in the former and a combination of neutron and γ dose, possibly in addition to trauma, in the latter. Trauma medicine should always predominate in the early evaluation of the patient, but ^{24}Na activation analysis early on can aid significantly in the determination of neutron dose.

The neutrophil (N) to lymphocyte (L) ratio, taken from the first complete blood count differential evaluated more than 4 hours post event can be a useful point of service triage tool since N/L rises from control values dramatically for acute dose greater than 2 Gy. The N/L control ratio is 2.10 ± 0.2 for 150 gender-matched controls. CRP is another widely available marker that has been shown in animal studies to be quite elevated when dose is greater than 2 Gy. In addition many laboratories are investigating rapid cytogenetic techniques using scoring of only 50 lymphocyte metaphases to triage less than 2 Gy or greater than 2 Gy. Hospitals will likely be stretched beyond capacity with patients in a major radiation event and collaborations are on-going to enlist assistance in reading cytogenetic slides from many laboratories around the world via the Internet (see Biological dosimetry for the clinician, pp. 361–362).

Medical treatment issues

If the accident is recent, the patient relatively asymptomatic, and the source term known, the patient may be followed with serial blood counts, with clinical support provided as necessary. In cases where a covert or unrecognized accident occurred 2–4 weeks previously, the treating medical team may see a patient with some or many aspects of the ARS and/or cutaneous syndromes:

• pancytopenia, immunodysfunction, sepsis, impaired wound healing, GI bleeding (ARS haemapoietic phase)
• malabsorption, ileus, fluid and electrolyte imbalance, acute kidney injury, cardiovascular failure (ARS gastrointestinal phase; 8–14 days post-accident)
• confusion and disorientation, hypotension, cerebral oedema, ataxia, convulsions/coma (ARS neurovascular phase; 1–2 days post accident).

Various authors have offered clinical advice helpful in determining the magnitude of the accident. For example, it has been noted that approximately 100% of patients with whole-body dose greater than the LD_{50} will have early nausea and vomiting, and many will exhibit altered deep tendon reflexes. In addition, an increased body temperature has been seen for effective whole-body dose greater than 2.5 Gy, and acute diarrhoea for dose greater than 9 Gy. These clinical details may be helpful in addition to information gained from the standard history and physical exam.

Consensus guidance on medical management of many patients with haematological ARS syndrome

An international consortium (see 'Further reading' at the end of this section) recently formulated guidelines for the treatment of ARS mass casualties using an evidence-based system. Studies were extracted using the Grading of Recommendations Assessment Development and Evaluation (GRADE) system. Based upon GRADE analysis and narrative review, a strong recommendation can be made for the administration of granulocyte colony-stimulating factor or granulocyte macrophage colony-stimulating factor and a weak recommendation for use of the use of erythropoiesis-stimulating agents or haematopoietic stem cell transplantation.

A strong recommendation was also made for the use of a serotonin-receptor antagonist prophylactically when the suspected exposure is greater than 2 Gy, and topical steroids, antibiotics, and antihistamines for radiation burns, ulcers, or blisters. Surgical excision and grafting of radiation ulcers or necrosis is necessary for patients with intractable pain. Medical personal should also provide supportive care to expectant patients with the neurovascular syndrome and administer fluid and electrolyte replacement therapy and sedatives to individuals with significant burns, hypervolemia, and/or shock. A strong recommendation is further made against the use of systemic steroids in the absence of a specific indication. A weak recommendation is made for the use of fluoroquinolones, bowel decontamination, loperamide, and enteral nutrition, and for selective oropharyngeal/digestive decontamination, blood glucose maintenance, and stress ulcer prophylaxis in critically ill patients.

Further reading

Dainiak N, Gent RN, Carr Z, et al. (2011). First global consensus for evidence-based management of the hematopoietic syndrome resulting from exposure to ionizing radiation. *Disaster Med Public Health Prep*, 5:202–12.

Dainiak N, Gent RN, Carr Z, et al. (2011). Literature review and global consensus on management of acute radiation syndrome affecting nonhematopoietic organ systems. *Disaster Med Public Health Prep*, 5:183–201.

Goans RE (2002). Clinical care of the radiation accident patient. In: Ricks RC, Berger ME, O'Hara M Jr (eds), *The Medical Basis for Radiation-Accident Preparedness. The Clinical Care of Victims*. Proceedings of the Fourth International REAC/TS Conference on the Medical Basis for Radiation Accident Preparedness, March 2001, Orlando, FL: Parthenon Publishing.

Treatment of internal contamination with radionuclides

Background
Internal contamination of individuals can occur any time radioactive materials are free to spread in an environment. The most common routes of industrial intakes are inhalation and absorption through wounds. The ingestion pathway is uncommon in industrial settings, but may become critical for the general public after an accidental release of airborne or liquid radioactive material into the environment.

Following an accidental intake of radioactive material, dose, toxicity, and treatment methods are dependent on various factors such as the identity of the radionuclide and its physical and chemical characteristics (physical and biological t½, particle size, chemical composition, solubility, etc.).

The fate of inhaled particles is critically dependent on particle physicochemical properties and the size of aerosol particles determines the region of the respiratory tract where most will be deposited. Highly insoluble particles may remain in the lung for long periods of time and a small fraction will be transported to the tracheobronchial lymph nodes by pulmonary macrophages. Insoluble particles may be swallowed and therefore excreted primarily in the faeces. General medical assessment in an inhalation accident should include initial attempts to determine the maximum credible accident.

In an inhalation accident, nasal swabs taken within a few minutes after an accident and analysed can aid in nuclide identification and in estimation of the amount of material inhaled. The initial problem for the health physicist and for the treating physician is to estimate the maximum credible accident. A rough rule of thumb from current lung models assumes that the combined activity of both nasal swipes is approximately 5–10% of deep lung deposition. Experience has shown that this is generally a very conservative overestimate, but useful for initial estimates, pending the results of bioassay and whole-body counting.

Health considerations
Industrial radiation physics considerations are therefore governed by current regulations on organ or whole-body dose. If there is evidence for significant intake, preparations may be made for 24-hour urine and faecal bioassay and whole-body or lung counting. Treatment considerations for decorporation therapy fall into six major categories:

1 Reduce and/or inhibit absorption of the isotope in the GI tract
2 Block uptake to the organ of interest
3 Utilize isotopic dilution
4 Alter the chemistry of the substance
5 Displace the isotope from receptors
6 Utilize traditional chelation techniques.

Medical issues with selected nuclides
(See also Alpha sources, pp. 363–366 and Beta sources, pp. 367–370.)

Tritium, ³H
Tritium is the only radioactive isotope of hydrogen, decaying to ³He with emission of an 18.6 KeV electron. Tritiated water, HTO, is taken easily into the body by inhalation, ingestion, or by transdermal absorption, and

it is assumed to be totally absorbed and mixed with body water. Dose to total body water is therefore the critical issue in the management of tritium accidents. The International Council on Radiological Protection (ICRP) model for tritium assumes two compartments with half-times of 10 and 40 days for adults. Age-dependent retention times are used for children and infants. For accident dosimetry purposes, a single exponential with a t½ of 10 days may approximate tritium retention.

Medical management of tritium intake is primarily directed to increasing body water turnover. Increasing oral fluid intake should treat single exposures. This has the dual value of diluting the tritium and increasing excretion by physiological mechanisms. An increase in oral fluids of 3–4 L/day reduces the biological t½ of tritium by a factor of 2–3 and therefore reduces whole-body dose in the same proportion. Bioassay is generally accomplished by 24-hour urine collections that are analysed by liquid scintillation counting. In high-level exposures, intravenous hydration, management of fluid intake and output, and use of diuretics is a possible modality for increasing turnover of body water, but, historically, this has rarely been necessary.

Strontium
⁹⁰Sr is the predominant isotope of interest, although other strontium isotopes are occasionally seen. ⁹⁰Sr decays by β emission to ⁹⁰Y, which also decays by β emission to stable ⁹⁰Zr. For most forms of strontium, except titanate, bone surface is the dose-limiting organ for both inhalation and ingestion. Because of the biologically significant rate of strontium transfer to the GI tract, it is also necessary to block intestinal absorption in those cases where intake is by inhalation. One or more of the following treatments may be used in the medical management of inhalation cases with strontium:

• IV calcium gluconate 2 g in 500 cc over 4–6 hours (competes for Sr at bone binding sites).
• Ammonium chloride (300 mg orally) to produce a moderate metabolic acidosis.
• Barium sulfate 300 g orally as soon as possible post-accident to block intestinal absorption.

Iodine
The dominant initial internal contaminant after a reactor accident, nuclear weapons test, or any incident involving *fresh* fission products is likely to be ¹³¹I. In addition, iodine is widely used in nuclear medicine for imaging studies. Occasionally, other isotopes, such as ¹²⁵,¹²⁹I are also encountered.

When iodine reaches the blood, approximately 30% is taken up by the thyroid and the remainder eventually excreted into the urine. Retention in the thyroid is described by a three-component exponential. For accident dosimetry, the effective t½ may be taken to be approximately 12 days. Methods of measurement for iodine isotopes include in vivo thyroid counting and γ-ray spectrometry on biological samples, such as urine.

The thyroid is the critical organ after intake of radioiodine. Thyroid blocking in adults is accomplished by administering 100–130 mg KI orally as soon as possible post-accident and one tablet daily for 7–14 days. For adolescents, the recommended dose is half of the adult dose, for children one-quarter of the adult dose and for infants, another dilution by two. Another convenient way to administer stable iodide is 5 or 6 drops of saturated solution of potassium iodide (SSKI; 1 g/mL). In addition, potassium perchlorate (200 mg) may be used in adult patients with iodine sensitivity.

The timing of iodine administration is immediate up to 6 hours post accident. However, in a situation with continuing exposure, stable I may be 50% effective even 5–6 hours after exposure to radioiodine.

Thyroid protection for pregnant women is crucial following a nuclear accident where material is released in a plume. In the first trimester, stable iodine will protect the mother and no fetal action is necessary. However, the fetal thyroid begins to function around the 12th week of gestation. Stable iodine should be given to all pregnant women in the near field of a radioactive incident for all trimesters and stable iodine to second and third trimester patients in the far field.

Caesium and thallium

^{137}Cs (physical t½, 30 years; biological t½, 109 days) is the dominant caesium radioisotope seen in industrial and laboratory settings. It is also usually the dominant radioisotope in *aged* fission products. ^{137}Cs decays by β decay to ^{137m}Ba. In addition, the characteristic 0.661 MeV gamma is seen. Similar chemically to caesium, thallium is rarely a problem in its radioactive form, but poisonings have occasionally occurred with stable thallium.

Systemic retention for caesium is often represented by a two exponential retention function with retention half-lives of approximately 2 days and approximately 110 days. However, a range of retention half-times have been noted. A urine to faecal ratio of 4:1 is assumed for material that has entered the blood. Measurement of ^{137}Cs is generally by whole-body counting, or direct *in vivo* γ counting of biological samples.

The most effective means for removing radioactive caesium is the oral administration of ferric ferrocyanate, Prussian Blue (PB). Insoluble PB, $Fe_4[Fe(CN)_6]_3$, is an orally administered drug that enhances excretion of isotopes of caesium and thallium from the body by means of ion exchange (interruption of enterohepatic cycling). 1g orally three times daily (titrated up to 3 g three times daily) for 2–3 weeks reduces the biological t½ of radiocaesium to about one-third of the normal value, and radiation dose by the same fraction. PB administration up to 15–20 g daily in divided doses is generally necessary for thallium decorporation therapy.

Uranium

The two most common uranium isotopes seen in research and in industry are ^{238}U and ^{235}U. Inhalation is the usual route of occupational exposure and acute toxicity is most closely related to chemical rather than radiological properties, particularly with regard to the renal system. Uranium has an overall biological t½ of 15 days and 85% of retained U resides in bone. It is assumed that all excretion occurs via the urine.

Kidney toxicity is the basis for current occupational exposure limits (for uranium enrichment <~15%). In acidic urine, the uranyl ion binds with renal tubular surface proteins, and some of the bound UO_2^{2+} is therefore retained in the kidney. Oral or intravenous infusion of sodium bicarbonate is the treatment of choice and

should be administered to keep the urine alkaline by frequent pH measurements. The non-toxic uranium carbonate complex is increased by 3–4 orders of magnitude in alkaline urine and promptly excreted.

The threshold for transient renal injury is estimated to be 0.058 mg U/kg body weight or intake of 4.06 mg in a 70 kg individual. Likewise, the threshold for permanent renal damage is estimated to be 0.3 mg U/kg body weight, or 21 mg U in a 70 kg person. From animal research, the 50% lethality level is estimated to be 1.63 mg/kg body weight, or 114 mg in a 70 kg person.

Actinides

The actinides are those heavy elements at the bottom of the periodic table beginning with actinium (89) and ending with the heaviest known elements. The primary actinides for consideration in radiation accidents are plutonium, americium, curium, and californium. ^{238}Pu and ^{239}Pu are the most commonly seen plutonium isotopes, while ^{241}Am and ^{244}Cm are the most commonly seen isotopes of americium and curium. All have long biological t½ and inhalation accounts for approximately 75% of industrial exposures. Soluble compounds eventually translocate from the lungs to ultimate disposition sites of bone and liver.

Ca-DTPA and Zn-DTPA chelation therapy is the treatment of choice for inhalation accidents involving actinides. DTPA belongs to the group of synthetic polyamino polycarboxylic acids that form stable complexes with a large number of metal ions. The drug effectively exchanges calcium or zinc for another metal of greater binding power and carries it to the kidneys where it is then excreted into the urine. The plasma t½ of DTPA is 20–60 minutes.

Ca-DTPA is thought to be more effective than Zn-DTPA for initial chelation of transuranics. Approximately 24 hours after exposure, Zn-DTPA is, for all practical purposes, as effective as Ca-DTPA. Each dose of Ca-DTPA should be 1 g and the route of administration may be either slow intravenous push of the drug over a period of 3–4 minutes, intravenous infusion (1 g in 100–250 mL D_5W, Ringer's lactate, or normal saline), or inhalation in a nebulizer (1:1 dilution with water or saline). The chelating efficacy is greatest immediately or within 6 hours of exposure. However, a post-exposure interval greater than 1 hour does not preclude the administration and effective action of Ca-DTPA. Ca-DTPA has been shown also to chelate trace elements and many physicians either alternate Ca-DTPA and Zn-DTPA or administrate vitamin supplements.

Further reading

Goans RE (2002). Clinical care of the radiation accident patient. In: Ricks RC, Berger ME, O'Hara M Jr (eds), *The Medical Basis for Radiation-Accident Preparedness. The Clinical Care of Victims.* Proceedings of the Fourth International REAC/TS Conference on the Medical Basis for Radiation Accident Preparedness, March 2001, Orlando, FL: Parthenon Publishing.

Johnson TE, Birky BK (2012). *Health Physics and Radiological Health,* 4th edition. Philadelphia, PA: Wolters Kluwer/ Lippincott and Williams & Wilkins.

National Council on Radiological Protection & Measurements (NCRP) (2008). *Management of Persons Contaminated with Radionuclides, Volumes I and II.* Report No. 161. Bethesda, MD: NCRP.

Occupational and industrial aspects of toxicology assessment

Principles of industrial hygiene and toxic hazards in the workplace

Background

Industrial hygiene is sometimes referred to as *occupational hygiene* and is the discipline of removing or separating people from unpleasant or deleterious situations or exposures in the workplace. In order to do this in the interest of the worker, and avoid unnecessary removal, it is often appropriate to monitor specific aspects of potential exposure.

Definitions

There are a number of variations on a theme in the worldwide definition and practice of occupational/industrial hygiene. Some definitions are given here but the key factors of anticipation, recognition, evaluation, prevention, and control are consistent throughout in some guise or other:

- Industrial hygiene: science and art devoted to the anticipation, recognition, evaluation, prevention, and control of those environmental factors or stresses arising in or from the workplace which may cause sickness, impaired health and well-being, or significant discomfort among workers or among citizens of the community (American Industrial Hygiene Association® (AIHA)).
- Occupational/industrial hygiene is the discipline of anticipating, recognizing, and evaluating and controlling health hazards in the working environment with the objective of protecting worker health and well-being and safeguarding the community at large (International Occupational Hygiene Association (IOHA)).
- Occupational hygiene is the practice of identifying hazardous agents—chemical, physical, and biological—in the workplace that could cause disease or discomfort, evaluating the extent of the risk due to exposure to these hazardous agents, and the control of those risks to prevent ill health in the long or short term. It is generally defined as the art and science dedicated to the anticipation, recognition, evaluation, communication and control of environmental stressors in, or arising from, the workplace that may result in injury, illness, impairment, or affect the well-being of workers and members of the community. These stressors are normally divided into the categories biological, chemical, physical, ergonomic and psychosocial (Australian Institute of Occupational Hygienists Inc. (AIOH)).
- Occupational hygiene is about the recognition, assessment, and control of health risks from workplace exposures to hazards such as chemicals, dusts, fumes, noise, vibration and extreme temperatures (British Occupational Hygiene Society (BOHS)).

The history of occupational and industrial hygiene

Occupational/industrial hygienists get involved at the interface of people and their workplaces. They use science and engineering to prevent ill health caused by the work environment. They are specialists in the assessment and control of risks to health from workplace exposure to hazards. Occupational/industrial hygienists can come from many backgrounds including: chemists, engineers, biologists, physicists, doctors, and nurses who have chosen to apply their skills to improving working practices and conditions. At their core is occupational/industrial hygiene in which science and engineering meet the human element of work.

There has been an awareness of occupational/industrial hygiene since antiquity. Hippocrates, who noted lead toxicity in the mining industry, recognized the environment and its relation to worker health as early as the 4th century BC. In the 1st century AD, Pliny the Elder, a Roman scholar, perceived health risks to those working with zinc and sulphur. He devised a facemask made from an animal bladder to protect workers from exposure to dust and lead fumes. In the 2nd century AD, the Greek physician, Galen, accurately described the pathology of lead poisoning and also recognized the hazardous exposures of copper miners to acid mists.

In the Middle Ages, guilds worked at assisting sick workers and their families. In 1556, the German scholar, Agricola, advanced the science of occupational/industrial hygiene even further when, in his book *De Re Metallica*, he described the diseases of miners and prescribed preventive measures. The book included suggestions for mine ventilation and worker protection, discussed mining accidents, and described diseases associated with mining occupations such as silicosis.

Occupational/industrial hygiene gained further respectability in 1700 when Bernardo Ramazzini, published in Italy the first comprehensive book on industrial medicine, *De Morbis Artificum Diatriba* (*The Diseases of Workmen*). The book contained accurate descriptions of the occupational diseases of most of the workers of his time. Ramazzini greatly affected the future of industrial hygiene because he asserted that occupational diseases should be studied in the work environment rather than in hospital wards.

Ulrich Ellenborg in 1743 published a pamphlet on occupational diseases and injuries among gold miners. Ellenborg also wrote about the toxicity of carbon monoxide, mercury, lead, and nitric acid.

In England in the 18th century, Percival Pott, as a result of his findings on the insidious effects of soot on chimney sweepers (e.g. as a causative factor in scrotal cancer), was a major force in getting the British Parliament to pass the Chimney Sweepers Act of 1788. The passage of the English Factory Acts beginning in 1833 marked the first effective legislative acts in the field of industrial safety. The Acts, however, were intended to provide compensation for accidents rather than to control their causes. Later, various other European nations developed workers' compensation acts, which stimulated the adoption of increased factory safety precautions and the establishment of medical services within industrial plants.

In the early 20th century in the USA, Alice Hamilton, led efforts to improve occupational/industrial hygiene. She observed industrial conditions first hand and startled factory managers, state officials, and mine owners with evidence that there was a correlation between worker illness and their exposure to toxins. She also presented definitive proposals for eliminating unhealthy working conditions.

Workplace risks

With good occupational/industrial hygiene science and practice, some occupational health risks have been eliminated and others brought under control. Thus, it is possible, today, to be a healthy miner; the ill health effects of working with or near to asbestos, and how to avoid these effects, are now understood; and the risk of silicosis has been eliminated in pottery workers who used to die from this lung disease. These are some of the major achievements of occupational/industrial hygiene and its scientists and practitioners.

Workplaces will continue to expose workers to health hazards, and the risks will always need to be properly understood and managed, e.g. man-made mineral fibres and elongate mineral particles have replaced asbestos in a large number of applications and are currently under extensive research scrutiny. Standards are still poor in many parts of the world, and new risks constantly emerge. The range of health risks in the workplace is more varied than ever including chemical hazards (see Chapters 9, pp. 205–264 and 10, pp. 265–288); physical hazards such as heat, cold, noise, vibration, and radiation (see Principles of radiation toxicology, Chapter 15, pp. 357–380), or ergonomic, biological, and psychological hazards. New and emerging technologies including nanotechnology and green technology are potentially changing ways of working and present new challenges.

Principles of occupational/industrial hygiene

The reader is directed to the 'Further reading' section for detailed information and a brief overview is given here. The principles include an understanding of the following:

- The nature and properties of workplace airborne contaminants including the sampling of aerosols, dusts, gases, and vapours.
- Principles of risk assessment (see Risk assessment and principles of occupational exposure assessment, pp. 28–29).
- Exposure assessment including noises, vibration, light and lighting, thermal environment, non-ionizing radiation (electromagnetic fields and optical radiation), ionizing radiation (including physics, measurement, biological effects, and control) (see Chapter 15, pp. 357–380), biological agents, psychological issues, ergonomics, and dermal.
- Biological monitoring.
- Epidemiology.
- Other allied issues that may be addressed also include occupational accident prevention.

An important aspect of occupational/industrial hygiene is targeted at the control of hazards, and would include:

- work organization and work-related stress
- control philosophy
- ventilation
- personal protective equipment (PPE)
- occupational health and hygiene management

This overview by its nature is limited and readers requiring further information are encouraged to look at the 'Further reading' section.

Toxic hazards in the workplace

These would include the following groups of hazards:

- inorganic chemicals
- organic chemicals
- toxic gases
- dusts and particles.

The importance of these exposures can be summarized in Table 16.1 and 16.2.

Inorganic chemicals

These would normally include metals such as lead, mercury, and cadmium. These and other metals are covered in detail in Chapter 10, pp. 265–288.

Organic chemicals

Examples would include benzene (C_6H_6), carbon disulphide (CS_2), and chlorinated hydrocarbons (see Common chemical poisonings, Chapter 9, pp. 205–264).

Toxic gases

These are normally thought of as three distinct groups.

Simple asphyxiants

An asphyxiant is a substance that can cause unconsciousness or death by suffocation due to oxygen deficit. Asphyxiants that have no other health effects are sometimes referred to as simple asphyxiants. Asphyxiation is an extreme hazard when working in enclosed spaces, e.g. sewers and storage tanks, where gases such as methane may displace oxygen from the atmosphere. Asphyxiants work by displacing so much oxygen from the ambient atmosphere (if the concentration falls <14%) that haemoglobin cannot pick up enough oxygen from the lungs to fully oxygenate the tissues. As a result, the victim slowly suffocates.

Common examples are nitrogen (N_2), helium (He), neon (Ne), argon (Ar), methane (CH_4), propane ($CH_3CH_2CH_3$), and carbon dioxide (CO_2).

Chemical asphyxiants

Chemical asphyxiants reduce the body's ability to absorb, transport, or utilize inhaled oxygen. They are often active at very low concentrations, a few parts per million (ppm).

Examples include carbon monoxide (CO), hydrogen cyanide (HCN), and hydrogen sulphide (H_2S) (see Common chemical poisonings, Chapter 9, pp. 205–264).

Irritants

The irritant gases cause either upper or lower airway compromise. This largely artificial distinction is due to solubility properties. Thus, the highly soluble gases—ammonia (NH_3), sulphur dioxide (SO_2), and chlorine (Cl_2) exert their irritant effect on the upper airways and unless the exposure is severe will save the lungs (see Common chemical poisonings, Chapter 9, pp. 205–264). Conversely, gases of low solubility—oxides of nitrogen and phosgene (CCl_2O)—have little effect on the upper airways and their effect tends to be delayed and the main damage is experienced in the lung tissue.

Dusts and particles

Many occupational hazards occur as airborne particles: dust, fibres, mists, fume, radioactive particles (see Principles of radiation toxicology, Chapter 15, pp. 357–380), bacteria, and viruses.

A dispersed suspension of liquid or solid particles in a gas (usually air in the workplace and environment) is known as an aerosol. The health risks from inhaling an aerosol depends on the type and size of the particles, their airborne concentration, and the part of the respiratory system they are deposited in. Particle size and the position in the lung are related.

A particle is assigned an aerodynamic diameter, which is defined as the diameter of a unit density sphere,

Table 16.1 Group 1 carcinogens as classified by IARC

Chemical (CAS number)	Human target organ(s)	Main industry/use
Acetaldehyde (75-07-0)	Digestive tract, upper; oesophagus	Consumption of alcoholic beverages
Acid mists, strong inorganic	Larynx	Steel making
Aflatoxins (1402-68-2)	Liver and bile duct	Foodstuffs
4-Aminobiphenyl (92-67-1)	Bladder	Rubber manufacture
Aristolochic acid (313-67-7)	Renal pelvis and ureter	Chinese herbal medicine
Arsenic (7440-38-2) and inorganic arsenic compounds	Lung, skin	Glass, metals, pesticides
Asbestos—all forms	Lung, pleura, peritoneum	Insulation, filter material, textiles
Azathioprine (446-86-6)	Skin, leukaemia, and/or lymphoma	Medicine
Benzene (71-43-2)	Leukaemia	Solvent, fuel
Benzidine (92-87-5)	Bladder	Dye/pigment manufacture, laboratory agent
Benzo[a]pyrene (50-32-8)	Colon	
Beryllium (7440-41-7) and beryllium compounds	Lung	Aerospace industry/metals
Bis(chloromethyl)ether (542-88-11)	Lung	Chemical intermediate/by-product
Busulfan (55-98-1)	Leukaemia and/or lymphoma	Medicine
1,3-Butadiene (106-99-0)	Leukaemia and/or lymphoma	Rubber manufacture
Cadmium (7440-43-9) and cadmium compounds	Lung	Dye/pigment manufacture
Chlorambucil (305-03-3)	Leukaemia and/or lymphoma	Medicine
Chloromethyl methylether (107-30-2)	Lung	Chemical intermediate/by-product
Chlornaphazine (494-03-1)	Urinary bladder	Medicine derived from nitrogen mustard
Chromium (VI) compounds	Nasal cavity, lung	Metal plating, dye/pigment manufacture
Coal-tar pitches (65996-93-2)	Skin, lung, bladder	Building material, electrodes
Coal-tars (8007-45-2)	Skin, lung	Fuel
Cyclophosphamide (50-18-0, 6055-19-2)	Urinary bladder, leukaemia, and/or lymphoma	Medicine
Cyclosporine (59865-13-3, 59865-13-3)	Skin, leukaemia, and/or lymphoma	Medicine
Diethylstilbestrol	Breast, vagina, uterine cervix	Medicine
Erionite (66733-21-9)	Mesothelium (pleura and peritoneum)	Naturally occurring fibrous mineral—environmental exposure
Ethanol (64-17-5)	Oral cavity, pharynx, oesophagus, colon and rectum, liver and bile duct, larynx	In alcoholic beverages
Ethylene oxide (75-21-8)	Leukaemia	Chemical intermediate, sterilizing agent
Etoposide (33419-42-0)	Leukaemia and/or lymphoma	Medicine
Formaldehyde (50-00-0)	Nasopharynx, leukaemia, and/or lymphoma	Preservative
Leather dust	Nasal cavity and paranasal sinus	Leather workers
Melphalan (148-82-3)	Leukaemia and/or lymphoma	Medicine
Methoxsalen (8-methoxypsoralen) (298-81-7)	Skin	Plus ultraviolet A radiation
Mineral oils, untreated and mildly treated	Skin	Lubricants
Mustard gas (sulphur mustard) (505-60-2)	Pharynx, lung	Chemical weapon
2-Naphthylamine (91-59-8)	Bladder	Dye/pigment manufacture
Nickel compounds	Nasal cavity, lung	Metallurgy, alloys, catalyst
Phenacetin (62-44-2)	Renal pelvis and ureter	Medicine
Semustine (13909-09-6)	Leukaemia and/or lymphoma	Medicine
Shale-oils (68308-34-9)	Skin	Lubricants, fuels
Silica dust, crystalline, in the form of quartz or cristobalite (14808-60-7)	Lung	Mining

(continued)

Table 16.1 Continued

Chemical (CAS number)	Human target organ(s)	Main industry/use
Soots	Skin, lung	Pigments, occupational exposure of chimney sweeps
Tamoxifen (10540-29-1)	Endometrium	Medicine
2,3,7,8-Tetrachlorodibenzo-para –dioxin (1746-01-6)	All cancer sites (combined)	Contaminant in chlorophenoxy herbicides
Thiotepa (52-24-4)	Leukaemia and/or lymphoma	Medicine
Tobacco	Leukaemia and/or lymphoma, oral cavity, pharynx, nasopharynx, oesophagus, stomach, colon and rectum, liver and bile duct, pancreas, nasal cavity and paranasal sinus, larynx, lung, uterine cervix, ovary, kidney, renal pelvis and ureter, urinary bladder	
Ortho-Toluidine (95-53-4)	Urinary bladder	Dye and glue manufacture
Treosulfan	Leukaemia and/or lymphoma	Medicine
Trichloroethylene (79-01-6)	Kidney	Degreasing
Vinyl chloride (75-01-4)	Liver, lung, blood vessels	Plastics, monomer
Wood dust	Nasal cavity	Wood industry

Data from International Agency for Research on Cancer, IARC Monographs, Volumes 1–108, IARC, Lyon, France, 2012. <http://monographs.iarc.fr/ENG/Classification/>.

Table 16.2 Examples of occupational groups at risk of cancer

Industry	Cancer site
Aluminium production workers	Lung
Asbestos workers	Lung, pleura, peritoneum
Auramine production	Urinary bladder
Vehicle mechanics exposed to engine exhaust, diesel	Lung, urinary bladder
Coal gasification	Lung
Coke production	Lung
Haematite mining (underground) due to radon exposure	Lung
Iron and steel founding (occupational exposure during)	Lung
Isopropyl alcohol manufacture using strong acids	Nasal cavity and paranasal sinus
Magenta production	Urinary bladder
Mining (silica exposure)	Lung
Painter (occupational exposure as a)	Urinary bladder
Rubber manufacturing industry	Lung, prostate, urinary bladder, leukaemia and/or lymphoma, oesophagus, stomach
Chimney sweeps	Lung, skin, urinary bladder
Carpenters (wood dust)	Nasal cavity and paranasal sinus, nasopharynx

i.e. water, which settles at the same velocity as the particle under investigation.

Examples of typical airborne particles

- Dusts: 1–75 μm diameter from cutting, grinding, sanding, finishing, transport, sieving, crushing, screening, blasting, etc.
- Fibres: 1:3 aspect ratio, various sources: natural mineral, e.g. asbestos; natural vegetable, e.g. cotton; synthetic mineral, e.g. glass fibre; synthetic organic, e.g. nylon.
- Fume: usually <1 μm: from the sublimation and oxidation of molten metal, e.g. lead, cadmium, chromium, iron, nickel (see Chapter 10, pp. 265–288).
- Mists: atmospheric: >20 μm; water droplets condensed on a particle nucleus from surfaces of open tanks.
- Smoke: mixture of particles and gases usually <1 μm; from combustion.
- Biological: bacteria, viruses, fungi.
- Radiation: radioactive particles, α and β (see Chapter 15, pp. 357–380).

Particle size and respiratory penetration

Ill health from the inhalation of aerosols can be divided in to three groups depending on anatomical deposition:

1 Extrathoracic (upper respiratory tract)—this includes some bacteria, fungi and allergens. Exposure leads to inflammation of the mucus membranes causing rhinitis, but in some cases going on to local cancer; examples include wood dust and nickel.

2 Thoracic (bronchi and bronchioles)—many particles that reach this area may lead to bronchoconstriction, bronchitis, and bronchial carcinoma. Toxic mechanisms include extrinsic allergen (e.g. occupational asthma from cotton fibres or isocyanates), local damage (dusts), and carcinogenesis (see Table 16.1).

3 Alveolar—many particles that reach this area may lead to pneumoconiosis, emphysema, alveolitis, and pulmonary carcinoma. These particles are known as respirable. Certain fibres (i.e. asbestos) may be carried to the pleura and lead to mesothelioma.

Biological monitoring

Biological monitoring is a way of assessing chemical exposures by measuring the chemical or its metabolite(s) in urine, blood, or breath (usually, although other samples such as hair are possible).

Biological monitoring is particularly useful where chemicals can be significantly absorbed through the skin and where controls rely upon the use of PPE, such as gloves and masks. The purpose is to determine the extent of systemic absorption for a chemical encountered in the workplace and this gives an indication of exposure. The merit of biological monitoring is that it takes into account all possible routes of absorption for the chemical under investigation.

A number of essential questions should be answered before performing biological monitoring:

- What is the chemical of interest?
- Is detection of the parent compound or the metabolite(s) required?
- If it is the metabolite, is it unique to the chemical of interest or can it be derived from different sources?
- When should the sampling take place? For example, end of shift?
- What should be collected? Urine, blood, or other samples?
- How much sample is needed?
- Are there special requirements for collection of the sample? For example, on ice?
- Are there special precautions for collection, packing, and dispatch of the samples?

Approved laboratories with adequate quality control mechanisms and sufficient experience in such analyses should be used. For the interpretation of such results, Biological Exposure Indices (BEIs®) are published annually by the American Conference of Governmental Industrial Hygienists (ACGIH). The BEIs®® are reference values intended to represent equivalent exposure to the Threshold Limit Values (TLVs®). In the UK the HSE has also started publishing annual biological monitoring guidance values (BMGVs). Examples for the UK are given in Table 16.3.

In Germany, the establishment of MAK values (maximum workplace concentrations) and BAT values (biological tolerance value for occupational exposure) for the classification of carcinogenic, embryotoxic/fetotoxic substances, and germ cell mutagens, and for the evaluation of measurement methods are similar to what is used in the USA and UK.

The MAK value is defined as the maximum concentration of a chemical substance (a gas, vapour, or particulate matter) in the workplace air which generally does not have known adverse effects on the health of employees nor causes irritation (e.g. noxious odour), even when a person is repeatedly exposed during long periods, usually for 8 hours daily but assuming on average a 40-hour working week. Known effects of a substance in man are given highest priority in the derivation of the MAK value, which is based on the 'no observed adverse effect level' (NOAEL) for the most sensitive effect with relevance to

Table 16.3 Biological monitoring guidance values (BMGVs)

Substance	Biological monitoring guidance values	Sampling time
Butan-2-one	70 micromol butan-2-one/L in urine	Post shift
2-Butoxyethanol	240 mmol butoxyacetic acid/mol creatinine in urine	Post shift
Carbon monoxide	30 ppm carbon monoxide in end-tidal breath	Post shift
Chromium VI	10 micromol chromium/mol creatinine in urine	Post shift
Cyclohexanone	2 mmol cyclohexanol/mol creatinine in urine	Post shift
Dichloromethane	30 ppm carbon monoxide in end-tidal breath	Post shift
N,N-Dimethylacetamide	100 mmol N-methylacetamide/mol creatinine in urine	Post shift
Glycerol trinitrate (nitroglycerin)	15 micromol total nitroglycols/mol creatinine in urine	At the end of the period of exposure
Lindane (gBHC(ISO))	35 nmol/L (10 micrograms/L) of lindane in whole blood (equivalent to 70 nmol/L of lindane in plasma)	Random
MbOCA (2,2' dichloro-4,4' methylene dianiline)	15 micromol total MbOCA/mol creatinine in urine	Post shift
Mercury	20 micromol mercury/mol creatinine in urine	Random
4-methylpentan-2-one	20 micromol 4-methylpentan-2-one/L in urine	Post shift
4,4'-Methylenedianimile (MDA)	50 micromol total MDA/mol creatinine in urine	Post shift for inhalation and pre-shift next day for dermal exposure
Polycyclic aromatic hydrocarbons (PAHs)	4 micromol 1-hydroxypyrene/mol creatinine in urine	Post shift
Xylene, o-, m-, p-, or mixed isomers	650 mmol methyl hippuric acid/mol creatinine in urine	Post shift

health. If a NOAEL cannot be derived from the available data, a MAK value is not established.

Biological effect monitoring (BEM) is the measurement and assessment of early biological effects caused by absorption of chemicals. It normally involves measuring biochemical responses (e.g. measuring plasma and erythrocyte cholinesterase activity in workers exposed to organophosphorus pesticides, or measuring increases in urinary protein following exposure to cadmium). These responses may have potential health implications for the individual, and may arise from causes other than occupational exposure.

Further reading

American Conference of Governmental Industrial Hygienists (ACGIH) (2012). *Biological Exposure Indices (BEIs®) and Threshold Limit Values (TLVs®).* <http://www.acgih.org/Products/beiintro.htm>.

Aw T-C, Gardiner K, Harrington JM (2006). *Pocket Consultant: Occupational Health*, 5th edition. Oxford: Wiley-Blackwell.

Baxter PJ, Aw T-C, Cockcroft A, et al. (eds) (2010). *Hunter's Diseases of Occupations*, 10th edition. London: Hodder.

Centers for Disease Control and Prevention National Institute for Occupational Safety and Health (2011). *Current Intelligence Bulletin 62. Asbestos fibers and other elongate mineral particles: state of the science and roadmap for research.* <http://www.cdc.gov/niosh/docs/2011-159/>.

Cherrie J, Howie R, Semple S (2010). *Monitoring for Health Hazards at Work*, 4th edition. Oxford: Wiley-Blackwell.

Gardner K, Harrington JM (2005). *Occupational Hygiene*, 3rd edition. Oxford: Blackwell.

HSE (2005). *EH40/2005 Workplace Exposure Limits.* <http://www.hse.gov.uk/pubns/priced/eh40.pdf>.

HSE (1997). *Biological Monitoring in the Workplace: A Guide to its Practical Application to Chemical Exposure.* HSG 167. <http://www.hse.gov.uk/pubns/books/hsg167.htm>.

Stellman J (ed) (1998). *Encyclopaedia of Occupational Health and Safety*, 4th edition, Vol. 1–4. Geneva: International Labour Organization.

Medical surveillance in the workplace

Background

Medical surveillance is the periodic clinical monitoring of workers exposed to hazardous substances. Medical surveillance indicates that some form of active examination, measurement, or monitoring is undertaken to identify early adverse health effects. The term health surveillance is often used synonymously, although in some countries this is restricted to documenting hazardous exposure. Occupational diseases and adverse health effects are preventable and medical surveillance is an essential step in the prevention process.

General principles

Medical surveillance in those exposed to chemicals in the workplace should only be undertaken after a suitable and sufficient risk assessment of the particular toxicological hazard. In many cases there is a statutory requirement to undertake medical surveillance. When taking account of control measures and PPE, there may remain a residual risk that determines the requirement for medical surveillance.

Prerequisites

Certain prerequisites are required before undertaking medical surveillance. These include:

- an identifiable adverse health effect or disease outcome linked to the work activity
- availability of suitable techniques which could identify adverse health effects or disease outcomes.

Whatever measurement or monitoring technique is chosen it should not be unduly invasive.

When a worker is exposed to a chemical substance, absorption into the body may occur via various routes. The effects may range from a temporary interference with the physiological or biochemical processes to more permanent and irreversible effects culminating in disease. Surveillance techniques can range from the assessment of exposure uptake, to the effect on these biological and physiological processes.

Types of medical surveillance

The main categories of medical surveillance are respiratory, dermatological, and serological. The latter is divided into biological monitoring and biological effect monitoring. Simplistically the former refers to the body's 'take up' of a toxic hazard and the latter, the effects on the biological systems. For example, in the case of lead exposure, biological monitoring can be by blood lead levels and biological effect monitoring by zinc protoporphyrin (ZPP) levels and haemoglobin (see also sections in Chapter 10, pp. 265–288). For some chemicals, particularly carcinogens, it may not be possible to establish a NOAEL of exposure. Biological monitoring in these circumstances provides feedback on the adequacy of workplace control measures. For example, the urinary measurement of 4,4'-methylenebis 2-chloroaniline (MBOCA) can reflect the effectiveness of workplace control measures in reducing exposure. Medical surveillance by lung function testing and skin inspection is now frequently used where there is exposure to an asthmagen or a skin sensitizing agent. Levels of respiratory surveillance are often tiered to the potential for sensitization. Lower-level surveillance by questionnaires to elicit symptoms of workplace-induced bronchospasm may be effective in the early detection of occupational asthma for less potent sensitizers. Higher-level surveillance using spirometry at periodic intervals (pre-placement, 6 weeks, 12 weeks, annually) is more appropriate for more potent sensitizing agents, e.g. isocyanates. Skin surveillance is commonplace in some countries, although this can often be undertaken by non-medical personnel, trained to detect the early signs of dermatitis. Despite the widespread use of this type of surveillance there is little evidence base to suggest appreciable prevention of occupational contact dermatitis.

Planning and ethical considerations

Once general principles and surveillance techniques have been decided, the next step is to prepare a workplace policy. This should include aspects of risk assessment, investigations, and outcome-based actions. Although a policy should cover issues of workplace controls and required PPE, it should address the potential need for medical surveillance and deal with the implications for the employee. This in turn will raise ethical considerations regarding ongoing exposure, temporary redeployment, and possible ongoing employability. There should be preliminary meetings between management and employee representatives or works councils to cover the employee relation aspects to delineate responsibilities and roles. Employee rights should not be abrogated and consent should always be embedded in medical surveillance programmes. Employees and their representatives often have to be reassured that medical surveillance and particularly biological monitoring will only include analysis of agreed chemical agents. All results should be treated as sensitive personal data, preserving individuals' confidentiality along with expert interpretation of the results. Workers need to feel confident that subjecting themselves to medical surveillance is in their best interest. The workers' informed consent will be required and refusal to participate should not affect their contract of employment. However, in many jurisdictions, some chemical substances dictate that medical surveillance is legally mandated and that employers and employees have a legal duty to participate.

Medical surveillance programmes

Most surveillance programmes will require initial surveillance at pre-employment or pre-placement. This will set baseline results and the identification of any individual susceptibility. The timing of surveillance and its periodicity should be informed by the latest peer-reviewed literature regarding respiratory and dermatological sensitizers and toxicokinetics of chemical substances. If possible, non-invasive techniques should be used such as questionnaires of symptoms. If sampling is required then breath and urine samples are preferable to blood sampling providing there is a valid analytical method. Workers with previously documented evidence of respiratory or skin sensitization should be restricted from working with those specific sensitizing agents. However, non-specific personal factors such as history of asthma, dermatitis, or atopy should not be used as broad exclusion criteria. There is a growing body of evidence that these exclusion criteria are not evidence based and each case should be treated separately. In practice, national guidance varies and country-specific legislation should always be referenced. Respiratory surveillance will normally take place at pre-placement, 6 weeks, 12 weeks, and annually, depending on the results. Skin surveillance may be carried out as required by a responsible and suitably trained person, at an appropriate frequency. A healthcare technician, or occupational health professional, will normally carry out biological monitoring in those requiring it. Procedures for safe handling of biological specimens must be understood with appropriate chain of custody for transportation of samples. Analytical laboratories should have appropriate quality assurance accreditation and operate to defined international standards.

Interpretation of results

The critical stage in any medical surveillance programme is the interpretation of results. If respiratory surveillance using spirometry is undertaken then levels of abnormality on screening tests should be set, i.e. FEV_1 less than 80% of predicted value corrected for age, sex, and height. These should be referred for further assessment with an occupational or respiratory physician who may undertake 2-hourly peak flow measurements. Similarly, those showing early signs of dermatitis should be referred to a specialist in dermatology and if a case of allergic contact dermatitis is suspected, undergo appropriate patch testing. Biological monitoring results should be referenced to appropriate recommended or statutory biological monitoring guidance values (See Principles of industrial hygiene and toxic hazards in the workplace pp. 382–387).

Management of the workplace and individuals

Depending on the results, individual and workplace factors should be reviewed. Viewing the workplace may suggest control measures are not being used to prevent exposure and unforeseen routes of absorption are apparent. Temporary redeployment may be necessary in some circumstances. In the case of clear work-related ill health or occupational diseases then permanent redeployment to alternative work is often required. Some conditions require statutory reporting to country health and safety enforcing authorities; there may also be specific legislative requirements for action to take place or suspension of the particular work activity. It should not be forgotten that the health surveillance programme

itself can be an opportunity to educate the individual worker of the requirements for appropriate PPE and working practices that minimize exposure. Once the individual results have been discussed and an individual management plan agreed, group results can be anonymized and reported to the employer.

Records

Medical surveillance programmes require the retention of a health record for individual results. This provides a historical record to compare with subsequent surveillance, actions taken, and details required by enforcing authorities. This health record can be either paper based or electronic. Country-specific legislation may mandate retention of these records for specified periods of time, particularly in the case of exposure to carcinogens, which may be for up to 50 years.

Further reading

Council Directive 89/391/EEC of 12 June 1989 on the introduction of measures to encourage improvements in the safety and health of workers at work; Section IV, miscellaneous provisions, Article 14, Health surveillance.

Fishwick D, Barber CM, Bradshaw LM, et al. (2008). Standards of care for occupational asthma. *Thorax*, **63**:240–50.

Health and Safety Executive (2013). *The Control of Substances Hazardous to Health Regulations 2002 (as amended). Approved Code of Practice and Guidance.* Regulation 11, paragraph (2)(b) L5, 6th edition. Sudbury: HSE Books.

Health and Safety Executive (2002). *Health Surveillance at Work.* Sudbury: HSE Books.

Health and Safety Executive (2002). *The Control of Lead at Work Regulations 2002. Approved Code of Practice, Regulations and Guidance*, L132, 3rd edition. Sudbury: HSE Books.

Health and Safety Executive (2012). *A Guide to the Reporting of Injuries, Diseases and Dangerous Occurrences Regulations 1995*, L73, 4th edition. London: HSE.

Nicholson PJ, Cullinan P, Burge PS, et al. (2010). *Occupational Asthma: Prevention, Identification & Management: Systematic Review & Recommendations.* London: The British Occupational Health Research Foundation.

Occupational Safety and Health Act Act of 1970. Section 5 (a) (1), *Occupational Safety and Health Standards.* Washington, DC: U.S Department of Labor Occupational Health and Safety Administration.

Nicholson PJ, Llewellyn D (eds) (2010). *Occupational Contact Dermatitis & Urticaria.* London: The British Occupational Health Research Foundation.

United Kingdom Accreditation Service (UKAS) for laboratory testing website: <http://www.ukas.org/testing/singlesearch.asp>.

Principles of air and water safety standards and their regulations

Background

It is often assumed that standards are necessary to control levels of toxicologically active chemicals in the environment. This is not entirely true. The Clean Air Act of 1956 (Ministry of Housing and Local Government, 1956) was probably the most effective policy development in the air pollution field in the 20th century and led to a very significant improvement in air quality in the UK. The Clean Air Act set no standards for air quality in general or for specific air pollutants. What the Act did do was to recognize that ambient levels of air pollutants were damaging to health, to locate the key source in towns and cities (coal burning), and to provide funds to allow cleaner fuel to be used. Political will, rather than standard setting, was the driving force.

In more recent times standards for concentrations of air pollutants have been set in the UK. Initially these were set on the basis of toxicological and epidemiological evidence of adverse effects and took no account of the likely costs of implementation. This has also been the approach adopted in the air pollution field in the USA. The assumption was made that if levels of air pollutants (expressed as a concentration and averaging time) could be reduced so as not to exceed the standards, no, or almost no, effects on health would occur. This is also the approach taken in the water area (World Health Organization, 2008). The approach thus assumes the existence of a threshold of effect: a common assumption in toxicological work. Of course for some pollutants, the genotoxic carcinogens, such an assumption was known to be likely to be invalid and variants of an 'as low as (practically) possible' approach have been adopted. The WHO has adopted the threshold assumption for non-genotoxic carcinogens in its publications (World Health Organization 1987, 2000, 2006).

Thresholds

Defining thresholds of effect involves assessing toxicological data and identifying such indices as the lowest observed adverse effect level (LOAEL) or, less often, the no-observed adverse effect level (NOAEL) (see also Basic mechanisms of poisoning, pp. 4–7). Recent developments in thinking have led to the concepts of benchmark dose and reference concentration (US Environmental Protection Agency, 2002). Safety factors (now known as assessment factors and until recently as uncertainty factors) are applied to some well-defined starting point, for example, a LOAEL. Standards derived in this way thus include a margin of safety and it is incorrect to assume, as is often done, that minor exceedance of a standard will, ipso facto, be associated with adverse effects on health. This is also the case with WHO guidelines values.

Establishing standards

Standard setting implies a means of ascertaining whether standards are being met. Monitoring of pollutant concentrations is needed and methods of monitoring, location of monitors, procedures for reporting the results, and for quality assurance/quality control (QA/QC) need to be defined. Location of monitors is a difficult issue in the air pollution field—less so in the water pollution area.

Consider, for example, the current European Commission (EC) limit value for nitrogen dioxide: 40 micrograms/m^3, annual average concentration. This is based on, indeed is identical with, the WHO air quality guidelines for nitrogen dioxide. The implication of the guideline is if exposure to nitrogen dioxide, expressed in terms of an annual average concentration, is kept below 40 micrograms/m^3 no adverse effects on health should be expected in the great majority of people. A question immediately arises: how is exposure linked to ambient concentration? This is imperfectly understood. It might also be asked: did the studies on which the guideline is based look at exposure or at concentration?

It will be understood that 'exposure' is the sum of the exposures (the concentration × time products) occurring in all the micro-environments through which people pass in a defined period. The studies, in fact, looked at indoor concentrations of nitrogen dioxide and sometimes used a proxy for concentrations (present or absence of a key source: gas as a fuel for cooking and heating) rather than measured concentrations. Monitoring concentrations of nitrogen dioxide at a busy road junction might be agreed to be a poor or at least imperfect proxy for exposure and debate about the need to meet the EC limit value at such locations is ongoing. In reality setting standards for air pollutants is less difficult than working out how the standards might most sensibly be applied.

Health effects

The effects on health of major air pollutants have been studied extensively by epidemiological methods. These include time series and cohort approaches and, to a lesser extent, panel studies.

Use of the time series and cohort methods has led to a startling conclusion. For pollutants including ozone, nitrogen dioxide, and sulphur dioxide and for particles monitored as PM10 and PM2.5 (the mass per m^3 of particles generally less than 10 and 2.5 μm aerodynamic diameter, respectively) no threshold of effect can be defined. How can this be explained? It seems counter-intuitive in terms of classical toxicology.

Current thinking suggests that the extreme sensitivity of these methods, combined with a perhaps unexpectedly wide range of individual sensitivity in the entire population and a wide range of actual exposure, makes demonstration of a threshold unlikely or, at least, very difficult. It should be recalled that modern methods allow very small increases in risk to be identified, for example, a 10 micrograms/m^3 increase in daily average PM10 is associated with about a 0.4% increase in risk of death. Details of actual risk estimates can be found in publications of the Committee on the Medical Effects of Air Pollutants (1998, 2001, 2009).

These findings have led to change in thinking about air quality standards. The 'new thinking' can be expressed as: progressive, cost–benefit tested, reductions in ambient concentrations. This approach has not yet been widely adopted and some would argue fo rmal standards are needed to encourage governments to take action. This view led to WHO recommending both coefficients (defining the slopes of concentration–response relationships) and numerical guidelines in the Global Update on Air Quality Guidelines published in 2006 (World Health Organization, 2006). Further developments in this area are expected.

Further reading

Committee on the Medical Effects of Air Pollutants (1998). *Quantification of the Effects of Air Pollution on Health in the United Kingdom*. London: The Stationery Office.

Committee on the Medical Effects of Air Pollutants (2001). *Statement and Report on Long-Term Effects of Particles on Mortality*. London: The Stationery Office.

Committee on the Medical Effects of Air Pollutants (2009). *Long-Term Exposure to Air Pollution: Effects on Mortality*. http://www.comeap.org.uk/documents/reports/39-page/linking/75-long-term-exposure-to-air-pollution-effect-on-mortality2.

Ministry of Housing and Local Government. (1956). *Clean Air Act*. London: HMSO. http://www.legislation.gov.uk/ukpga/Eliz2/4-5/52/enacted.

US Environmental Protection Agency (2002). *A Review of the Reference Dose and Reference Concentration Processes*. EPA/630/P-02/002F. Washington, DC: US Environmental Protection Agency, Risk Assessment Forum. http://www.epa.gov/raf/publications/review-reference-dose.htm.

World Health Organization (1987). *Air Quality Guidelines for Europe*. WHO Regional Publications, European Series, No 23.Copenhagen: WHO Regional Office for Europe.

World Health Organization (2000). *Air Quality Guidelines for Europe*, 2nd edition. WHO Regional Publications, European Series, No. 91. Copenhagen: WHO Regional Office for Europe. http://www.euro.who.int/en/health-topics/environment-and-health/air-quality/publications/pre2009/who-air-quality-guidelines-for-europe,-2nd-edition,-2000-cd-rom-version.

World Health Organization (2006). *Air Quality Guidelines. Global Update 2005. Particulate Matter, Ozone, Nitrogen Dioxide and Sulfur Dioxide*. Copenhagen: WHO Regional Office for Europe. http://whqlibdoc.who.int/hq/2006/WHO_SDE_PHE_OEH_06.02_eng.pdf.

Index

Where a heading has multiple entries, page numbers in **bold** indicate major coverage of the topic. Page numbers in *italics* refer to figures and tables.